AF478478

Targeted Therapy for Cancer

Oxford University Press makes no representation, express or implied, that the drug dosages in this book are correct. Readers must therefore always check the product information and clinical procedures with the most up to date published product information and data sheets provided by the manufacturers and the most recent codes of conduct and safety regulations. The authors and the publishers do not accept responsibility or legal liability for any errors in the text or for the misuse or misapplication of material in this work.

Targeted Therapy for Cancer

Edited by

KONSTANTINOS N. SYRIGOS
Assistant Professor of Oncology in Medicine
Consultant Medical Oncologist
Head, Oncology Unit
3rd Department of Medicine
Athens Medical School
Sotiria General Hospital
Athens
Greece

and

KEVIN J. HARRINGTON
Molecular Medicine Program
Mayo Clinic
Rochester, Minnesota
USA
&
Targeted Therapy Laboratory
Institute of Cancer Research
London
UK

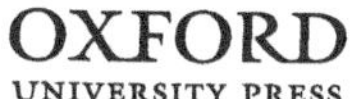

OXFORD
UNIVERSITY PRESS

*This book has been printed digitally and produced in a standard specification
in order to ensure its continuing availability*

OXFORD
UNIVERSITY PRESS

Great Clarendon Street, Oxford OX2 6DP

Oxford University Press is a department of the University of Oxford.
It furthers the University's objective of excellence in research, scholarship,
and education by publishing worldwide in

Oxford New York

Auckland   Cape Town Dar es Salaam Hong Kong Karachi
Kuala Lumpur Madrid Melbourne Mexico City Nairobi
New Delhi Shanghai Taipei Toronto
With offices in
Argentina Austria Brazil Chile Czech Republic France Greece
Guatemala Hungary Italy Japan South Korea Poland Portugal
Singapore Switzerland Thailand Turkey Ukraine Vietnam

Oxford is a registered trade mark of Oxford University Press
in the UK and in certain other countries

Published in the United States
by Oxford University Press Inc., New York

© Oxford University Press, 2003

Not to be reprinted without permission
The moral rights of the author have been asserted
Database right Oxford University Press (maker)

Reprinted 2007

ISBN 978-0-19-850896-0

Preface

The quest for therapeutic specificity is implicit in all branches of medicine. In cancer treatment, where the therapeutic modality is a cytotoxic agent such as radiotherapy or chemotherapy, such specificity is of paramount importance. The relative levels of cell death occurring in the malignant and critical normal tissue compartments as a result of the administration of a cytotoxic treatment dictate the therapeutic index. Unfortunately, in most solid tumour types the therapeutic indices of radiotherapy and chemotherapy are relatively low and cure rates have remained essentially static for the last two decades, despite massive investment in research. The growing realisation that current therapeutic options are likely to yield no more than incremental improvements in outcome has fuelled the search for more active targeted approaches. In its ultimate embodiment as the mythical 'magic bullet', targeted therapy offers the prospect of fulfilling the twin goals of maximal therapeutic efficacy with minimal adverse effects.

Exactly what constitutes targeted therapy is a moot point. We have applied a fairly liberal definition in an attempt to draw on examples from a number of different disciplines. In general terms, we have included those approaches that seek to exploit a difference between the biology of the tumour and the adjacent or distant normal tissues. As expected, archetypal systemic targeted therapies, such as those employing monoclonal antibodies or liposomes, receive significant attention in this volume but we have also been keen to include those strategies, such as photodynamic therapy and boron neutron capture therapy, that rely on direct physical targeting of disease. Furthermore, the explosion in our understanding of the molecular biology of cancer in recent years has led to the identification of a number of new potential therapeutic targets. Indeed, such has been the pace of research that new targets have been identified at a rate that has exceeded our ability to investigate them. Furthermore, it is likely that the data from the Human Genome Project and the so-called Cancer Genome Projects will highlight many more potential therapeutic targets over the next few years. The intensity of interest in this field of research is exemplified by the fact that in a relatively short period of time the fledgling science of cancer gene therapy has become established and the first series of clinical trials has been completed. Further significant clinical activity in this arena is anticipated in the coming years with the very real prospect that gene therapy approaches may find an established role in the standard treatment of some of the common cancers.

We believe that the next decade will be a very exciting time in the field of targeted therapy research. We predict that there will be progress in the implementation of clinical protocols incorporating these new agents with the possibility that they may yield significant clinical gains.

A comprehensive textbook is inevitably not fully up to date at the time of publication and this applies particularly in the areas where advances have been more rapid. It is therefore a tribute to our distinguished contributors and to the publisher, Oxford University Press, that this edition has appeared within 2 years of its initiation. Our thanks are due to their staff, as well as to our contributors who have been most patient during the gestation of the volume.

Finally this volume is dedicated to the memory of the late Nikolaos K. Syrigos (1934–1992) and to Poulia D. Barlami, parents of one of the editors, as well as to Marcella Harrington, and to the memory of the late Gregory Lynch (1923–2002), mother and uncle of the other editor.

<table>
<tr><td>Konstantinos N. Syrigos, MD, PhD
Assistant Professor of Athens Medical School</td><td>Kevin J Harrington, MRCP, FRCR
CRC Center for Cell and Molecular Biology
October 2002</td></tr>
</table>

Contents

Contributors

Arap, Wadih, MD
Department of Genitourinary Medical Oncology and Cancer Biology, The University of Texas MD Anderson Cancer Center, Houston, Texas, USA

Bagshawe, K.D., CBE, FRS
Emeritus Professor of Medical Oncology, Imperial College of Science and Medicine, Charing Cross Campus, London, UK

Bateman, Andrew, PhD
Molecular Medicine Program, Mayo Clinic, Rochester, Minnesota, USA

Batra, Surinder K., PhD
Associate Professor, Department of Biochemistry and Molecular Biology, Eppley Institute for Research in Cancer and Allied Diseases, University of Nebraska Medical Center, Omaha, Nebraska, USA

Begent, Richard H.J., PhD
Professor of Medical Oncology, Cancer Research Campaign Targeting and Imaging Group, Department of Oncology at Royal Free Campus of Royal Free, University College Medical School, London, UK

Buchsbaum, Donald J., PhD, MD
Professor and Director, Division of Radiation Biology, Department of Radiation Oncology, University of Alabama at Birmingham, Birmingham, Alabama, USA

Cardó-Vila, Marina, MD
Department of Genitourinary Medical Oncology and Cancer Biology, The University of Texas MD Anderson Cancer Center, Houston, Texas, USA

Chong, Heung, PhD
Molecular Medicine Program, Mayo Clinic, Rochester, Minnesota, USA

Coderre, Jeffrey A., PhD
Medical Department, Brookhaven National Laboratory, Upton, New York, USA

Colcher, David, PhD
Director, Radioimmunotherapy Research, Coulter Pharmaceutical Inc, San Francisco, California, USA

Culp, Lloyd A., MD, PhD
Department of Molecular Biology and Microbiology, Case Western Reserve University School of Medicine, Cleveland, Ohio, USA

Cunningham, David, MD, FRCP
Head of Gastrointestinal and Lymphoma Units, Royal Marsden Hospital, Down Road, Sutton, Surrey, UK

Diaz, Rosa Maria, PhD
Molecular Medicine Program, Mayo Clinic, Rochester, Minnesota, USA

Francis, Roslyn J.
Cancer Research Campaign Targeting and Imaging Group, Department of Oncology at Royal Free Campus of Royal Free, University College Medical School, London, UK

Goel, Apollina, PhD
Research Associate, Department of Biochemistry and Molecular Biology, University of Nebraska Medical Center, Omaha, Nebraska, USA

Hamblin, Michael R., PhD
Assistant Professor of Dermatology, Harvard Medical School, Massachusetts General Hospital, Boston, Massachusetts, USA

Harrington, Kevin J., MRCP, FRCR
Molecular Medicine Program, Mayo Clinic, Rochester, Minnesota, USA & Targeted Therapy Laboratory, Institute of Cancer Research, London, UK

Holleran, Julianne L., PhD
Department of Molecular Biology and Microbiology, Case Western Reserve University School of Medicine, Cleveland, Ohio, USA

Judware, Raymond, PhD
Department of Molecular Biology and Microbiology, Case Western Reserve University School of Medicine, Cleveland, Ohio, USA

Kleinman, Nanette R., PhD
Department of Molecular Biology and Microbiology, Case Western Reserve University School of Medicine, Cleveland, Ohio, USA

Kogerman, Priit, PhD
Department of Molecular Biology and Microbiology, Case Western Reserve University School of Medicine, Cleveland, Ohio, USA

Lahdenranta, Johanna, MD
Department of Genitourinary Medical Oncology and Cancer Biology, The University of Texas MD Anderson Cancer Center, Houston, Texas, USA

Lin, Wen-Chang, PhD
Department of Molecular Biology and Microbiology, Case Western Reserve University School of Medicine, Cleveland, Ohio, USA

Melcher, Alan, MD, PhD
Molecular Medicine Program, Mayo Clinic, Rochester, Minnesota, USA

Miller, Carson J., PhD
Department of Molecular Biology and Microbiology, Case Western Reserve University School of Medicine, Cleveland, Ohio, USA

Morris, Gerard M., PhD
Research Institute, University of Oxford, Churchill Hospital, Oxford, UK

Pandha, Hardev S., MB, ChB, PhD, MRCP, FRACP
Hon. Simon Weinstock Senior Lecturer in Tumour Immunology, Department of Medical Oncology, St. George's Hospital Medical School, London, UK

Pasqualini, Renata, MD
Department of Genitourinary Medical Oncology and Cancer Biology, The University of Texas MD Anderson Cancer Center, Houston, Texas, USA

Pavlinkova, Gabriela, RNDR
Instructor, Department of Biochemistry and Molecular Biology, University of Nebraska Medical Center, Omaha, Nebraska, USA

Raben, David, MD
Assistant Professor, Department of Radiation Oncology, University of Colorado, Denver, Colorado, USA

Rigg, Anne, BSc, MB, BS, MRCP, PhD
Department of Medicine, Royal Marsden Hospital, London, UK

Rowlinson-Busza, Gail, PhD
Antisoma Research Ltd, St George's Hospital Medical School, London, UK

Schecheter, Bilha, MD
Department of Immunology, The Weizmann Institute of Science, Rehovot, Israel

Sela, Michael, MD
Department of Immunology, The Weizmann Institute of Science, Rehovot, Israel

Syrigos, Konstantinos N., MD, PhD
Assistant Professor of Oncology in Medicine, Consultant Medical Oncologist, Head, Oncology Unit, 3rd Department of Medicine, Athens Medical School, Sotiria General Hospital, Athens, Greece

Vidal, Claudia, MD
Department of Genitourinary Medical Oncology and Cancer Biology, The University of Texas MD Anderson Cancer Center, Houston, Texas, USA

Vile, Richard G., PhD
Molecular Medicine Program, Mayo Clinic, Rochester, Minnesota, USA

Waters, Justin, MD
Department of Medicine, Royal Marsden Hospital, Down Road, Sutton, Surrey, UK

Yarden, Yosef, MD, PhD
Department of Biological Regulation, The Weizmann Institute of Science, Rehovot, Israel

Abbreviations

AAV	adeno-associated virus
AC	anthracycline/cyclophosphamide
ACTH	adrenocorticotrophic hormone
ADCC	antibody-directed cell-mediated cytotoxicity
ADEPT	antibody-directed enzyme prodrug therapy
AEC	mAb–enzyme conjugate
AFP	alpha fetoprotein
Ag	antigen
AGENT	antibody-guided enzyme nitrile therapy
AHSCS	autologous hemopoietic stem cell support
AIDS	autoimmune disease syndrome
ALA	5-aminolevulinic acid
ALL	acute lymphoblastic leukemia
AMIRACS	antimetabolite with inactivation of rescue agent at cancer sites
AML	acute myeloid leukemia
AO	antisense oligonucleotides
AP	alkaline phosphatase
APC	antigen-presenting cells
APL	acute promyelocytic leukemia
APTT	activated partial thromboplastin time
ATP	adenosine 5′-triphosphate
Ara-C	cytosine arabinoside
ARCA	attenuated replication-competent adenovirus
AUC	area under curve
AV	adenovirus
BBB	blood–brain barrier
BCG	bacille Calmette–Guérin
bFGF	basic fibroblast growth factor
BMRR	Brookhaven Medical Research Reactor
BNCT	boron neutron capture therapy
BPA	p-(dihydroxyboryl)-phenylalanine
BPD	benzoporphyrin derivative
b-ricin	biotinyl-S,S,-ricin
BSH	sulfhydryl borane $Na_2B_{12}H_{11}SH$
C	constant chain
C_H	constant heavy chain
C_L	constant light chain
CAR	coxsackie and adenovirus receptor
CAT	chloramphenicol acetyltransferase
CBE	compound biological effectiveness
CDase	cytosine deaminase
CDK4	cyclin-dependent kinase 4 (gene)
CDR	complement-determining regions

CEA	carcinoembryonic antigen
CGT	cancer gene therapy
CHART	continuous hyperfractionated accelerated radiotherapy
CML	chronic myelogenous leukemia
CMV	cytomegalovirus
CPG2	carboxypeptidase G2
CRAbs	chelating recombinant antibodies
CT	computerized tomography
CTL	cytotoxic T lymphocyte
DC	dendritic cell
DCIS	ductal carcinoma *in situ*
DMEM	Dulbecco's modified Eagle's medium
DMPC	dimyristoyl phosphatidylcholine
DMPG	dimyristoyl phosphatidylglycerol
DMXAA	dimethylxanthenone-4 acetic acid
DOTA	1,4,7,10-tetraazacyclododecane-N,N',N'',N''' tetraacetic acid
dsFv	disulfide-stabilized Fv
DSPC	distearoyl phosphatidylcholine
DTH	delayed-type hypersensitivity (response)
DTPA	diethylenetriaminepentaacetic acid
EBRT	external beam radiation therapy
EBV	Epstein–Barr virus
ECM	extracellular matrix
ED_{50}	median effective dose
EGF	epidermal growth factor
ELISA	enzyme-linked immunosorbent assay
epi-glu	epirubicin–glucuronide
EPR	enhanced penetration and retention (effect)
FAA	flavone-8 acetic acid
Fab	antigen-binding fragment of molecule
FACS	fluorescence-activated cell sorting
FasL	Fas ligand
FasR	Fas receptor
Fc	constant chain fragment of molecule
5FC	5-fluorocytosine
FDG	18-fluorodeoxyglucose
FGF	fibroblast growth factor
FISH	fluorescence *in situ* hybridization
FIV	feline immunodeficiency virus
FMG	fusogenic membrane glycoproteins
FMPA	fusion-protein-mediated prodrug activation
FPC	fission plate converter
FR	folate receptor
5FU	5-fluorouracil
Fv	variable chain fragment of molecule
GCV	ganciclovir
GDEPT	gene sequence-directed enzyme prodrug therapy
GELA	Groupe d'Etude des Lymphomes de l'Adulte
GFP	green fluorescent protein
GM-CSF	granulocyte–macrophage colony-stimulating factor
GPAT	genetic prodrug activation therapy

GTP	guanosine 5′-triphosphate
GUS	β-glucuronidase
GVHD	graft-versus-host disease
HA	hyaluronan
HAMA	human anti-mouse antibodies
HARA	human anti-ricin antibodies
HB-EGF	heparin-binding epidermal growth factor
HCC	hepatocellular carcinoma
HCG	human chorionic gonadotrophin
HDL	high-density lipoprotein
HIV-1	human immunodeficiency virus 1
HLA	human leukocyte antigen
HMFG	human milk fat globulin
HPI	hydrogenated phosphatidylinositol
HPMPA	N-(2-hydroxyupropyl) methacrylamide
HPV	human papilloma virus
HmR	hammerhead ribozyme
HOG	high-osmolarity glycerol
HP	hematoporphyrin
HPD	hematoporphyrin derivative
HpR	hairpin ribozyme
HRE	hypoxia response element
HSP	heat shock protein
HSV	herpes simplex virus
HSV-DISC	HSV-disabled infectious single cycle
HSVtk	HSV thymidine kinase
HTN	hemorrhagic tumor necrosis
HVJ	hemagglutinating virus of Japan
IAP	immunosuppressive acidic protein
IC$_{50}$	injected drug concentration corresponding to 50 per cent cell survival
ICAM	intercellular adhesion molecule
ICE	IL-1β-converting enzyme
i.d.	injected dose
ID	intradermal
IDDM	insulin-dependent diabetes mellitus
IFN-γ	interferon γ
IGF-1R	insulin-like growth factor receptor 1
IL-2	interleukin 2
IMRT	intensity-modulated radiation therapy
IP	intraperitoneal
IPC27	immediate–early protein 27
ISS	immunostimulatory sequences
ITR	inverted terminal repeat
IV	intravenous
KI	knock-in
KLH	keyhole limpet hemocyanin
KO	knock-out
LC	Langerhans cells
LCAA	lung-cancer-associated antigen
LCM	laser-capture microdissection
LDL	low-density lipoprotein

LET	linear energy transfer
LPD	lipid–protamine–DNA
LPS	lipopolysaccharide
LTR	long terminal repeat
LUV	large UV
mAb	monoclonal antibody
MAP	mitogen-activated protein
MAPK	mitogen-activated protein kinase
MBS	maleimidobenzoyl-*n*-hydroxysuccinimide ester
MCSF	macrophage colony-stimulating factor
MDEPT	macromolecule-directed enzyme prodrug therapy
MDR-1	multidrug resistance 1
MHC	major histocompatibility complex
MIBG	meta-iodobenzyl guanidine
MLV	multilamellar vesicles
MMAC1/PTEN	mutated in multiple advanced cancers 1/phosphatase and tensin homolog
MMP	matrix metalloproteinase
MMP	metalloproteinase inhibitor
MMTV	mammary tumor virus
MOI	multiplicity of infection
MoMLV	Moloney murine leukemia virus
MPEG	methoxypolyethylene glycol
MPEG-DSPE	MPEG-derivatized phosphatidylethanolamine
MRI	magnetic resonance imaging
MTD	maximum tolerated dose
mTHPC	*meta*-tetrahydroxyphenylchlorin
$^1n_{th}$	thermal neutron
NADH	nicotinamide adenine dinucleotide, reduced
NADPH	nicotinamide adenine dinucleotide phosphate, reduced
NAT	noradrenaline (norepinephrine) transporter
NCA	nonspecific cross-reacting antigen
NCAM	neural cell adhesion molecule
NDDP	*cis*-bis-neodecanoato *trans*-R, R-1,2 diaminocyclohexane platinum
NGF	nerve growth factor
NHL	non-Hodgkin's lymphoma
NIS	sodium iodide symporter
NK	natural killer
NOD	non-obese diabetic
NSCLC	non-small cell lung cancer
PAP	placental alkaline phosphatase
PBL	peripheral blood lymphocyte
PBS	phosphate-buffered saline
PC	phosphatidylcholine
PC	phthalocyanine
PCA	prostate carcinoma
PDEPT	polymer-directed prodrug therapy
PDGF	platelet-derived growth factor
PDGFR	PDGF receptor
PDT	photodynamic theory
PE	phosphatidylethanolamine
PEG	polyethylene glycol

PEG–PE	polyethylene glycol-conjugated phosphatidylethanolamine
PEM	polymorphic epithelial mucin
PET	positron emission tomography
PGA	polyglutamic acid
Ph	Philadelphia chromosome
PIC	photoimmunoconjugate
PI3K	phosphatidyl inositol 3-kinase
PKC	protein kinase C
PML	promyelocytic leukemia
PPE	plantar–palmar erythrodysesthesia
PPIX	protoporphyrin
PS	photosensitizer
PSA	prostate-specific antigen
PSMA	prostate-specific membrane antigen
PT	prothrombin time
PV	pox virus
PVA	penicillin-V amidase
PVA	polyvinyl alcohol
RA	retinoic acid
RAID	radioimmunodetection
RBE	relative biological effectiveness
RCAV	replication-competent adenoviruses
RDAV	replication-defective adenoviruses
RES	reticuloendothelial system
RGD	arginine–glycine–aspartate
RI	radiolocalization index
RIA	radioimmunoassay
RIGS	radioimmunoguided surgery
RIT	radioimmunotherapy
ROS	reactive oxygen species
RTOG	Radiation Therapy Oncology Group
RT-PCR	reverse transcriptase polymerase chain reaction
RV	retrovirus
SA	streptavidin
SC	subcutaneously
scFv	single-chain Fv
sc(Fv)$_2$	covalent dimeric scFv
[sc(Fv)$_2$]$_2$	noncovalent tetrameric scFV
SCID	severe combined immunodeficiency (mouse)
SCN-Bz-DTPA	isothiocyanatobenzyldiethylenetriamine-pentaacetic acid
SEREX	serological identification of antigens by recombinant expression cloning
SIV	simian immunodeficiency virus
SPECT	single-photon emission computer tomography
SPR	surface plasmon resonance
SUV	small unilamellar vesicle
SVA40	simian virus 40 gene A
TAA	tumor-associated antigen
TAG-72	tumor-associated glycoprotein-72
TAP	transporter-associated protein
TBI	total body irradiation
TCC	transitional cell carcinoma

TCR	T-cell receptor
TFO	triplex-forming oligonucleotide
TGF	transforming growth factor
Th	T helper cell
TIL	tumor-infiltrating lymphocyte
TNF	tumor necrosis factor
TRAIL	TNF-related apoptosis-inducing ligand
TSP	tissue-specific promoter
UV	unilamellar vesicle
V	variable chain
V_H	variable heavy chain
V_L	variable light chain
VCAM	vascular cell adhesion molecule
VDEPT	viral vector-directed prodrug therapy
VEGF	vascular endothelial growth factor
VLDL	very low-density lipoprotein
VLS	vascular leak syndrome
VPC	vector producer cells
VPF	vascular permeability factor

Section I

1 | *The history of targeted therapy for cancer*

K.D. Bagshawe

Introduction

Like many other areas of scientific development, targeted cancer therapy has many roots and many trunks each with its own array of branches. As a consequence, a strictly chronological account is not possible, nor is it possible to review every approach that can claim to be a form of targeting. Although many ideas on specific forms of therapy can be traced back to the beginning of the twentieth century the incentive to try to develop selective therapy for cancer in the last three decades began with the recognition of two fundamental facts. One was a realization that metastatic cancer, which constitutes the main threat of cancer to life, requires therapeutic means that can access neoplastic cells wherever in the body they are located. By the 1960s the limitations of surgery and external beam radiotherapy had become apparent despite great advances in their techniques in the years following the Second World War. The second fact was the failure in clinical practice of an increasing range of cytotoxic drugs to discriminate effectively between neoplastic and normal cells. Cells in the process of replication proved most vulnerable to cytotoxic action but it was replication in normal cell renewal systems that defined the limits of tolerance so that only a few of the less common cancers could be eradicated whilst the majority of the common cancers eventually proved resistant to tolerable dosage.

Conventional drugs of all types are used to achieve selective effects by virtue of the expression of specific ligands on certain types of cell. The drug therefore has the function of delivering itself to certain sites and of providing an effector mechanism at those sites. In the absence of specific ligands for cancer cells the essence of the targeting approach is to recognize that the delivery function and the effector function of a therapy system are distinct entities that require different characteristics even if they are incorporated in a single molec-ular structure. It is also appropriate to recognize that the design of 'conventional' drugs has undergone a revolutionary change in recent years so that the design of new drugs is frequently based on the three-dimensional structure of the tumor target thus providing improved binding affinities. The difference between targeted therapy and conventional drugs has therefore become blurred and this process can be expected to continue.

The concept of targeting in cancer therapy can be seen to have two related objectives. One is to achieve a greater degree of functionality at cancer sites than has been achieved by conventional means. Underpinning much of the field is evidence that, *in vitro*, the cell killing potential of antitumor agents is dose- and time-dependent and that exposure to sublethal concentra-tions can evoke resistance mechanisms. The second objective is that this should be achieved with minimal toxicity to normal host tissues.

Given that the delivery function and the effector function are distinct entities, their evolution can be viewed separately. The components used for delivery of effectors to tumors include antibodies, other molecules for which receptors exist on cancer cells, and tumor blood vessels and macromolecules. Effectors include radioisotopes, drugs, toxins, enzymes, antibodies them-selves, and immune cells.

The first phase of development conformed to the concept that the delivery component and the effector component should be a single molecular structure. Later it came to be recognized that more complex systems would be required to achieve the desired selec-tivity. For simplicity of presentation, targeting based on single molecular or molecular constructs is reviewed first and the more complex multistep systems are reviewed later, although, inevitably, there is consider-able chronological overlap. Targeting with immune cells is omitted because it would require a full review of the large and complex field of tumor immunology.

One-stage targeting

Targeting with antibodies

Identification of tumor-associated antigens

The earliest observations on tumor-associated substances preceded the evolution of protein chemistry. Bence Jones (1) is associated with the first recognition of such a substance in 1847, and almost a century went by before Brown (2) in 1928 described what is now known as the ectopic hormone syndrome associated with carcinomas secreting adrenocorticotrophic hormone (ACTH). Zondek (3) in 1929 described the first tests for human chorionic gonadotrophin (HCG) produced by normal and malignant trophoblast, ACTH was identified by Cushing (4) in 1932, and the association of acid phosphatase with prostatic cancer by Gutman and Gutman occurred in 1938 (5).

Identification of these substances depended on a variety of methods including bioassay and conventional chemistry. Between 1930 and 1960 a great array of bioassays was described for the detection of gonadotrophic and other hormones using toads, mice, rats, and rabbits. During the 1930s also came the first evidence for the production of antibodies to hormones (6), and protein chemistry developments resulted in the purification of prolactin and thyrotropin. Prodigious amounts of these hard-won substances were used to immunize rabbits, and the antisera obtained gave precipitin reactions (7). Insulin had been recognized as a protein 30 years before Stavitsky and Arquilla (8) developed the first anti-insulin antisera in 1953.

The development of immunoassays was one of the earliest practical applications of these antisera which began in the late 1950s and it acted as a spur to other developments. Antigen-coated erythrocytes, latex particles, and bentonite were agglutinated by antisera to human growth hormone (9, 10), to HCG (11), and to thyroglobulin (12). Complement fixation was described for HCG (13). Hemagglutinin inhibition became a widely used method before the principles of radioimmunoassay were put forward by Yallow and Berson in 1959 (14). The technique of radiolabeling proteins advanced with the chloramines T method of Hunter and Greenwood (15). If antibodies could be used to identify and bind to tumor products *in vitro*, could they be used *in vivo*?

The beginnings of targeted therapy

Gorer (16) had reported in 1942 that an antitumor antiserum could suppress the growth of that tumor in an animal. This work preceded recognition of transplantation antigens and the antibodies may have been directed at these rather than tumor-associated antigens, but his work was confirmed by others (17–19). It was also found that the suppressive effect was limited to fairly small numbers of tumor cells (19), and the view gained ground that native antisera were relatively impotent against established cancers. There was some evidence that antibodies could actually stimulate tumor growth (20). It therefore seemed logical to attach a 'warhead' to anticancer antibodies.

In fact, *in vivo* application of antisera directed at tumor products had anticipated these developments and had already been begun by Pressman and Korngold (21) in 1953 and Bale *et al.* (22) in 1955. Following this, there was a hiatus until 1967 when Ghose *et al.* (23) used ^{131}I-labeled antibodies in both diagnostic and therapeutic roles. Anti-HCG antibodies were shown to localize in choriocarcinoma xenografts growing in the hamster cheek pouch (24). This hiatus is in retrospect all the more surprising since the discipline of nuclear medicine was in its formative years and the developments with radiolabeled antibodies came, with some notable exceptions, from outside that discipline.

Meanwhile, interest in tumor markers was accelerated by the discovery of carcinoembryonic antigen (CEA) by Gold and Freeman (25) in 1965. Affinity purification of crude antisera was used by Mach *et al.* (26) in 1974 with anti-CEA antisera, and this group and that of Goldenberg *et al.* (27) in 1978 pioneered immunoscintigraphy using ^{131}I-labelled polyclonal antisera and the gamma camera. However, rabbit and sheep antisera had their limitations and it was only the advent of monoclonal antibodies (28) that converted these interesting experiments into a practical clinical methodology. By 1980 several groups had confirmed that antibodies to CEA and HCG localized in human cancers expressing those antigens *in vivo* (26, 27, 29–31).

These studies showed that the amount of antibody that localized in tumors, both as xenografts in mice and as naturally occurring tumors in man, was quite small and that most of the antibody remained in the circulation. Various techniques were introduced to overcome this limitation in order to increase the contrast between tumor and background including double isotope subtraction techniques and accelerated clearance. Accelerated clearance adopted a technique first used in double antibody radioimmunoassay, that is, a second antibody directed at the first antitumour antibody was administered after the first had localized at tumor sites. This resulted in the formation of immune complexes (antibody–antibody) which were then cleared from the blood by the reticuloendothelial systems. When first used there was the fear that immune complex formation would induce pulmonary or renal complications and the second antibody was loaded into liposomes to minimize the risk but subsequent studies showed it was unnecessary (32).

If antibodies directed at tumor products could be shown to localize preferentially at tumor sites *in vivo* for diagnostic purposes, then the interest in whether they could be used therapeutically would gather momentum. In fact, the incentive to develop new and more selective forms of cancer therapy ensured that the earliest approaches anticipated the more sophisticated developments in the diagnostic field. Inevitably, Paul Ehrlich's vision of magic bullets (33), perhaps borrowed from Weber's opera, *Der Freischutz*, has been exploited by the popular media to burden the field with unrealistic expectations.

Although radioisotopes were the first 'warheads' to be attached to antibodies, other toxic elements followed in the early 1970s. In 1970, Moolten and Cooperbrand (34) reported that mouse kidney cells bearing antigens induced by the mumps virus were lysed selectively by diphtheria toxin conjugated to an antibody directed at mumps antigens. This quite remarkable paper anticipated some of the potential problems that were only fully recognized years later. The improved cytotoxic potential of diphtheria toxin-antibody conjugates was confirmed (35, 36). Thus the field of antibody–toxin conjugates, later known as immunotoxins, was born.

In a somewhat similar fashion came the origins of antibody–drug conjugates. In 1972 Ghose and Nigam (37) reported the attachment of chlorambucil to antibodies directed at the Ehrlich's ascites tumor and it was claimed that this conjugate was a more effective inhibitor of the tumor both *in vitro* and *in vivo* than either the native antibody or chlorambucil alone.

At about the same time, we saw the emergence of the concept of delivering an enzyme to tumor sites by conjugation to an antibody and using the tumor-located enzyme to generate a cytotoxic moiety from a substance (glucose) present in tissue (38). This anticipated the much later development of antibody-directed enzyme prodrug therapy (ADEPT) in which an enzyme conjugated to an antitumor antibody is used to convert an administered low-toxicity prodrug to a highly cytotoxic compound (39).

Recognition of the problems of targeting with antibodies

From the developments in the early 1970s emerged the obstacles that had to be overcome in the antibody-based targeting approach. It began to be realized that 'tumor antigens' were not truly specific. Those most widely used for targeting were also expressed on at least some normal tissues and, for the most part, tumors simply overexpressed some normal tissue markers. Perhaps more important was the recognition that not all clonogenic cells in tumors expressed the targeted antigen. This heterogeneity factor applied more to the carcinomas than to the hemopoietic malignancies and it indicated that not all of a carcinoma could be destroyed even with potent toxins if that toxin had to be internalized through antibody–antigen interaction on the cell membrane of every clonogenic cell. This led to recognition of the necessity for a 'bystander effect', in which cells lacking the target antigen would be accessed by the cytotoxic component. It was also realized that big molecules such as intact antibodies diffuse more slowly through a tumor mass than small molecules. Even the best intact antibodies or large antibody fragments were found to deliver only a small percentage of administered dose to tumor sites and 99 per cent or more was present in blood and normal tissues. Clearance of such molecules from blood proved to be slow so that positive tumor to blood ratios were only achieved, if at all, after several days. Antibodies could only be loaded with a limited number of drug molecules before losing their antigen-binding ability. Although the means to humanize murine monoclonal antibodies became available in the 1990s, antibody-bacterial enzyme conjugates, immunotoxins, and possibly antibody-drug conjugates remained as potential immunogens with the host antibody response able to terminate therapies using these components after comparatively brief exposure to them.

Developments with radiolabeled antibodies

Despite the fact that antibodies deliver only a very small fraction of a radiolabel to tumor sites they have, nevertheless, entered clinical practice. In general, the problem with radiolabeled antibodies is similar to that with cytotoxic drugs in that their effects on hemopoietic tissue in particular limit dosage to a level below that necessary to eradicate solid cancers. On the other hand, radiolabeled antibodies have a positive bystander effect through their cross-fire, which has the potential to overcome the problems of heterogeneity of antigen expression. Not all of the cells in a tumor need to bind the radiolabeled antibody, although it is notable that there is less heterogeneity of antigen expression in lymphomas, the main area of success for radiolabeled antibodies, than there is in the carcinomas. The main factor in susceptibility to radiolabeled antibodies appears to be that of radiosensitivity.

Lymphomas are amongst the most radiosensitive malignancies, and radiolabeled antibodies directed at CD20 have been approved for the treatment of some lymphomas in the USA in conjunction with cytotoxic drugs.

The limitation of radiolabeled antibodies may be overcome in special situations such as that following apparently successful surgical removal of stage 1 ovarian carcinomas where there is a statistical certainty of relapse in a high percentage of patients. The administration of ^{131}I-labelled anti-MUC (mucin) antibodies takes advantage both of the small number of cancer cells in the peritoneum and the limited space of the peritoneal cavity into which the antibody is delivered.

Drug–antibody conjugate

The late 1970s and early 1980s witnessed a flurry of activity in conjugating various cytotoxic agents to antibodies directed at tumor-associated antigens. Some of the problems encountered were referred to in the previous section. Additional issues were rapid catabolism resulting in poor pharmacokinetics, poor endocytosis, and release of drug and heterogeneity of antigen expression, which limited efficacy. Nevertheless, there were claims of superiority for drug–antibody conjugates compared with free drug when used in preclinical testing (40). By the mid-1980s enthusiasm was beginning to wane. Drug delivery by liposomes and attached to polymers are discussed later.

Targeting to non-antigenic receptors

Iodine and other agents

The relationship of iodine to the thyroid gland has been known since the middle of the nineteenth century. The lack of iodine in the soil in goitrous districts had been demonstrated before Caleb Parry (41) described thyrotoxicosis in 1825.

Radioiodine became available from cyclotrons in the late 1930s and was soon applied to clinical problems of the thyroid gland. Attempts to quantify ^{131}I-iodine uptake began in the 1940s using Geiger–Müller (GM) detectors, which were very inefficient at detecting gamma rays. Nevertheless, in 1950 Veall (42) was able to use a collimated GM detector to obtain images but it was the advent of the photomultiplier tube soon after the Second World War that transformed radionuclide detection. ^{99m}Tc-Pertechnetate had been the most widely used thyroid imaging agent for some years. It can be claimed that iodine was the first targeting agent and that ^{131}I-iodine the first targeted therapeutic agent.

It is well known that hormones secreted by endocrine organs are transported to the same organ or other organs that express receptors for those hormones. Tumors arising from hormone receptor tissues may continue to express those receptors. An early attempt to exploit these receptors was the development of 'Estracyt', an estra-mustine phosphate (oestradiol-3-N bis-2-chloroethyl-carbamate-17 phosphate). ^{131}I-labeling of this drug was claimed to be useful in imaging cancers of prostate and ovary (43).

A range of compounds have been found to be taken up selectively by certain cancers. Pheochromocytomas of the adrenal medulla, neuroblastomas, and medullary thyroid cancer have been detected by [^{131}I]-meta-iodobenzyl guanidine (MIBG) (44–46). It was also proposed that, because the pancreas synthesized enzymes from amino acids, ^{75}Se-L-selenomethionine would accumulate in this organ (47), but pancreatic scintigraphy with it was not highly successful and has been superseded by computerized tomography (CT). Another selenium compound, 6-methyl [^{75}Se] selenomethyl-19-norcholest-5 (10)-en-3β-o1, has been available in the UK as an adrenal gland imaging agent (75(Se)-norcholesterol).

There has been considerable interest in compounds that act as photosensitizers and that accumulate in tumors and that may also accumulate in liver, spleen, and kidneys. These include porphyrin derivatives, chlorins, and phthalocyanins. Porphyrins are phosphatases that are activated by visible light which is not damaging to biomolecules. Photosensitizers have been linked to antibodies (48) and later to polymers. Such an approach is obviously limited by the ability of light to penetrate tissues from accessible anatomical sites.

A selective retention of rhodamine 123 by the mitochondria of carcinoma cells was reported (49) and a therapeutic effect was observed at the maximum tolerated dose using Ehrlich ascites tumor. The effect was potentiated by 2-deoxyglucose, which inhibits glycolysis.

Enzyme inhibitors

Interest in enzymes secreted by tumor cells has a long history. The element of invasion by neoplastic cells and their ability to colonize distant tissues suggested that they secreted enzymes facilitating these processes. It is clear that invasion of tissues by cancer cells has to overcome various barriers in which pressure, locomotion, and lytic action may all play a part. The macromolecular components of the extracellular matrix are proteoglycans, glycoproteins including fibronectin, collagen, and elastin. Proteoglycans are formed by covalent binding of polysaccharide chains to a protein core. Proteolysis occurs under the influence of several proteinases, notably pepsin, cathepsin G, cathepsin D, trypsin, and elastases (50).

As the characteristics of these enzymes emerged, so the possible application of enzyme inhibitors was realized and their synthesis or extraction from tissues began (51–53). Proteinase inhibitors comprise 10 per cent of human plasma proteins and α_2 macroglobulin has the broadest spectrum of inhibition. Interest has therefore focused on matrix metalloproteinase inhibitors (MMPs), a family of zinc-dependent endoproteinases. These are linked by a core of common domain structures and by a link with tissue inhibitors of metalloproteinases. Proteinases remove physical barriers to cellular invasion by degrading collagens, laminins, and proteoglycans. They can also modulate cell adhesion, and metalloproteinase action on plasminogen is now known to produce the angiogenesis inhibitor angiostatin (54, 55).

Utilization of enzymes overexpressed by cancers

It was recognized in the 1960s that if tumors overexpressed enzymes they might be used to activate prodrugs. Despite intensive searching no enzyme was found to be present in tumors that was not present in significant amounts in normal tissues. However, in recent years enzymes in the nitro reductase class have been found to be overexpressed in tumors. DT diaphorase (NQ01) has been used to activate diaziridinyl-benzoquinine analog (56) with therapeutic results in mice. Another recently identified enzyme human NQ02 has been found to convert a monofunctional alkylating agent CB1954 to its hydroxylamine, which is more than 1000 times more toxic in association with a cofactor (57). A further example of overexpression is thymidine phosphorylase (identical to platelet-derived endothelial cell growth factor), an enzyme with multiple actions including the promotion of angiogenesis and the reduction of thymidine to thymine and of 5′-deoxy-5-fluorouridine to 5-fluorouracil (58). Whether such systems will form practical clinical therapies will depend on the amount of enzyme in normal tissues and whether this will result in normal tissue toxicity.

Folic acid receptors

The identification of folic acid and its role in cell replication goes back to the discovery of pteridines in butterfly wings in 1898 by Hopkins (59). In the 1930s Lucy Wills, a British physician working in India, observed the response of macrocytic anemias to 'Marmite' and crude liver (60, 61). In 1940 Woods (62) identified p-aminobenzoic acid as the structure in sulfonamide responsible for its bacteriostatic action and in 1946 Angier *et al.* (63) showed that folic acid was *para*-aminobenzoic acid linked to a pteridine ring and glutamic acid. It was related that folic acid given to leukemic children appeared to accelerate their disease and this led to the proposal to make the folate antagonists, which were introduced by Farber *et al.* (64, 65). The first of these was aminopterin and it was soon followed by amethopterin (methotrexate), which remains an important cytotoxic compound in wide clinical use.

Since 1980 there has been increasing interest in folate receptors. At first, these were studied in terms of folate transport across the intestinal wall and placenta (66, 67) but soon interest turned to the influence of folate receptors on the uptake of folate analogs including methotrexate (68). Since then, at least 270 papers have appeared on the subject. The main outcome of these studies is confirmation that the cellular accumulation of folate and folate analogs is dependent on such receptors. Folic acid appears to enter cells either through a carrier protein known as the reduced folate carrier or through the folate receptor (FR), which mediates endocytosis. Folate–drug conjugates are not substrates for the reduced carrier but can enter cells via the folate receptor. When a drug is covalently linked to the gamma-carboxyl of folic acid the binding affinity of the receptor remains unchanged and endocytosis proceeds.

Evidence has been presented that FR is overexpressed by human tumors including those of ovary, kidney, uterus testis, brain, colon, lung, and myelocytic blood cells. The high binding affinity (dissociation constant, $K_d = 10^{-10}$ M) of folate receptors makes them an attractive target for radiopharmaceuticals such as ^{111}In-DTPA-folate (DTPA, diethylenetriainepentaacetic acid), MRI contrast agents, radiotherapeutic agents, liposomes with entrapped drugs, antisense oligonucleotides, ribozymes, and immunotherapeutic agents, including a fusion protein with interleukin 2 (IL-2). Most of these relate to preclinical studies. Clearly, folate receptors are not unique to malignant cells and uptake by cell renewal populations limits the specificity of folic acid conjugates. Nevertheless, the folate receptor is one of the more favored non-antigenic receptors and it can be assumed that ingenuity will be applied to its exploitation.

Tumor vasculature as a target

The capillary network of tumors was described by Virchow (69) in 1863, and it has been recognized since the beginning of the twentieth-century that an essential requirement for the growth of grafted tumors is the vascular contribution of the host (70). Studies of the vasculature with dyes followed and in 1939 Duran Reynolds (71) demonstrated the hyperpermeability of tumor blood vessels. He concluded that 'the findings are interpreted as indicating that newly formed capillaries of tumors are, in general, more permeable than the capillaries of any normal tissue'. In 1945 Algire and Chalkey (72) suggested that it was a characteristic of tumor cells to elicit growth of capillary endothelium *in vivo* but, as so often, the challenge thrown down by these observations was not taken up for several years until in 1972 Folkman (73) opened the field with studies aimed at identifying angiogenic factors. It was suggested that 'inhibition of angiogenesis might arrest solid tumors at a tiny diameter of a few millimetres'.

Since then the structure of tumor blood vessels, their permeability, tumor blood flow, angiogenic factors, and inhibitors of tumor blood vessel growth have been the subject of numerous studies. The consequences of tumor blood vessel permeability is discussed in the next section but here we consider the diverse developments relating to angiogenesis. The absence of muscle fibers from tumor blood vessels is one factor in their response to vasoactive agents. The recognition of antigenic markers on new blood vessels and of growth factors and the receptors for them has led to a new research industry.

One line of reasoning was that, if necrosis, a common factor of most tumors, results from hypoxia and inadequate blood supply, then diminishing blood flow would increase the amount of necrosis. Agents that lowered systemic blood pressure were studied in the 1980s. Hydrallazine induced a reduction in tumor blood flow and increased the efficacy of co-administered cytotoxic drugs (74). However, it was found that propranolol, a widely used hypotensive agent, had only a modest effect on tumor blood flow and did not modify the biodistribution of an antitumor antibody (75).

Tumor necrosis factor (TNF) and TNF-inducing agents

Tumor necrosis factor (TNF) was first described (76) in 1975, although it seems possible that the successes claimed for Coley's toxin in the nineteenth century were due to its induction. TNF is a 17 000 molecular weight protein produced by macrophages and lymphocytes in response to bacterial infection, and it induces hemorrhagic necrosis in transplantable murine tumors (77). Although it may have a direct reaction on tumor cells, hemorrhagic necrosis is probably mediated by its ability to produce vascular congestion and blockage of blood flow within 1–2 hours (78). It was found to have multiple effects, some of which are mediated through the immune system. Although effective against murine tumors, side-effects were marked in clinical trials and limited the dosage that could be given (79). Agents that induced TNF were sought.

Flavone-8-acetic acid (FAA), a synthetic flavonoid, showed activity against an experimental murine tumor and its activity was enhanced by co-administering IL-2 (80, 81). In the human, FAA with or without IL-2 failed to show activity (82, 83). The action of FAA in mice was found to be inhibited by antibodies to TNF and it failed to induce TNF in human cells, although it caused hypotension.

The process of interfering with tumor blood supply took a further step with the development of dimethylxanthenone-4-acetic acid (DMXAA) which was found to induce TNF by some human cell lines and was substantially more potent than FAA (84). DMXAA causes irreversible cessation of tumor blood flow within 4 hours of administration, resulting in hemorrhagic necrosis comparable to that produced by TNF. In contrast to FAA, it was found to be effective in human cancer xenografts.

It was reported (85) that angiogenesis was also markedly inhibited by a non-anticoagulating derivative of heparin conjugated to a corticosteroid with a C20 ketone but not C3 ketone. Angiogenesis has also been inhibited by a dextran derivative in a breast tumor model (86).

Vascular endothelial growth factor (VEGF), also described as vascular permeability factor (VPF), was identified as a multifunctional cytokine that was originally discovered as a tumor-secreted protein (87). Soon after it was found that VEGF acts directly on cultured endothelial cells, inducing transient accumulation of calcium, change in cell shape, cell division, and migration as well as angiogenesis and increased permeability *in vivo* (88).

Inhibitors of angiogenesis

Recognition of factors promoting angiogenesis was followed in the 1990s by identification of two important inhibiting factors. Metalloproteinases were found to convert human plasminogen to the angiogenesis inhibitor angiostatin (89, 90). Another factor, described as endostatin, was found to be formed by catalytic action on collagen.

Together, these substances have provided a prospect of control of tumor growth and metastasis by inhibiting the proliferation of vascular endothelium. Their potential has not escaped the attention of the media but it is clear that early experiments have not always been repeated successfully. Nevertheless, they represent important progress in our understanding of the mechanisms of neoplasia and they will no doubt establish a place in the control of malignancy.

Antibodies directed at tumour endothelial cells

Thorpe and his colleagues (91) reported that a murine monoclonal antibody (TEC-11) recognized endoglin, an antigenic marker on human endothelial cells. Whereas tumor endothelial cells stained strongly, only weak staining was found with most endothelial cells in normal tissues and this was related to the proliferative activity of endothelial cells. Using an immunotoxin based on this antibody, proliferating cells were found to be much more sensitive than confluent cultures.

This group has also targeted the VEGF receptor complex with antibodies. Two antibodies localized selectively on tumor xenograft endothelium and one of them blocked VEGF-mediated endothelial cell growth. They also showed (92) that thrombosis of tumor blood vessels could be achieved by targeting the extracellular domain of a tissue factor by an antibody to an experimentally induced marker on tumor vascular endothelium. They went on to show that a monoclonal antibody to VCAM-1, a vascular cell adhesion molecule expressed in Hodgkin's and other solid tumors and covalently linked to the extracellular domain of human tissue factor, caused thrombosis in tumor blood vessels. Although VCAM is expressed in the heart and lungs of mice it did not induce thrombosis there, apparently as a result of differences in phosphatidylserine expression in VCAM-1.

Another approach to attacking tumor vasculature has also been directed at the VEGF receptor. A small-molecule inhibitor of the VEGF receptor has been shown to arrest the growth of a range of tumor xenografts in immunodeficient mice, and inhibition of growth persisted as long as the VEGF inhibitor was administered (93). A small-molecule inhibitor has obvious advantages over antibodies and is potentially of great value.

Tubulin-binding agents

The induction of tumor vascular collapse has also resulted from various tubulin-binding agents, the first of which was colchicine. Compounds isolated from the stem wood of the South African tree, *Combretum caffoune*, have structural similarity to the colchicine-binding site on tubulin (94). *In vitro* combretastatin A-4 produced profound effects on proliferating endothelial cells and, with *in vivo* models, vascular shutdown was maximal by 6 hours and persisted for 12 hours resulting in hemorragic necrosis. These effects were obtained at less than one-tenth of the maximum tolerated dose for combretastatin A4 (95).

Liposomes

The characteristics of liquid crystals (liposomes) of phosphatidyl choline and phosphatidic acid began to be described in the late 1960s (96, 97), although there had been earlier studies with dispersions of phospholipids. Early studies were in terms of their potential use as carriers of proteins including enzymes (98). Their use as drug carriers followed (99, 100).

Early forms tended to be cleared quickly from the circulation and to be delivered to the liver and reticuloendothelial system and this was a major obstacle to their use in tumor therapy. Liposomes lend themselves to a vast number of potential versions and by the 1980s numerous attempts were being made to tailor their characteristics to specific requirements. Attempts to improve their delivery to specific target cells included the incorporation of polyclonal antibodies (101), and later monoclonal antibodies (102). Small liposomes were found to be better than large ones for delivery *in vitro* (103). Adjustment of liposome size and selective compositional change increased their circulation time and reduced uptake by liver and spleen and increased uptake by tumors (104). pH-sensitive liposomes were devised for release at low pH in tumors (105). In a further embodiment they were used for arterial chemoembolization of a range of cancers (106).

There is a long history for the use of liposomes as immunological adjuvants (107, 108). More recently, liposomes incorporating methoxypolyethylene glycol and linked to periodate oxidized chimerized mouse IgG antihuman epidermal growth factor receptor exhibited prolonged circulation time and marked immunogenicity. Other formulations of liposomes coated with polyethylene glycol (PEG) have become known as 'stealth' liposomes for their low immunogenicity and prolonged circulation time.

Tumor hydrodynamics

Two lines of research merge in this area. The study of tumor blood vessel permeability and the emergence of polymers as potential drug carriers were independent areas of research but in recent years their interdependence has emerged.

Reference has been made to the time gap between the first recorded observation of the hyperpermeability of tumor blood vessels in 1939 (71) and the interest awakened by Folkman in 1972 (73). The study of tumor hemodynamics by Jain's group has contributed to sharper understanding of the many factors involved (109). It is clear that any effector, whether a cell or a soluble molecule, must utilize the vasculature, then escape from the vasculature into the extracellular space of the tumor, and finally make contact with tumor cell membrane and in many cases be internalized by the target cell. The size, shape, and charge of a cell or molecule are obviously involved in these processes as are its diffusion characteristics and deformability. In the same way tumors may be seen as ecosystems, however disorganized they may appear. Tumor blood vessel morphology varies in terms of tortuosity, diameter, length, numbers, permeability, and rate of blood flow. Whereas the center of a tumor tends to be poorly vascularized, the main network tends to be peripheral. The vascular pressure within vessels is countered by the interstitial pressure within the tumor and determines the hydraulic conductivity of molecules into a tumor. The vascular concentration of a solute and its interstitial concentration determine its diffusion behavior into tumor extracellular space.

Within extracellular space, diffusion and convection are determined by concentration gradients and pressure gradients, respectively.

The transport of molecules into tumors is clearly influenced by the pore size of the fenestrated tumor vessel endothelium. Using sterically stabilized liposomes it has been estimated that these vessels were permeable to liposomes up to 400 nm in diameter (109). This is a surprisingly large figure and it was shown by the same authors that much smaller tracer molecules in the molecular weight range of 25 000–160 000 entered tumors at different rates. They also found (110) that the effective permeability of tumor vessels to liposomes was six times less than that to bovine serum albumin.

Macromolecules as targeting agents

Although the permeability of tumor blood vessels to macromolecules has been known for 60 years, it is unclear whether knowledge of this was the motivation for studies using polymers as drug delivery vehicles. It seems more likely that polymers were used simply because they were there.

In 1975 Ringsdorf (111) suggested that a water-soluble polymer with a biodegradale linker could be used to release a drug at cancer sites. This has been followed by a substantial development of pollymer–drug conjugates. The rationale for the accumulation of polymers at cancer sites has been summarized as a combination of tumor blood vessel permeability and deficient lymphatic drainage, described in 1986 by Matsumura and Maeda (112) as the enhanced penetration and retention effect (EPR). The effect of molecular weight of a soluble co-polymer (N-(2-hydroxypropyl) methacrylamide) (HPMA) in the molecular-weight range 22 000–778 000 was reported in 1995 by Seymour *et al.* (113). Polymers larger than the renal threshold showed progressive tumour accumulation up to 50 hours postadministration with tumor-to-muscle ratios of 6–12 and up to 10 per cent of injected dose per gram of tumor. The only normal tissue to show accumulation of the high-molecular-weight polymers was skin. Tumors-to-blood ratios suggest that tumor levels tend to equate with blood levels and that tumor accumulation is a function of blood concentration. A wide range of polymer–drug conjugates has been reported and is reviewed by Duncan *et al.* (114).

Multistep targeting systems

ADEPT

Antibody-directed enzyme prodrug therapy (ADEPT) was first proposed in 1987 by Bagshawe (39). The idea was to localize an enzyme in tumors by conjugating it to an antibody directed at a tumor-associated antigen. This is then used to convert a nontoxic prodrug to a highly cytotoxic drug. The cytotoxic drug, being of low molecular weight, is able to diffuse through the tumor much more readily than the high-molecular-weight antibody–enzyme conjugate and, therefore, has a good bystander effect. The immunogenicity of murine antibodies was beginning to be resolved by the late 1980s by humanization techniques and later by the development of human antibodies. The choice of enzyme, however, presented an interesting conflict in the sense that high specificity could be conferred by using bacterial enzymes that have no human analog, whereas human enzymes risk prodrug activation at nontumor sites.

Human enzymes such as alkaline phosphatase (115) that were present in blood had obvious limitations. But, with antibody–enzyme conjugates, slow clearance of the enzyme from blood presented a similar problem and methods for clearing enzyme from blood were used at an early stage in ADEPT development. A second antibody directed at the enzyme proved very effective and its penetration into tumors was limited by galactosylation which resulted in its rapid clearance via hepatic galactose receptors in liver. In a clinical trial tumor and liver biopsies showed the enzyme level in tumor to be > 10 000 higher than that in normal liver and blood (116). An alternative method in mice is to galactosylate the antibody–enzyme conjugate and to block the galactose receptors temporarily with bovine sialo submaxillary mucin. (117)

Alkylating agent prodrugs were selected as the most appropriate choice partly as a result of their cytotoxicity being concentration-dependent and partly because they are less prone to resistance mechanisms, but doxorubicin and other prodrugs have also been used. For a fuller discussion of prodrug development the reader is referred to Melton and Knox (118).

Further developments of ADEPT systems have included the use of high-affinity single-chain antibody variable chain fragments (scFv) used to make fusion proteins with enzymes. Human enzymes have been modified by molecular engineering techniques so as to be specific for particular enzyme substrates.

Macromolecules in the form of polyethylene glycol have been substituted for antibodies as the enzyme delivery model (macromolecule-directed enzyme prodrug therapy, MDEPT). Whereas antibodies are applicable only to tumors expressing the corresponding antigen, a PEG–enzyme conjugate can localize in a wide range of cancer xenografts.

VDEPT and GDEPT

It was proposed in 1991 by Huber *et al.* (119) that tumor cells could be induced to synthesize the necessary enzyme by introducing the corresponding gene sequence via a viral vector. This has become known as VDEPT (viral vector-directed enzyme prodrug therapy) or GDEPT (gene-sequence-directed enzyme prodrug therapy) and has had a wide following. By restricting the expression of the enzyme to cells expressing a tumor marker it was expected that selectivity would be achieved. However, gene delivery exclusively to tumors has continue to present obstacles.

A further variant known as PDEPT (polymer-directed enzyme prodrug therapy) employs a polymer (hydroxypolymethacrylate) to deliver a drug to tumor sites. Drug not at tumor sites quickly clears and clearance is followed by an enzyme–polymer conjugate that cleaves the drug from its carrier (120).

Antimetabolite with inactivation of rescue agent at cancer sites (AMIRACS)

Tumor-located enzyme can be used in a somewhat different fashion in conjunction with antimetabolite cytotoxic drugs. Antimetabolites that act to block DNA synthesis are well known to be bypassed by co-administration of a metabolite that acts downstream on the DNA synthesis pathway. Probably the best known example of this is the antagonism of antifolates such as methotrexate by folinic acid. In the system known as AMIRACS, the tumor-located enzyme is used to degrade the rescue agent, whereas, in the blood, the rescue agent protects normal tissues from the action of the antimetabolite.

When this system was first described (121), the only suitable antimetabolite in clinical use was trimetrexate. Trimetrexate is an antifolate that lacks the terminal glutamate of classical folates and antifolates. The enzyme carboxypeptidase G2 (CPG2) inactivates glutamated folates and antifolates by cleaving the terminal glutamates. Thus the action of trimetrexate is unaffected by CPG2 but folinic acid is degraded by it (121).

In recent years there has been a flurry of new antimetabolite compounds. These include thymidine synthetase inhibitors and inhibitors of glycinamide ribonucleotide transferase inhibitors. Rescue agents for these are thymidine and hypoxanthine, respectively. One of the problems with preclinical studies of AMIRACS is the fact that folate and thymidine levels in mice are some 10 times higher than in the human. A two patient study showed that it was possible to give 12–14 times the maximum tolerated dose of trimetrexate without toxicity and with some evidence of efficacy (121).

Avidin, streptavidin, and biotin

The very high binding affinity (K_d = 10^{-15} M)of streptavidin (SA) and avidin for the vitamin biotin was reported in 1975 by Green (122). Since then numerous attempts have been made to exploit the phenomenon both in diagnosis and in therapy. Early studies linked SA or avidin directly to antitumor monoclonal antibodies. The problem here was the prolonged retention of the conjugates in blood and accumulation in liver and kidney. Two- and three-step approaches were, therefore, evolved to reduce background levels of radiolabeled biotin. The pre-targeting concept required the initial injection of SA-antibody, which circulates and accumulates at tumor sites, and this was followed by a clearing agent to remove circulating SA antibody followed by radiolabeled biotin (123). A three-step approach consisted of biotinylated antibody, followed by avidin and then radiolabeled biotin (124). A further development has been to use galactosylated streptavidin–antibody conjugates, which have a much faster clearance rate from blood (125).

Advantages of multistep targeting systems

The indications are that multistep targeting systems can achieve greater specificity than is generally possible with simple conjugates. The disadvantage of complexity is sometimes argued against them but they are not more complex than multidrug therapy with conventional agents. At the same time there are opportunities for simplification of administration, which can be achieved by refinement of the components of multistep therapies.

One consideration relating to these multistep systems and to some single-step approaches is that they may not be effective against all metastases. Antigen-negative metastases may arise from antigen-negative cells in an otherwise antigen-positive cancer. Vascular permeability only becomes available in metastases big enough to have evoked a vascular network.

Immunogenicity and immune tolerance

The use of immunogenic substances in targeting is a serious obstacle to repeated therapy. In the original ADEPT trial it was found that patients who received a conjugate comprising a murine monoclonal antibody and a bacterial enzyme had antibodies in the blood to both components 10 days later. Antibody titers rose rapidly and were still detectable almost a year later (121). The immune response was delayed till 20–21 days by co-administration of cyclosporin A starting 48 hours before the conjugate. Co-administration of cyclosporin with the ADEPT drugs increased toxicity (126).

The host antibody response was anticipated from the results obtained in preclinical testing (127). It is apparent that the humanization of the antibody component can largely eliminate the response to the immunoglobulin component but it would be disadvantageous to lose the benefit of specificity provided by bacterial enzymes.

One approach has been to use molecular engineering to substitute the epitopes on a bacterial enzyme that evoke the immune response in humans. Clearly, this would be a labour-intensive approach when applied to all potential enzymes (128).

A further approach has been to start with a human enzyme and a prodrug and to modify the substrate specificity of the enzyme and to modify the prodrug substrate so that the mutant acts on the modified prodrug whereas the native enzyme does not. This is perhaps a less laborious approach than engineering out the active epitopes of enzyme and has the advantage of giving rise to enzymes able to activate multiple prodrugs (129).

A more general approach to the issue is the induction of immune tolerance. One approach has been to use monoclonal antibodies directed at various key epitopes on subpopulations of lymphocytes (130). It has been known for many years that conjugation of polyethylene glycol-291 (PEG) to proteins can reduce their immunogenicity (131). It was later shown that pegylation could render allergenic proteisn non-immunogenic and could induce tolerance. Similar reduction in immunogenicity was achieved with L-asparaginase, and immune tolerance was induced with uricase, another bacterial enzyme (132). Tolerance induced to immunoglobulins was found to be transferable to non-tolerized mice by T cells and T-cell extracts (133).

Although the significance of inducing tolerance to foreign proteins has not received the attention it appears to merit, its potential has been shown in studies in mice with antibody–enzyme conjugates known to be potent immunogens. It was found that a conjugate comprising a murine monoclonal antibody A5B7 and the bacterial enzyme CPG2 could induce tolerance in normal mice only when the PEG–protein ratio was at or near the maximum that could be achieved. Tolerance to repeated challenge with native conjugate was demonstrated and was transferable to naive mice with spleen cell transfer (134). The practicability of inducing immune tolerance to such conjugates has yet to be demonstrated in the clinic but if the pre-clinical evidence is substantiated it could provide a general solution to the use of immunogenic proteins.

References

1. Bence Jones H. Papers on chemical pathology. Lancet 1847, **2**, 254–7.
2. Brown WH. A case of pluriglandular syndrome: diabetes of a bearded woman. Lancet 1928, ii, 1022.
3. Zondek B. Hypophysenvorderlappen und Schwangerschaft. Endocrinologie 1929, **5**, 425–34.
4. Cushing H. The basophil adenomas of the pituitary body and their clinical manifestations (pituitary basophilism). Bull Johns Hopkins Hosp 1932, **50**, 137–95.
5. Gutman AB, Gutman EB. 'Acid' phosphatase occurring in serum of patients with metastatising carcinoma of the prostate gland. J Clin Invest 1938, **17**, 473–8.
6. Collip JB, Andersen EM. Serum inhibitory to the thyrotropic hormone. Lancet 1934, **226**, 76.
7. Young FG. Identity and mechanism of action of glycotropic (anti-insulin) substance of anterior pituitary gland. Biochem J 1938, **32**, 1521–39.
8. Stavitsky AB, Arquilla ER. Estimation of insulin and antibodies to insulin *in vitro* by hemagglutinin and hemolysis of insulin treated red cells and inhibitions of these reactions. Fed Proc 1953, **12**, 461.
9. Read CH, Stone DR. An immunological assay for minute amounts of human pituitary growth hormone. Am J Dis Child 1958, **96**, 538.
10. Hartog M, Fraser R. The immunological assay of growth hormone in human serum. J Endocrinol. 1961, **22**, 101–6.
11. Wide L, Gemzell CA. An immunological pregnancy test. Acta Endocrinol (Copenhagen) 1960, **35**, 261–7.
12. Roitt IM, Campbell PN, Doniach D. The nature of the thyroid autoantibodies present in patients with Hashimoto's thyroiditis (lymphadenoid goiter). Biochem J 1958, **69**, 248–56.
13. Brody S, Carlstrom G. Estimation of human chorionic gonadotrophin in biological fluids by complement fixation. Lancet 1960, ii, 99.
14. Yallows RS, Berson SA. Assay of plasma insulin in human subjects by immunological methods. Nature 1959, **184**, 1648–9.
15. Hunter WM, Greenwood FC. Preparation of iodine-131 labelled human growth hormone of high specific activity. Nature 1962, **192**, 495.
16. Gorer PA. The role of antibodies in immunity to transplanted leukaemia in mice. J Pathol Bacteriol 1942, **54**, 51.
17. Winn HJ. Immune mechanisms in homotranslantation. J Immunol 1960, **84**, 530.
18. Motta PE, Fagiani MB, Dolcetti A, *et al.* Passive immunotherapy of leukaemia and other cancer. Adv Cancer Res 1971, **14**, 161–79.
19. Shin HS, Pasternak GR, Economiou JS, *et al.* Immunotherapy of cancer with antibody. Science 1976, **194**, 327.
20. Shearer WT, Philpott GW, Parker CW. Stimulation of cells by antibody. Science 1973, **182**, 1537.
21. Pressman D, Korngold L. The *in vivo* localisation of anti-Wagner osteogenic sarcoma antibodies. Cancer 1953, **6**, 619–23.
22. Bale WF, Spar II, Goodland RL, *et al. In vivo* and *in vitro* studies of labeled antibodies against rat kidney and Walker carcinoma. Proc Soc Exp Biol Med 1955, **1**, 564–8.
23. Ghose T, Cerini M, Carter M, *et al.* Immunoradioactive agent against cancer. Br Med J 1967, **1**, 90–3.
24. Quinones J, Mizejewski G, Beierwaltes WH. Choriocarcinoma scanning using radiolabelled antibody to chorionic gonadotrophin. J Nucl Med 1971, **12**, 69–75.
25. Gold P, Freedman SO. Specific carcinoembryonic antigens of the human digestive system. J Exp Med 1965, **122**, 467–9.
26. Mach JP, Buchegger F, Forni M. Radiolabelled monoclonal anti-CEA antibodies for the detection of human colon carcinoma by external photoscanning and immunoscintigraphy. Immunol Today 1981, **2**, 239–49.
27. Goldenberg DM, Deland F, Kim E, *et al.* Use of radiolabelled antibodies to carcinoembryonic antigen for the detection and localisation of diverse cancers by external photoscanning. New Engl J Med 1978, **298**, 1384–8.
28. Kohler H, Milstein C. Continuous cultures of fused cells secreting antibodies of predefined specificity. Nature 1975, **256**, 495.
29. Dykes PW, Hine KR, Bradwell AR, *et al.* Localisation of tumour deposits by external scanning after injection of radiolabelled anti-CEA antigen. Br Med J 1980, **280**, 220.
30. Searle F, Bagshawe KD, Begent RJH, *et al.* Radioimmunolocalisation of tumours by external scintigraphy after administration of ^{131}I antibody to CEA. Nucl Med Commun 1980, **1**, 131–9.

31. Begent RHJ, Searle F, Stanway G, *et al.* Radioimmunolocalisation of tumour by external scintigraphy after administration of ^{131}I antibody to human chorionic gonadotrophin: preliminary communication. J R Soc Med 1980, **73**, 624.

32. Begent RHJ, Green AJ, Bbagshawe KD, *et al.* Liposomally entrapped second antibody improves tumour imaging with radiolabelled (first) antitumour antibody. Lancet 1982, **ii**, 739.

33. Ehrlich P. Collected studies on immunology, Vol. II. John Wiley, New York, 1906, 442–7.

34. Moolten FL, Cooperbrand SR. Selective destruction of target cells by diphtheria toxin conjugated to antibody directed against antigens on the cells. Science 1970, **169**, 68.

35. Philpott GW, Bower RJ, Parker CW. Selective iodination and cytotoxicity of tumour cells with an antibody–enzyme conjugate. Surgery 1973, **74**, 51.

36. Thorpe PE, Ross WCJ, Cumber AJ, *et al.* Toxicity of diphtheria toxin for lymphoblastoid cells is increased by conjugation to anti-lymphocytic globulin. Nature 1978, **271**, 752–4.

37. Ghose T, Nigam SP. Antibody as carrier of chlorambucil. Cancer 1972, **29**, 1398–400.

38. Philpott GW, Bower RJ, Parker CW. Improved selective cytotoxicity with an antibody–diphtheria toxin conjugate. Surgery 1973, **73**, 928.

39. Bagshawe KD. Antibody directed enzymes revive anticancer prodrugs concept. Br J Cancer 1987, **56**, 531.

40. Reisfeld RA, Sell S. Monoclonal antibodies and cancer therapy, UCL Symposium in Molecular and Cellular Biology, New Series Vol. 27. Alan R. Liss Inc, New York, 1985, 207–57.

41. Parry C. Collected works. London, 1825.

42. Veall, NL. Diagnostic and therapeutic uses of radioactive isotopes. Br J Radiol 1950, **23**, 527.

43. Szendrol Z, Kocsar L, Tottossy B, *et al.* Perspectives in scintigraphic detection of gynaecologic tumors using labeled estrogen. Neoplasma 1975, **22**, 535–7.

44. Sisson JC, Frager MS, Ross D *et al.* Scintigraphic localisation of phaeochromocytoma. New Engl J Med 1981, **305**, 12.

45. Hadley GP, Rabe E. Scanning with iodine[131] MIBG in children with solid tumours. J Nucl Med 1986, **27**, 620.

46. Endo K, Shiomi K, Kasagi K, *et al.* Imaging of medullary thyroid cancer with ^{131}I-MIBG. Lancet 1984, **ii**, 233.

47. Haynie TP, Miale A. The pancreas. In: Clinical scintillation imaging, 2nd edn (ed. LM Freeman, PM Johnson). Grune and Stratton, New York, 1971, 601–22.

48. Mew D, Wat CK, Towers GHN, *et al.* Photoimmunotherapy: treatment of animal tumours with tumor-specific monoclonal antibody–haematoporphyrin conjugates. J Immunol 1983, **130**, 1473–7.

49. Bernal SD, Lampidis TJ, McIsaac RM, *et al.* Anticarcinoma activity *in vivo* of Rhodamine[123] a mitochondrial-specific dye. Science 1983, **22**, 169.

50. Strauli P, Barrett AJ, Baici A. Proteinases and tumor invasion, EORTC monograph series No. 6. Raven Press, New York, 1980, 1–210.

51. Udaka K, Hayashi H. Further purification of a protease inhibitor from rabbit skin with healing inflammation. Biochem Biophys Acta 1965, **97**, 251–62.

52. Keilova H, Tomasek V. Effect of papian inhibitor from chicken egg white on cathepsin NB. Biochem Biophys Acta 1974, **334**, 179–86.

53. Breith J, Miesch F, Metais P. Enzymatic and immunologic inhibitors of proteases in the CSF. Clin Chim Acta 1969, **24**, 203–9.

54. Kleiner DE, Stetler Stevenson WG. Matrix metalloproteinases and metastasis. Cancer Chemother Pharmacol 1999, Suppl. 43, 542–51.

55. Cornelius LA, Nehring LC, Harding E, *et al.* Matrix metalloproteinases generate angiostatin. J Immunol 1998, **161**, 6845–52.

56. Hargreaves RHJ, Winski SL, Ross D. *et al.* RHI, preclinical studies [abstract]. Br J Cancer 1999, Suppl. 12, 95A.

57. Knox RJ, Jenkins T, Hobbs SM, *et al.* Bioactivation of CB1954 by human NQ02 a novel co-substrate mediated prodrug therapy. Cancer Res 2000, **60**, 4179–86.

58. Patterson AV, Zhang H, Moghaddam A, *et al.* Increased sensitivity to the prodrug 5'-deoxy-5-fluorouridine and modulation of 5-fluoro-2'-deoxyuridine sensitivity in MCF-7 cells transfected with thymidine phosphorylase. Br J Cancer 1995, **72**, 669–75.

59. Hopkins FG. Note on yellow pigment in butterflies [abstract]. Paper presented to The Chemical Society. Nature 1898, **40**, 335.

60. Wills L. Nature of haemopoietic factor in Marmite. Lancett 1933, **1**, 1283.

61. Wills L, Clutterbuck PN, Evans PDF. A new factor in the production of cure of macrocytic anaemias and its relationship to other haemopoietic principles curative in pernicious anaemia. Biochem J 1933, **31**, 2136.

62. Woods DD. Relationship of *p*-aminobenzoic acid to the mechanism of action of sulphanamide. Br J Exp Pathol 1940, **21**, 74.

63. Angier RB, Boothie JH, Hutchings BL, *et al.* Structure and function of liver L casei factor. Science 1946, **103**, 667.

64. Farber S, Cutler EC, Hawkins B, *et al.* Action of pteroylglutamic conjugates in man. Science 1947, **106**, 619–21.

65. Farber S, Diamond LK, Mercer RD, *et al.* Temporary remissions in acute leukaemia in children produced by folic acid antagonist. New Engl J Med 1948, **238**, 789–93.

66. Strum WB. Intestinal folate transport: binding characteristics of the folate receptor from human placenta. Cancer Res 1980, **28**, 30A.

67. Antony AC, Utley C, Van Horne KC, *et al.* Isolation and characterisation of folate receptor from human placenta. J Biol Chem 1981, **256**, 9684–92.

68. Kane MA, Elwood PC, Portillo RM, *et al.* The interrelationship of the soluble and membrane associated folate-binding proteins in human KB cells. J Biol Chem 1986, **261**, 15625–31.

69. Virchow R. Die Krankhaften Geschiwulste. August Hirschwald, Berlin, 1863.

70. Bradford EF, Russel BRG, *et al.* 1908–1912 Scientific reports. Imperial Cancer Research Fund, London.

71. Duran-Reynolds F. Studies in the localisation of dyes and foreign proteins in normal and malignant tissues. Am J Cancer 1939, **35**, 98.

72. Algire GH, Chalkey HW. Vascular reactions of normal and malignant tissues *in vivo*: vascular reactions of mice to wounds and to normal and neoplastic transplants. J Natl Cancer Inst 1945, **6**, 73.

73. Folkman J. Anti-angiogenesis: new concept for the therapy of solid tumors. Ann Surg 1972, **175**, 409–16.

74. Chaplin DJ. Hydralazine-induced tumor hypoxia: a potential target for cancer chemotherapy. J Natl Cancer Inst 1989, **81**, 618.

75. Pimm MV. An examination of the influence of vasoactive drugs in blood flow and localisation of a monoclonal antibody in human tumour xenografts. Br J Cancer 1990, **62**, 69.

76. Carswell EA, Old LJ, Kassel RL, *et al.* An endotoxin-induced serum factor that causes necrosis of tumors. Proc Natl Acad Sci, USA 1975, **25**, 3666.

77. Old LJ. Tumor necrosis factor (TNF). Science (Washington DC) 1985, **230**, 630.

78. Watanabe N, Niitsu Y, Umeno H, *et al.* Toxic effect of tumor necrosis factor on tumor vasculature in mice. Cancer Res 1988, **48**, 2179.

79. Creaven PJ, Brenner DE, Cowens JW, *et al.* A phase I clinical trial of recombinant human tumor necrosis given daily for five days. Cancer Chemotherapy Pharmacol 1990, **23**, 186.

80. Plowman J, Narayan VL, Dykes V, *et al.* Flavone acetic acid: a novel agent with preclinical antitumor activity against colon adenocarcinoma. Cancer Treat Rep 1986, **70**, 631.

81. Wiltrout RH, Boyd MR, Back TC, *et al.* Flavone-8-acetic acid augments systemic natural killer cell activity and synergises with IL 2 for treatment of murine renal cancer. J Immunol 1988, **140**, 3261.

82. Kaye SB, Clavel M, Didion P, *et al.* Phase II trials with flavone acetic acid in patients with advanced carcinoma of the breast, colon, head and neck and melanoma. Invedst New Drugs 1990, **8**, 595–9.

83. Thomsen LL, Baguley BC, Rustin GJS, *et al.* Flavone acetic acid (FAA) with recombinant interleukin-2 (TIL-2) advanced malignant melanoma ii: induction of nitric acid production. Br J Cancer 1992, **66**, 723–7.

84. Wayne RJ, Cao Z, Mountjoy KG, *et al.* Stimulation of tumors to synthesise tumor necrosis factor-α *in situ* using 5, 6-dimethylxanthone-4-acetic acid: a novel approach to cancer therapy. Cancer Res 1999, **59**, 633–8.

85. Derbyshire EJ, Yang YC, Li SH, *et al.* Heparin–steroid conjugates lacking glucocorticoid or mineral corticoid activities inhibit the proliferation of vascular endothelial cells. Biochem Biophys Acta 1996, **1310**, 86–96.

86. Bagheri-Yarmand R, Kourbali Y, Rath AM, *et al.* Carboxymethyl benzylamide dextran blocks angiogenesis of MDA-MB435 breast carcinoma xenografted in fat pad and its lung metastases in nude mice. Cancer Res 1999, **59**, 507–15.

87. Clauss M, Gerlach M, Gerlach H, *et al.* Vascular permeability factor: a tumor derived polypeptide that induces endothelial cell and monocyte procoagulant activity and promotes and promotes monocyte migration. J Exp Med 1990, **172**, 1535–45.

88. Conn G, Soderman DD, Schaeffer M-T, *et al.* Purification of a glyoprotein vascular endothelial cell mitogen from a rat glioma-derived cell line. Proc Natl Acad Sci, USA 1990, **87**, 1323–5.

89. Gateley S, Twardowski P, Stack MS, *et al.* Human prostate carcinoma cells express enzymatic activity that converts human plasminogen to the angiogenesis inhibitor angiostatin. Cancer Res 1996, **56**, 4887–90.

90. O'Reilly MS, Holmgren L, Shin Y, *et al.* A novel angiogenesis inhibitor that mediates the suppression of metastases by a Lewis lung carcinoma. Cell 1994, **79**, 315–28.

91. Burrows FJ, Derbyshire EJ, Tazzxari PL, *et al.* Up-regulation of endoglin on vascular endothelial cells in human solid tumours: implications for diagnosis and therapy. Clin Cancer Res 1995, **1**, 1623–34.

92. Ran WS, Gao BN, Duffy S, *et al.* Infarction of solid Hodgkin's tumour in mice by antibody directed targeting of tissue factor to tumour vasculature. Cancer Res 1998, **58**, 4646–53.

93. Wedge S, Ogilvie DJ, Dukes M. 2 D4190: An orally active inhibitor of VEGF receptor tyrosine kinase activity. Br J Cancer 1999, **80** (Suppl. Z), 254A.

94. Pettit GR, Singh SB, Hamel E, *et al.* Isolation and structure of the strong cell growth and tubulin inhibitor combretastatin A-4. Experimenta 1989, **45**, 209–11.

95. Dark GG, Hill SA, Prise VE, *et al.* Combretastatin A-4: an agent that displays potent and selective toxicity toward tumor vasculature. Cancer Res 1997, **57**, 1829–35.

96. Bangham AD, Standish M, Watkins JC. Diffusion of univalent ions across the lamella of swollen phospholipids. J Mol Biol 1965, **13**, 238.

97. Papahadjopoulos D, Watkins JC. Phospholipid model membranes. ii Permeability properties of hydrated liquid crystals. Biochem Biophys Acta 1967, **133**, 839.

98. Gregoriadis G, Ryman NBE. Fate of protein containing liposomes injected into rats. An approach to the treatment of storage diseases. Eur J Biochem 1971, **24**, 485–91.

99. Gregoriadis G. Drug entrapment in liposomes. FEBS Lett 1973, **36**, 292–6.

100. Gregoriadis G, Neerunjun ED. Treatment of tumour bearing mice with liposome entrapped antinomycin D prolong their survival. Res Commun Chem Pathol Pharmacol 1975, **10**, 351–61.

101. Gregoriadis G. Homing of liposomes to target cells. Biochem Soc Transact 1975, **3**, 613–18.

102. Leserman LD, Machy P, Barbet J. Cell specific drug transfer from lipsome bearing monoclonal antibodies. Nature 1981, **293**, 226–8.

103. Machy P, Leserman LD. Small liposomes are better than large liposomes for specific drug delivery *in vitro*. Biochim Biophys Acta 1983, **730**, 313–29.

104. Gabizon A, Papahadjopoulos D. Liposome formulations with prolonged circulation time in blood and enhanced uptake by tumors. Proc Natl Acad Sci, USA 1988, **85**, 6949–53.

105. Yatvin MB, Kreutz W, Horwitz BA. pH sensitive liposomes: possible clinical implications. Science 1980, **210**, 1253–4.

106. Kato T, Nemoto R, Mori H, *et al.* Arterial chemoembolisation with mitomycin C microcapsules in the treatment of primary and secondary carcinoma of the

kidney, liver, bone and intrapelvic organs. Cancer 1981, **48**, 674–80.

107. Allison AC, Gregordiadis G. Liposomes as immunological adjuvants. Nature 1974, **252**, 252.

108. Fogler WE, Talmadge JE, Fidler IJ. The activation of tumoricidal properties in macrophages of endoxin responder and nonresponder mice by liposome-encapsulated immunomodulators. Res J Reticuloendothel Soc 1983, **33**, 165–74.

109. Yuan F, Dellian M, Fukumara D, *et al*. Vascular permeability in a human tumor xenograft: molecular size dependence and cut off size. Cancer Res 1995, **55**, 3752–6.

110. Yuan F, Lennig M, Huang SK, *et al*. Microvascular permeability and interstitial penetration of sterically stabilized (stealth) liposomes in a human tumor xenograft. Cancer Res 1994, **54**, 3352–6.

111. Ringsdorf H. Structure and properties of pharmacologically active polymers. J Polym Sci Polymer Symp 1975, **51**, 135–53.

112. Matsumura Y, Maeda H. A new concept for macromolecular therapeutics in cancer therapy: mechanism of tumoritropic accumulation of proteins and the antitumor agent, SMANCS. Cancer Res 1986, **46**, 6387–92.

113. Seymour LW, Miyamoto Y, Maeda H, *et al*. Influence of molecular weight on passive tumour accumulation of a soluble macromolecular carrier. Eur J Cancer 1995, **31A**, 766–70.

114. Duncan R, Dimitoijevic S, Evagaron EG. The role of polymer conjugates in the diagnosis and treratment of cancer. STP Pharma Sci 1996, 6(4), 237–63.

115. Senter PD, Saulnier MG, Schreiber GJM, *et al*. Antitumor effects of antibody–alkaline phosphatase conjugate combination with etoposide phosphate. Proc Natl Acad Sci, USA 1988, **85**, 4842–6.

116. Napier MP, Sharma SK, Springer CJ, *et al*. Antibody-directed enzyme prodrug therapy (ADEPT): efficacy and mechanism of action in colorectal carcinoma. Clin Cancer Res 2000, **6**, 765–72.

117. Sharma SK, Bagshawe KD, Burke PJ, *et al*. Antibody directed enzyme prodrug therapy (ADEPT): a three phase system. Dis Markers 1991, **9**, 225–31.

118. Melton RG, Knox RJ. (Eds.). Enzyme–prodrug strategies for cancer therapy. Kluwer Academic/Plenum Publishers, 1999, 417–28.

119. Huber BE, Richards CA, Krenitsky TA. Retroviral-mediated gene therapy for the treatment of hepatocellular carcinoma: An innovative approach for cancer therapy. Proc Natl Acad Sci, USA 1991, **88**, 8039–43.

120. Satchi R, Duncan R. PDEPT: Polymer directed enzyme prodrug therapy. Proceedings of 3rd International Symposium on Polymer Therapeutics. School of Pharmacy, University of London, January 1988, p. 58.

121. Bagshawe KD. ADEPT and related concepts. Cell Biophys 1994, **24/25**, 91–3.

122. Green NM. Avidin. Advan Protein Chem 1975, **29**, 85–133.

123. Goodwin DA, Meares CF, McCall MJ, *et al*. Pretargeted immunoscintigraphy of murine tumors with indium-III labeled bifunctional haptens. J Nucl Med 1988, **29**, 226–34.

124. Paganelli G, Magnani P, Zito F, *et al*. Three step monoclonal antibody tumor targeting in carcinoembryonic antigen positive patients. Cancer Res 1991, **51**, 5960–6.

125. Rosebrough SF, Hashmi M. Galactose-modified streptavidin–GC4 antifibrin monoclonal antibody conjugates: application for two-step thrombus/embolus imaging. J Pharmacol Exp Ther 1996, **276**, 770–5.

126. Bagshawe KD. Developments with targeted enzymes. Tumor Targeting 1998, **3**, 21–4.

127. Ledermann JA, Begent RHJ, Bagshawe KD. Cyclosporin A prevents the anti-murine antibody response to a monoclonal anti-tumour antibody in rabbits. Br J Cancer 1988, **58**, 562–6.

128. Spencer DIR, Robson L, Bhatia J, *et al*. Identifying immunogenic sites on ADEPT enzyme CPG2 using a SCFV phage library and SELDI™-AMS [abstract]. Br J Cancer 1999, **80** (suppl. 2), 254a.

129. Wolfe LA, Mullin RJ. Laethem R, *et al*. Antibody directed enzyme prodrug therapy with T268G mutant of arboxypeptidase A1: *in vitro* and *in vivo* studies with prodrugs of methotrexate and the thymidylate synthetase inhibitors GW1031 and GW1843. Bioconj Chem 1999, **10**, 38–48.

130. Waldmann H, Hale G, Clark M, *et al*. Monoclonal antibodies for immunosuppression. Prog Allergy 1988, **45**, 16–30.

131. Albuchowski A, van Es T, Palczuk C, *et al*. Alteration of immunological properties of bovine serum albumin by covalent attachment of polyethylene glycol. J Biol Chem 1979, **252**, 3578–81.

132. Savoka KV, Davis FF, Palczuk NC. Induction of tolerance in mice by uricase and monomethroxypolyethylene glycol-modified uricase. Int Arch Allergy Appl Immunol 1984, **75**, 58–67.

133. Wilkinson IM, Chung JA, Jackson C, *et al*. Tolerance induction in mice by conjugate of monoclonal immunoglobulins and monomethoxypolyethylene glycol. Transfer of tolerance by T cells and T cell extracts. J Immunol 1987, **139**, 326–31.

134. Bagshawe KD, Sharma SK, Knox RJ, Ammoquaye E. Studies with polymer enzyme conjugate and AMIRACS. In: Advances in the Application of Monoclonal Antibodies in Clinical Oncology [abstract]. Samos, Greece, May 1999.

2

Preclinical models for the study of targeted therapy

Gail Rowlinson-Busza

Introduction

When monoclonal antibodies were first produced (1), there was immense interest in their clinical application, as it was anticipated that they would be the 'magic bullets' that would specifically target cancer cells. However, the uptake of monoclonal antibodies in tumors in patients was found to be disappointingly low (2) and very few cases of successful immunotherapy with antibodies were reported. Over the last 20 years, much has been learnt about the difficulties associated with antibody therapy and ways to overcome them. In particular, advances in the field of protein engineering have allowed modifications to antibodies to improve their pharmacokinetics and to convey upon them novel tumoricidal properties (3). This technology has also been utilized to humanize murine antibodies to render them less immunogenic and allow repeated treatments (4).

Although the most widely used, antibodies are not the only means of targeting tumors. Liposomes have been shown to localize selectively in xenografts (5) and an improved therapeutic index of liposomally encapsulated drugs compared with free drug has been reported (6). The two technologies have been combined with the development of immunoliposomes, that is, liposomes with monoclonal antibodies on their surface to improve their tumor-targeting capacity (7).

Many factors may influence the uptake of targeting molecules in tumors, some of which are dependent on the molecule itself and some on the tumor. In the case of radiolabeled monoclonal antibodies, characteristics such as antibody affinity, whether the antibody is the whole immunoglobulin molecule or a fragment (for example, $F(ab')_2$, Fab, or other small antigen-binding molecules that can be constructed), route of administration, choice of radioisotope, and method of labeling may be important determinants of successful targeting. For liposomal targeting of tumors, the size of the lipo-

some is significant, as is whether or not it is modified, for example, with polyethylene glycol (PEG). Other influences on uptake are different properties of the tumor, such as site, size, vasculature, and antigen density on the tumor cell surface. Animal models for studying these parameters are usually based on transplanted tumors in mice or rats. In this chapter, various tumor model systems will be described with some discussion of what data can be obtained using them.

Tumor xenografts

Background

It is not a novel concept to transplant tumors into foreign hosts. However, it was not until the beginning of the twentieth century that it was realized that this was most successful if the donor animal was related to the recipient (8). This led to the proposal of a theory of inheritable susceptibility to tumor transplantation (9), but the nature of the process was unknown. Initially, it was supposed that host antibodies were responsible for tumor rejection. A significant development was the introduction of inbred strains of mice, in which many generations of sibling matings yielded animals all of which were homozygous for the same genes. This allowed the allotransplantation of tumors and other tissues from one animal to another in these genetically homogeneous mice, and also to F_1 hybrids of the pure line and a different strain. This led Haldane (10) to propose that there were distinct antigens on all tissues, similar to blood group antigens. Medawar (11) demonstrated, in skin-grafting experiments in rabbits, that a second allograft to the same recipient from the same donor was rejected more quickly than the first.

The immunological function of the thymus was elucidated in 1961 by Miller (12), who demonstrated that neonatally thymectomized mice tolerated skin grafts from a different mouse strain for up to 2 months, but that intact mice and thymectomized mice, which were then grafted with thymuses, rejected the grafts within 2 weeks. Therefore, if successful transplantations of human tumors into experimental animals were to be achieved, it would be necessary to find a method of overcoming immunological rejection.

Originally, it was found that immunologically-privileged sites were capable of supporting the growth of tumor xenografts. For example, it was possible to grow rat sarcomas in the outer membrane of chick embryos (13) and successful transplants of some human tumors in the anterior chamber of the eye in rabbits and guinea pigs were also reported (14), but most tumors regressed or did not grow at all. Of 20 different human tumors implanted intracranially into the brains of mice, growth of three of these tumors was observed in some of the mice (15), although a higher success rate was reported with human tumors that had first been grown in the eye prior to transfer to the brain in experimental animals (16). When reviewing his attempts between 1939 and 1950 to transplant tumors into the anterior chamber of the eye, Greene (17) noted that metastatic tumors grew in many more cases than did primary tumors.

Immune-deprived animals

Hamsters treated with cortisone were used as hosts for xenograft studies and it was found that 26 of 68 tested human tumors survived as viable nodules in the hamsters' cheek pouches, although only 10 of the tumors actually grew (18). It was also determined that human tumors could be serially transplanted as subcutaneous xenografts in rats and hamsters treated with cortisone in addition to X-irradiation (19). Tumors grown in immunologically privileged sites, or in animals treated to make them less able to reject foreign tissue, were used for a number of studies of therapeutic agents (20). However, tumors did not grow reliably in these animals, and it was difficult to measure tumor growth in privileged sites, such as the hamster cheek pouch, although it was possible to use this model to study the localization of radiolabeled polyclonal antibody by photoscanning (21). A major drawback of this strategy is that animals treated with drugs to render them immunologically incompetent regain their immunity after a period of time, and the resulting tumor rejection could be misinterpreted as tumor regression following experimental therapy.

More consistent hosts for engraftment of human tumors were produced by neonatal thymectomy fol-

lowed either by anti-thymocyte serum or by potentially lethal total-body irradiation with reconstitution of the bone marrow by injection of syngeneic bone marrow cells (22). This technique was later refined to remove the need for bone marrow reconstitution by protecting the mice with an injection of cytosine arabinoside (Ara-C) 2 days prior to irradiation (23). Mice treated in this way were found to be good hosts for human tumor xenografts, which retained the characteristics of the original tumors in terms of chromosome analysis, histology, and antigen expression (24). Human colorectal tumors established in these immune-suppressed mice were used in growth delay experiments following chemotherapy, and a correlation of the response of the xenograft with that of the original tumor in the patient was reported (25). However, immune-deprived mice are unsuitable for long-term experiments as they may regain their immunity after a period of time.

Immunodeficient mice

Immunodeficient mice are widely recognized as the optimum host for human tumor xenografts. They have the advantage of permanent lack of immunity, although this makes animal husbandry difficult, since all food, water, and bedding must be sterile. This problem is minor, however, compared with the enormous advantage these animals have brought to cancer research.

Nude mice

The hairless mutant 'nude' (*nu/nu*) was first described in 1966 (26), and it was observed that the majority of the mice died before weaning and that those that survived grew slowly, were poorly fertile, and developed a fatal liver disease before the age of 6 months. It was also concluded that the lack of hair was caused by abnormal keratinization of the hair and not by absence of follicles. It was another 2 years before it was reported that the *nu/nu* homozygote (nude phenotype) was essentially athymic, although heterozygous (phenotypically normal) litter-mates had a normally developed thymus (27). In addition, blood leukocyte counts were very low both in *nu/nu* homozygotes and in heterozygotes. In 1969, Rygaard and Povlsen (28) were the first to grow human tumors in nude mice, using a surgical specimen of a resected colon tumor. The same group later demonstrated that serial transplantation of human tumors was possible in these mice (29). Nude mice have now become established as the primary host for human tumor xenografts for targeted therapeutic studies.

Not all human tumors will grow in nude mice, however, with surgical specimens taken directly from the patient being less successful than cell lines established in tissue culture (30). As discovered in early experiments in immunologically privileged sites (17), xenografts were more easily established from metastases than from primary tumors (31). Fogh *et al.* (32) reported that 78 per cent of 162 cultured human tumor cell lines grew as xenografts in nude mice and retained the histopathology of the original tumor. Almost all reports of the successful establishment of a xenograft line report that the histological characteristics of the original human tumor are maintained, although the degree of differentiation may alter (33). This change usually occurs during transfer from human to mouse, the xenograft then remaining stable in subsequent passages from mouse to mouse (34). Chromosome analysis of xenografts has shown that they retain their human karyotype (35). In addition, it has been reported that biochemical parameters, such as the presence of intracellular enzymes, are maintained in xenografts, for example, in melanomas and pancreatic adenocarcinomas (36). A comparison of tumor vasculature in human squamous cell carcinoma xenografts and the original tumors revealed that the qualitative histology of the tumors was preserved in the xenografts, with proliferation of tumor cells concentrated around blood vessels (37). The median distance between interphase tumor cells and blood vessels in the xenograft was shorter than in the original tumor, as were the distances between blood vessels.

SCID mice

The severe combined immunodeficiency mutation, *scid*, was first described in 1983 (38) as an autosomal mutation in CB17 mice that greatly impairs lymphopoiesis. The SCID mouse lacks both humoral and cellular immunity owing to a lack of mature B and T lymphocytes. This absence of an adaptive immune system is caused by the inability of mice homozygous for the *scid* gene mutation to express rearranged antigen receptors (39), but it does not impair myeloid, erythroid, or natural killer (NK) cell development. However, a proportion of mice develop a limited number of B and T cells at about 3–9 months of age, a phenomenon termed 'leakiness' (40). This effect has been shown to be age- and strain-dependent, with detectable levels of serum immunoglobulin measured in

79 per cent of CB17 SCID mice, while only 15 per cent of C3H SCID mice were found to be leaky (41). Leaky SCID mice are able to reject allogeneic skin grafts, a T-cell-dependent reaction, and approximately 40 per cent of leaky mice develop thymic lymphomas.

SCID mice have been shown to be suitable hosts for human tumor xenografts, including several Hodgkin's lymphoma cell lines that could not be established in nude mice (42). Sensitivity to chemotherapeutic agents has been compared in xenografts implanted in nude or SCID mice and consistent results were found in over 90 per cent of experiments. However, a human T-cell lymphoma growing in nude mice was resistant to cyclophosphamide, although it was sensitive to the same treatment if the tumor was xenografted in SCID mice (43). These experiments suggest that the genetic immune background of the host mouse should not be ignored as a factor affecting the growth and therapy of xenografts.

Lymphomagenesis can also be studied in the SCID mouse. Epstein–Barr virus (EBV) can lead to lymphoproliferative disease in immunosuppressed patients. Injection of peripheral blood lymphocytes (PBLs) from EBV-positive patients into SCID mice induces a lymphoproliferative disease in the mice that closely resembles that in posttransplant patients (44). This model can then be used in the assessment of novel therapies. The model may also be useful in autoimmune disease syndrome (AIDS) research, as SCID mice injected with human PBLs can be infected with human immunodeficiency virus 1 (HIV-1) (45).

SCID mice have been grafted with lymphoid tissue, using murine bone marrow cultures, and a functional immune system was restored (46). An interesting extension of this model is to reconstitute the immune system with human bone marrow or umbilical cord blood (47) or human PBLs (48). These mice were shown to have circulating human B and T cells. A superior host for engraftment of a human immune system is the NOD–SCID mouse, in which the *scid* mutation is backcrossed on to the non-obese diabetic (NOD) mouse (49). The SCID mouse is deficient in B and T cells, but has higher than normal NK-cell activity, presumably in compensation. The NOD mouse has a functional deficit of NK cells, but is susceptible to T-cell-mediated autoimmune insulin-dependent diabetes mellitus (IDDM). The NOD–SCID mouse demonstrates multiple adaptive and innate immunodeficiency and, owing to a lack of T cells, does not develop IDDM. Due to their multiple immunological deficiencies, NOD–SCID mice have been shown to be superior to nude or SCID mice for xenotransplantation of human leukemia and lymphoma (50). The model has been used for targeted therapy of non-Hodgkin's lymphoma implanted intraperitoneally (51). The NOD–SCID model also has advantages for studies of human stem cells, as it can sustain the growth of human lymphoid and myeloid stem cells at higher levels than any other mouse model (52). This mouse has been used as a model for acute lymphoblastic leukemia (ALL) by intravenous injection of primary leukemic cells from patients (53). Engraftment was more successful in the NOD–SCID mice than in SCID mice, providing a system for the study of the biology and treatment of ALL.

Factors affecting the growth of tumors

The growth of human tumors in immunodeficient mice is influenced by several factors. The strain of mouse can affect the growth rate of xenografts (54). The age of the animal at the time of tumor inoculation can influence the incidence of tumors, a higher proportion of 'takes' occurring in younger animals, with a faster growth rate (55). The site of tumor implantation has also been shown to affect the growth of syngeneic murine tumors in mice, tumors implanted nearer the head growing 2–3 times more rapidly than those implanted more caudally (56). It has also been demonstrated that human tumor xenografts implanted on the right flank grew significantly more slowly than those on the left flank (57). It was suggested that these differences were caused by morphogenic gradients similar to those believed to control differentiation during ontogeny.

The cancer type also affects the success rate of establishing xenografts in nude mice; for example, human lymphoid tumors have proved more difficult to grow than many other tumors. Hormone-dependent tumors, such as those of breast, ovary, or prostate, can also be difficult to establish in mice, since the murine hormones may not be recognized by the human receptors in the tumor. It has been shown that primary infiltrating ductal breast carcinoma implants grew aggressively and metastasized in 100 per cent of female SCID mice, but in only 33 per cent of male SCID mice (58). In this case, implantation of slow-release human hormone pellets can facilitate the engraftment of these tumors (59). Alternatively, inoculation of tumor cells suspended in Matrigel rather than culture medium has been shown

to produce tumors from cell lines that would not otherwise grow in mice, including both prostate (60) and breast (61). Matrigel is a mixture of basement membrane components, which is a liquid at 4°C but forms a solid gel at 37°C (62).

In the context of comparing different targeting strategies *in vivo*, the immunodeficient mouse provides a convenient model, since genetically identical tumors can be induced in several animals, allowing direct comparisons to be made. However, for the reasons outlined above, when using xenograft models for targeted therapy research, it is important to use the same strain of mouse of the same sex and of approximately the same age throughout each experiment. Tumors should be implanted at the same location in the mice. In this way, the variability between repeats of experiments is minimized.

Antibody localization in xenografts

Targeting of radiolabeled antibodies began with the work of Pressman and Keighley (63), who demonstrated that radiolabeled rabbit antiserum raised against normal rat kidney could localize in the kidneys following intravenous injection into normal rats. The same group later targeted radiolabeled rabbit antisera to a rat osteogenic sarcoma (64). Specific localization was confirmed by the use of the dual-label technique (65). In these experiments, specific antitumor antiserum was radiolabeled with ^{131}I and co-injected with ^{133}I-labeled normal serum immunoglobulin into rats bearing syngeneic lymphosarcoma, resulting in a tumor uptake of the antitumor antiserum higher than that of the normal immunoglobulin.

Following the pioneering work of Pressman and Korngold (64) in targeting tumors with radiolabeled antitumor antiserum, the discovery of antigens that are more specific for tumors led to the development of tumor-associated antibodies. Many of these antigens are either inappropriately expressed, for example, fetal proteins in adult tissues, or are aberrant forms of normal proteins, which may be truncated or incorrectly glycosylated, or may be oncogene products. For example, Gold and Freedman (66) identified carcinoembryonic antigen (CEA) in colonic carcinomas, but not in normal adult tissues. Human tumor xenograft models were developed to study the localization of polyclonal antibodies against CEA *in vivo*; these demonstrated specific uptake by the tumor using both immunoscintigraphy and γ-counting of tissues (67). These, and many similar studies, showed that it was feasible to target human tumors with radiolabeled antibodies against tumor-associated antigens, and that a specific antibody localized at higher levels in tumor than did an irrelevant control antibody. Sharkey *et al.* (68) compared tumor localization of a purified goat polyclonal and four mouse monoclonal anti-CEA antibodies and found that the monoclonals generally showed better uptake. The advent of monoclonal antibody technology has allowed the production of highly specific antibodies, which have been studied extensively in human tumor xenograft systems in immunodeficient mice.

Factors affecting targeting in xenografts

Several factors have been reported to affect the localization of radiolabeled monoclonal antibodies in xenografts. Tumor vascular permeability has been shown to correlate with the uptake of antibody in two different human tumors in nude mice (69). Variables relating to the tumor target (antigen expression levels, vascular volume, and permeability) have been shown to be important factors in determining antibody accumulation in tumors, whereas differences in antibody affinity for the antigen varying by 100-fold had little effect on tumor uptake (70). Even within the same tumor and antibody model, differences in the host animal can affect antibody uptake. It has been reported that tumor size was inversely proportional to uptake (measured as per cent injected dose per gram tumor weight, % i.d. g^{-1})) of ^{75}Se endogenously labeled, as well as ^{125}I- and ^{111}In-labeled, specific antibody in three different xenografts (71). This is probably due to tumor necrosis in larger tumors and a decrease in blood flow. Similar findings have been reported for the uptake of ^{111}In-labelled liposomes in xenografts (72). The uptake of antibody in xenografts also depends on the administered protein dose. A direct correlation was seen between the radioiodinated antibody dose and the amount localized in the tumor, although tumor-bound antibody could not be displaced by a subsequent injection of a large amount of unlabeled antibody (73).

Models of metastasis

Metastatic spread is uncommon following subcutaneous implantation of human tumors into nude mice. Sharkey and Fogh (74) found dissemination in only 14 of 801 mice (1.7 per cent) bearing subcutaneous xenografts, representing 10 per cent of 106 different primary tumors implanted without prior culture *in vitro*. This percentage is similar to that usually found in other such studies. However, Neulat-Duga *et al.* (75) reported a much higher incidence (13.2 per cent of mice having metastases) in a series of 831 nude mice bearing a total of 63 different malignant tumors. These authors found secondary deposits in lungs, and to a lesser extent in lymph nodes, but these were small and, therefore, usually only detectable microscopically. In addition, they found that metastatic human tumors exhibited higher metastatic potential in nude mice (46 per cent of metastases formed secondary deposits compared with only 13 per cent of primary tumors). These factors could account for the discrepancy between this and other studies, as well as the fact that many mice are killed for experiment before the appearance of detectable metastases.

Intraperitoneal, rather than subcutaneous, inoculation of tumor cells significantly increases the incidence of metastases (76) and intrasplenic injection of tumor cells is a useful technique for inducing liver metastases in nude mice for the study of the metastatic potential of different tumors (77). This model of experimental liver metastases has also been employed for studying the efficacy of targeted radioimmunotherapy combined with fractionated radiotherapy (78). Although not true metastatic spread, intravenous injection of tumor cells can result in the formation of lung colonies (77). SCID mice injected intravenously with human lung tumor cells developed primary tumor nodules in the lung, which subsequently metastasized to the liver and adrenal glands (79). This model was used to study the potential of targeted therapy using doxorubicin-loaded immunoliposomes, which were found to prevent metastatic spread of the primary lung tumors.

Orthotopic inoculation of the xenograft (that is, into the animal organ from which the human tumor was originally derived) increases the incidence of metastatic spread. For example, human renal cell carcinoma cells were found to metastasize to lungs and all peritoneal organs following implantation into the renal subcapsule of nude mice (80), the growth of human bladder tumors in the bladders of nude rats resulted in metastatic spread to distant organs in 25 per cent of cases (81), and human colon cancers transplanted into the cecum of nude mice were frequently locally invasive and developed liver metastases (82). It has further been shown that, following intradermal injection of melanoma cells in nude mice, the organ-specific metastatic spread of the xenografts to lung, lymph nodes, or brain reflected the pattern of the distant metastases in the donor patients (83).

Other models of targeting

Antigen-coated polymer beads have been implanted into normal animals as an artificial target for antibody localization, either subcutaneously, intraperitoneally, or intravenously; in the latter case the particles are sequestered in the lung capillary bed (84). This approach has the major disadvantage that there is no tumor vasculature and so is very far removed from the human tumor situation. However, it is relatively cheap as an initial test of antigen-binding *in vivo* or as a test of two-step targeting, for example using avidin or biotin conjugated to agarose beads (85). This model does have the advantage that the amount of antigen present is known and can be varied and therefore it can be used in quantitative studies of antibody uptake as well as for the comparison of different antibodies and fragments in immunocompetent animals. A refinement of this technique is the implantation of a micropore diffusion chamber containing antigen-coated particles (86). The chamber walls allow free diffusion of proteins, but the pores do not allow host immune cells to enter and possible destroy the antigen. The model has even been used with human tumor cells inside the diffusion chamber implanted into the peritoneal cavity of immunocompetent mice (87).

Other models used for cancer research include allotransplantation of syngeneic tumors in normal mice. Some of these murine tumors have been shown to have biological behavior similar to that of the equivalent human tumor (88). Although these mice have the advantage of being immunocompetent, the tumor is of murine origin and most monoclonal antibodies are raised again human antigens, so they may be of limited use for targeted therapy studies. It is possible to use murine cell lines transfected with a human antigen, such as the human polymorphic epithelial mucin (PEM) associated with breast and other epithelial cancers (89). However, these cell lines are not always stable and may not be as tumorigenic in the mice, owing to their foreign component.

Spontaneous tumors most closely resemble the human cancer situation, but this is not a reliable model for cancer research, as the animals are usually too old before tumors develop. If a spontaneous tumor does develop in a rodent, it can be serially transplanted to other animals of the same strain to establish a murine tumor line. Carcinogens can be employed to generate tumors fairly rapidly and predictably (90). Surprisingly, considering the lack of immunity in nude mice and the hypothesis of immunological surveillance, the incidence of spontaneous tumors in these animals is very low (91).

Transgenic mice

Genetically modified, transgenic mice are mice that have had a foreign gene stably inserted into their genome. Genetically modified mice have made it possible to study the functions, expression, and regulatory mechanisms of genes involved in disease in an *in vivo* model. They have also been developed as experimental models to reproduce human diseases in order to test therapeutic molecules or gene therapy. The most commonly used and successful method of producing transgenic mice is microinjection of DNA into the one-cell embryo (pro-nuclear injection). These mice have one extra gene, or transgene, inserted at random into the mouse genome. A refinement is the development of knock-in (KI) and knock-out (KO) mice, which are produced by means of embryonic stem cells, using a technique based on homologous recombination. This allows the insertion (in KI mice) or deletion (in KO mice) of the extra gene at a precise location in the genome of the embryonic stem cells. For example, a murine protein could be replaced by the equivalent human protein.

The first account of transgenic mice associated with the development of cancer was in 1984 (92), when mouse embryos were microinjected with plasmids containing the early region of the simian virus 40 (SV40) chromosome, whose gene product has been shown to transform cells in culture (93). Nearly every animal that carried the transgene developed spontaneous brain tumors of the choroid plexus. This is not the case with all transgenic mice, in which transgene expression alone is not sufficient for tumorigenesis. Transgenic mice have been produced carrying the *c-myc* oncogene under the control of a hormonally inducible mouse mammary tumor promoter (94). Only multiparous females developed mammary tumors at around 4–5 months of age. In fact, multistep tumorigenesis can be studied in similar transgenic mice (95).

Transgenic mice can be made susceptible to spontaneous tumor growth by the incorporation of an oncogene (96) or by the mutation of the p53 tumorsuppresser gene (97). Mice deficient in p53 are extremely susceptible to tumors induced by radiation (98). There are several advantages of transgenic mice for cancer research, but there are also many disadvantages compared with xenograft models. A major advantage is that spontaneously occurring tumors in immunocompetent animals more closely resemble human cancers. Metastases should occur in these mice in the same manner as in patients. The main disadvantage is the inefficiency of production of tumors in transgenic mice. Only around 10 per cent of mice born from injected embryos carry the injected DNA incorporated into the genome and there is no way of knowing from the phenotype of the mice which are transgenic. Screening for the transgene is time-consuming and labor-intensive. In addition, not all transgenic mice will develop tumors and, in those that do, the tumors will occur at different times and possibly at different sites. This makes the spontaneous tumor in the transgenic mouse a very expensive model, and unsuitable for routine screening of new tumor-targeting therapies.

Particularly useful models for research into monoclonal antibody localization are those in which a human tumor-associated antigen is expressed in transgenic mouse tissues. Transgenic mice have been produced that express the human MUC1 gene product, PEM, in a tissue-specific manner with a very similar profile to that seen in humans (99). PEM is overexpressed and aberrantly glycosylated in many tumors of epithelial origin, such as breast cancer. Antibodies against the core protein of the human mucin were shown to stain the mouse tissue, although they do not react with tissues of normal mice, owing to the lack of homology between the human and mouse mucin. Syngeneic murine tumors can be transfected with the same human antigen and implanted into the transgenic mice as a tumor-targeting model (89).

The model has been taken one stage further by developing mice transgenic for human CEA, which is expressed by a variety of human adenocarcinomas, such as those of colon (100). These mice were subsequently crossed with mice genetically predisposed to tumor development, resulting in F_1 mice that developed CEA-positive tumors of the small intestine and colon. These mice represent a good model for targeted therapy using anti-CEA antibodies or immunoliposomes, since the damage to CEA-expressing normal tissues can be assessed. Since these mice are immunocompetent and also tolerant to human CEA, they could be used as a model for passive immunotherapy studies that would not be possible in immunodeficient mice.

Limitations and benefits of human tumor xenografts

Undoubtedly, human tumor xenografts in nude or SCID mice have their limitations as a model of targeted therapy of human cancer. The tumor is the only human component in the mouse, so that there will be no cross-reactivity with human antigens, such as CEA or non-specific cross-reacting antigen (NCA) in normal colon mucosa, as would be found in patients (101). The absolute uptake of antibody by xenografts is at least 10 % i.d. g^{-1}, around 1000-fold higher than that found in tumors in patients (2). This is probably due to the small blood volume in the mouse in relation to the size of the tumor, and may give misleading results if experimental therapy of xenografts is attempted. In addition, the nude mouse has an abnormal immune system, which allows the growth of human tumors, but which also implies that immune complexes will not be formed, so that clearance of the antibody may differ from that in an immunocompetent patient. For the same reason, the nude mouse model cannot be used for vaccination studies or, for example, in strategies aimed at recruiting effector functions, such as antibody-directed cell-mediated cytotoxicity (ADCC) or T cells, for tumor cell killing.

Nonetheless, the human tumor xenograft model is valuable for comparing, within the system, various different strategies to improve tumor targeting *in vivo*, in a physiological system that mimics the human disease. Factors affecting antibody uptake that can be studied in this model include: intact monoclonal antibodies versus enzymatically generated fragments or recombinantly produced antigen-binding molecules (for example, single-chain Fv regions), the choice of radioisotope and its stability *in vivo*, antibody affinity, injected protein dose, route of administration (systemic or locoregional), the use of biological response modifiers (for example, cytokines), and two-step pre-targeting approaches (for example, the avidin/biotin system). In addition, studies can be carried out to compare different therapeutic strategies, such as ADEPT (antibody-directed enzyme prodrug therapy), drugs entrapped within liposomes compared with free drug, antibody–toxin conjugates, etc.

Care must be taken in interpreting results of targeted therapy experiments, as the relative uptake of monoclonal antibodies and other targeting molecules is very much higher in xenografted tumors than in human tumors in clinical trials. However, as a proof of principle, xenograft models can provide useful information. For the foreseeable future, the human tumor xenograft model in nude or SCID mice is likely to continue to be the most commonly used for tumor localization studies using monoclonal antibodies and other targeted therapies for cancer. Most of these therapeutic molecules undergoing clinical trials will first have been tested in this preclinical model for stability, their ability to localize to tumors, and for efficacy *in vivo*.

References

1. Köhler G, Milstein C. Continuous cultures of fused cells secreting antibody of predefined specificity. Nature 1975, **256**, 495–7.
2. Epenetos AA, Snook D, Durbin H, *et al*. Limitations of radiolabeled monoclonal antibodies for localization of human neoplasms. Cancer Res 1986, **46**, 3183–91.
3. Linardou H, Epenetos AA, Deonarain MP. A recombinant cytotoxic chimera based on mammalian deoxyribonuclease-1. Int J Cancer 2000, **86**, 561–9.
4. Jones PT, Dear PH, Foote J, *et al*. Replacing the complementarity-determining regions in a human antibody with those from a mouse. Nature 1986, **321**, 522–5.
5. Harrington KJ, Rowlinson-Busza G, Syrigos KN, *et al*. Biodistribution and pharmacokinetics of ^{111}In-DTPA-labelled pegylated liposomes in a human tumour xenograft model: implications for novel targeting strategies. Br J Cancer 2000, **83**, 232–8.
6. Gabizon AA. Selective tumor localization and improved therapeutic index of anthracyclines encapsulated in long-circulating liposomes. Cancer Res 1992, **52**, 891–6.
7. Park JW, Hong K, Carter P, *et al*. Development of anti-p185[HER2] immunoliposomes for cancer therapy. Proc Natl Acad Sci, USA 1995, **92**, 1327–31.
8. Tyzzer EE. A study of inheritance in mice with reference to their susceptibility to transplantable tumors. J Med Res 1909, **21**, 519–73.
9. Little CC, Tyzzer EE. Further experimental studies on the inheritance of susceptibility to a transplantable tumor, carcinoma (J.w.A.) of the Japanese waltzing mouse. J Med Res 1916, **33**, 393–453.
10. Haldane JBS. The genetics of cancer. Nature 1933, **132**, 265–7.
11. Medawar PB. The behaviour and fate of skin autografts and skin homografts in rabbits. J Anat 1944, **78**, 176–99.
12. Miller JFAP. Immunological function of the thymus. Lancet 1961, **2**, 748–9.
13. Murphy JB. Transplantability of malignant tumors to the embryos of a foreign species. J Am Med Assoc 1912, **59**, 874–5.
14. Greene HSN. Heterologous transplantation of mammalian tumors. II. The transfer of human tumors to alien species. J Exp Med 1941, **73**, 475–86.
15. Chesterman FC. Intracranial heterotransplantation of human tumours. Br J Cancer 1955, **9**, 541–61.
16. Greene HSN. The transplantation of tumors to the brains of heterologous species. Cancer Res 1951, **11**, 529–34.
17. Greene HSN. The significance of the heterologous transplantability of human cancer. Cancer 1952, **5**, 24–44.
18. Handler AH, Davis S, Sommers SC. Heterotransplantation experiments with human cancers. Cancer Res 1956, **16**, 32–6.
19. Toolan HW. Transplantable human neoplasms maintained in cortisone-treated laboratory animals: H.S.#1; H.Ep.#1; H.Ep.#2; H.Ep.#3; and H.Emb.Rh.#1. Cancer Res 1954, **14**, 660–6.
20. Teller MN, Merker PC, Palm JE, *et al*. The human tumor in cancer chemotherapy in the conditioned rat. Ann NY Acad Sci 1958, **76**, 742–51.
21. Goldenberg DM, Preston DF, Primus FJ, *et al*. Photoscan localization of GW-39 tumors in hamsters using radiolabeled anticarcinoembryonic antigen immunoglobulin G. Cancer Res 1974, **34**, 1–9.
22. Stanbridge EJ, Boulger LR, Franks CR, *et al*. Optimal conditions for the growth of malignant human and animal cell populations in immunosuppressed mice. Cancer Res 1975, **35**, 2203–12.
23. Steel GG, Courtenay VD, Rostom AY. Improved immune-suppression techniques for the xenografting of human tumours. Br J Cancer 1978, **37**, 224–30.
24. Selby PJ, Thomas JM, Monaghan P, *et al*. Human tumour xenografts established and serially transplanted in mice immunologically deprived by thymectomy, cytosine arabinoside and whole body irradiation. Br J Cancer 1980, **41**, 52–61.
25. Nowak K, Peckham MJ, Steel GG. Variation in response of xenografts of colo-rectal carcinoma to chemotherapy. Br J Cancer 1978, **37**, 576–84.
26. Flanagan SP. 'Nude', a new hairless gene with pleiotropic effects in the mouse. Genet Res 1966, **8**, 295–309.
27. Pantelouris EM. Absence of thymus in a mouse mutant. Nature 1968, **217**, 370–1.
28. Rygaard J, Povlsen CO. Heterotransplantation of a human malignant tumour to 'nude' mice. Acta Pathol Microbiol Scand 1969, **77**, 758–60.
29. Povlsen CO, Rygaard J. Heterotransplantation of human adenocarcinomas of the colon and rectum to the mouse mutant nude. A study of nine consecutive transplantations. Acta Pathol Microbiol Scand 1971, **79**, 159–69.
30. Schmidt M, Deschner EE, Thaler T, *et al*. Gastrointestinal cancer studies in the human to nude mouse heterotransplant system. Gastroenterology 1977, **72**, 829–37.
31. Fogh J, Orfeo T, Tiso J, *et al*. Establishment of human colon carcinoma lines in nude mice. Exp Cell Biol 1979, **47**, 136–44.
32. Fogh J, Fogh JM, Orfeo T. One hundred and twenty-seven cultured human tumor cell lines producing tumors in nude mice. J Natl Cancer Inst 1977, **59**, 221–6.
33. Hajdu SI, Lemos LB, Kozakewich H, *et al*. Growth pattern and differentiation of human soft tissue sarcomas in nude mice. Cancer 1981, **47**, 90–8.
34. Fogh J, Orfeo T, Tiso J, *et al*. Twenty-three new human tumor lines established in nude mice. Exp Cell Biol 1980, **48**, 229–39.

35. Giovanella BC, Yim SO, Stehlin JS, *et al.* Development of invasive tumors in the 'nude' mouse after injection of cultured human melanoma cells. J Natl Cancer Inst 1972, **48**, 1531–3.

36. Grant AG, Duke D, Hermon-Taylor J. Establishment and characterization of primary human pancreatic carcinoma in continuous cell culture and in nude mice. Br J Cancer 1979, **39**, 143–51.

37. Lauk S, Zietman A, Skates A, *et al.* Comparative morphometric study of tumor vasculature in human squamous cell carcinomas and their xenotransplants in athymic nude mice. Cancer Res 1989, **49**, 4557–61.

38. Bosma GC, Custer RP, Bosma MJ. A severe combined immunodeficiency mutation in the mouse. Nature 1983, **301**, 527–30.

39. Lieber MR, Hesse LE, Lewis S, *et al.* The defect in murine severe combined immune deficiency:joining of signal sequences but not coding segments in V(D)J recombination. Cell 1988, **55**, 7–16.

40. Bosma GC, Fried M, Custer RP, *et al.* Evidence of functional lymphocytes in some (leaky) scid mice. J Exp Med 1988, **167**, 1016–33.

41. Nonoyama S, Smith FO, Bernstein ID, *et al.* Strain-dependent leakiness of mice with severe combined immune deficiency. J Immunol 1993, **150**, 3817–24.

42. von Kalle C, Wolf J, Becker A, *et al.* Growth of Hodgkin cell lines in severely combined immunodeficient mice. Int J Cancer 1992, **52**, 887–91.

43. Yoshimura M, Endo S, Hioki k, *et al.* Chemotherapeutic profiles of human tumors implanted in SCID mice showing appreciable inconsistencies with those in nude mice. Exp Anim 1997, **46**, 153–6.

44. Fuzzati-Armentero MT, Duchosal MA. hu-PBL-SCID mice: an in vivo model of Epstein–Barr virus-dependent lymphoproliferative disease. Histol Histopathol 1998, **13**, 155–68.

45. Mosier DE. Adoptive transfer of human lymphoid cells to severely immunodeficient mice: models for normal human immmune function, autoimmunity, lymphomagenesis, and AIDS. Advan Immunol 1991, **50**, 303–25.

46. Dorshkind K, Denis KA, Witte ON. Lymphoid bone marrow cultures can reconstitute heterogeneous B and T cell-dependent responses in severe combined immunodeficient mice. J Immunol 1986, **137**, 3457–63.

47. Arakawa-Hoyt J, Dao MA, Thielmann F, *et al.* The number and generative capacity of human B lymphocyte progenitors, measured *in vitro* and *in vivo*, is higher in umbilical cord blood than in adult or pediatric bone marrow. Bone Marrow Transplant 1999, **24**, 1167–76.

48. Mosier DE, Gulizia RJ, Baird SM, *et al.* Transfer of a functional immune system to mice with severe combined immunodeficiency. Nature 1988, **335**, 256–9.

49. Shultz LD, Schweitzer PA, Christianson SW, *et al.* Multiple defects in innate and adaptive immunologic function in NOD/LtSz–scid mice. J Immunol 1995, **154**, 180–91.

50. Hudson WA, Li Q, Le C, *et al.* Xenotransplantation of human lymphoid malignancies is optimized in mice with multiple immunologic defects. Leukemia 1998, **12**, 2029–33.

51. Bertolini F, Fusetti L, Mancuso P, *et al.* Endostatin, an antiangiogenic drug, induces tumor stabilization after chemotherapy or anti-CD20 therapy in a NOD/SCID mouse model of human high-grade non-Hodgkin lymphoma. Blood 2000, **96**, 282–7.

52. Cashman J, Bockhold K, Hogge DE, *et al.* Sustained proliferation, multi-lineage differentiation and maintenance of primitive human haemopoietic cells in NOD/SCID mice transplanted with human cord blood. Br J Haematol 1997, **97**, 1026–36.

53. Steele JPC, Clutterbuck RD, Powles RL, *et al.* Growth of human T-cell lineage acute leukemia in severe combined immunodeficiency (SCID) mice and non-obese diabetic SCID mice. Blood 1997, **90**, 2015–19.

54. Maruo K, Ueyama Y, Hoiki K, *et al.* Strain-dependent growth of a human carcinoma in nude mice with different genetic backgrounds. Selection of nude mouse strains useful for anticancer agent screening system. Exp Cell Biol 1982, **50**, 115–19.

55. Maruo K, Ueyama Y, Kuwahara Y, *et al.* Human tumour xenografts in nude rats and their age dependence. Br J Cancer 1982, **45**, 786–9.

56. Auerbach R, Morrissey LW, Sidky YA. Regional differences in the incidence and growth of mouse tumors following intradermal or subcutaneous inoculation. Cancer Res 1978, **38**, 1739–44.

57. Pimm MV, Morris TM. Growth rates of human tumours in nude mice. Eur J Cancer 1990, **26**, 764–5.

58. Visonneau S, Cesano A, Torosian MH, *et al.* Growth characteristics and metastatic properties of human breast cancer xenografts in immunodeficient mice. Am J Pathol 1998, **152**, 1299–311.

59. Huseby RA, Maloney TM, McGrath CM. Evidence for a direct growth-stimulating effect of estradiol on human MCF-7 cells *in vivo*. Cancer Res 1984, **44**, 2654–9.

60. Pretlow TG, Delmoro CM, Dilley GG, *et al.* Transplantation of human prostatic carcinoma into nude mice in Matrigel. Cancer Res 1991, **51**, 3814–17.

61. Mullen P, Ritchie A, Langdon SP, *et al.* Effect of Matrigel on the tumorigenicity of human breast and ovarian carcinoma cell lines. Int J Cancer 1993, **67**, 816–20.

62. Kleinman HK, McGarvey ML, Hassell JR, *et al.* Basement membrane complexes with biological activity. Biochemistry 1986, **25**, 312–18.

63. Pressman D, Keighley G. The zone of activity of antibodies as determined by the use of radioactive tracers: the zone of activity of nephritoxic antikidney serum. J Immunol 1948, **59**, 141–6.

64. Pressman D, Korngold L. The *in vivo* localization of anti-Wagner-osteogenic-sarcoma antibodies. Cancer 1953, **6**, 619–23.

65. Pressman D, Day ED, Blau M. The use of paired labeling in the determination of tumor-localizing antibodies. Cancer Res 1957, **17**, 845–50.

66. Gold P, Freedman SO. Specific carcinoembryonic antigens of the human digestive system. J Exp Med 1965, **122**, 467–81.

67. Mach J-P, Carrel S, Merenda C, *et al. In vivo* localisation of radiolabelled antibodies to carcinoembryonic antigen in human colon carcinoma grafted into nude mice. Nature 1974, **248**, 704–6.

68. Sharkey RM, Primus FJ, Shochat D, *et al.* Comparison of tumor targeting of mouse monoclonal and goat poly-

clonal antibodies to carcinoembryonic antigen in the GW-39 human tumor–hamster host model. Cancer Res 1988, **48**, 1823–8.

69. Sands H, Jones PL, Shah SA, *et al.* Correlation of vascular permeability and blood flow with monoclonal antibody uptake by human Clouser and renal cell xenografts. Cancer Res 1988, **48**, 188–93.

70. Shockley TR, Lin K, Sung C, *et al.* A quantitative analysis of tumor specific monoclonal antibody uptake by human melanoma xenografts: effects of antibody immunological properties and tumor antigen expression levels. Cancer Res 1992, **52**, 357–66.

71. Hagan PL, Halpern SE, Dillman RO, *et al.* Tumor size: effect on monoclonal antibody uptake in tumor models. J Nucl Med 1986, **27**, 422–7.

72. Harrington KJ, Rowlinson-Busza G, Syrigos KN, *et al.* Influence of tumour size on uptake of ^{111}In-DTPA-labelled pegylated liposomes in a human tumour xenograft model. Br J Cancer 2000, **83**, 684–8.

73. Pimm MV, Baldwin RW. Quantitative evaluation of the localization of a monoclonal antibody (791T/36) in human osteogenic sarcoma xenografts. Eur J Cancer Clin Oncol 1984, **20**, 515–24.

74. Sharkey FE, Fogh J. Metastasis of human tumors in athymic nude mice. Int J Cancer 1979, **24**, 733–8.

75. Neulat-Duga I, Sheppel A, Marty C, *et al.* Metastases of human tumor xenografts in nude mice. Invasion Metastasis 1984, **4**, 209–24.

76. Kyriazis AP, DiPersio L, Michael GJ, *et al.* Growth patterns and metastatic behavior of human tumors growing in athymic mice. Cancer Res 1978, **38**, 3186–90.

77. Giavazzi R, Campbell DE, Jessup JM, *et al.* Metastatic behavior of tumor cells isolated from primary and metastatic human colorectal carcinomas implanted into different sites in nude mice. Cancer Res 1986, **46**, 1928–33.

78. Vogel C-A, Galmiche MC, Buchegger F. Radioimmunotherapy and fractionated radiotherapy of human colon cancer liver metastases in nude mice. Cancer Res 1997, **57**, 447–53.

79. Sugano M, Egilmez NK, Yokota SJ, *et al.* Antibody targeting of doxorubicin-loaded liposomes suppresses the growth and metastatic spread of established human lung tumor xenografts in severe combined immunodeficient mice. Cancer Res 2000, **60**, 6942–9.

80. Naito S, von Eschenbach AC, Giavazzi R, *et al.* Growth and metastasis of tumor cells isolated from a human renal cell carcinoma implanted into different organs in nude mice. Cancer Res 1986, **46**, 4109–15.

81. Russell PJ, Ho Shon I, Boniface GR, *et al.* Growth and metastasis of human bladder cancer xenografts in the bladder of nude rats. A model for intravesical radioimmunotherapy. Urol Res 1991, **19**, 207–13.

82. Pocard M, Tsukui H, Salmon RJ, *et al.* Efficiency of orthotopic xenograft models for human colon cancers. In Vivo 1996, **10**, 463–9.

83. Rofstad EK. Orthotopic human melanoma xenograft model systems for studies of tumour angiogenesis, pathophysiology, treatment sensitivity and metastatic pattern. Br J Cancer 1994, **70**, 804–12.

84. Otsuka FL, Welch MJ, McElvany KD, *et al.* Development of a model system to evaluate methods for radiolabeling monoclonal antibodies. J Nucl Med 1984, **25**, 1343–9.

85. Hnatowich DJ, Virzi F, Rusckowski M. Investigations of avidin and biotin for imaging applications. J Nucl Med 1987, **28**, 1294–302.

86. Fjeld JG, Benestad HB, Stigbrand T, *et al. In vivo* evaluation of radiolabelled antibodies with antigen-coated polymer particles in diffusion chambers. J Immunol Methods 1988, **109**, 1–7.

87. Fjeld JG, Bruland ØS, Benestad HB, *et al.* Radioimmunotargeting of human tumour cells in immunocompetent animals. Br J Cancer 1990, **62**, 573–8.

88. Ziegler MM, Ishizu H, Nagabuchi E, *et al.* A comparative review of the immunobiology of murine neuroblastoma and human neuroblastoma. Cancer 1997, **79**, 1757–66.

89. Lalani E-N, Berdichevsky F, Boshell M, *et al.* Expression of the gene coding for a human mucin in mouse mammary tumor cells can affect their tumorigenicity. J Biol Chem 1991, **266**, 15420–6.

90. Taguchi O, Michael SD, Nishizuki Y. Rapid induction of ovarian granulosa cell tumors by 7,12-dimethylbenz(*a*)anthracene in neonatally estrogenized mice. Cancer Res 1988, **48**, 425–9.

91. Rygaard J, Povlsen CO. The nude mouse vs. the hypothesis of immunological surveillance. Transplant Rev 1976, **28**, 43–61.

92. Brinster RL, Chen HY, Messing A, *et al.* Transgenic mice harboring SV40 T-antigen genes develop characteristic brain tumors. Cell 1984, **37**, 367–79.

93. Tegtmeyer P. Function of simian virus 40 gene A in transforming infection. J Virol 1975, **15**, 613–18.

94. Stewart TA, Pattengale PK, Leder P. Spontaneous mammary adenocarcinomas in transgenic mice that carry and express MTV/*myc* fusion genes. Cell 1984, **38**, 627–37.

95. Hanahan D. Dissecting multistep tumorigenesis in transgenic mice. Annu Rev Genet 1988, **22**, 479–519.

96. Thomas H, Balkwill FR. Oncogene transgenic mice as therapeutic models in cancer research. Eur J Cancer 1994, **30A**, 533–7.

97. Donehower LA, Harvey M, Slagle BL, *et al.* Mice deficient for p53 are developmentally normal but susceptible to spontaneous tumours. Nature 1992, **356**, 215–21.

98. Kemp CJ, Wheldon T, Balmain A. p53-deficient mice are extremely susceptible to radiation-induced tumorigenesis. Nat Genet 1994, **8**, 66–9.

99. Peat N, Gendler S, Lalani E-N, *et al.* Tissue-specific expression of a human polymorphic epithelial mucin (MUC1) in transgenic mice. Cancer Res 1992, **52**, 1954–60.

100. Thompson JA, Eades-Perner A-M, Ditter M, *et al.* Expression of transgenic carcinoembryonic antigen (CEA) in tumor-prone mice: an animal model for CEA-directed tumor immunotherapy. Int J Cancer 1997, **72**, 197–202.

101. Kodera Y, Isobe K, Yamauchi M, *et al.* Expression of carcinoembryonic antigen (CEA) and nonspecific cross-reacting antigen (NCA) in gastrointestinal cancer; the correlation with degree of differentiation. Br J Cancer 1993, **68**, 130–6

Section II

3

Monoclonal antibody targeting therapy: an overview

Roslyn J. Francis and Richard H.J. Begent

Introduction

Monoclonal antibody targeted therapy has the promise of the 'magic bullet' proposed by Paul Ehrlich almost a century ago. The aim is to develop a system that will target therapeutic agents to specific tissues such as tumors to maximize effect, while at the same time reducing systemic toxicity. Since the 1980s monoclonal antibodies, either alone or conjugated to therapeutic agents such as radionuclides, drugs, toxins, enzymes, or growth factors, have become exciting novel agents for the diagnosis and treatment of cancer.

Antibody therapy for cancer was used as early as 1895 when Hericourt and Richet immunized animals with human tumor extracts and gave the serum to patients resulting in some tumor responses (1). Polyclonal antibodies were used from the 1940s, and were shown to react with tumor antigens (2). However, the development of hybridoma technology in 1975 by Köhler and Milstein allowed for the first time the generation of monoclonal antibodies with defined specificities (3). More recently, techniques such as the development of phage technology for generating large libraries of monoclonal antibodies with the ability to select for desired characteristics has further expanded the possibilities of monoclonal antibody therapy (4).

Monoclonal and polyclonal antibodies

A normal immune response to a foreign antigen involves the activation of B lymphocytes to secrete antibodies that bind to various epitopes of the antigen. This polyclonal antibody response has heterogeneous specificities and affinities. Each 'batch' of polyclonal antiserum made to an antigen is also variable. Monoclonal antibodies, however, bind to the antigen (a defined epitope) with one specificity and one affinity, and can be produced reproducibly in large amounts in the laboratory under standard conditions. This 'uniformity' makes them more suitable for therapeutic use.

Monoclonal antibodies—production and design

Monoclonal antibody production

The two main methods of generating monoclonal antibodies are hybridoma technology and combinatorial phage libraries. Köhler and Milstein developed the hybridoma technique in 1975 (3). It involves the immunization of mice against a target antigen and then immortalizing the antibody-producing B cells by fusing with myeloma cells to produce a hybridoma. The resultant hybridoma produces uniform antibodies of a single specificity. The hybridoma can potentially produce a large quantity of antibody indefinitely. However, the method has the limitation that only a small amount of an antibody repertoire can be examined because each clone must be studied separately for its specificity.

Combinatorial phage libraries have developed more recently as a result of the ability to purify antibody variable region genes from populations of B cells by polymerase chain reaction (PCR) using specific primers. cDNA encoding Fab or V_H and V_L, joined by a synthetic linker, is cloned into a bacteriophage genome where it encodes the antibody protein. If filamentous phage are used, the protein product can be displayed on the cell surface, therefore allowing the bacteriophage to be used directly to select for required specificity and binding characteristics (4–6) (Fig. 3.1). Table 3.1 lists the advantages of phage libraries over hybridoma techniques.

Human antibodies have also been more recently produced using immunization of transgenic mice that carry

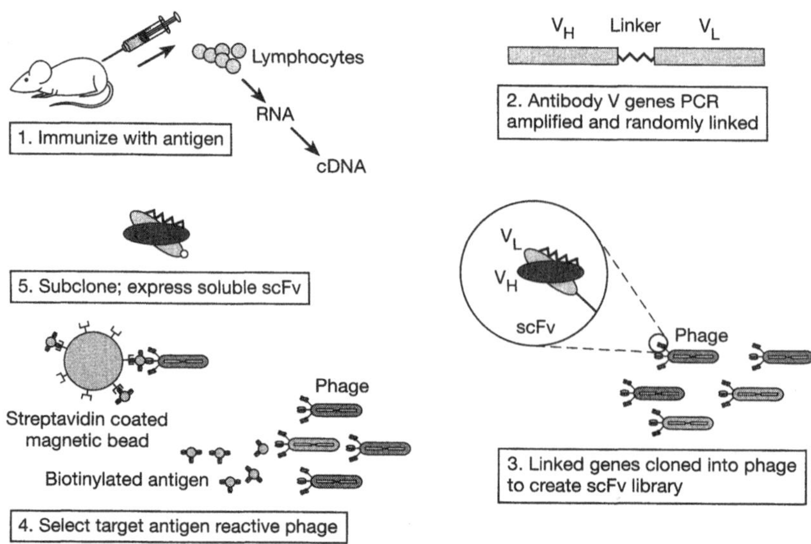

Fig. 3.1   Diagrammatic representation of generation of an scFv using a combinatorial phage library.

Table 3.1   Advantages of combinatorial phage libraries for producing monoclonal antibodies

Able to produce large quantities ($> 10^{12}$) of antibody clones (hybridoma 10^3–10^4)

V_H and V_L are randomly recombined in scFv, giving a potentially broader repertoire than that occurring naturally

Selection for a desired characteristic can be made from the whole library, whereas hybridomas are screened clone by clone

Production is commonly via bacterial or yeast cells and not by mammalian cells eliminating the risk of mammalian virus and DNA contamination

Production is relatively low cost

Antibodies are cloned facilitating generation of engineered antibodies and fusion proteins

the human immunoglobulin locus (7). These mice have had their immunoglobulin locus 'knocked out' and human immunoglobulin genes inserted, so human immunoglobulins are formed after immunization. Monoclonal antibodies are then made using the hybridoma technique mentioned previously. At present, there are three different transgenic mice strains commercially available for human antibody production.

Antibody design

Genetic engineering has allowed the design of various antibody-derived molecules (8). A whole IgG antibody has a molecular weight of 150 kDa and consists of 2 variable light chains (V_L), 2 variable heavy chains (V_H), 2 constant light chains (C_L), and 6 constant heavy chains ($2 \times C_H1$, $2 \times C_H2$, $2 \times C_H3$; see Fig. 3.2). The domains of V_L, V_H, C_L, and C_H1 make up the antigen-binding end of the molecule (Fab). The C_H2 and C_H3 domains comprise the Fc portion, which is important in recruitment of the host immune response and persistence of the antibody in the circulation. Smaller antibody fragments may penetrate tumor better and have a favorable tumor to normal tissue ratio. Fvs are the smallest antibody fragment retaining full antibody specificity, but only remain stable if the V_H and V_L chains are joined by a small polypeptide linker to form a single-chain Fv (scFv) or a disulfide bond to form a disulfide-stabilized Fv (dsFv) (9, 10). An scFv has a molecular weight of 27 kDa. scFvs can also be produced as bispecific antibodies such as diabodies and chelating recombinant antibodies (CRAbs). Diabodies can be formed by shortening the polypeptide linker that joins the V_H and V_L chains. CRAbs are two scFvs with specificities for different epitopes on the same molecule joined by linkers. These antibody fragments each have unique characteristics that may be important in the development of useful therapeutic systems (Fig. 3.3).

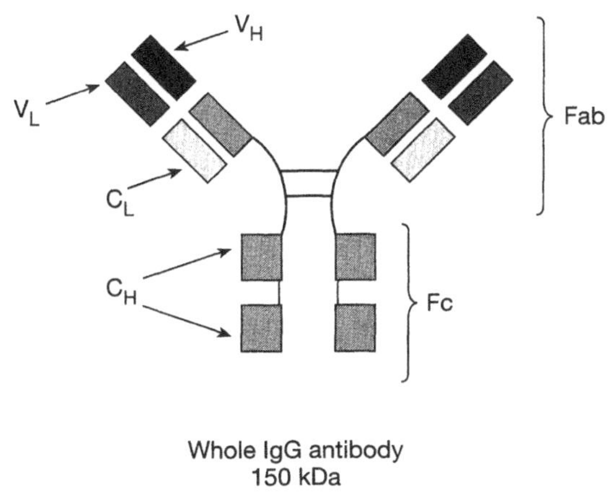

V_H: Variable heavy chain V_L: Variable light chain

C_H: Constant heavy chain C_L: Constant light chain

Fig. 3.2　Diagrammatic representation of IgG antibody.

Factors that influence antibody targeting

The ability to produce an effective therapeutic system using antibody therapies is influenced by many factors. These include the nature of the target antigen, the features of the targeting antibody, and tumor and host characteristics.

Target antigen

The choice of target antigen is essential in the design of any antibody targeting based system. The ideal characteristics of a target antigen would include high and homogeneous tumor expression, minimal expression in normal tissues, little or no soluble form, and accessibility to the circulation (8, 11).

To overcome heterogeneous antigen expression within a tumor, antibody therapies frequently employ a 'bystander effect', which involves destruction of neighboring cells as well as the cell binding the antigen. If an antibody therapy has a bystander effect, not every cell needs to express the antigen and not every cell need to be accessible to the antibody. This theoretically improves the likelihood of cure.

Specificity is also very important, as cross-reactivity to normal tissues will limit therapeutic ratio. Cross-reactivity with a tissue that is not easily accessible may be acceptable. For example, carcinoembryonic antigen (CEA) is expressed on the luminal surface of normal intestinal glands as well as on colorectal tumors. The inaccessibility of the normal intestinal luminal surface to antibodies, coupled with the abundance in tumor compared with normal tissues, means that, despite this cross-reactivity, CEA remains a good antigen target (11). Tumor vasculature is becoming an increasingly attractive target, as it is readily accessible and is essential for tumor growth (8, 11). New targets are continuing to be identified from the study of mutations, altered gene expression, and as a result of proteomic studies (12–14).

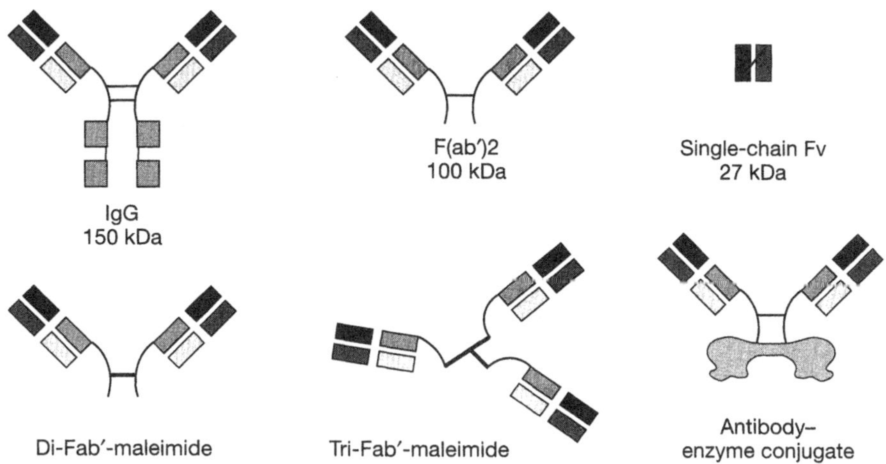

Fig. 3.3　Diagrammatic representation of antibody fragments and conjugates

Antibody characteristics

Antibody size

The molecular weight of an antibody directly influences both the penetration of the antibody into a tumor and the rate of clearance from the circulation. Whole antibodies (IgG) have a molecular weight of 150 kDa. These penetrate tumor relatively slowly, and tend to remain in peripheral areas of the tumor, close to blood vessels (15). They are initially retained in the circulation, resulting in low tumor:blood ratios over the first 24–72 hours after administration. This may not be ideal for some therapies that require early high tumor:blood ratios and good tumor penetration. This has led to the design of antibody fragments such as $F(ab)_2$ (100 kDa) and scFvs (27 kDa). These fragments generally penetrate tumors better and clear the circulation more rapidly (16). However, the rapid clearance by the circulation results in less total antibody available for tumor binding and lower absolute tumor antibody levels. The choice of whether whole antibody or antibody fragments are used therefore depends on the therapeutic system chosen.

Affinity

Affinity describes the interaction between antigen and antibody. This interaction is influenced by kinetic 'on rate' and 'off rate'. High affinity is important for targeting, especially when antigen concentration is low within a tumor.

Avidity

This typically describes a univalent interaction; however natural antibodies are polyvalent (that is, have more than one binding site), which results in a much more stable interaction. Avidity is used to describe a monovalent or polyvalent interaction; the latter can result in a large improvement in functional affinity. For example, IgG, which is a bivalent molecule, has an approximately 1000-fold increase in functional affinity in comparison to a single Fab fragment (8). Genetic engineering has allowed the development of di-Fab and tri-Fab antibodies, which seem to have increased avidity and have resulted in increased levels of antibody at the tumor and high tumor:blood ratios compared with those of single Fab fragments (17, 18).

Stability

For the antibody to be an effective therapeutic strategy it must be stable in production, storage, reconstitution, the circulation, and in the tumor.

Immunogenicity

Murine antibodies are immunogenic in humans and in the presence of an intact immune system lead to the production of human anti-mouse antibodies (HAMA). Repeat administration results in a progressively shorter circulating half-life of the antibody, with poor tumor localization and retention. It may also lead to immune reactions such as anaphylaxis and serum sickness. The development of chimeric antibodies with murine variable regions and human constant regions has greatly reduced problems of immunogenicity. Chimeric antibodies are formed using protein engineering techniques, whereby the murine complement-determining regions (CDR) are grafted on to human variable region framework linked to human constant regions (19, 20). 'Reshaped' or 'humanized' antibodies have also been developed, in which only the antigen binding site, rather than the whole variable domain, is transplanted from rodent antibodies on to human antibodies, with the advantage of potentially even further reduced immunogenicity (21).

Chimeric or humanized antibodies can be given repeatedly with no significant reduction in circulating half-life. The half-life of chimeric antibodies in humans is much longer than that of murine antibodies, with half-lives in serum of 10 days or longer being reported (22, 23). It also appears that having a human effector Fc arm of the antibody results in better recruitment of the host immune response, in particular, cell-mediated immunity. It is possible to develop human antibodies to chimeric antibodies—either to the murine variable region (anti-idiotypic antibodies) or to the human constant regions, although in clinical practice to date this has not frequently been a significant problem.

Other methods of reducing immunogenicity to murine antibodies include using smaller antibody fragments, adding polyethylene glycol (PEG) or glycosylations to the antibody, or suppressing the immune system with drugs such as cyclosporin.

Attachment of polyethylene glycol (PEG) or glycosylations of antibodies

Attachment of PEG to or glycosylation of antibodies may alter their pharmacological properties by increasing plasma circulation time and reducing immunogenicity, which may benefit tumor targeting (15). PEG modification of an Fab or f(ab′)$_2$ fragment of an anti-CEA antibody resulted in animal models having a prolonged plasma half-life and increased tumor uptake when compared to the non-PEGylated fragment (24, 25). It has also been shown that PEGylation can reduce immunogenicity or induce tolerance in animal models (26, 27).

Antibodies produced in yeast or plant systems are usually glycolsylated. This may result in increased clearance from the circulation and alterations in the stability and immunogenicity of the antibody.

Radiolabeling

Antibodies may be labeled with radioactive isotopes for diagnostic purposes, therapeutic purposes, or for identification of antibody localization as part of a therapeutic strategy. Isotopes of iodine are labeled by attachment to tyrosine in the antibody. This can cause problems if the antigen-binding site contains tyrosine, as antigen binding can be disrupted. To overcome this site-specific labeling with the incorporation of a macrocycle or a peptide that binds a radionuclide can be performed. The radioactive metal ions, technetium-99m, indium-111, and yttrium-90, can be coupled to antibodies by chelating molecules. This may, however, result in normal tissue binding (especially liver) and *in vivo* transchelation where the radioisotope is transferred to nonspecific serum proteins. Current chelation chemistry techniques aim to limit these problems.

Conjugation—chemical or genetic

Conjugation to a protein is required for some therapeutic strategies. For example, in antibody-directed enzyme prodrug therapy (ADEPT), an antibody–enzyme conjugate is administered. This conjugation can be performed either chemically or by genetic fusion. Chemical conjugation often produces a heterogeneous population of products, whereas genetic fusion produces a more homogeneous and reproducible protein product. With both methods there may be problems as the conjugation technique may lead to a reduction in purity and yield.

The tumor

Tumors are heterogeneous, rapidly outgrowing their blood supply. This results in viable well-vascularized areas and slow-growing and necrotic poorly vascularized areas. Tumor vasculature is 'leakier' than normal tissue vasculature, which is probably an advantage for antibody-targeted systems. However, flow in tumor vessels is erratic and high pressure tends to develop in the center of tumor masses. The penetration of an antibody into a tumor depends on size and affinity of the antibody, and the vascularity of the tumor, which determines the accessibility of the antibody to the cancerous cells. Small antibody fragments such as scFv penetrate better than large antibodies such as IgG. Nonspecific antibodies pass through the tumor into the necrotic center, whereas antibodies with a reasonable affinity will be retained in the viable areas (28). This is shown using an animal model in Fig. 3.4. The effect of therapeutic modalities, in particular, radioisotopes involved in radioimmunotherapy and many DNA-interacting drugs, is severely impaired in hypoxic, poorly vascularized areas. Understanding the complex environment of the tumor is vital for developing effective treatments for cancer.

Host factors

Host factors are important determinants of the success of antibody therapies. The biodistribution of antibodies in humans is influenced by many factors. These include metabolism/catabolism of the antibody, excretion (renal or hepatic), immune complex formation, and cross-reactivity with normal tissues. Renal excretion from filtration increases rapidly with antibodies or antibody fragments with molecular weights of less than 50 kDa (15). The isoelectric charge of the amino acids that constitute the antibody may have an effect on renal uptake, and lead to unwanted renal retention of antibody. This and other characteristics of the antibody may be manipulated by genetic engineering.

As previously mentioned, murine antibodies are recognized as 'foreign' by an intact human immune system. This will result in the generation of human

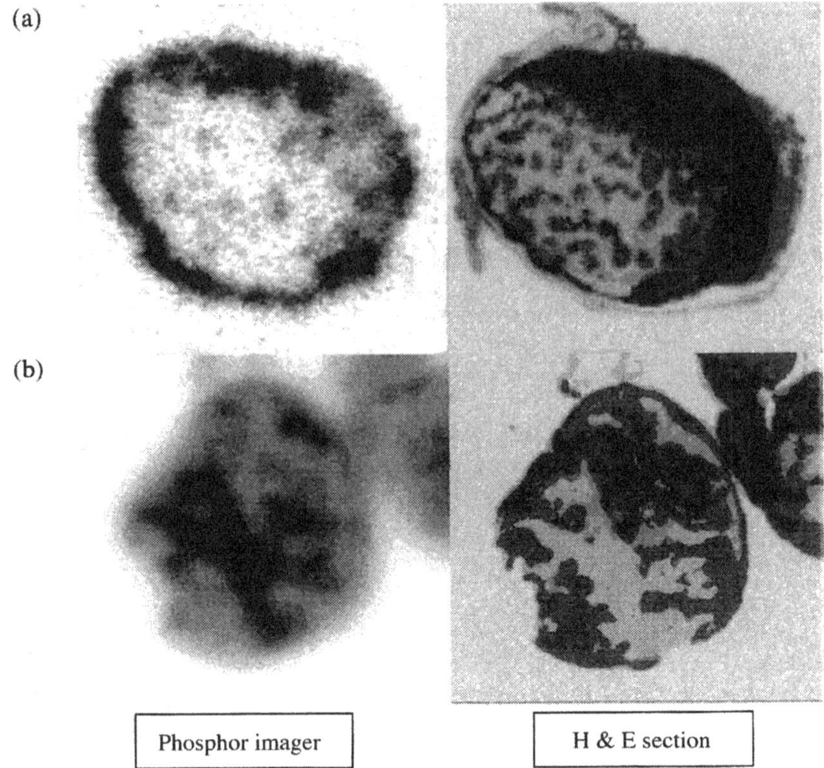

Fig. 3.4 Phosphor imager and hematoxylin and eosin (H & E) stain of antibody distribution in a human xenograft model of (a) a specific antibody and (b) a nonspecific antibody. The specific antibody is retained in the viable tumor rim. The nonspecific antibody collects in the nonviable necrotic center of the tumor. (See also 'Plates' section.)

anti-mouse antibodies (HAMA) after repeated administration, which will then result in a significantly shortened circulating half-life of the antibody, with poor tumor localization and retention. Even chimeric or humanized antibodies may result in an immune reaction against the antigen-binding site (anti-idiotypic antibodies) which will have an effect on biodistribution.

The ability to label antibodies with trace amounts of radioactivity and assess their biodistribution using gamma camera imaging can aid in the assessment of the safety and possible efficacy of *in vivo* use. Techniques of analysis such as quantitative assessment of single-photon emission computerized tomography (SPECT) images further increase the potential usefulness of gamma camera imaging (29).

Therapeutic strategies

Monoclonal antibodies can be used in many different ways to try and achieve therapeutic effect (Table 3.2).

Some of these strategies will be reviewed in more detail in the following chapters.

Natural effector mechanisms

Most of these therapeutic strategies utilize the Fc portion of the antibody molecule to activate the host immune system to achieve antitumor effects. This can be through activation of antibody-dependent cellular cytotoxicity (ADCC), activation of complement cascade, or direct cytotoxicity. The antibody is used to

Table 3.2 Therapeutic strategies and licensed antibodies for cancer therapy

Therapeutic strategy	Licensed antibody
Natural effector mechanism/ADCC	Rituximab, herceptin, panorex
Radioimmunotherapy	
Immunotoxins	Myelotarg
Pretargeting systems	
Combined therapies	

target the host immune response to the tumor cells, and the Fc part of the antibody directs the immune response. There are three monoclonal antibodies that utilize natural effector mechanisms of action that are currently licensed for therapy and these will be discussed below.

Two other related novel experimental approaches also utilize natural effector mechanisms in a different way. These are monoclonal antibodies used to generate anti-idiotypic cancer vaccines and control of growth of cancer cells via monoclonal antibodies targeted to membrane-mediated signal transduction pathways. Both of these new approaches will be covered briefly here; however they are covered in more detail in later chapters.

Anti-CD20 antibody (rituximab, mabthera, IDEC-C2B8) for B-cell lymphoma

CD20 is a cell surface antigen expressed on more than 90 per cent of B-cell non-Hodgkin's lymphomas (NHL) (30). Normal B cells from the pre-B-cell stage of differentiation through to mature B-cell development also express CD20, but it is not present on early pre-B-cells, stem cells, or antigen-presenting dendritic cells. The CD20 is a cell surface antigen that does not internalize and is not shed from the cell surface into the circulation (31). Rituximab is a chimeric antibody with murine variable domains and human constant regions, with the human constant regions mediating normal host effector functions, providing a longer half-life and reduced immunogenicity, allowing for repeat dosing (32). *In vitro* rituximab induces ADCC and complement-dependent cytotoxicity. In some cell lines it inhibited proliferation and directly induced apoptosis (33). Between April 1995 and March 1996, 166 patients with relapsed low-grade or follicular lymphoma from 31 centers in the USA and Canada were entered into a pivotal trial for rituximab (32). They received infusions of rituximab weekly for 4 weeks. All patients had been

Table 3.3 Toxicity of rituximab in 166 patients with relapsed low-grade or follicular lymphoma

Toxicity	Incidence (% of patients)
Fever	43
Chills	28
Nausea	18
Pruritis	13
Rash	10
Angioedema	14
Tumor-related pain	11
Hypotension	10

previously treated with chemotherapy (97 per cent), radiotherapy (25 per cent), or bone marrow transplant (14 per cent). The median number of prior treatments was three. The overall response rate achieved with rituximab was 48 per cent of which 6 per cent were complete responses and 42 per cent partial responses. The mean time to progression was 13 months. The side-effects experienced were mostly mild and usually occurred with the first course of treatment. Table 3.3 lists the main toxicities reported in the study. Rituximab is now licensed in the USA and Europe for patients with follicular lymphoma who are resistant to relapse or are in their second or subsequent relapse following antilymphoma treatment. There have, however, been several deaths reported which appear to be due to cytokine release syndrome and features of tumor lysis syndrome. Patients with high tumor burden and a high number of circulating malignant cells appear to be particularly at risk. Rituximab, in spite of this, remains an important advance in the treatment of follicular lymphoma.

17-1A Antibody (panorex) in colorectal cancer

This is a murine IgG2a antibody directed against a cell surface glycoprotein expressed on gastrointestinal and other carcinomas as well as normal epithelial cells (34). Its mode of action is thought to be via ADCC (34). In adjuvant therapy of Dukes stage C carcinoma after a median follow-up of 7 years it produced a 32 per cent reduction in mortality ($p = 0.01$ by log rank) and a 23 per cent reduction in recurrence rate ($p = 0.07$ by log rank) compared to no treatment (35). The patients who had 17-1A had a significantly reduced risk of distant metastasis ($p = 0.004$) but not of local relapses ($p = 0.52$) (35). This reduction in relapses and deaths is comparable to that with cytotoxic chemotherapy but with less toxicity. The toxicities associated with 17-1A therapy included, in 1–2 per cent of infusions, fever/chills, malaise, dizziness, fatigue, flushing, rash, nausea/vomiting, or diarrhea (34). In 4 of 371 infusions an anaphylactic reaction occurred, which was controlled by intravenous steroids and did not result in hospital admission (34). Eighty per cent of patients developed HAMA after the second or third infusion; however, initial titers were low and reached their maximum after the fifth infusion (34). As a result of this study, 17-1A is licensed for adjuvant therapy of colorectal carcinoma in Germany and is in multinational clinical trials comparing it with conventional adjuvant chemotherapy.

Anti-HER2/neu antibody (herceptin, trastuzumab) in breast cancer

HER2/*neu* (c-erbB2) is an oncogene that is a member of the epidermal growth factor receptor family and codes for a transmembrane tyrosine kinase (36). It is overexpressed in many solid tumors including breast, ovarian, lung, gastric, and oral cancers (36). HER2/*neu* overexpression has been shown to be a poor prognostic sign for survival in breast and ovarian cancer (37–41). Murine monoclonal antibodies for the extracellular domain of HER2 were generated, and the most potent growth-inhibitory antibody, muMAb 4D5, was humanized for therapeutic purposes (42, 43). This antibody is herceptin (trastuzumab). Clinical trials (phase I/II/III) have been performed mainly on patients with advanced breast cancer and have used herceptin either alone or in combination with cisplatin or other chemotherapies. In preclinical studies herceptin alone appears to downregulate HER2, causing apoptosis and stimulating ADCC. In combination with cisplatin, herceptin appears to interfere with the DNA repair that occurs after cisplatin administration, therefore promoting cisplatin cytotoxicity in a synergistic fashion (44). Preclinical models have also demonstrated that herceptin causes a marked enhancement of paclitaxel antitumor activity and a moderate enhancement in combination with doxorubicin (45). This effect only occurs in HER2/*neu*-overexpressing cells; it does not have an effect on cells without this overexpression (44).

The results of the efficacy studies of herceptin alone for previously treated metastatic breast cancer are summarized in Table 3.4. H0551g was a phase II trial of 10 weekly infusions of herceptin alone in 46 patients with HER2/*neu*-overexpressing metastatic breast cancer (46). Toxicity was minimal and no anti-herceptin antibodies were detected. There was an overall response rate of 11.6 per cent from 43 assessable patients (46). A larger multinational phase II trial of herceptin alone (H0649g) recruited 222 patients with HER2-overexpressing metastatic breast cancer who had had one or two previous chemotherapy regimes. Preliminary results reviewed by an independent com-

mittee determined that the overall response rate was 15 per cent (42, 47). Nine patients had a reduction in ejection fraction—all had either prior anthracycline chemotherapy or pre-existing cardiac disease (42). Toxicity was otherwise minimal.

Herceptin was used in combination with cisplatin in a phase II trial (H0552g) of patients with pretreated metastatic breast cancer overexpressing HER2 published in 1998 (48). Thirty-nine patients were entered into the trial and 37 were assessable for response. 24.3 per cent of patients had a partial response, with the toxicities of the combined treatment being no greater than those with cisplatin alone (48). A phase III trial examining the combination of herceptin and first-line chemotherapy for HER2-overexpressing metastatic breast cancer (H0648g) recruited 469 patients (42, 49). The chemotherapy regimens used included anthracycline/cyclophosphamide (AC) regime or paclitaxel. Herceptin was added for half the patients. Preliminary results reveal an improvement in response rates with the addition of herceptin without an increase in overall severe adverse events (42, 49). However, there was an increase in cardiac dysfunction similar to that observed with anthracyclines, which occurred more commonly when herceptin was added to AC (18 per cent for grade 3/4) than with AC alone (3 per cent) and with paclitaxel plus herceptin (2 per cent) and not with paclitaxel alone (0 per cent) (43, 49).

These clinical trial results are very encouraging and show that targeting growth factor receptors can induce regression in some cancers. Herceptin is currently approved for use in the USA for patients with HER2/*neu*-overexpressing advanced breast cancer.

Monoclonal antibodies as cancer vaccines (anti-idiotypic cancer vaccines)

The general principle of this form of therapy is that an antibody is made against the idiotype of an antitumor antibody. This mimics a tumor antigen and can induce an immune response against the tumor. Evidence of tumor recognition has been demonstrated in some

Table 3.4   Phase II clinical studies of single-agent herceptin for patients with Her2neu-positive previously treated advanced breast cancer

Study	Number of patients	Number (%) showing response		
		Overall response	Complete response	Partial response
H0551g	46 (43 assessable)	5 (11.6)	1 (2.3)	4 (9.3)
H0649g	222	33 (15)	8 (4)	25 (11)

patients and clinical trials are ongoing to determine the efficacy of this approach (50). Monoclonal antibodies as cancer vaccines are covered in more detail in Chapter 7.

Monoclonal antibodies targeted to membrane-mediated signal transduction pathways

Antibodies are being developed to membrane signal transduction proteins, which may have effects due to downstream signaling. These include antibodies to c-erbB3, epithelial growth factor receptor, and vascular endothelial growth factor (VEGF) receptor. Herceptin (see above) is thought to act, in part, through a signal transduction effect.

Radioimmunotherapy

Radioimmunotherapy uses an antitumor antibody to target radiation to a tumor. Radionuclides with γ emissions are used for imaging and β emissions are used for therapy. α-Emitting radioisotopes are also being explored for therapy; however, they are difficult to prepare in a suitable chemical form (51).

The antibody is usually targeted against a cell surface antigen, and the energy of the emissions for therapy ensures that there is a bystander effect locally. Radionuclides emitting medium- to high-energy β particles are suitable as they deposit their energy over a relatively wide area without requiring binding to each individual cell or internalization for therapeutic effect. The most common radioisotopes used include iodine-131 (γ and β emitter) and yttrium-90 (β emitter only). Iodine-131 has the advantage of being able to be used for dosimetry and therapy, due to its γ radiation. This does, however, lead to problems with radiation protection for staff and family. Yttrium-90 therapy has the advantage of being essentially an outpatient therapy, as the lack of γ emissions prevents radioprotection problems for staff and family. Indium-111 is usually used as a substitute for yttrium for dosimetry studies. When iodine-131 radiolabeled antibody is broken down in the tumor environment, iodine is released into the circulation and rapidly cleared. Yttrium-90, however, is retained within cells (51).

The path length of the β emissions produced is important when choosing a suitable radionuclide for therapy. Radionuclides that can be used for radioimmunotherapy are outlined in Table 3.5 (52).

Radioimmunotherapy can be administered via intravenous, intraarterial, and intracavitary routes. Therapy depends on the ability of the radionuclide to produce DNA strand-breaks at a rate that is faster than repair. The bone marrow, lungs, and heart are particularly vulnerable to side-effects from exposure to circulating radiolabeled antibody.

Radioimmunotherapy has been particularly successful in the treatment of relapsed lymphoma. High-dose radioimmunotherapy with autologous bone marrow

Table 3.5   Common radionuclides for radioimmunotherapy and their characteristics

Radionuclide	Decay mode*	Physical half-life	Max. range (mm)†	Advantages‡	Disadvantages
^{67}Cu	β, γ	62 hours	2.2	Imaging, long retention in tumor	Scarce
^{177}Lu	β, γ	6.7 days	2.2	Imaging	Scarce, bone seeker
^{131}I	β, γ	8.0 days	2.4	Iodine chemistry, inexpensive	Dehalogenation, radiation safety concerns
^{186}Re	β, γ, EC	91 hours	5.0	Similar to ^{99m}Tc chemistry	Scarce
^{90}Y	β	64 hours	11.9	Metal chemistry, outpatient therapy	Doesn't image well, bone seeker
^{188}Re	β	17 hours	11.1	Images, metal chemistry	Scarce, short half-life
^{212}Bi	β, α	1 hour	0.09	High RBE, hypoxia less important, short range	Doesn't image well, short half-life, unstable daughter product
^{211}At	α, EC	7 hours	0.09	High RBE, hypoxia less important, short-range	Doesn't image well, short half-life, unstable daughter product
^{125}I	EC	60 days	0.02	Short-range	Doesn't image, long half-life

* EC, Electron capture.
† Maximum range of particulate energy in tissue.
‡ RBE, Relative biological effectiveness.

rescue using an iodine-131 labeled anti-CD20 antibody produced a complete response rate of 84 per cent and a partial response rate of 10 per cent in 19 patients with relapsed B-cell lymphoma (53). Many of these patients were heavily pretreated, and the responses were often sustained, with a progression-free survival of 62 per cent after 2 years. These results suggest that some of the patients may have been cured by the high-dose therapy, which clearly illustrates the potential of radioimmunotherapy.

Zevalin (yttrium-90 ibritumomab tiuxetin) is an yttrium-90 radiolabeled murine IgG monoclonal antibody against CD20. This antibody is the murine antibody from which rituximab was derived. Favorable results have been seen in phase I/II trials of relapsed or refractory, low- or intermediate-grade CD20-positive NHL. Overall response rates of 64–67 per cent have been seen at doses of radioimmunotherapy that were non-myeloablative (54, 55). Phase III trials are now underway with zevalin.

A recently published phase I/II clinical trial of 67Cu-2IT-BAT-Lym-1 for patients with chemotherapy-resistant NHL had a response rate of 58 per cent (7/12) (56). Lym-1 is a mouse monoclonal antibody that preferentially targets malignant lymphocytes. Cu-67 has beta emissions comparable to those of iodine-131 but has gamma emissions more favorable for imaging. No significant nonhematological toxicity was observed. Hematological toxicity, especially thrombocytopenia, was dose-limiting.

Radioimmunotherapy for the treatment of common solid tumors has generally been associated with response rates lower than those associated with hematological malignancy. However, trials have shown definite evidence of localization of antibody to tumors and response rates between 5 and 40 per cent have been seen. In advanced colorectal carcinoma a 10 per cent response rate was seen in pretreated patients with bulk disease using an iodine-131-labeled murine monoclonal anti-CEA antibody (57). Response rates of up to 26 per cent have been reported when patients with small-volume colorectal cancer, with a total tumor bulk of less than 2.5 cm, were treated with an iodine-131-labeled murine monoclonal anti-CEA antibody (58, 59). This response rate is comparable with current chemotherapy options for colorectal cancer and is associated with fewer side-effects.

Locoregional radioimmunotherapy has also been shown to be promising. Iodine-131-radiolabeled anti-tenascin murine monoclonal antibodies were infused intratumorly into patients with high-grade malignant gliomas (60). Responses were seen in both bulky recurrent disease and minimal residual disease (60–63). Patients' median survival and time to relapse were also extended. Patient benefit was most likely with limited extension of the tumor at the time of therapy (60). Systemic and local toxicities were minimal (60–63).

Ovarian cancer has also been treated in early clinical trials with locoregional radioimmunotherapy. Intraperitoneal administration of radiolabeled antibodies has led to some clinical responses, particularly in patients with minimal residual disease (64–70). The therapy has generally been well tolerated. Further trials are ongoing to assess the efficacy of this approach for the future.

Immunotoxins

Immunotoxins consist of an antibody linked to a cellular toxin, which is usually plant- or animal-derived. The toxins most commonly used for clinical trials are ricin A, saporin, and *Pseudomonas* exotoxin. The toxin's normal cell binding and internalization domains are replaced by an antibody in order to allow specific targeting of the toxin to cancerous cells. The immunotoxin must be internalized into the cell for therapy as the toxin acts on intracellular targets such as ribosomes (71). Extracellularly, the toxins have no effect. These toxins have a very high potency and only a few molecules need to be internalized for effect. There is, however, no bystander effect, so theoretically each tumor cell must be targeted in order to produce 'cure'.

A phase I study of RFB4-SMPT-dgA (anti-CD22 murine antibody linked to deglycosylated ricin A) was performed in 26 patients with refractory B-cell lymphoma (72). In 24 evaluable patients there was one complete response and five partial responses at 1 month (overall response rate, 25 per cent). The main side-effects were vascular leak syndrome (VLS) and myalgia. The VLS was dose-limiting. Responses were rapid (37.5 per cent of patients had a > 50 per cent reduction in size of tumours at 1 week) but generally not sustained (30–78 days for responders at 1 month). VLS can be a serious problem, particularly when it involves the lungs and causes pulmonary edema, which may be fatal.

Other early-phase clinical trials have been performed with immunotoxins in hematological malignancies (73–81) and solid tumors (82–89). Response rates to date, however, remain variable and therapy is limited by biodistribution, toxicities, and the formation of HAMA and human anti-ricin antibodies (HARA) (71).

Genetic engineering with the development of recombinant immunotoxins appears to be more promising. Several agents are being developed and early results in clinical trials are encouraging; however, further trials are ongoing (10, 90–92).

Bispecific antibodies have also been used as part of immunotoxin therapy. An antibody is developed that has a dual specificity for the toxin and the target cell. This has the advantage of reducing the likelihood of damage to the toxin or to the antibody during the process of chemical conjugation (93). The disadvantage is that the relatively weak noncovalent bonds may lead to dissociation of the toxin in the circulation. Several bispecific antibodies are currently undergoing preclinical and clinical trials (93–96).

Immunotoxins may also be formed by the conjugation of an antibody to a cytotoxic agent rather than to a plant or animal toxin. Initially, it was hoped that this would improve the specificity of commonly used cytotoxics; however, clinical trials to date have not been encouraging (97–99). Results with immunoconjugates using high-potency cytotoxics, such as calicheamicin, have, however, been more promising. CMA-676 (gemtuzumab zogamicin, Mylotarg ^{TM}) is an immunoconjugate of a humanized anti-CD33 antibody with calicheamicin, which has been shown in clinical trials to produce responses in patients with refractory acute myeloid leukemia (AML) (100, 101). It has recently been licensed for use in the USA for the treatment of relapsed CD33-positive AML in patients aged over 60. CD33 is expressed on the cell surface of AML blast cells in approximately 90 per cent of patients (101). CMA-676 was shown *in vitro* to be rapidly internalized into the CD33-expressing cells (102). A phase I clinical trial in 40 patients with refractory or relapsed AML established the dose for further trials to be 9mg/m^2 every 2 weeks for 2 doses (101). The toxicities experienced included fever/chills postinfusion, hypotension, elevated liver function tests, and grade 4 myelosuppression (101). Three pooled phase II studies consisting of 142 patients in total showed an overall remission rate of 26 per cent (21/80 patients) in patients aged 60 and older with CD33-positive AML in first relapse (103). The toxicities of the treatment were similar to those of the phase I trial, with no significant difference in toxicities for patients < 60 years old compared to those > 60 years old (103). This is the first antibody conjugate to be licensed anywhere in the world.

Pretargeting systems

Two- or three-stage pretargeting systems are designed to improve therapeutic ratios between tumor and normal tissues and therefore achieve high tumor uptake of a therapeutic molecule with minimal nontarget normal tissue uptake. This is achieved in several steps. First, a nontoxic antibody is administered and accumulates in the tumor. The antibody clears from the circulation by itself, or a second clearing antibody can be introduced to accelerate systemic clearance. When tumor to normal tissue ratios are favorable, a therapeutic molecule is given which is bound to or activated by the antibody, which is localized in the tumor. High concentrations of the therapeutic molecule are therefore generated specifically in the tumor with reduced levels in normal tissues.

In a two-step system, the first antibody is allowed to clear by itself and, in the three-step system, a 'chaser' is given to accelerate systemic clearance of the antibody. Without the use of a 'chaser' the antibody may take 5–12 days to clear to sufficient levels to administer the second molecule (104). Several pretargeting systems have been developed for therapy, some of which will be discussed in more detail in later chapters (105).

Avidin–biotin systems

Avidins are small oligomeric proteins consisting of four identical subunits, each with a binding site for biotin. Binding to biotin occurs with extremely high affinity (dissociation constant of 10^{15}) and is virtually 'irreversible'(104). Biotin has a 'head' region that binds to avidin and a carboxyl 'tail' that can be used to bind to a monoclonal antibody, without altering its ability to bind avidin (104). This system has been used in both preclinical and clinical settings in a three-step system that involves the initial injection of a biotinylated monoclonal antibody to target the tumor, followed by avidin 'chase' and then administration of radiolabeled biotin (104). The three-step avidin–biotin system is being developed both for therapy and for immunoscintography and radioimmunoguided surgery (106–115). Magnani *et al.* demonstrated in patients undergoing enucleation for uveal melanoma using SPECT imaging that the three-step avidin–biotin system resulted in an increased tumor-to-nontumor ratio of 3.1 versus 1.5 for conventional radioimmunoscintigraphy (110).

Although the avidin–biotin three-step pretargeting system does have the advantage of reducing background levels of the therapeutic agent, therefore improving tumor:normal tissue ratios, it has the disadvantage of the immunogenicity of avidin and the complexity of the system, which requires precise timing for maximal effect (104).

Streptavidin–biotin systems

Streptavidin–biotin systems are commonly used in two-step pretargeting strategies, which may consist of either a biotinylated monoclonal antibody followed by radiolabeled streptavidin, or a streptavidinylated antibody followed by radiolabeled biotin (104). Several studies have demonstrated, either in models or preclinical settings, that a tumor to normal tissue ratio can be achieved with this two-step targeting system that is improved compared to that achieved with one-step radioimmunotargeting (116–118).

Antibody-directed enzyme prodrug therapy (ADEPT)

ADEPT utilizes the pretargeting strategy in an enzyme–prodrug system. An antibody–enzyme conjugate is administered as the first step to localize the enzyme to the tumor. This is followed by the administration of a prodrug, which is converted to an active cytotoxic by the enzyme at the tumor. A chaser ('clearing antibody') can be used as an extra step prior to prodrug administration. This consists of a galactosylated anti-enzyme antibody that will clear remaining enzyme from the circulation. ADEPT has the advantages of having a bystander effect (adjacent tumor cells are destroyed by the activated cytotoxic) and an amplification effect (one enzyme can activate multiple prodrug molecules). The disadvantages of this system include problems with immunogenicity, enzyme selection, and the complexity of this targeting system (119). The enzyme cannot be a naturally systemically available enzyme or nonspecific activation would occur; therefore, non-human enzymes are commonly used, such as the bacterial enzyme carboxypeptidase G2 (CPG2).

Early clinical trials conducted with ADEPT in 1990 established the feasibility of this system in a pilot scale clinical study of 24 patients with advanced colorectal cancer (120, 121). Partial responses were observed and doses of conjugate and prodrug established. A detailed mechanistic clinical study was then performed in 1994–95 in 10 patients with advanced colorectal cancer. High tumor to normal tissue ratios of the antibody–enzyme conjugate were demonstrated (> 10 000:1), and evidence of efficacy again seen (122). Repeated therapy was possible in both trials with the addition of immunosuppression using cyclosporin; however, a maximum of three courses could be given before the development of HAMA and human antibodies to the CPG2 enzyme (120, 122).

ADEPT is discussed in more detail in Chapter 4.

Combined therapies

The efficacy of antibody-targeted therapies for advanced cancers may be further improved by combining them with other agents. Combining an antibody therapy with a conventional chemotherapy may improve efficacy without producing additive side-effects. Clinical trials are already ongoing with herceptin and rituximab in combination with chemotherapy, and the early results appear promising (42, 44, 48, 49, 123).

The combination of radioimmunotherapy and ADEPT with the new antivascular agents 5,6-dimethylxanthenone-4-acetic acid (DMXAA) and combretastatin has shown impressive preclinical results. The heterogeneity of solid tumor structure, physiology, and blood supply limits the effectiveness of antibody therapies alone. Using phosphor image technology it has been shown that specific antibodies and their larger fragments tend to localize in the outer, well vascularized area of the tumor, leaving the poorly vascularized inner areas untreated by, or untreatable by, antibody-directed therapies (28). Antivascular therapies such as DMXAA and combretastatin cause specific destruction of tumor vasculature, but current strategies frequently fail to destroy all functional vessels, especially those around the periphery of the tumor. Central necrosis results, but a viable rim survives and the tumor continues to grow (124, 125). It has been shown that combining DMXAA and radioimmunotherapy in a xenograft model produced cures in 85 per cent of mice (124). The optimal time for administration of DMXAA was 48 hours after radioimmunotherapy to allow maximal accumulation of antibody in the tumor before shutting down the blood supply (126). Combining DMXAA with ADEPT also resulted in higher enzyme–prodrug accumulation and greater therapeutic effect (127). Similar results were found when combretastatin was combined with radioimmunotherapy, resulting in a significantly greater therapeutic effect than was seen after radioimmunotherapy alone. There was no increase in toxicity from the combined treatment, and it was demonstrated that 2–3 times the normal amount of therapeutic antibody could be trapped within the tumor without increasing the levels in normal tissues. This combination therapy is an exciting prospect for the future.

Issues in the design of clinical trials of novel antibody-targeted anticancer therapies

Understanding the complexity of an antibody-targeted strategy in a clinical setting allows the development of rational modifications to occur in the laboratory. The design of 'mechanistic', phase I trials, which incorporate measurements of mechanism as well as the conventional endpoints of side-effects, pharmacokinetics, and maximum dose achieved, are now being more widely used in order to improve our understanding of antibody therapies in patients. This results in fewer patients being required in phase I trials, where, unfortunately, the realistic chance of direct benefit to the patient often remains relatively small.

Radiolabeling antibodies with gamma-emitting tracers such as iodine-131, technetium-99m, and indium-111 allows dosimetry studies to be performed from gamma camera scans. This may result in a quantifiable measurement of dose to tumor and to normal tissues of the radiolabeled antibody (29). It is then assumed that the 'cold' unlabeled antibody will have the same biodistribution as the radiolabeled antibody. It must therefore be shown prior to administration that the antigen-binding characteristics of the labeled antibody remain as unaltered as possible during the radiolabeling process.

Tumor biopsies may provide important information in the understanding of the mechanism of an antibody system. This is particularly important in complex therapeutic systems such as ADEPT where tumor biopsies have provided valuable information for the understanding of this system in humans (122, 128).

18-Fluorodeoxyglucose positron emission tomography (FDG-PET) can be used to quantify the metabolic activity of tumors. It is becoming increasingly used in the assessment of response to conventional chemotherapy, as it may provide an earlier and more reliable indi-

cation of response (129–136). FDG-PET may become particularly important in the assessment of efficacy of novel therapies, as the patient groups studied are usually heavily pretreated and may only achieve subtle responses. Using conventional radiological assessments of response therapies may be discarded as ineffective, but with the additional of a functional assessment with FDG-PET a better understanding of metabolic change with therapy may be achieved.

Finally, to complete the understanding of a novel antibody therapy it is important to develop a mathematical model of the system. This will help integrate knowledge about targeting. The model aids conceptual appreciation of the mechanisms of action, helps to define design priorities, and permits hypothetical investigation of changes before making or investigating new products

A mathematical model of antibody targeting can be built by collecting quantitative data about the behavior of targeting systems and describing the system in terms of compartments interconnected by equations defining the passage of targeting agents between them (137, 138). Hypothetical questions can be asked so that the effect of a putative change can be analyzed. This gives a robust, versatile platform for research into antibody targeting and a flexible approach to making effective targeted therapeutics for common cancers.

Conclusions

Monoclonal antibody-targeted therapy for cancer is an exciting and rapidly developing area in oncology. The targeted approach has the theoretical advantages of reducing nonspecific side-effects from therapies and increasing the chance of cure by concentrating treatments on tumor alone. Antibody therapies may be used alone or in combination with other treatments, where the therapeutic effects may be complementary without additional side-effects.

Integral to the development of successful therapies to attain the ultimate aim of cure is an understanding of the complex host–tumor environment and antibody interaction in this setting. This understanding must occur in both the preclinical and clinical settings. Mechanistic clinical trial designs are important in broadening this understanding and focusing research and therapeutic developments for the future.

Promising advances in antibody therapies for cancer have already occurred in the last decade and look certain to be part of our routine clinical practice in the future.

References

1. Hericourt J, Richet C. De la serotherapie dans le traitment du cancer. C R Acad Sci 1895, **121**, 567–9.

2. Boschoff C, Begent R. Tumor markers. In: Essential general surgical oncology (ed. I Taylor, T Cook, and P Guillou). Churchill Livingstone, Edinburgh, 1996, 131–40.

3. Köhler G, Milstein C. Continuous cultures of fused cells secreting antibody of predefined specificity. Nature 1975, **256**, 495–7.

4. Huse WD, Sastry L, Iverson SA, *et al*. Generation of a large combinatorial library of the immunoglobulin repertoire in phage lambda. Science 1989, **246**, 1275–81.

5. McCafferty J, Griffiths AD, Winter G, *et al*. Phage antibodies: filamentous phage displaying antibody variable domains. Nature 1990, **348**, 552–4.

6. Chester KA, Begent RH, Robson L, *et al*. Phage libraries for generation of clinically useful antibodies. Lancet 1994, **343**, 455–6.

7. Bruggemann M, Taussig MJ. Production of human antibody repertoires in transgenic mice. Curr Opin Biotechnol 1997, **8** (4), 455–8.

8. Hawkins RE, Chester KA. Antibody technology has been transformed. In: Molecular biology for oncologists (ed. J Yarnold, M Stratton, and T McMillan). Chapman & Hall, London, 1996, 250–60.

9. Huston J, Levinson D, Mudgett-Hunter M, *et al*. Protein engineering of antibody binding sites: recovery of specific activity in an anti-digoxin single chain Fv analogue produced in *Escherichia coli*. Proc Natl Acad Sci, USA 1988, **85** (16), 5879–83.

10. Reiter Y, Brinkmann U, Lee B, *et al*. Engineering antibody Fv fragments for cancer detection and therapy: disulfide-stabilized Fv fragments. Nat Biotechnol 1996, **14** (10), 1239–45.

11. Chester KA, Hawkins RE. Clinical issues in antibody design. Tibtech 1995, **13**, 294–300.

12. Vogelstein B, Lane D, Levine AJ. Surfing the p53 network. Nature 2000, **408** (6810), 307–10.

13. Alizadeh AA, Eisen MB, Davis RE, *et al*. Distinct types of diffuse large B-cell lymphoma identified by gene expression profiling. Nature. 2000, **403** (6769), 503–11.

14. Martin KJ, Kritzman BM, Price LM, *et al*. Linking gene expression patterns to therapeutic groups in breast cancer. Cancer Res 2000, **60** (8), 2232–8.

15. Pedley BR. Pharmacokinetics of monoclonal antibodies. Clin Immunother 1996, **6** (1), 54–67.

16. Begent R, Verhaar M, Chester K, *et al*. Clinical evidence of efficient tumor targeting based on single-chain Fv antibody selected from a combinatorial library. Nat Med 1996, **2** (9), 979–84.

17. King DJ, Turner A, Farnsworth AP, *et al*. Improved tumor targeting with chemically cross-linked recombinant antibody fragments. Cancer Res 1994, **54**, 6176–85.

18. Casey JL, Pedley RB, King DJ, *et al*. Dosimetric evaluation and radioimmunotherapy of anti-tumour multivalent Fab fragments. Br J Cancer 1999, **81** (6), 972–80.

19. Boulianne GL, Hozumi N, Shulman MJ. Production of functional chimeric mouse/human antibody. Nature 1984, **312**, 643–6.

20. Neuberger M, Williams G, Mitchell E, *et al*. A hapten-specific chimeric IgE antibody with human physiological effector function. Nature 1985, **314**, 268–70.

21. Riechmann L, Clark M, Waldmann H, *et al*. Reshaping human antibodies for therapy. Nature 1988, **332**, 323–7.

22. Begent R, Ledermann J, Bagshawe K, *et al*. Chimeric B72.3 antibody for repeated radioimmunotherapy of colorectal cancer. Antibody Immunoconj Radiopharmaceut 1990, **3**, 86.

23. Amlot PL, Rawlings E, Fernando ON, *et al*. Prolonged action of a chimeric interleukin-2 receptor (CD25) monoclonal antibody used in cadaveric renal transplantation. Transplantation 1995, **60**, 748–56.

24. Pedley R, Boden J, Boden R, *et al*. The potential for enhanced tumor localization by poly(ethylene glycol) modification of anti-CEA antibody. Br J Cancer 1994, **70**, 1126–30.

25. Delgado C, Pedley R, Herraez A, *et al*. Enhanced tumor specificity of an anti-carcinoembrionic antigen Fab fragment by poly(ethylene glycol) (PEG) modification. Br J Cancer 1996, **73**, 175–82.

26. Marshall D, Pedley R, Boden J, *et al*. Polyethylene glycol modification of a galactosylated streptavidin clearing agent: effects on immunogenicity and clearance of a biotinylated anti-tumor antibody. Br J Cancer 1996, **73**, 565–72.

27. Kitamura K, Takahashi T, Yamaguchi T, *et al*. Chemical engineering of the monoclonal antibody A7 by polyethylene glycol for targeted cancer therapy. Cancer Res 1991, **51**, 4310–15.

28. Flynn AA, Green AJ, Boxer GM, *et al*. A novel technique, using radioluminography, for the measurement of uniformity of radiolabelled antibody distribution in a colorectal cancer xenograft model. Int J Rad Oncol Biol Phys 1999, **43**, 183–9.

29. Green AJ, Dewhurst SH, Begent RH, *et al*. Accurate quantification of 131-I distribution by gamma camera imaging. Eur J Nucl Med 1990, **16**, 361–5.

30. Anderson KC, Bates MP, Slaughenhoupt BL, *et al*. Expression of human B cell-associated antigens on leukemias and lymphomas: a model of human B cell differentiation. Blood 1984, **63** (6), 1424–33.

31. Press OW, Appelbaum F, Ledbetter JA, *et al*. Monoclonal antibody IF5 (anti-CD20) serotherapy of human B cell lymphoma. Blood 1987, **69** (2), 584–91.

32. McLaughlin P, Grillo-Lopez AJ, Link BK, *et al*. Rituximab chimeric anti-CD20 monoclonal antibody therapy for relapsed indolent lymphoma: half of patients respond to four-dose treatment program. J Clin Oncol 1998, **16** (8), 2825–33.

33. Maloney DG, Grillo-Lopez AG, White CA, *et al*. IDEC-C2B8 (Rituximab) anti-CD20 monoclonal antibody

therapy in patients with relapsed low-grade non-Hodgkin's lymphoma. Blood 1997, **90** (6), 2188–95.

34. Riethmuller G, Schneider-Gadicke E, Schlimock G, *et al.* Randomized trial of monoclonal antibody for adjuvant therapy of resected Duke's C colorectal carcinoma. Lancet 1994, **343**, 1177–83.

35. Riethmuller G, Holz E, Schlimock G, *et al.* Monoclonal antibody therapy for resected Duke's C colorectal cancer: seven year outcome of a multicenter randomized trial. J Clin Oncol 1998, **16** (5), 1788–94.

36. Hung M-C, Lau Y-K. Basic science of HER-2/neu: a review. Sem Oncol 1999, **26** (4, suppl. 12), 51–9.

37. Slamon DJ, Godolphin W, Jones LA, *et al.* Studies of the HER-2/neu proto-oncogene in human breast and ovarian cancer. Science 1989, **244** (4905), 707–12.

38. Slamon DJ, Clark GM. Amplification of c-erbB-2 and aggressive human breast tumors? Science 1988, **240** (4860), 1795–8.

39. Slamon D, Clark G, Wong S. Human breast cancer: correlation of relapse and survival with amplification of the HER-2/neu oncogene. Science 1987, **235**, 177–82.

40. Slamon DJ, Clark GM, Wong SG, *et al.* Human breast cancer: correlation of relapse and survival with amplification of the HER-2/neu oncogene. Science 1987, **235** (4785), 177–82.

41. Berchuck A, Kamel A, Whitaker R, *et al.* Overexpression of HER-2/neu is associated with poor survival in advanced epithelial ovarian cancer. Cancer Res 1990, **50** (13), 4087–91.

42. Shak Steven for the Herceptin Multinational Investigator Study Group. Overview of the trastuzumab (Herceptin) anti-HER2 monoclonal antibody clinical program in HER2-overexpressing metastatic breast cancer. Sem Oncol 1999, **26** (4, suppl. 12), 71–7.

43. Carter P, Presta L, Gorman C. Humanization of an anti-p185HER2 antibody for human cancer therapy. Proc Natl Acad Sci, USA 1992, **89**, 4285–9.

44. Pegram MD, Slamon DJ. Combination therapy with trastuzumab (Herceptin) and cisplatin for chemoresistant metastatic breast cancer: evidence for receptor-enhanced chemosensitivity. Sem Oncol. 1999, **26** (4, suppl. 12), 89–95.

45. Baselga J, Norton l, Albanell J, *et al.* Recombinant humanized anti-HER2 antibody (Herceptin) enhances the anti-tumor activity of paclitaxel and doxorubicin against HER2/*neu* overexpressing human breast cancer xenografts. Cancer Res 1998, **58**, 2825–31.

46. Baselga J, Tripathy D, Mendelsohn J, *et al.* Phase II study of weekly intravenous recombinant humanized anti-p185HER2 monoclonal antibody in patients with HER2/*neu*-overexpressing metastatic breast cancer. J Clin Oncol 1996, **14** (3), 737–44.

47. Cobleigh M, Vogel C, Tripathy D, *et al.* Efficacy and safety of Herceptin (humanized antiHER2 antibody) as a single agent in 222 women with HER2 overexpression who relapsed following chemotherapy for metastatic breast cancer. Proc Am Soc Clin Oncol, USA 1998, **17**, 97A.

48. Pegram MD, Lipton A, Hayes DF, *et al.* Phase II study of receptor-enhanced chemosensitivity using recombinant humanized anti-p185HER2/neu monoclonal antibody plus cisplatin in patients with HER2/neu-overexpressing metastatic breast cancer refractory to chemotherapy treatment. J Clin Oncol 1998, **16** (8), 2659–71.

49. Slamon D, Leyland-Jones B, Shak S, *et al.* Addition of Herceptin (humanized anti-HER2 antibody) to first line chemotherapy for HER2 overexpressing metastatic breast cancer (HER2+/MBC) markedly increases anti-cancer activity: a randomized multinational phase III trial. Proc Am Soc Clin Oncol, USA 1998, **17**, 98A.

50. Yao T-J, Meyers M, Livingston PO, *et al.* Immunization of melanoma patients with BEC2-keyhole limpet hemocyanin plus BCG intradermally followed by intravenous booster immunizations with BEC2 to induce anti-GD3 ganglioside antibodies. Clin Cancer Res 1999, **5**, 77–81.

51. Dykes P, Bradwell A, Chapman C, *et al.* Radioimmunotherapy of cancer: clinical studies and limiting factors. Cancer Treat Rev 1987, **14**, 87–106.

52. Wilder RB, DeNardo GL, DeNardo SJ. Radioimmunotherapy: recent results and future directions. J Clin Oncol. 1996, **14** (4), 1383–400.

53. Press OW, Eary J, Appelbaum F, *et al.* Radiolabelled antibody therapy of B-cell lymphoma with autologous bone marrow support. New Engl J Med 1993, **329**, 1219–24.

54. Witzig TE, White CA, Wiseman GA, *et al.* Phase I/II trial of IDEC-Y2B8 radioimmunotherapy for treatment of relapsed or refractory CD20 (+) B-cell non-Hodgkin's lymphoma. J Clin Oncol 1999, **17** (12), 3793–803.

55. Wiseman GA, White CA, Witzig TE, *et al.* Radioimmunotherapy of relapsed non-Hodgkin's lymphoma with zevalin, a 90Y-labeled anti-CD20 monoclonal antibody. Clin Cancer Res 1999, **5** (10 suppl.), 3281s–6s.

56. O'Donnell RT, DeNardo GL, Kukis DL, *et al.* A clinical trial of radioimmunotherapy with 67Cu-2IT-BAT-Lym-1 for non-Hodgkin's lymphoma. J Nucl Med 1999, **40** (12), 2014–20.

57. Lane D, Eagle K, Begent R, *et al.* Radioimmunotherapy of metastatic colorectal tumours with iodine-131-labelled antibody to carcinoembryonic antigen: phase I/II study with comparative biodistribution of intact and F(ab)$_2$ antibodies. Br J Cancer 1994, **70**, 521–5.

58. Behr T, Salib A, Liersch T, *et al.* Radioimmunotherapy of small volume disease of colorectal cancer metastatic to the liver: preclinical evaluation in comparison to standard chemotherapy and initial results of a phase I clinical study. Clin Cancer Res 1999, **5** (10 suppl.), 3232s–42s.

59. Behr T, Liersch T, Canelo R, *et al.* Radioimmunotherapy of small volume disease of colorectal cancer: results of a clinical phase I/II trial [abstract]. Eur J Cancer 1999, **35** (suppl. 5), S51.

60. Riva P, Franceschi G, Arista A, *et al.* Local application of radiolabeled monoclonal antibodies in the treatment of high grade malignant gliomas: a six-year clinical experience. Cancer 1997, **80** (12 suppl.), 2733–42.

61. Riva P, Arista A, Franceschi G, *et al.* Local treatment of malignant gliomas by direct infusion of specific monoclonal antibodies labeled with 131I: comparison of the results obtained in recurrent and newly diagnosed tumors. Cancer Res. 1995, **55** (23 suppl.), 5952s–6s.

62. Riva P, Arista A, Tison V, *et al.* Intralesional radioimmunotherapy of malignant gliomas. An effective treatment in recurrent tumors. Cancer 1994, **73** (3 suppl.), 1076–82.

63. Riva P, Arista A, Sturiale C, *et al.* Treatment of intracranial human glioblastoma by direct intratumoral administration of 131I-labelled anti-tenascin monoclonal antibody BC-2. Int J Cancer 1992, **51** (1), 7–13.

64. Rosenblum MG, Verschraegen CF, Murray JL, *et al.* Phase I study of 90Y-labeled B72.3 intraperitoneal administration in patients with ovarian cancer: effect of dose and EDTA coadministration on pharmacokinetics and toxicity. Clin Cancer Res 1999, **5** (5), 953–61.

65. Juweid M, Swayne LC, Sharkey RM, *et al.* Prospects of radioimmunotherapy in epithelial ovarian cancer: results with iodine-131-labeled murine and humanized MN-14 anti-carcinoembryonic antigen monoclonal antibodies. Gynecol Oncol. 1997, **67** (3), 259–71.

66. Alvarez RD, Partridge EE, Khazaeli MB, *et al.* Intraperitoneal radioimmunotherapy of ovarian cancer with 177Lu-CC49: a phase I/II study. Gynecol Oncol 1997, **65** (1), 94–101.

67. Meredith RF, Partridge EE, Alvarez RD, *et al.* Intraperitoneal radioimmunotherapy of ovarian cancer with lutetium-177-CC49. J Nucl Med 1996, **37** (9), 1491–6.

68. Jacobs AJ, Fer M, Su FM, *et al.* A phase I trial of a rhenium 186-labeled monoclonal antibody administered intraperitoneally in ovarian carcinoma: toxicity and clinical response. Obstet Gynecol 1993, **82** (4 pt. 1), 586–93.

69. Hird V, Maraveyas A, Snook D, *et al.* Adjuvant therapy of ovarian cancer with radioactive monoclonal antibody. Br J Cancer 1993, **68** (2), 403–6.

70. Nicholson S, Gooden CS, Hird V, *et al.* Radioimmunotherapy after chemotherapy compared to chemotherapy alone in the treatment of advanced ovarian cancer: a matched analysis. Oncol Rep 1998, **5** (1), 223–6.

71. Byers V, Baldwin RW. Therapeutic strategies with monoclonal antibodies and immunoconjugates. Immunology 1988, **65**, 329–35.

72. Amlot P, Stone M, Cunningham D, *et al.* A phase I study of an anti-CD22-deglycosylated ricin A chain immunotoxin in the treatment of B-cell lymphomas resistant to conventional therapy. Blood 1993, **82** (9), 2624–33.

73. Falini B, Bolognesi A, Flenghi L, *et al.* Response of refractory Hodgkin's disease to monoclonal anti-CD30 immunotoxin. Lancet 1992, **339**, 1195–6.

74. Grossbard M, Freedman A, Ritz J, *et al.* Serotherapy of B-cell neoplasms with anti-B4-blocked ricin: a phase I trial of daily bolus infusions. Blood 1992, **79** (3), 576–85.

75. Multani PS, O'Day S, Nadler LM, *et al.* Phase II clinical trial of bolus infusion anti-B4 blocked ricin immunoconjugate in patients with relapsed B-cell non-Hodgkin's lymphoma. Clin Cancer Res 1998, **4** (11), 2599–604.

76. Grossbard ML, Gribben JG, Freedman AS, *et al.* Adjuvant immunotoxin therapy with anti-B4-blocked ricin after autologous bone marrow transplantation for patients with B-cell non-Hodgkin's lymphoma. Blood 1993, **81** (9), 2263–71.

77. Grossbard ML, Lambert JM, Goldmacher VS, *et al.* Anti-B4-blocked ricin: a phase I trial of 7-day continuous infusion in patients with B-cell neoplasms. J Clin Oncol 1993, **11** (4), 726–37.

78. LeMaistre CF, Meneghetti C, Rosenblum M, *et al.* Phase I trial of an interleukin-2 (IL-2) fusion toxin (DAB486IL-2) in hematologic malignancies expressing the IL-2 receptor. Blood 1992, **79** (10), 2547–54.

79. Grossbard ML, Freedman AS, Ritz J, *et al.* Serotherapy of B-cell neoplasms with anti-B4-blocked ricin: a phase I trial of daily bolus infusion. Blood 1992, **79** (3), 576–85.

80. LeMaistre CF, Rosen S, Frankel A, *et al.* Phase I trial of H65-RTA immunoconjugate in patients with cutaneous T-cell lymphoma. Blood 1991, **78** (5), 1173–82.

81. Vitetta ES, Stone M, Amlot P, *et al.* Phase I immunotoxin trial in patients with B-cell lymphoma. Cancer Res 1991, **51** (15), 4052–8.

82. LoRusso PM, Lomen PL, Redman BG, *et al.* Phase I study of monoclonal antibody–ricin A chain immunoconjugate Xomazyme-791 in patients with metastatic colon cancer. Am J Clin Oncol 1995, **18** (4), 307–12.

83. Gonzalez R, Salem P, Bunn PA, Jr, *et al.* Single-dose murine monoclonal antibody ricin A chain immunotoxin in the treatment of metastatic melanoma: a phase I trial. Mol Biother 1991, **3** (4),192–6.

84. Oratz R, Speyer JL, Wernz JC, *et al.* Antimelanoma monoclonal antibody–ricin A chain immunoconjugate (XMMME-001-RTA) plus cyclophosphamide in the treatment of metastatic malignant melanoma: results of a phase II trial. J Biol Response Mod 1990, **9** (4), 345–54.

85. Weiner LM, O'Dwyer J, Kitson J, *et al.* Phase I evaluation of an anti-breast carcinoma monoclonal antibody 260F9-recombinant ricin A chain immunoconjugate. Cancer Res 1989, **49** (14), 4062–7.

86. Durrant LG, Byers VS, Scannon PJ, *et al.* Humoral immune responses to XMMCO-791-RTA immunotoxin in colorectal cancer patients. Clin Exp Immunol 1989, **75** (2), 258–64.

87. Spitler LE, del Rio M, Khentigan A, *et al.* Therapy of patients with malignant melanoma using a monoclonal antimelanoma antibody–ricin A chain immunotoxin. Cancer Res 1987, **47** (6), 1717–23.

88. Spitler LE. Immunotoxin therapy of malignant melanoma. Med Oncol Tumor Pharmacother 1986, **3** (3–4), 147–52.

89. Pai-Scherf LH, Villa J, Pearson D, *et al.* Hepatotoxicity in cancer patients receiving erb-38, a recombinant immunotoxin that targets the erbB2 receptor. Clin Cancer Res 1999, **5** (9), 2311–15.

90. Kuska B. First responses seen in cancer patients to a recombinant immunotoxin. J Natl Cancer Inst 1999, **91** (23), 1997.

91. Kreitman RJ, Wilson WH, Robbins D, *et al.* Responses in refractory hairy cell leukemia to a recombinant immunotoxin. Blood 1999, **94** (10), 3340–8.

92. Reiter Y, Pastan I. Antibody engineering of recombinant Fv immunotoxins for improved targeting of cancer:

disulfide-stabilized Fv immunotoxins. Clin Cancer Res. 1996, **2** (2), 245–52.

93. Antonietta Bonardi M, French R, Amlot P, *et al.* Delivery of saporin to human B-cell lymphoma using bispecific antibody targeting via CD22 but not CD19, CD37, or immunoglobin results in efficient killing. Cancer Res 1993, **53**, 3015–21.

94. Duke-Cohan JS, Morimoto C, Schlossman SF. Targeting of an activated T-cell subset using a bispecific antibody–toxin conjugate directed against CD4 and CD26. Blood 1993, **82** (7), 2224–34.

95. Sforzini S, Bolognesi A, Meazza R, *et al.* Differential sensitivity of CD30+ neoplastic cells to gelonin delivered by anti-CD30/anti-gelonin bispecific antibodies. Br J Haematol 1995, **90** (3), 572–7.

96. Duke-Cohan JS, Morimoto C, Schlossman SF. Depletion of the helper/inducer (memory) T cell subset using a bispecific antibody–toxin conjugate directed against CD4 and CD29. Transplantation 1993, **56** (5), 1188–96.

97. Elias DJ, Hirschowitz L, Kline LE, *et al.* Phase I clinical comparative study of monoclonal antibody KS1/4 and KS1/4–methotrexate immunoconjugate in patients with non-small cell lung carcinoma. Cancer Res 1990, **50** (13), 4154–9.

98. Tjandra JJ, Pietersz GA, Teh JG, *et al.* Phase I clinical trial of drug–monoclonal antibody conjugates in patients with advanced colorectal carcinoma: a preliminary report. Surgery 1990, **107** (3), 261–5.

99. Tolcher AW, Sugarman S, Gelmon KA, *et al.* Randomized phase II study of BR96–doxorubicin conjugate in patients with metastatic breast cancer. J Clin Oncol 1999, **17** (2), 478–84.

100. Bernstein ID. Monoclonal antibodies to the myeloid stem cells: therapeutic implications of CMA-676, a humanized anti-CD33 antibody calicheamicin conjugate. Leukemia 2000, **14** (3), 474–5.

101. Sievers EL, Appelbaum FR, Spielberger RT, *et al.* Selective ablation of acute myeloid leukemia using antibody-targeted chemotherapy: a phase I study of an anti-CD33 calicheamicin immunoconjugate. Blood 1999, **93** (11), 3678–84.

102. van der Jagt R, Badger C, Appelbaum F, *et al.* Localization of radiolabeled antimyeloid antibodies in a human acute leukemia xenograft tumor model. Cancer Res 1992, **52**, 89.

103. Sievers E, Larson R, Estey E, *et al.* Comparison of the efficacy and safety of Gemtuzumab Ozogamicin (CMA-676) in patients < 60 and ≥ 60 years of age with AML in first relapse. Proc Am Soc Clin Oncol, USA 2000, **19**, 23A.

104. Stoldt H, Aftab F, Chinol M, *et al.* Pretargeting strategies for radio-immunoguided tumor localization and therapy. Eur J Cancer 1997, **33** (2), 186–92.

105. Goodwin DA, Meares CF. Pretargeting. Cancer 1997, **80**, 2675–80.

106. Paganelli G, Grana C, Chinol M, *et al.* Antibody-guided three-step therapy for high grade glioma with yttrium-90 biotin. Eur J Nucl Med 1999, **26** (4), 348–57.

107. Paganelli G, Orecchia R, Jereczek-Fossa B, *et al.* Combined treatment of advanced oropharyngeal cancer with external radiotherapy and three-step radioimmunotherapy. Eur J Nucl Med 1998, **25** (9), 1336–9.

108. Chinol M, Paganelli G, Sudati F, *et al.* Biodistribution in tumor-bearing mice of two 90Y-labelled biotins using three-step tumor targeting. Nucl Med Commun 1997, **18** (2), 176–82.

109. Magnani P, Paganelli G, Songini C, *et al.* Pretargeted immunoscintigraphy in patients with medullary thyroid carcinoma. Br J Cancer 1996, **74** (5), 825–31.

110. Magnani P, Paganelli G, Modorati G, *et al.* Quantitative comparison of direct antibody labeling and tumor pretargeting in uveal melanoma. J Nucl Med 1996, **37** (6), 967–71.

111. Paganelli G, Stella M, Zito F, *et al.* Radioimmunoguided surgery using iodine-125-labeled biotinylated monoclonal antibodies and cold avidin. J Nucl Med 1994, **35** (12), 1970–5.

112. Paganelli G, Magnani P, Zito F, *et al.* Pre-targeted immunodetection in glioma patients: tumor localization and single-photon emission tomography imaging of [99mTc]PnAO-biotin. Eur J Nucl Med 1994, **21** (4), 314–21.

113. Paganelli G, Magnani P, Zito F, *et al.* Three-step monoclonal antibody tumor targeting in carcinoembryonic antigen-positive patients. Cancer Res 1991, **51** (21), 5960–6.

114. Paganelli G, Pervez S, Siccardi AG, *et al.* Intraperitoneal radio-localization of tumors pre-targeted by biotinylated monoclonal antibodies. Int J Cancer 1990, **45** (6), 1184–9.

115. Pervez S, Paganelli G, Epenetos AA, *et al.* Localization of biotinylated monoclonal antibody in nude mice bearing subcutaneous and intraperitoneal human tumour xenografts. Int J Cancer Suppl 1988, **3**, 30–3.

116. Zhu H, Jain RK, Baxter LT. Tumor pretargeting for radioimmunodetection and radioimmunotherapy. J Nucl Med 1998, **39** (1), 65–76.

117. Saga T, Weinstein JN, Jeong JM, *et al.* Two-step targeting of experimental lung metastases with biotinylated antibody and radiolabeled streptavidin. Cancer Res 1994, **54** (8), 2160–5.

118. Sung C, van Osdol WW. Pharmacokinetic comparison of direct antibody targeting with pretargeting protocols based on streptavidin-biotin binding. J Nucl Med 1995, **36** (5), 867–76.

119. Sharma S. Immune Response in ADEPT. Advanced Drug Deliv Rev 1996, **22**, 369–76.

120. Bagshawe K, Sharma S, Springer C, *et al.* Antibody directed enzyme prodrug therapy: a pilot scale clinical trial. Tumour Targeting 1995, **1**, 17–30.

121. Bagshawe K, Sharma S, Springer C, *et al.* Antibody directed enzyme prodrug therapy (ADEPT): clinical report. Dis Markers 1991, **9**, 233–8.

122. Napier M, Sharma S, Springer C, *et al.* Antibody-directed enzyme prodrug therapy (ADEPT): efficacy and mechanism of action in colorectal cancer. Clin Cancer Res 2000, **6**, 765–72.

123. Czuczman MS. CHOP plus rituximab chemoimmunotherapy of indolent B-cell lymphoma. Sem Oncol 1999, **26** (5 suppl. 14), 88–96.

124. Pedley R, Begent R, Boden J, *et al.* Enhancement of radioimmunotherapy by drugs modifying tumor blood flow in a colonic xenograft model. Int J Cancer 1994, **57**, 830–5.

125. Dark G, Hill S, Prise V, *et al*. Combretastatin A4, an agent that displays potent and selective toxicity toward tumor vasculature. Cancer Res 1997, 57, 1829–34.

126. Pedley RB, Boden JA, Boden R, *et al*. Ablation of colorectal xenografts with combined radioimmunotherapy and tumor blood flow-modifying agents. Cancer Res 1996, **56**, 3293–300.

127. Pedley RB, Sharma SK, Boxer GM, *et al*. Enhancement of antibody-directed enzyme prodrug therapy in colorectal xenografts by an antivascular agent. Cancer Res 1999, **59** (16), 3998–4003.

128. Begent RHJ, Bagshawe KD. Biodistribution Studies. Advanced Drug Deliv Rev 1996, **22**, 325–9.

129. Jansson T, Westlin J, Ahlstrom H, *et al*. Positron emission tomography studies in patients with locally advanced and/or metastatic breast cancer: a method for early therapy evaluation? J Clin Oncol 1995, **13**, 1470–7.

130. Schulte M, Brecht-Krauss D, Werner M, *et al*. Evaluation of neoadjuvant therapy response of osteogenic sarcoma using FDG PET. J Nucl Med 1999, **40** (10), 1637–43.

131. Higashi T, Sakahara H, Torizuka T, *et al*. Evaluation of intraoperative radiation therapy for unresectable pancreatic cancer with FDG PET. J Nucl Med 1999, **40** (9), 1424–33.

132. Kitagawa Y, Sadato N, Azuma H, *et al*. FDG PET to evaluate combined intra-arterial chemotherapy and radiotherapy of head and neck neoplasms. J Nucl Med 1999, **40** (7), 1132–7.

133. Sakamoto H, Nakai Y, Ohashi Y, *et al*. Monitoring of response to radiotherapy with fluorine-18 deoxyglucose PET of head and neck squamous cell carcinomas. Acta Otolaryngol Suppl 1998, **538**, 254–60.

134. Couper GW, McAteer D, Wallis F, *et al*. Detection of response to chemotherapy using positron emission tomography in patients with esophageal and gastric cancer. Br J Surg 1998, **85** (10), 1403–6.

135. Lowe VJ, Dunphy FR, Varvares M, *et al*. Evaluation of chemotherapy response in patients with advanced head and neck cancer using [F-18]fluorodeoxyglucose positron emission tomography. Head Neck 1997, **19** (8), 666–74.

136. Wahl RL, Zasadny K, Helvie M, *et al*. Metabolic monitoring of breast cancer chemohormonotherapy using positron emission tomography: initial evaluation. J Clin Oncol 1993, **11** (11), 2101–11.

137. Baxter LT, Zhu H, Mackensen DG, *et al*. Biodistribution of monoclonal antibodies: scale-up from mouse to human using a physiologically based pharmacokinetic model. Cancer Res 1995, **55**, 4611–22.

138. Baxter LT, Jain RK. Pharmacokinetic analysis of the microscopic distribution of enzyme-conjugated antibodies and prodrugs: comparison with experimental data. Br J Cancer 1996, **73**, 447–56.

4 | Antibody-directed enzyme prodrug therapy (ADEPT)

Konstantinos N. Syrigos and Kevin J. Harrington

Introduction

Although the management of cancer by exploiting properties distinguishing neoplastic and normal cells has always been an attractive concept, it was the development of hybridoma technology and the resulting tumour-associated monoclonal antibodies (mAbs) (1, 2) that offered new prospects for this strategy. Twenty years later, some of the applications of mAbs in oncology are now part of everyday diagnosis and treatment (for example, immunohistochemistry, radioimmunodetection), while others are the subject of intensive investigation. With regard to the development of new therapeutic strategies for cancer, several techniques have been developed to exploit the suitability of mAbs as carriers of cytotoxic agents. These agents could be conventional cytotoxic drugs, radioisotopes, or toxins derived from plants (ricin, abrin) or bacteria (Diphtheria, Pseudomonas) that inhibit protein synthesis. Although the systemic toxicity was reduced, with the application of the above techniques, the therapeutic results were very poor, mainly because of the inadequate uptake of the conjugate by the tumor cells and the consequent failure to administer a cytotoxic dose to the tumor.

Since selective delivery of a toxic agent exclusively to the tumor site has proven to be elusive, attempts have been made to generate an active drug from an inactive precursor, by the action of an enzyme present predominantly at the tumor site. Central to this approach is the concept of a prodrug, a molecule that is not active itself, but that can be converted to a cytotoxic agent by enzymatic activation *in vivo*. The criteria of the ideal prodrug were set by Connors and Whisson (3–5) more than 30 years ago and, although they can only be applied with limitations, they still provide guidelines for the design and choice of the optimal chemotherapeutic agent. They are listed below.

- The prodrug must be nontoxic, while its active derivative should be highly cytotoxic.
- Tumors should contain the enzyme, which activates the prodrug in considerably higher concentrations in the tumor than in normal tissues.
- The enzyme–prodrug system should be functional *in vivo*.
- The active drug should not produce major toxicity to normal organs.

The chemotherapeutic agents initially used in line with these guidelines were cyclophosphamide, dacarbazine, and mitozolamide, activated in the liver by the mixed-function oxidase system (6). They have been used for the treatment of a range of malignancies with some success (7), but without significantly reducing toxicity, since the activating enzymes are general ubiquitous metabolic enzymes.

Ideally, the activation of a prodrug should be restricted to the site of treatment. Up to now, few prodrugs that can be activated by tumor cell enzymes have been described. One such prodrug is nitrogen mustard, which can be reduced in the presence of the xanthine oxidase system present in high amounts in some hepatocellular carcinomas (5, 8). The reduction results in the formation of highly toxic aniline and *p*-phenylenediamine derivatives, which are extremely potent alkylating agents with established antitumor activity. Unfortunately, as neoplastic tissues usually share the enzyme repertoire of normal tissues (8), conventional prodrug chemotherapy systems depend on activation by general metabolic enzymes (6).

Since the use of a tumor-associated antibody as carrier of a prodrug is not satisfactory, Philpott and colleagues exploited the idea of using the antibodies to carry enzymes to the tumor sites (9, 10). This concept was further developed and described by Bagshawe *et al.* (11, 12) and Senter *et al.* (13, 14). This two-step approach, is known as antibody-directed enzyme prodrug therapy (ADEPT). Tumor-associated antibodies are linked to enzymes, delivered to tumor sites, and allowed to clear from normal tissues. Subsequently, a prodrug is administered. This is converted by the enzyme into an active cytotoxic agent. The interval between the two administrations is optimized to achieve minimal systemic toxicity by accomplishing satisfactory accumulation of the conjugate in the tumor and clearance from blood and normal tissues. In addition, as the active drug diffuses throughout the tumor, it provides a bystander effect, killing antigen-negative cells.

This approach has two advantages compared with other applications of monoclonal antibodies in oncology:

1. *Reduced toxicity* because the systemic effect is minimized by optimizing the interval between the two steps. One can also use enzymes not present in humans to minimize the release of cytotoxic agent at sites other than the tumor.

2. *Amplification*. These systems can, theoretically, overcome the problem of low absolute uptake of antibody by the tumor, because a single molecule of enzyme can activate more than one prodrug molecule. This is of particular interest because of the poor localization of immunoconjugates in humans (15). It has also been shown that the drug generated at the surface of tumor cells is more effective than equivalent concentrations of free drug (16).

Target antigen

The optimal target antigen (Ag) for ADEPT must be easily accessible to the antibody. It should therefore be either expressed on the tumor cell membrane, or secreted into the extracellular matrix of the tumor (17). It has been speculated that membrane-bound Ags offer longer residence times for the immunoconjugates, but their superiority in ADEPT has not been established, since secreted Ags accumulated in the tumor interstitial space result in high levels of conjugate at the tumor sites. In addition, secreted Ags are not subject to modulation and downregulation after prolonged exposure to antibodies, as is the case with some membrane-bound Ags (18). On the other hand, secreted Ags are often present in the plasma and, when their concentration is

high, they compete with the tumor cells for binding of the conjugate. In this way they may interfere with the clearance and localization of the antibody–enzyme conjugates (19, 20). The same problem may also arise when activation of the prodrug results in tumor lysis and release of Ags. It is unlikely, however, that there would be significant concentrations of immunoconjugate in the circulation at that time, unless repeated cycles of therapy were administered.

Selection of a target Ag whose expression is restricted to cancer cells is very important. If this is not possible then the expression of the target Ag in normal tissues should be as low as possible, with regard both to the volume of the tissue and the density of antigen expression. In particular cross-reactivity with Ags expressed on critical normal organs and rapidly renewing tissues should be avoided.

Heterogeneous Ag expression by the tumor is undesirable, but it is very common in epithelial tumors (21). Although most of the cells should express the Ag, this is not an absolute requirement, because of the bystander effect of the mAb–enzyme conjugate (17). Heterogeneity of Ag expression in cancers of the same histological type, occurring in different individuals, should also be examined. Radioimmunoscintigraphy studies have demonstrated that the level of Ag expression varies considerably amongst individuals with tumors of the same histological type (22, 23). It is expected, therefore, that the method will be more successful in tumors with the highest level of Ag expression. Furthermore, it would be preferable to choose an Ag expressed by a wide range of tumors. Finally, the tumor heterogeneity could be circumvented with the application of a 'cocktail' of conjugates constructed with the same enzyme and a variety of antibodies directed against different tumor-associated Ags (24).

Several groups of antigens have been considered as potential ADEPT targets. These include oncogene products with an extracellular domain, such as c-myc (25) or c-erbB-2 (26), overexpressed gene products, growth factor receptors, transmembrane adhesive molecules, such as carcinoembryonic antigen (CEA), or mucins, such as polymorphic epithelial mucin (PEM).

The antibody

In order that ADEPT might succeed, the optimal antibody must be identified and delivered. High affinity of the monoclonal antibody (dissociation constant,

$K_d > 10^{-10}$) is essential, since it facilitates binding of the antibodies in the periphery of tumor masses. The class of immunoglobulin is not important, but their size should be taken into consideration. IgM is usually avoided for ADEPT studies, because of its low penetration, while IgG1 and IgG2 are more commonly used for systemic administration. However, recent preliminary results of animal studies suggest that IgM radioconjugates, when administered via the intraperitoneal route, have an early and high (29 per cent injected dose per gram of tumor (% i.d./g)) tumor uptake, as well as prolonged retention, with a biological half-life of 4 days. Furthermore, as the peritoneal membrane acts as a barrier delaying the diffusion of the large IgM molecule into the circulation, the uptake by normal organs is reduced and the toxicity significantly attenuated (27). The above findings are of particular interest if ADEPT is to be administered locally, that is, intraperitoneally, in patients with ovarian cancer, or intravesically in patients with bladder cancer.

It is now recognized that whole antibodies penetrate tumors poorly (28–30). The best access is in the tumor periphery, while cells located in the center of the tumor may be inaccessible to the immunoconjugate, even though they express the antigen. Since smaller molecules penetrate tumors better, to increase further tumor penetration of the conjugate, antibody fragments rather than intact antibodies have been used: F(ab′)₂; Fab; single-chain antibodies; recombinant antigen-binding proteins. Unfortunately, the potential benefit of these molecules is hampered by the size of the enzyme used and the cost of their construction. One should also bear in mind that small-sized molecules have a rapid blood clearance (31). Although this is highly desirable

after localization of the conjugate at the tumor site, the rapid plasma clearance results in diminished absolute levels of tumor uptake and therefore greater total amounts of antibody–enzyme conjugate need to be administered.

When ADEPT studies initially began in 1985, at Charing Cross Hospital, the mAbs W14 and SB10 to human b chorionic gonadotrophin and the antibody A5B7 to CEA, were used. Since then a wide range of antibodies have been successfully used for *in vitro* and *in vivo* trials of ADEPT, as is demonstrated in Table 4.1.

The prodrug–drug system

The main purpose of ADEPT is to deliver an enzyme to the tumor site that is capable of catalyzing the conversion of an inactive chemical (prodrug) into an active drug. Therefore, the main requirement for the prodrug is to be a suitable substrate for the enzyme used, under physiological conditions. In addition, a large toxicity differential between the prodrug and the active drug is an advantage. Ideally, a very potent drug with a very short half-life offers the optimal combination since the amount of drug diffusing from the tumor and reaching the circulation would be negligible. On the other hand, the prodrug must be substantially less toxic than the activated agent and should not be converted by host enzymes.

As has already been mentioned, the mAb–enzyme conjugate (AEC) may be immunogenic. If this is the case, then, within 10 days of the initial administration of the AEC, circulating host anti-AEC antibodies may interfere with the treatment. Therefore, the action of

Table 4.1   The antibody-directed enzyme prodrug systems (ADEPT) that have been tried for the treatment of cancer *in vitro* and *in vivo*

Enzyme*	Antibody	Antigen†	Active drug
CPG2	W14	HCG	Benzoic acid
	A5B7	CEA	Benzoic acid
Carboxypeptidase A	KS1/4	LCAA	Methotrexate
AP	L6	TAA	Etoposide, mitomycin C, doxorubicin
PVA	L6	LCAA	Doxorubicin, melphalan
Penicillin-G amidase	L6	LCAA	Doxorubicin, melphalan
CDase	L6	LCAA	5-Fluorouracil
β-lactamase	L6	LCAA	Nitrogen mustard
GUS	BW431	CEA	Doxorubicin, epirubicin
Nitroreductase	BW431	CEA	CB1954
β-glucosidase	H17E2	hPLAP	Cyanide

* CPG2, Carboxyhpeptidase G2; AP, alkaline phosphatase; PVA, penicillin-V amidase; CDase, cytosine deaminase; GUS, β-glucoronidase.
† HCG, Human chorionic gonadotrophin; CEA, carcinoembryonic antigen; LCAA, lung cancer-associated antigen; TAA, tumour-associated antigen; hPLAP, human placental alkaline phosphatase.

the drug chosen should be dose-dependent and independent of the cell cycle stage. It should also be able to achieve total cell killing in a very limited number of treatments. Finally, drug resistance should also be taken into consideration when the prodrug system is chosen (32).

The enzyme

The enzyme's function in the ADEPT strategy is to convert, *in vivo*, an inactive prodrug into the active drug. Therefore, the first criterion for the enzyme is to be able to exert its activity under physiological conditions of pH and temperature and preferably to have an optimum pH close to the pH of the tumor extracellular fluid. An enzyme with pH optimum beyond the physiological range, could still be used, provided that it retains sufficient activity at pH 7.0–7.4 (33). Enzymes with high K_{cat}, high V_{max}, and low K_m require smaller amounts of enzyme for comparable rates of substrate conversion and are therefore preferable. Enzymes that require a cofactor not present in the tumor extracellular fluid have a disadvantage because they require the administration of an additional component.

It is crucial for the ADEPT strategy that prodrug activation is restricted solely to the tumor site. Therefore, enzymes that are widely present in human tissues (for example, alkaline phosphatase) lack the specificity needed. On the other hand, enzymes of non-human origin (for example, from bacteria or plants, such as carboxypeptidase G2 and β-glucosidase) have the advantage of specificity, but have been shown to be immunogenic. A challenging option is the use of human placental enzymes (provided that they are not expressed in normal adult tissues) or of enzymes restricted to intracellular sites only, such as β-glucuronidase (provided that the prodrugs used cannot cross the cell membrane). The techniques, currently under consideration, that aim to minimize the immunogenicity of enzymes of non-human origin, will be discussed later. Finally, one should pay special attention when enzymes found in the intestinal flora, are used, since they may activate any prodrug excreted via the gut. If such enzymes are used, sterilization of the gut by antibiotics during antineoplastic therapy may be useful.

Several enzyme systems have been developed and tried for ADEPT (Table 4.1), the most important of which are briefly described.

Carboxypeptidase G2 (CPG2)

The first ADEPT system, proposed by Bagshawe (11) used carboxypeptidase G2 (CPG2), a zinc metalloenzyme originally isolated from *Pseudomonas* species. The enzyme is not found in mammalian cells (34) and has been cloned into *Escherichia coli* (35). This enzyme cleaves a glutamate moiety from a benzoic acid mustard (36).

Several prodrugs have been used in combination with mAb–CPG2 conjugates. Two tumor-associated mAbs have been conjugated to CPG2: W14, which recognizes b-human-chorionic gonadotrophin (b-HCG), and A5B7, which recognizes CEA (37). CGP2 was covalently attached to F(ab′)₂ fragments of W14 using maleimidobenzoyl-*n*-hydroxysuccinimide ester (MBS) (38) and administered to nude mice bearing CC3 human choriocarcinoma tumor xenografts that strongly express β-HCG. Biodistribution studies showed that F(ab′)₂ W14–CPG2 can localize at tumor sites as effectively as native W14 (39). Clearance of the conjugate was faster than that of native W14, resulting in lower uptake by normal organs. *In vivo* stability of conjugates was satisfactory (39). The prodrug was administered by three consecutive injections starting 56 hours after the administration of the conjugate. The conjugate was shown to be active *in vivo* and there was marked suppression of tumor growth in mice receiving both conjugate and prodrug (12, 40). Unfortunately, retention of the conjugate at nontumor sites resulted in the generation of active drug in the plasma and normal organs (40) and, as the half-life of the active drug is long, systemic toxicity was common (12).

Preliminary clinical studies using the CPG2–mustard prodrug had encouraging results even in patients with advanced cancer. CPG2 was conjugated to the F(ab′)₂ fragments of the mAb A5B7 directed against CEA. Patients had either elevated plasma CEA levels or immunohistological confirmation of CEA in their tumor tissue. AEC of approximately 20 000 U/m² was administered intravenously, followed 72 hours later by the prodrug administration as a series of bolus injections over 1–5 days, while a group of patients received the prodrug only. The prodrug alone was found to be nontoxic, while objective response was observed in most of the patients who were given the full course of treatment (41).

Carboxypeptidases A and B

Bovine pancreatic carboxypeptidase A and porcine pancreatic carboxypeptidase B can remove alanine residues from a-peptidyl methotrexate derivatives (42), producing the active methotrexate molecule. This molecule, which is almost 200-fold more active than its precursor, is an anticancer drug with a broad spectrum of activity. Conjugates of these enzymes with mAbs have shown some cytotoxicity in an ADEPT system in the L1210 leukemia cells and the UCLA-P3 lung adenocarcinoma cell line (16).

Alkaline phosphatase (AP)

This system utilizes phosphorylated derivatives of many established chemotherapeutic agents, such as mitomycin, etoposide, and doxorubicin, as prodrugs (13, 43, 44). These prodrugs are activated in the presence of alkaline phosphatase, an enzyme that hydrolytically removes phosphates and is found in mammalian cells. Conjugates of this enzyme with tumor-specific mAbs have been used both in *in vitro* and *in vivo* cytotoxicity studies. There was a 100-fold increase in the cytotoxic activity of the prodrugs, significant specific antitumor activity, and prolonged antitumor responses (45). The mitomycin combination was the most effective, resulting in 99 per cent elimination of tumor cells, while combinations of conjugate with two prodrugs resulted in higher toxicity (14). However, this system is not ideal for therapy because of the high levels of endogenous AP present in many normal tissues and the slow clearance from the circulation. On the other hand, human alkaline phosphatase conjugated with a humanized mAb may result in a conjugate with reduced immunogenicity (43).

Penicillin-V amidase (PVA)

This enzyme can be used to hydrolyse the phenoxyacetamide group of doxorubicin- and melphalan-amide derivatives to release doxorubicin and melphalan, respectively (46). *In vitro* experiments have shown that the combination of specific AEC and doxorubicin prodrug resulted in considerable cytotoxicity to H2981 cells (46). This did not occur with melphalan, probably because the conjugate hydrolyzed the melphalan prodrug at a 25-fold slower rate than the unmodified enzyme. The above observation highlights the importance of using an enzyme with a high turnover with each substrate in order to generate high concentrations of active drug.

Penicillin-G amidase

This *E. coli* enzyme has been shown to activate the phenylacetamido deratives of doxorubicin and melpha-

lan (46, 47). For the melphalan compound a 20-fold differential in IC_{50} (injected drug concentration that results in 50 per cent cell survival) between drug and prodrug was demonstrated *in vitro* (48).

Cytosine deaminase (CDase)

This enzyme hydrolyzes the conversion of cytosine into uracil and, therefore, it can catalyze the hydrolysis of 5-fluorocytosine (5FC), which is an antifungal agent, into 5-fluorouracil (5FU), a well established chemotherapeutic agent used in a wide range of human malignancies. The advantages of this system are that, unlike AP, CDase is not present in any mammalian tissue and that both the prodrug and the active drug have well known pharmacological properties.

CDase has already been used in experimental models in order to convert 5FC into 5FU, with encouraging results (49). *In vitro* studies with H2981 lung adenocarcinoma cells have demonstrated that the 5FC prodrug is nontoxic at up to 200 mM, whereas 5FU has an IC_{50} of 20 mM. *In vivo* experiments have shown that the combination of specific immunoconjugate and 5FC could result in a cytotoxic effect similar to that of 5FU alone (50, 51). Further experiments with the same system, but with the additional use of a second antibody-clearing agent, further enhanced the tumor-to-nontumor ratios of CDase, leading to a 17-fold increase in the area under the curve for targeted therapy, compared with that for systemic drug administration (46, 49).

β-Lactamases

These enzymes from *E. coli* and *Enterobacter cloacae* (52) can hydrolyse a series of cephalosporin carbamates releasing the cephalosporin group from a wide range of prodrugs, including nitrogen mustard and vinca alkaloid deratives (53). In addition, as this enzyme is not present in eukaryotic cells, the prodrug is subject to only minimal interference from endogenous enzyme systems. *In vitro* use of this system with the L6 mAb has shown good targeted prodrug activation (54, 55). The released active drug was 50-fold more toxic than the prodrug. The antigen CEA has also been used as target of the above system (56).

β-glucuronidase (GUS)

As this enzyme is found in humans, it provides the advantage of not being immunogenic. Furthermore, in humans it is mainly found intracellularly in lysosomes and microsomes and, therefore, should not cause systemic toxicity after *in vivo* prodrug administration. In addition, as the pH microenvironement around the tumor is acid to neutral, it is much more suitable for β-glucuronidase (*E. coli* GUS pH optimum at 6.8; human GUS pH optimum at 5.4), than for enzymes such as alkaline phosphatase. Epirubicin–glucuronide (epi-glu), a natural compound occurring as a result of the metabolism of epirubicin in humans (57), has been isolated from the urine of patients treated with epirubicin and used as the prodrug. It is 100- to 1000-fold less toxic than its active drug and, in the presence of an mAb–*E. coli*-derived β-glucuronidase conjugate, epirubicin was released and entered cells growing in culture. This increased the toxicity of the prodrug to levels similar to those of the active drug (58). The *E. coli* enzyme has also been used in conjunction with aniline mustard prodrugs, which are over 500-fold less toxic than the corresponding drug (59, 60).

A human anti-CEA Fab'–human GUS fusion protein has been constructed and expressed in baby hamster kidney transfectomas (61). When this protein was used with doxorubicin–glucuronide as a prodrug in mice bearing tumor xenografts, a significant tumor growth delay was observed (62, 63).

Nitroreductase

The reductase group of enzymes has the disadvantage that these enzymes require a cofactor, usually NADH (nicotinamide adenine dinucleotide, reduced) or NADPH (nicotinamide adenine dinucleotide phosphate, reduced), for activity. Nevertheless, the discovery that the sensitivity of Walker carcinoma to the alkylating agent CB1954 (a dinitrobenzamide) was due to the presence of the reductase DT diaphorase that activates CB1954, raised new hopes. Some human colon tumor cell lines have also been found to have a degree of diaphorase and nitroreductase activity, enough to make them sensitive to drugs. The *E. coli* nitroreductase can catalyze the same reaction with great efficiency and *in vitro* data suggest that the combination of prodrug plus enzyme plus NADH was 10 000-fold more toxic, compared with the use of prodrug plus enzyme or prodrug plus NADH (64–66).

β-glucosidase

The subgroup of glucosidases comprises enzymes that catalyze the hydrolysis of glucosides. Several enzymes are listed under the name β-glucosidase but, when they are isolated from different sources, they may have variable properties and specific activities. In mammals, several β-glucosidases have been extracted and identified, including enzymes from bovine spleen and liver (67), from human spleen, and from human skin fibroblasts (68, 69), but it is generally accepted that these enzymes do not catalyze the hydrolysis of naturally occurring glucosides. The hydrolysis of amygdalin, in particular, by the enzyme β-glucosidase results in the release of the powerful metabolic poison cyanide. The amygdalin–β-glucosidase system exploits the activation of the naturally occurring cyanogenic glucoside amygdalin, instead of using a modified chemotherapeutic agent, and it has several theoretical advantages compared with the other ADEPT systems: With regard to the enzyme, β-glucosidase, it has been shown that it can be activated under physiological conditions. The active drug cyanide is of low molecular weight and, therefore, it can easily diffuse through several cell layers, kill cells away from where the conjugate is localized, and provide a bystander effect. Furthermore, as cyanide has a very short half-life, the possibility of escaping back to the circulation is limited. There is, nevertheless, a naturally occurring detoxifying system in mammals, through the sulfuration route, with the use of rhodanase, a widely distributed human enzyme. Most of the detoxification takes place in the liver providing an additional advantage of this concept. Since no resistance to cyanide has been reported, it has the potential of circumventing the problem of tumor resistance. In addition, cyanide toxicity is autonomous of cell cycle stage and, therefore, it should be able to achieve total tumor cell killing in a few consecutive treatments, before human anti-mouse antibody (HAMA) response develops. Finally, as amygdalin has been used, unsuccessfully, in the past for the treatment of human malignancies (70), its pharmacokinetics is well known.

The above system is known as antibody-guided enzyme nitrile therapy (AGENT). It has already been tried *in vitro* with promising results. In fact, the prodrug, amygdalin, proved cytotoxic to HT1376 bladder cancer cells only at high concentrations, while the combination of amygdalin with the mAb–enzyme conjugate enhanced the cytotoxic effect of amygdalin by 36-fold and the toxic effect was dose-dependent. In addition to the cytotoxic effect, specificity was demonstrated as well (71). Based on the above observations, preliminary clinical trials to study the feasibility of the above system are now in progress (72).

Future prospects

Preliminary clinical trials of ADEPT have been very encouraging, but they have also illustrated the problems of its clinical application, which should form the focus of future research.

The circulating levels of AEC are a crucial aspect of ADEPT. Although a high AEC plasma concentration results in higher tumor uptake, this concentration should be very low at the time that the prodrug is administered, in order to avoid activation of the prodrug in plasma and the subsequent occurrence of dose-limiting toxicities (20, 73). Clinical studies have demonstrated that adequate clearance of AEC from the plasma requires 7 days before the prodrug may be administered safely. Unfortunately, by that time, the enzyme activity at the tumor site is also very low and inadequate to activate sufficient prodrug to cause satisfactory cell killing. To accelerate the removal of enzyme activity from the plasma, without affecting the enzyme activity at tumor sites, a third step (AEC + clearing agent + prodrug) has been used with the administration of a galactosylated anticonjugate antibody (SB43-gal). The galactosylated antibody can react with the conjugate in the circulation, decreasing its blood levels, but cannot be extravasated to reach the conjugate at the tumor sites. To further augment its effect, this antibody could also enzymatically inactivate the conjugate, being directed against the active site of the enzyme. The antibody–conjugate immune complexes are rapidly cleared by the hepatic galactose receptors. Unfortunately, the whole procedure makes ADEPT much more complicated, changing it to a three-step system, while the penetration of the tumor by the additional antibody cannot be ruled out (41, 73, 74). An alternative option would be to add galactose residues to the enzyme conjugate, which would accelerate their clearance via the galactose receptors of hepatocytes (73, 75).

An approach complementary to the clearing systems is the administration of agents that increase the tumor localization of the conjugate, such as tumor necrosis factor α (TNFα), or increase the antigenic expression by the malignant cells, such as interferon, butyrate, glucocorticoids, and transforming growth factor (39).

To further increase the specificity of ADEPT, the use of an enzyme cascade system has been proposed (33). This system applies two target antigens with different distribution in the normal tissues and two conjugates (with different antibodies and enzymes). The prodrug is activated in two stages at the tumor sites, where both conjugates are bound. Normal tissues, on the other hand, would localize only one of the conjugates (depending on the antigen expression) and therefore the drug would not be activated. Although this system has the advantage of specificity, it is very complicated and has not been tested *in vivo* yet.

The main problem of ADEPT is the immunogenicity of the antibody–enzyme conjugate, which limits the application of ADEPT to a few chemotherapy cycles only. The application of genetic engineering techniques could in future provide some solutions, such as humanized proteins, fusion proteins with dual biological activity (of the antibody and the enzyme), and the development of antibodies with catalytic function, known as 'abzymes' (76). These bifunctional proteins, with both tumor targeting and catalytic function, also have the potential of being 'humanized'. Immunogenicity of the foreign enzymes can also be reduced by conjugation to polyethylene glycol (77), or by concomitant administration of immunosuppression (for example, cyclosporin) (33, 41). Rapamycin, FK506, and anti-CD4 antibodies, which are nonspecific immunosuppressives, appear to delay further the host–antibody response. Finally, the consecutive use of a combination of different enzyme conjugates and prodrugs could provide a possible solution to the host immune response, as well as to the problem of the tumor drug resistance.

In conclusion, ADEPT holds the potential of being an effective, relatively nontoxic treatment of cancer, and *in vitro*, animal, and preclinical studies are very promising. The strategy has its limitations and problems, which could be circumvented through various manipulations aiming to increase its specificity and reduce its immunogeneity and toxicity, at the cost of some complexity. It is expected that further research, which is in progress, will make ADEPT an important element of the anticancer armament.

References

1. Köhler G, Milstein C. Continuous cultures of fused cells secreting antibody of predefined specificity. Nature 1975, **256**, 495–7.
2. Köhler G, Milstein C. Derivation of specific antibody-producing tissue culture and tumor lines by cell fusion. Eur J Immunol 1976, **6**, 511–19.
3. Whisson ME, Connors TA. Cure of mice bearing advanced plasma cell tumours with aniline mustard. Nature 1965, **206**, 689–91.
4. Connors TA, Farmer PB, Foster AB, Gilsenan AM, Jarman M, Tisdale MJ. Metabolism of aniline mustard

(N,N-di-(2-chloroethyl)aniline). Biochem Pharmacol 1973, **22**, 1971–80.

5. Connors TA, Foster AB, Gilsenan AM, Jarman M, Tisdale MJ. Chemical trapping of a reactive metabolite. The metabolism of the AZO-mustard 2'-carboxy-4-di-(2-chloroethyl)amino-2-methylazo-benzene. Biochem Pharmacol 1972, **21**, 1309–16.

6. Wilman DE. Prodrugs in cancer chemotherapy. Biochem Soc Trans 1986, **14**, 375–82.

7. Newlands ES, Blackledge G, Slack JA, Goddard C, Brindley CJ, Holden L, Stevens MF. Phase I clinical trial of mitozolomide. Cancer Treat Rep 1985, **69**, 801–5.

8. Connors TA, Cumber AJ, Ross WC, Clarke SA, Mitchley BC. Regression of human lung tumor xenografts induced by water-soluble analogs of hexamethylmelamine. Cancer Treat Rep 1977, **61**, 927–8.

9. Philpott GW, Bower RJ, Parker CW. Selective iodination and cytotoxicity of tumor cells with an antibody–enzyme conjugate. Surgery 1973, **74**, 51–8.

10. Philpott GW, Shearer WT, Bower RJ, Parker CW. Selective cytotoxicity of hapten-substituted cells with an antibody–enzyme conjugate. J Immunol 1973, **111**, 921–9.

11. Bagshawe KD. Antibody directed enzymes revive anti-cancer prodrugs concept. Br J Cancer 1987, **56**, 531–2.

12. Bagshawe KD, Springer CJ, Searle F, Antoniw P, Sharma SK, Melton RG, Sherwood RF. A cytotoxic agent can be generated selectively at cancer sites. Br J Cancer 1988, **58**, 700–3.

13. Senter PD Saulnier MG Schreiber GJ Hirschberg DL Brown JP Hellstrom I Hellstrom KE. Anti-tumor effects of antibody–alkaline phosphatase conjugates in combination with etoposide phosphate. Proc Natl Acad Sci, USA 1988, **85**, 4842–6.

14. Senter PD, Schreiber GJ, Hirschberg DL, Ashe SA, Hellstrom KE, Hellstrom I. Enhancement of the *in vitro* and *in vivo* antitumor activities of phosphorylated mitomycin C and etoposide derivatives by monoclonal antibody–alkaline phosphatase conjugates. Cancer Res 1989, **49**, 5789–92.

15. Begent RH. Recent advances in tumour imaging. Use of radiolabelled antitumour antibodies. Biochim Biophys Acta 1985, **780**, 151–66.

16. Haenseler E, Esswein A, Vitols KS, Montejano Y, Mueller BM, Reisfeld RA, Huennekens FM. Activation of methotrexate-alpha-alanine by carboxypeptidase A–monoclonal antibody conjugate. Biochemistry 1992, **31**, 891–7.

17. Mason DW, Williams AF. The kinetics of antibody binding to membrane antigens in solution and at the cell surface. Biochem J 1980, **187**, 1–20.

18. Gordon J, Anderson VA, Robinson DS, Stevenson GT. The influence of antigen density and a comparison of IgG and IgM antibodies in the anti-complementary modulation of lymphocytic surface immunoglobulin. Scand J Immunol 1982, **15**, 169–77.

19. Begent RH, Searle F, Stanway G, Jewkes RF, Jones BE, Vernon P, Bagshawe KD. Radioimmunolocalization of tumours by external scintigraphy after administration of 131I antibody to human chorionic gonadotrophin. preliminary communication. J R Soc Med 1980, **73**, 624–30.

20. Bagshawe KD. Towards generating cytotoxic agents at cancer sites. Br J Cancer 1989, **60**, 275–81.

21. Primus FJ, Kuhns WJ, Goldenberg DM. Immunological heterogeneity of carcinoembryonic antigen: immunohistochemical detection of carcinoembryonic antigen determinants in colonic tumors with monoclonal antibodies. Cancer Res 1983, **43**, 693–701.

22. Begent RH, Ledermann JA, Green AJ, Bagshawe KD, Riggs SJ, Searle F, Keep PA, Adam T, Dale RG, Glaser MG. Antibody distribution and dosimetry in patients receiving radiolabelled antibody therapy for colorectal cancer. Br J Cancer 1989, **60**, 406–12.

23. Boxer GM, Begent RH, Kelly AM, Southall PJ, Blair SB, Theodorou NA, Dawson PM, Ledermann JA. Factors influencing variability of localisation of antibodies to carcinoembryonic antigen (CEA) in patients with colorectal carcinoma—implications for radioimmunotherapy. Br J Cancer 1992, **65**, 825–31.

24. Tagliabue E, Porro G, Barbanti P, Della Torre G, Menard S, Rilke F. Improvement of tumor cell detection using a pool of monoclonal antibodies. Hybridoma 1986, **5**, 107–15.

25. Chan SY, Evan GI, Ritson A, Watson J, Wraight P, Sikora K. Localisation of lung cancer by a radiolabelled monoclonal antibody against the c-myc oncogene product. Br J Cancer 1986, **54**, 761–9.

26. Park JW, Hong K, Carter P, Asgari H, Guo LY, Keller GA, Wirth C, Shalaby R, Kotts C, Wood WI. Development of anti-p185HER2 immunoliposomes for cancer therapy. Proc Natl Acad Sci, USA 1995, **92**, 1327–31.

27. Quadri SM, Malik AB, Tang XZ, Patenia R, Freedman RS, Vriesendorp HM. Preclinical analysis of intraperitoneal administration of ^{111}In-labeled human tumor reactive monoclonal IgM AC6C3-2B12. Cancer Res 1995, **55**, 5736–42.

28. Cobb LM, Humphreys JA, Harrison A. The diffusion of a tumour-specific monoclonal antibody in lymphoma infiltrated spleen. Br J Cancer 1987, **55**, 53–5.

29. Moshakis V, McIlhinney RA, Neville AM. Cellular distribution of monoclonal antibody in human tumours after i.v. administration. Br J Cancer 1981, **44**, 663–9.

30. Moshakis V, McIlhinney RA, Raghavan D, Neville AM. Localization of human tumour xenografts after i.v. administration of radiolabeled monoclonal antibodies. Br J Cancer 1981, **44**, 91–9.

31. Boucher Y, Baxter LT, Jain RK. Interstitial pressure gradients in tissue-isolated and subcutaneous tumors. implications for therapy. Cancer Res 1990, **50**, 4478–84.

32. Baldini N. Multidrug resistance—a multiplex phenomenon. Nature Med 1997, **3**, 378–80.

33. Bagshawe KD, Sharma SK, Springer CJ, Rogers GT. Antibody directed enzyme prodrug therapy (ADEPT). A review of some theoretical, experimental and clinical aspects. Ann Oncol 1994, **5**, 879–91.

34. Sherwood RF, Melton RG, Alwan SM, Hughes P. Purification and propeties of carboxypeptidase G2 from *Pseudomonas* sp strain RS-16. Use of a novel triazine dye affinity method. Eur J Biochem 1985, **148**, 447–53.

35. Minton NP, Atkinson T, Bruton CJ, Sherwood RF. The complete nucleotide sequence of the *Pseudomonas* gene coding for carboxypeptidase G2. Gene 1984, **31**, 31–8.

36. Springer CJ, Bagshawe KD, Sharma SK, Searle F, Boden JA, Antoniw P, Burke PJ, Rogers GT, Sherwood RF, Melton RG. Ablation of human choriocarcinoma xenografts in nude mice by antibody-directed enzyme prodrug therapy (ADEPT) with three novel compounds. Eur J Cancer 1991, **27**, 1361–6.

37. Searle F, Partridge CS, Kardana A, Green AJ, Buckley RG, Begent RH, Rawlins-GA. Preparation and properties of mouse monoclonal antibody (W14A) to human chorionic gonadotropin. Int J Cancer 1984, **33**, 429–34.

38. Searle F, Bier C, Buckley RG, Newman S, Pedley RB, Bagshawe KD, Melton RG, Alwan SM, Sherwood RF. The potential of carboxypeptidase G2-antibody conjugates as anti-tumour agents. I. Preparation of antihuman chorionic gonadotrophin–carboxypeptidase G2 and cytotoxicity of the conjugate against JAR choriocarcinoma cells *in vitro*. Br J Cancer 1986, **53**, 377–84.

39. Melton RG, Searle F, Sherwood RF, Bagshawe KD, Boden JA. The potential of carboxypeptidase G2. antibody conjugates as antitumour agents. *In vivo* localisation and clearance properties in a choriocarcinoma model. Br J Cancer 1990, **61**, 420–4.

40. Antoniw P, Springer CJ, Bagshawe KD, Searle F, Melton RG, Rogers GT, Burke PJ, SherwoodRF. Disposition of the prodrug 4-(bis (2-chloroethyl) amino) benzoyl-L-glutamic acid and its active parent drug in mice. Br J Cancer 1990, **62**, 909–14.

41. Bagshawe KD, Sharma SK, Springer CJ, Antoniw P. Antibody directed enzyme prodrug therapy: a pilot-scale clinical trial. Tumour Targeting 1995, **1**, 17–19.

42. Kuefner U, Lohrmann U, Montejano YD, Vitols KS, Huennekens FM. Carboxypeptidase-mediated release of methotrexate from methotrexate alpha-peptides. Biochemistry 1989, **28**, 2288–97.

43. Senter PD, Su PC, Katsuragi T, Sakai T, Cosand WL, Hellstrom I, Hellstrom KE. Generation of 5-fluorouracil from 5-fluorocytosine by monoclonal antibody–cytosine deaminase conjugates. Bioconjug Chem 1991, **2**, 447–51.

44. Wallace PM, SenterPD. *In vitro* and *in vivo* activities of monoclonal antibody–alkaline phosphatase conjugates in combination with phenol mustard phosphate. Bioconjug Chem 1991, **2**, 349–52.

45. Wallace PM, Senter PD. Selective activation of anticancer prodrugs by monoclonal antibody–enzyme conjugates. Methods Find Exp Clin Pharmacol 1994, **16**, 505–12.

46. Kerr DE, Senter PD, Burnett WV, Hirschberg DL, Hellstrom I, Hellstrom KE. Antibody–penicillin-V-amidase conjugates kill antigen-positive tumor cells when combined with doxorubicin phenoxyacetamide. Cancer Immunol Immunother 1990, **31**, 202–6.

47. Bignami GS, Senter PD, Grothaus PG, Fischer KJ, Humphreys T, Wallace PM. N-(4′-hydroxyphenylacetyl)palytoxin: a palytoxin prodrug that can be activated by a monoclonal antibody–penicillin G amidase conjugate. Cancer Res 1992, **52**, 5759–64.

48. Vrudhula VM, Senter PD, Fischer KJ, Wallace PM. Prodrugs of doxorubicin and melphalan and their activation by a monoclonal antibody–penicillin-G amidase conjugate. J Med Chem 1993, **36**, 919–23.

49. Wallace PM, MacMaster JF, Smith VF, Kerr DE, Senter PD, Cosand WL. Intratumoral generation of 5-fluorouracil mediated by an antibody–cytosine deaminase conjugate in combination with 5-fluorocytosine. Cancer Res 1994, **54**, 2719–23.

50. Senter PD. Activation of prodrugs by antibody–enzyme conjugates: a new approach to cancer therapy. FASEB J 1990, **4**, 188–93.

51. Senter PD, Wallace PM, Svensson HP, Kerr DE, Hellstrom I, Hellstrom KE. Activation of prodrugs by antibody–enzyme conjugates. Adv Exp Med Biol 1991, **303**, 97–105.

52. Galleni M, Lindberg F, Normark S, Cole S, Honore N, Joris B, Frere JM. Sequence and comparative analysis of three *Enterobacter cloacae* ampC beta-lactamase genes and their products. Biochem J 1988, **250**, 753–60.

53. Vrudhula VM, Svensson HP, Kennedy KA, Senter PD, Wallace PM. Antitumor activities of a cephalosporin prodrug in combination with monoclonal antibody–beta-lactamase conjugates. Bioconjug Chem 1993, **4**, 334–40.

54. Svensson HP, Vrudhula VM, Emswiler JE, MacMaster JF, Cosand WL, Senter PD, Wallace PM. *In vitro* and *in vivo* activities of a doxorubicin prodrug in combination with monoclonal antibody–beta-lactamase conjugates. Cancer Res 1995, **55**, 2357–65.

55. Svensson HP, Wallace PM, Senter PD. Synthesis and characterization of monoclonal antibody–beta-lactamase conjugates. Bioconjug Chem 1994, **5**, 262–7.

56. Meyer DL, Jungheim LN, Mikolajczyk SD, Shepherd TA, Starling JJ, Ahlem CN. Preparation and characterization of a beta-lactamase–Fab′ conjugate for the site-specific activation of oncolytic agents. Bioconjug Chem 1992, **3**, 42–8.

57. Haisma HJ, Boven E, van Muijen M, de Jong J, van der Vijgh WJ, Pinedo HM. A monoclonal antibody–beta-glucuronidase conjugate as activator of the prodrug epirubicin–glucuronide for specific treatment of cancer. Br J Cancer 1992, **66**, 474–8.

58. Haisma HJ, van Muijen M, Pinedo HM, Boven E. Comparison of two anthracycline-based prodrugs for activation by a monoclonal antibody–beta-glucuronidase conjugate in the specific treatment of cancer. Cell Biophys 1994, **24–25**, 185–92.

59. Roffler SR, Wang SM, Chern JW, Yeh MY, Tung E. Anti-neoplastic glucuronide prodrug treatment of human tumor cells targeted with a monoclonal antibody–enzyme conjugate. Biochem Pharmacol 1991, **42**, 2062–5.

60. Wang SM, Chern JW, Yeh MY, Ng JC, Tung E, Roffler SR. Specific activation of glucuronide prodrugs by antibody-targeted enzyme conjugates for cancer therapy. Cancer Res 1992, **52**, 4484–91.

61. Bosslet K, Czech J, Lorenz P, Sedlacek HH, Schuermann M, Seemann G. Molecular and functional characterisation of a fusion protein suited for tumour specific prodrug activation. Br J Cancer 1992, **65**, 234–8.

62. Bosslet K, Czech J, Hoffmann D. Tumor-selective prodrug activation by fusion protein-mediated catalysis. Cancer Res 1994, **54**, 2151–9.

63. Bosslet K, Czech J, Seemann G, Monneret C, Hoffmann D. Fusion protein mediated prodrug activation (FMPA) *in vivo*. Cell Biophys 1994, **24–25**, 51–63.

64. Knox RJ, Boland MP, Friedlos F, Coles B, Southan C, Roberts JJ. The nitroreductase enzyme in Walker cells that activates 5-(aziridin-1-yl)-2,4-dinitrobenzamide (CB 1954) to 5-(aziridin-1-yl)-4-hydroxylamino-2-nitrobenza-

mide is a form of NAD(P)H dehydrogenase (quinone) (EC 1.6.99.2). Biochem Pharmacol 1988, **37**, 4671–7.

65. Knox RJ, Friedlos F, Boland MP. The bioactivation of CB 1954 and its use as a prodrug in antibody-directed enzyme prodrug therapy (ADEPT). Cancer Metastasis Rev 1993, **12**, 195–212.

66. Anlezark GM, Melton RG, Sherwood RF, Wilson WR, Denny WA, Palmer BD, Knox RJ, Friedlos F, Williams A. Bioactivation of dinitrobenzamide mustards by an *E. coli* B nitroreductase. Biochem Pharmacol 1995, **50**, 609–18.

67. Weinreb NJ, Brady RO, Tappel AL. The lysosomal localization of sphingolipid hydrolases. Biochim Biophys Acta 1968, **159**, 141–6.

68. Mueller OT, Rosenberg A. Beta-glucoside hydrolase activity of normal and glucosylceramidotic cultured human skin fibroblasts. J Biol Chem 1977, **252**, 825–9.

69. Mueller OT, Rosenberg A. Activation of membrane-bound glucosylceramid:. beta-glucosidase in fibroblasts cultured from normal and glucosylceramidotic human skin. J Biol Chem 1979, **254**, 3521–5.

70. Moertel CG, Fleming TR, Rubin J, Kvols LK, Sarna G, Koch R, Currie VE, Young CW, Jones SE, Davignon JP. A clinical trial of amygdalin (Laetrile) in the treatment of human cancer. New Engl J Med 1982, **306**, 201–6.

71. Syrigos KN, Rowlinson-Busza G, Epenetos AA. *In vitro* cytotoxicity following specific activation of amygdalin by β-glucosidase conjugated to a bladder cancer-associated monoclonal antibody. Int J Cancer, 1998, **78**, 712–19.

72. Syrigos KN, Khawaja M, Krausz T, Williams G, Epenetos AA. Intravesical administration of radiolabelled tumour associated monoclonal antibody in bladder cancer. Acta Oncol, 1999, **38**, 379–82.

73. Sharma SK, Bagshawe KD, Burke PJ, Boden JA, Rogers GT, Springer CJ, Melton RG, Sherwood RF. Galactosylated antibodies and antibody-enzyme conjugates in antibody-directed enzyme prodrug therapy. Cancer 1994, **73**, 1114–20.

74. Sharma SK, Bagshawe KD, Springer CJ, Burke PJ, Rogers GT, Boden JA. Antibody directed enzyme prodrug therapy (ADEPT): a three phase system. Dis Marker 1991, **9**, 225–31.

75. Mattes MJ. Biodistribution of antibodies after intraperitoneal and intravenous injection and effect of carbohydrate modification. J Natl Cancer Inst 1987, **79**, 855–63.

76. Shokat KM, Leumann CJ, Sugasawara R, Schultz PG. A new strategy for the generation of catalytic antibodies. Nature 1989, **338**, 269–71.

77. Wilkinson I, Jackson CJ, Lang GM, Holford-Strevens V, Sehon AH. Tolerance induction in mice by conjugates of monoclonal immunoglobulins and monomethoxypolyethylene glycol. Transfer of tolerance by T cells and by T cell extracts. J Immunol 1987, **139**, 326–31.

Monoclonal antibody targeted radionuclide therapy

Surinder K. Batra, Apollina Goel, Gabriela Pavlinkova, and David Colcher

Introduction

The pivotal work by Köhler and Milstein (1) on the development of hybridoma technology has made the production of an unlimited supply of monoclonial antibody (mAb) molecules possible. A wide range of mAbs has been generated for applications in research and health care. mAbs have made an impact in clinical medicine for the treatment of cancer, infectious diseases, and the immunomodulation of transplant rejection. These 'natural drugs' can be used in their native form to cause the death of bacteria, cells, or viruses by antibody-dependent cellular toxicity, or by complement-mediated lysis, or by the inhibition of viral cellular functions. Alternatively, mAbs can be used to deliver cytotoxic agents such as radionuclides, enzymes, genes, drugs or toxins to the target cell. The most striking characteristic of antibody molecules is their remarkable specificity and ability to discriminate between similar molecular structures. Gene technology has now revolutionized the use of mAbs for clinical medicine. Antibody genes can be cloned and expressed to yield antibody-based reagents with reduced immunogenicity, improved affinity and avidity, altered size, and distinct effector functions (2, 3).

For cancer treatment, several modalities, including surgery, radiation, and chemotherapy, have been used either alone or in combination with only modest success in most malignancies (4). External beam radiotherapy can be employed for a locally advanced disease at conformed sites; however, normal tissue toxicity can limit the optimal dose required for curative treatment. Because of their inherent specificity, mAbs directed against tumor-associated antigens (TAAs) are ideal agents for delivering radionuclides to a specific tissue or malignant cell population. Such radioimmunoconjugates can be used for the radioimmunodetection (RAID) of cancer using external imaging techniques and can also be useful for radioimmunotherapy

(RIT) (5–7). RIT combines the advantages of the specific tumor targeting of anti cancer mAbs with the cytotoxic properties of therapeutic radionuclides. Besides targeting both known and occult malignant lesions, RIT permits the maximum eradication of cancer cells through a bystander radiation effect and may be effective in drug-resistant cases (multiple drug resistance). Therefore, RIT is an attractive concept as a form of specifically targeted therapy.

Complete clinical responses have been observed with the use of RIT in hematological diseases such as non-Hodgkin's lymphoma. Indeed, RIT is crossing the threshold to become a standard mode of treatment (7). However, partial responses have been reported in solid tumors, due primarily to poor accessibility and the lower radiosensitivity of these tumor types (6, 8, 9). RIT of solid tumors, therefore, requires a high radiation doses that can lead to a significant nonspecific uptake by normal tissue with secondary toxicity, especially to the hemopoietic system. mAbs have not proven to be the 'magic bullet' optimistically envisioned by early workers in the field, mainly because of their long persistence in circulation, leading to hematological toxicities, while only limited quantities are delivered to tumors (10). Furthermore, intact mAbs show poor diffusion from the vasculature into and through the tumor (11). Some limitations of traditional murine mAbs as therapeutic agents are being addressed by the application of techniques of molecular cloning and genetic engineering.

This chapter is intended as a review of the use of mAbs linked to radioinuclides for the therapy of malignancies, particularly solid tumors. The initial portion of the chapter will discuss tumor-associated mAbs, choice of radioisotopes, the principle of radioimmunotherapy, and clinical trials using radio labeled mAbs in solid tumors. Lastly, the chapter will describe the pitfalls encountered with radio labeled-antibody-based therapy and strategies for overcoming biological problems using genetically engineered antibodies.

Tumor-associated antigens (TAAs) and their monoclonal antibodies

Oncogene-associated and/or cell surface products have been proposed as tumor-associated target molecules for several tumor types. They can provide an opportunity for the design of novel radioimmunotherapy and vaccine strategies. Although more than 100 TAAs have been cataloged, only a handful of immunologically detected molecules have been considered viable candidates as targets for immunotherapeutic intervention (5). The candidate molecules include altered or overexpressed oncogene products (platelet-derived growth factor (PDGF)) and their receptors (PDGFR), the epidermal growth factor receptor (EGFR) family, vascular endothelial growth factor receptor (VEGFR), developmentally related or cell lineage-related epitopes (neural cell adhesion molecule (NCAM), L1 gangliosides), matrix metalloproteinases (MMPs), epitopes with an extracellular matrix location (tenascin, gp40), carcinoembryonic antigen (CEA), prostate-specific membrane antigen (PSMA), and high-molecular-weight glycoprotein mucins. Tumor-associated epitopes on mucins including the human milk fat globulin (HMFG) have been implicated extensively in the pathogenesis of many cancers (12–14). However, most antigens fail to express preferentially in tumors over normal tissues when measured by either quantitative or qualitative analyses, therefore limiting the clinical efficacy of mAb-directed therapy.

One of the most extensively studies groups of mAbs for RIT in solid tumors, B72.3 (Oncoscint OV/CR) and CC49, is reactive with the high-molecular-weight mucin, tumor-associated glycoprotein-72 (TAG-72). This mucin is expressed on a wide range of carcinomas including gastrointestinal, breast, ovary, endometrium, prostate, and non-small lung tumors but has an uncommon expression in the normal tissues except for the secretory endometrium (15–17). Several other clinically useful antibodies (DF3, SM3, anti-HMFG, DU-PAN2), originally generated against tumors of secretory epithelial cell origin from the pancreas, breast, colon, and lung, recognize epitopes on MUC1 mucin. Another mAb, 7E11-C5.3 (CYT-356), recognizes PSMA in prostate cancer patients and is marketed as ProstaScint® (Capromab Pendetide) by Cytogen

Corporation (18). mAb 17.1A is one of the first mAbs studied for gastrointestinal cancers (19). Other pancarcinoma antigens have been described by mAbs B3 and NR-LU-10 and have entered clinical trials for cancer therapy (20, 21). mAb A33 reacts with a glycoprotein homogeneously expressed by > 95 per cent of colon cancers and in the colon mucosa but not other epithelial tissues. The A33 antigen is on the cell surface and a fraction of membrane-bound mAb A33 is usually internalized (22).

A few common antibodies for RIT of hemopoietic antigens include anti-CD20 (B1 and 2B8), anti-CD22 (LL2), anti-CD33 (M195), anti-CD37 (MB1), and Lym-1 for B-cell lymphoma and leukemia (reviewed by DeNardo *et al.* (7)).

Radionuclides and their choice for radioimmunotherapy

Depending on several clinical and physical factors, a range of radioisotopes has been proposed for RIT (23, 24). Some of the radioisotopes with therapeutic applications are listed in Table 5.1. Radioisotopes undergo radioactive decay due to the inherent instability of their nuclei with a characteristic half-life (time needed for 50 per cent of the atoms in a pure sample of a particular radioisotope to undergo radioactive decay) and the release of radioactive emissions. Each of these emissions has a characteristic pattern of energy deposition in tissue, which should be considered when planning a particular radioisotope–antibody conjugate for RIT. For clinical purposes, the most important types of emissions are alpha, beta, gamma, and electron capture. In general, long- or intermediate-range beta-emitting radioisotopes have been chosen for preclinical and clinical trials. Therefore, depending upon the radioisotope characteristics, radioactivity can both kill distant non-targeted and targeted cells and be used for targeting heterogeneous tumors.

The gamma rays emitted by a radioisotope like iodine-131 are quite energetic and penetrate and deposit their energy over greater distances. Gamma rays have no direct role in therapy, but with their longer range of energy they can be detected from outside the patient's body. Consequently, external scintigraphic imaging can be used to determine the biodistribution of radiolabeled antibodies. In contrast, beta particles travel only a few millimeters or centimeters in tissue, and consequently deposit their energy

Table 5.1 Properties of selected radionuclides suitable for clinical use with mAbs

Radionuclide	Emission	Energy		Half-life (hours)
		E_{max} (KeV)	Frequency (%)	
Actinium-225 (^{225}Ac)	Alpha	6000	100	240
Astatine-211 (^{211}At)	Alpha	6000	42	7
	Gamma	80	19	
Bismuth-212 (^{212}Bi)	Alpha	6000	36	1
	Beta	492	64	
Copper-67 (^{67}Cu)	Beta	395	45	61
	Beta	484	35	
	Beta	570	20	
	Gamma	184	47	
Iodine-131 (^{131}I)	Beta	606	86	193
	Gamma	364	82	
Lutetium-177 (^{177}Lu)	Beta	497	79	161
	Beta	384	9	
	Beta	176	12	
	Gamma	208	11	
	Gamma	113	6	
Radium-223 (^{223}Ra)	Alpha	6000	100	274
	Gamma	80	40	
	Gamma	270	14	
Rhenium-186 (^{186}Rh)	Beta	1077	73	90
	Beta	939	21	
	Gamma	137	9	
Rhenium-188 (^{188}Rh)	Beta	2120	79	17
	Beta	1985	20	
	Gamma	155	15	
Scandium-47 (^{47}Sc)	Beta	600	100	82
	Gamma	160	68	
Yttrium-90 (^{90}Y)	Beta	2270	100	64

in the vicinity of the point of decay. Beta particles are emitted from the nucleus, have the mass of an electron, and are released with a spectrum of energies. The energy of these particles determines, in part, the distance over which the radiation effects will occur. Recent evidence suggests that medium-energy beta particles like those emitted by ^{131}I can deposit their energy effectively over tumor deposits the size of small cell clusters. Beta emissions from radioisotopes such as ^{131}I, ^{90}Y, ^{177}Lu, or ^{67}Cu directly target the antigen-positive tumor cells as well as killing the nearby antigen-negative tumor cells through a 'cross-fire-effect'. For highly cellular tumors with little connective tissue, such as lymphomas, this cross-fire effect increases the chances of tumor regression.

Iodine-131 was selected initially and continues to be used for RIT because of its straightforward radiochemistry, greater availability, and lower cost, thus ensuring a consistent supply. However, ^{131}I can be enzymatically eliminated by dehalogenation from tumors before it can deposit all its energy. Furthermore, the dehalogenation of iodinated antibodies is primarily a problem if the targeted antigen undergoes modulation (that is, internalization following antibody binding). Small iodinated peptides and free iodine, for the most part, are excreted via the kidneys; however, some iodine is concentrated in the thyroid, salivary glands, and stomach. Yttrium-90 is a pure beta emitter with a high energy of 2.29 MeV. The greater energy of ^{90}Y provides it with a longer path length of energy transfer and the potential to provide therapeutic effects over a distance up to 1 cm in most tissues, which is an advantage in treating bulky disease sites in solid tumors. A disadvantage of ^{90}Y is that, in its free form, the radioisotope accumulates in cortical bone. Lutetium-177 and copper-67 are very suitable for RIT and have a sufficiently long half-life, emit beta particles, and do not accumulate in bone. However, ^{67}Cu and ^{177}Lu are not regularly available.

Some radioisotopes decay by emitting alpha particles, basically a helium nucleus consisting of two patrons and two neutrons, which are huge relative to beta particles. This particle discharges very large amounts of energy over a much shorter distance in tissue than beta particles (range of 50 to 100 μm). Alpha particles are more efficient in cell killing than beta emitters on the basis of cells killed per disintegration. A single 'hit' to the nucleus from an alpha particle emitter is usually sufficient to kill a cell. Alpha emitters proposed for use include Bi-212, Bi-213, and At-211. Because they do not kill nearby normal cells or adjacent non-target tumor cells, α-emitters are useful for targeting homogeneously expressing antigen in tumors.

Radioisotopes such as ^{125}I have the shortest range of radioactive emissions, and decay by electron capture or internal conversion. In this mode of decay, the radioactive nucleus is relatively proton- or neutron-rich. The nucleus captures one of its own orbital electrons, or converts a neutron to a proton and an electron. The decay process results in the emission of a large number of Auger electrons of 30 keV. The tumor-killing effect by electron capture emission requires intranuclear deposition.

The synthesis of radioisotope–antibody conjugates requires conditions that prevent any alterations of antigen–antibody binding properties (immunoreactivity). The majority of therapy studies have been conducted with ^{131}I, which was originally selected for its ease of labeling by simple direct methods using Iodogen or chloramine-T. Iodine-125 or ^{131}I are covalently linked to antibodies at tyrosine residues. Radioisotopes like ^{90}Y, ^{177}Lu, or ^{67}Cu cannot be covalently attached by direct binding and must be linked to antibodies by an intermediary molecule called a chelate. The epsilon amino group of lysine or sulfhydryl-residues are frequently involved in chelation. A number of chelation methods for coupling radioisotopes with mAbs are now available (25, 26). Chemical chelate conjugates such as cyclic anhydride of isothiocyanatobenzyldiethylenetriamine-pentaacetic acid (SCN-Bz-DTPA) were initially used. Recently, new chelates have been developed that show strong bond formation between radioisotope and antibodies (27, 28). Chelates such as isothiocyanatobenzyl DTPA show decreased liver uptake. Larger chelating agents such as 1,4,7,10-tetraazacyclododecane-$N,N(x'),N'',N'''$ tetraacetic acid (DOTA) are also available. However, a few studies have claimed that some of the macrocyclic chelating agents may be immunogenic. This could be a major problem in treatment strategies requiring multiple dose administrations using certain macrocycle chelate conjugates.

The principle of radioimmunotherapy

RIT is based on the fundamental principle of using antibodies as carriers of selected radionuclides for the targeted destruction of tumor cells. RIT is particularly advantageous for tumors that are not amenable to surgery, recurrence, and distant metastases. The success of RIT relies on the concentration of radioactivity in tumors over a long duration. Radiation damage is the result of ionization along the emitted particle track that disrupts critical biomolecules in the cells. In addition to causing double-strand breaks in DNA (29), the cytotoxic effects of radiation are also exerted by cellular perturbations affecting the growth factors and signal transduction pathways (30–32), induction of apoptosis (33), and changes in cell cycle regulation (34).

RIT is unique because it has more potential for delivering increased radiation specifically to a tumor than external beam radiation therapy, and dose distribution can be easily determined. This modality is in the early stages of development, and preliminary data from the clinical trials are encouraging.

Clinical trials using radioimmunoconjugates

Preclinical studies in animal models have shown that features of the mAb (isotype, specificity, size, affinity) may be potentially important for a successful RIT trial. Generally, the development of any therapy for malignancy involves a logical progression through phase I (safety, toxicity, and definition of maximum tolerated dose and optimum biological end point), phase II (efficacy), and phase III (comparative efficacy) trials. For RIT, an additional step (pre-phase I trials) is appropriate involving the *in vivo* localization of radiolabeled mAbs. In many cases, radionuclide localization is visualized by simple gamma scan imaging studies, correlating positive images with routine radiolabeled antibodies to document the absolute amount of radioactivity delivered to the tumor site at a single point in time. For example, ^{131}I-mAb B72.3 IgG was demonstrated in biodistribution studies to localize selectively in tumors (35). Biopsy studies compared the percentage of the injected dose of mAb per gram in tumor (% i.d./g) with that found in the normal tissues from the same patient, providing a relative radiolocal-

Table 5.2　Radioimmunotherapy for hematological malignancies using murine intact immunoglobulins

Tumor type*	Phase	Agent†	Antigen	Response‡	Ref.
NHL	I	^{131}I-IF-5	CD20	1/1 PR	99
NHL	I/II/III	^{131}I-Anti-B1	CD20	4/9 CR, 2/9 PR	100
				16/21 CR, 2/21 PR	39
				20/53 CR, 22/53 PR	101
NHL	I/II	^{90}Y-2B8	CD20	13/51 PR, 21/51 CR	102
NHL	I	C2B8-SA, ^{131}Y-B	CD20	2/7 CR,2/7 PR	103
NHL	I	^{131}I-OKB-7	CD21	1/18 PR, 12/18 MR	104
NHL	I/II	^{131}I-nti-LL2	CD22	1/8 CR, 2/8 PR, 2/8 MR	105
NHL	I/II	^{131}I-Anti-MB1	CD37	5/6 CR, 1/6 PR	106
				6/9 CR	107
				6/6 CR	99
NHL	I/II	^{131}I-Lym-1	HLA-DR10	3/30 CR, 14/30 PR	108
				7/21 CR, 4/21 PR	109
NHL	I	^{131}I/^{90}Y-Anti-Ferritin	Ferritin	1/37 CR, 14/37 PR	110
				4/8 CR	111
APL	I/II	^{131}I-anti CD33, RA	CD33	4/7 PR	112
				2/7 PR	113

* NHL, Non-Hodgkin's lymphoma; APL, acute promyelocytic leukemia.
† B, Biotin; SA, streptavidin; RA, all-*trans* retinoic acid.
‡ PR, Partial response; CR, complete response; MR, mixed response.

ization index (RI) for each lesion). Of the tumor lesions examined, 70 per cent had an RI of at least 3 (that is, 3 times greater uptake per gram than adjacent normal tissue) and 31 per cent of the tumor lesions had RIs of over 10. Only 12 of 210 (6 per cent) histologically normal tissues had RIs greater than 3. Generally, antibodies that fail to localize in the majority of tumor sites based on imaging studies or that produces a low ratio of tumor to normal tissue uptake should not be selected for therapy trials (35).

In advanced hematological malignancies like lymphoma and leukemia, RIT has resulted in a 'partial' to 'complete' cure (Table 5.2). This is primarily due to the radiosensitive nature of these tumor types, vascular accessibility, and a high expression of tumor-specific antigen. The lineage-specific antigens, such as the pan-B-cell differentiation antigens like CD20, CD37, or CD22 widely expressed on the surface of B cells, have been used for immunotherapy-based treatments (36, 37). Rituximab (IDEC-C2B8), a chimeric anti-CD20 mAb, has shown a response rate of 48 per cent and a complete response of 6 per cent in 166 patients with relapsed low-grade or follicular non-Hodgkin's lymphoma (38). The anti-B1 (Bexxar™, Coulter Pharmaceutical Incorporated, Palo Alto, CA) and anti-CD22 (Lymphocide™, Immunomedics Incorporated, Morris Plains, New Jersey) antibodies have shown excellent results in phase I/II trial studies in non-Hodgkin's lymphoma (39, 40).

Table 5.3 summarizes various clinical trials using radiolabeled murine mAbs in other solid tumors such as breast, colorectal, brain, liver, ovary, prostate, and kidney. Overall, response in patients with these tumors varied from 'no objective response' to 'partial', with the stabilization of disease in many trials. This is mainly due to the hematological toxicity rendered by the long circulation half-life of mAbs, which limits the maximum tolerated dose and further dose escalation. Intact mAbs have practical limitations of biodistribution to normal organs (41), low quantitative delivery to tumors, and poor diffusion of mAb from the vasculature into the tumor (42). Antibodies can be dissected by specific proteases into individual domains or groups of domains (Fig. 5.1). The antibody is cleaved at the hinge region to generate divalent or monovalent Fab fragments. While F(ab')$_2$ or Fab fragments generated by proteolytic digestion help to improve specific localization, it is often difficult to generate these forms of immunoglobulins in a manner that retains their immunoreactivity. Fabs are normally obtained from whole antibodies by enzyme digestion, but the process is tedious and has to be optimized for each antibody (43). In spite of the problems, clinical trials using antibody fragments have been encouraging (Table 5.4).

Human mAbs would presumably be superior to those of other species when administered to patients because the human mAbs might be more compatible with the recipient's effector cells and may be less

Table 5.3   Radioimmunotherapy for solid tumors using murine intact immunoglobulins

Tumor type*	Phase	Agent[†]	Antigen[‡]	Response[§]	Ref.
Breast	I	^{90}Y/^{111}In-mBrE-3	MUC-1	6/9, PR	114
				3/6 MR	115
	I	^{111}In/^{90}Y-170, cyclosporin	MUC-1	1/3 PR, 1/SD	116
Colorectum	I	131I-F19	FAP	17, MR	117
	II	131I-CC49, IFNα	TAG-72	15, NR	118
				4/14 SD, 10/14 NR	119
	I	^{125}I-A33	HMW glycoprotein	4/23 MR	120
	II	^{90}Y-B, NR-LU-10, SA	Ep-CAM	2/25 PR, 4/25 SD	121
Epithelial tissue	I	^{111}In/^{90}Y-B3	Lewis Y carbohydrate	26, MR	122
Hepatocellular	I/II	131I-Hepama-1, surgery	anti-hepatocellular	32, MR	123
Glioma	I/II	131I-3F8	GD2	2/7 PR, 3/8 MR	124
	I	131I-81C6	Tenascin	MR	125
	I/II	131I-81C6	Tenascin	Dosimetry study	126
				1/31 PR, 13/31SD	127
Ovary	I	^{177}Lu-CC49	TAG-72	1/8 PR	128
				1/13 PR	129
	I/II	^{90}Y-HMFG1, chemotherapy	MUC-1	18/25 PR	130
	I	^{90}Y-B72.3	TAG-72	38, MR	131
Prostate	II	131I-CC49, α-IFN	TAG-72	2/6 MR; 5/6 PR	132
RCC	I/II	131I-G250	G250	17/33 SD, 2/33 CR	133

* RCC, Renal cell carcinoma.

[†] α-IFNα, Alpha interferon; SA, streptavidin; B, biotin.

[‡] FAP, Fibroblast activation protein.

[§] CR, Complete response; PR, partial response; MR, mixed response; NR, no response; SD, stabilized disease.

immunogenic. However, very few human mAbs are available due to low clonal frequency, low production levels, and cell line stability. Clinical trials with murine mAbs (Tables 5.2 and 5.3) have shown that the administration of a single systemic dose can elicit human anti-mouse antibodies (HAMA) responses in 50–80 per cent of patients (44), with the exception of lymphoma patients who are less prone to develop an immune response to the murine antibody. Two to three mAb administrations have led to a HAMA response in more than 90 per cent of patients (54). The HAMA response is usually directed against most or all mouse immunoglobulin classes (anti-isotypic), although a significant idiotypic response is often detected. The HAMA responses can reduce the efficacy of treatment by removing the circulating mAb and altering the pharmacokinetic properties (rates of blood and whole body clearance) of the antibody. These HAMA responses may also cause immune complex hypersensitivity or allergic reactions that may be harmful to the patients. Due to these drawbacks, many clinical trials were based on a single therapeutic administration strategy, which has its own limitations of providing a suboptimal dose administration schedule. Therefore, it is of great interest to use less immunogenic antibody forms to permit multiple administration over a prolonged time period. This would more closely approximate fractionated external beam radiotherapy, a routine technique used to minimize normal tissue toxicity and allow for a higher dose to tumor (46). This technique has been successful in preclinical studies using mAbs B72.3 and CC49 (47–49).

In an attempt to further minimize the immunogenicity of mouse antibody in humans, recombinant DNA technology has been used to generate the chimeric antibody by joining the variable regions of mouse antibody to the constant regions of human immunoglobulin. A number of mouse/human chimeric antibodies against TAAs have been generated (50, 51). The mouse/human chimeric antibodies retain the same specificity and equivalent affinity as those of the mouse hybridoma from which the variable region genes are isolated. A schematic structure for the mouse–human chimeric antibody is shown in Fig. 5.2. Gillies and Wesolowski (52)

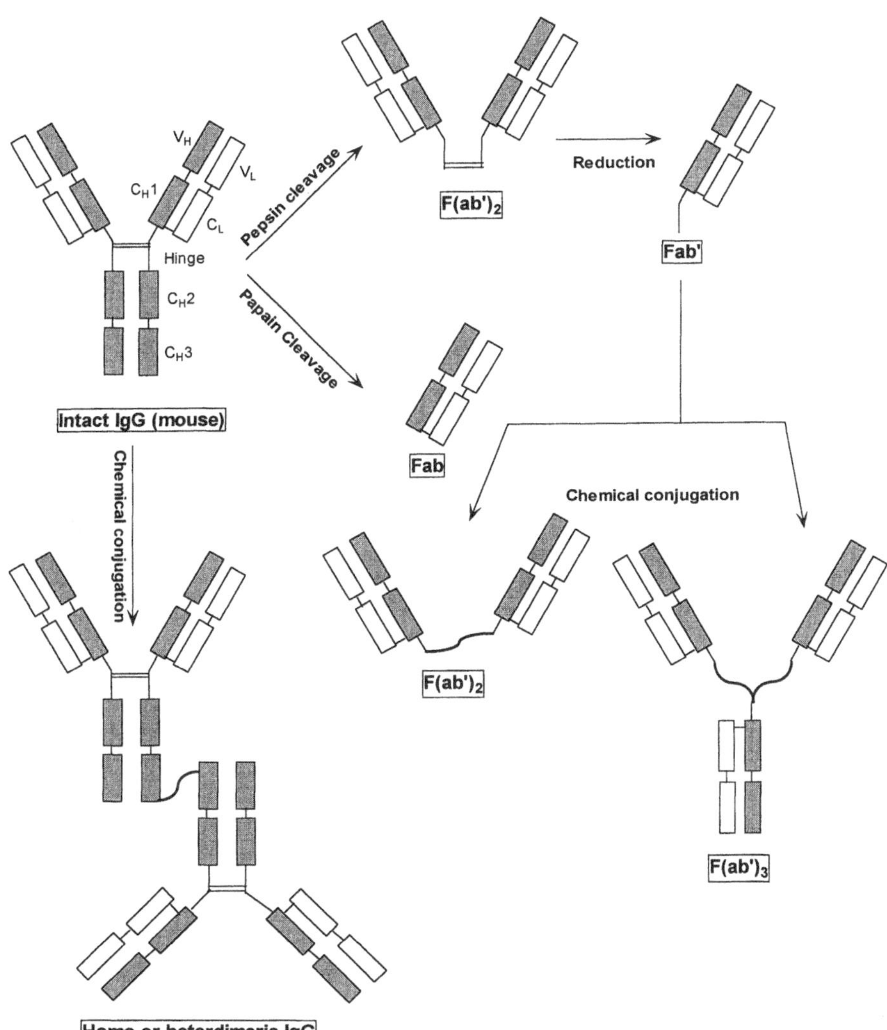

Fig. 5.1 Chemically modified antibody fragments evaluated for preclinical radioimmunotherapeutic efficacy. The bivalent F(ab')$_2$ fragment is generated by the hydrolysis of antibody with pepsin, while papain generates the monovalent Fab fragment. Fab' fragments are obtained by mild reduction of F(ab)'$_2$. mAbs have also been dimerized by thioether bonds (149). Chemically linked divalent and trivalent Fab'ΔCys fragments (92) or Fab'(150) have been prepared by using a stable bis maleinide linker. Disulfide bonds are depicted by straight lines and thioether bonds are shown by curved lines. V$_L$ and V$_{H'}$ denote variable regions and C$_L$ and C$_H$ denote constant regions of light and heavy chains, respectively.

Table 5.4 Radioimmunotherapy for solid tumors using murine immunoglobulin fragments

Tumor type	Phase	Agent	Antigen	Response*	Ref.
Colorectum	I/II	^{131}I anti CEA F(ab')$_2$	CEA	1/9 CR, 1/10 PR	134
Glioma	I	^{131}I-Me1-14 F(ab')$_2$	Proteoglycan chondroitin sulfate-associated protein	4/5 PR	135
Thyroid	I	^{131}I-MN-14 F(ab')$_2$	CEA	1/12 PR, 1/MR, 10/12 SD	136

* CR, Complete response; PR, partial response; MR, mixed response; SD, stabilized disease.

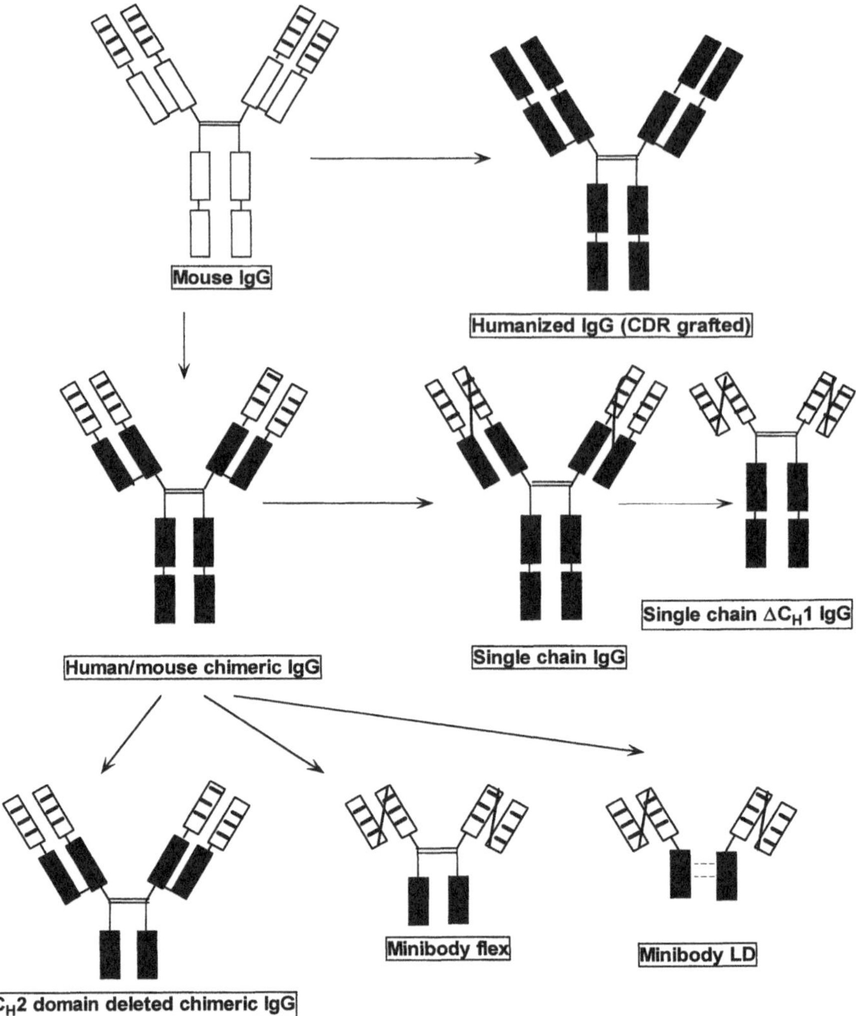

Fig. 5.2 The engineering of humanized forms of murine IgG. The murine IgG is represented by white, while the black areas represent the human IgG framework. The complement-determining (CDR) of the murine IgG are depicted by gray areas. Humanized CC49 IgG was constructed by grafting the murine CC49 hypervariable regions to V_L and V_H regions to human mAbs LEN and 21/28′CL, respectively (151), while chimeric B72.3 was generated by combining the murine variable region and a human gamma 1 constant region (152). To simplify the *in vivo* gene inoculation as well as the *ex vivo* transfection of patients' lymphocytes for immunotherapy protocols, single-chain (sc)CC49 IgG and scΔC$_H$1CC49 were developed by Lee *et al.* (153). Chimeric ΔC$_H$2CC49 was generated and assessed for tumor targeting and pharmacokinetic properties in xenografted mice (55). The T84.66/212 minibody (Flex and LD) was generated by joining the V_L and V_H to C$_H$3 using two different linkers (154).

demonstrated that direct genetic engineering of an F(Ab′)$_2$ fragment of the chimeric mAb 14.18 resulted in an unstable complex of covalently bonded Fab′ fragments. However, the C$_H$2 domain deletion mutant, ch14.18 ΔC$_H$2, exhibited significantly higher antigen binding activity as compared to that of the intact chimeric antibody (Fig. 5.2). Mueller *et al.* (53) showed that this ch14.18 ΔC$_H$2 was cleared from the blood of tumor-bearing mice with the same kinetics as human

F(ab′)$_2$ and much faster than the corresponding intact chimeric IgG antibody. A similar, but improved, C$_H$2-deletion mutant construct for chimeric antibody B72.3 was prepared by Slavin-Chiorini *et al.* (54). The C$_H$2 domain was replaced by a 10-amino-acid linker peptide, gly–gly–gly–ser–ser–gly–gly–gly–ser–gly, which provided relative stability to the cB72.3ΔC$_H$2 construct in comparison with the ch14.18ΔC$_H$2. Humanized mAb CC49 (as shown in Fig. 5.2) was modified further with the deletion of the second constant region of the heavy chain of IgG (55). The hCC49ΔC$_H$2 antibody has not yet entered clinical trials. However, studies in non-human primates have shown that the humanized form of this antibody construct is less immunogenic and has a somewhat shorter half-life than the parental murine mAb CC49 (55). Furthermore, hCC49ΔC$_H$2 has a more rapid blood clearance than intact huCC49mAb. Chester *et al.* (56) reported the production and characterization of recombinant chimeric Fab for mAb A5B7 to CEA. Biodistribution and therapeutic ratios for recombinant Fab' A5B7 were better for the intact murine antibody.

Studies using antibody fragments have shown that the C$_H$2 domain plays an important role in effector function, and aglycosylated IgG lacking carbohydrate in the C$_H$2 domain was unable to activate complement (57). Using domain-switched chimeric antibodies, Tao *et al.* (58) showed that the structure responsible for the differential ability of human IgG1 and IgG4 to activate complement is located in the carboxy terminal part of the C$_H$2 domain. Hand *et al.* (59) demonstrated no difference in the plasma clearance of an aglycosylated aGcB72.3 and a chimeric cB72.3 mAb in primates after intravenous inoculation; however, a rapid peritoneal clearance was observed in mice with an aGcB72.3. This study demonstrates that comparative analyses in more than one system are required to understand the pharmacokinetic of an mAb construct.

Encouraging results have been obtained in phase I clinical trails using human/mouse chimeric or human-ized radiolabeled antibodies (Table 5.5). The chimeric mAb L6 showed a complete response in 1 of 3 breast cancer patients (60). The poor tumor penetration of mAb usually results in the localization of only 0.0001–0.01 per cent of the injected dose per gram (i.d./g) of tumor (11). To achieve complete and lasting responses, more intensive dosing is required. However, in many cases only 'partial' or 'no' responses were observed. If chimeric or human mAbs remain in circulation for an extended time, they can increase the radiation dose delivered to normal tissues. Further approaches to enhance the therapeutic windows using antibody fragments or domain-deleted antibodies are currently under investigation.

New generation of recombinant Fvs

A new generation of recombinant antibody fragments called genetically engineered antibodies are about to enter clinical trials for cancer therapy (61, 62). Innovative technology has enabled researchers to engineer small fragment antibodies for the desired pharmacokinetics and biodistribution. The smallest-sized functional module of antibodies required for binding to an antigen are Fv fragments, consisting of the variable light (V$_L$) chain domain and the variable heavy (V$_H$) chain domain of IgGs (Fig. 5.1). Their smaller size makes them potentially more useful than whole anti-

Table 5.5 Radioimmunotherapy using chimeric immunoglobulins

Tumor type*	Phase	Agent	Antigen	Response†	Ref.
Breast	I	^{131}I-chimeric L6	L6	6/10 MR	137
		[90]Y/^{111}In chimeric L6		1/3 CR	60
	I	^{90}Y-chimeric T84.66	CEA	1/7 SD, 4/7 MR	138
Colorectum	I	^{131}I-chimeric B72.3	TAG-72	4/12 SD	139
	I	[186]Re-chimeric NR-LU-13	Ep-CAM	9, NR	140
	I	^{111}In-chimeric T84.66	CEA	13, dose escalation trial	141
Ovary	I	^{131}I-humanized MN-14	CEA	1/14 CR, 1/12 PR	142
	I	^{131}I-chimeric MOv18	Folate binding protein	15, NR	143
				8, Dosimetric study	144
RCC	I	^{131}I-chimeric G250	G250	1/12 SD, 1/12 PR	145
NHL	I	^{90}Y-hLL2	CD22		40
APL	I/II	^{90}Y-HuM195	CD33	8/12 MR	146
		[213]Bi-HuM195		13/18 MR	147

* RCC, Renal cell carcinoma; NHL, non-Hodgkin's lymphoma; APL, acute promyelocytic leukemia.
† CR, Complete response; PR, partial response; MR, mixed response; NR, no response; SD, stabilized disease.

body for clinical applications of diagnosis (imaging) and therapy (pretargeting). There are relatively few reports of successful isolation of Fv fragments by proteolytic digestion of intact antibody molecules due to practical limitations in reproducibility. However, the application of recombinant technology enabled the production of Fv fragments in *E. coli*, yeast, virus, and myeloma cells (63–66). Fv fravments of antibodies may dissociate at low protein concentrations and often are too unstable for many applications at physiological temperatures. Options available to stabilize Fv fragments include chemical cross-linking, disulfide bond engineering (disulfide-stabilized Fv, dsFv), and genetic linking by a peptide linker (single-chain Fv, scFv) (67). The scFv have demonstrated a 10-fold increase in stability over the natural Fv fragment, while the greatest stability, up to 60-fold, was achieved with the dsFv (68). Stabilization of the V_L and V_H fragments together with a peptide linker has proven the most popular approach. The scFv recombinant protein for a given mAb can be prepared by connecting genes encoding for heavy chains and light chains at the DNA level by an appropriate oligonucleotide (69, 70). The resulting translation product forms a single chain with a linker peptide bridging the two variable domains. A number of different linkers have been used to join the variable regions, including synthetic oliogomers of Gly_4Ser (70) and natural sequences derived from the protein of a known three-domensional structure (69). The length of the linkers affects the folding of the scFv polypeptide, and a joining peptide of 14–15 amino acids seems to be optimal.

Compared to intact mAbs and more conventional F(ab′)₂ and Fab fragments, scFv molecules offer several advantages as carriers for the selective delivery of radionuclides to tumors. First, the rate of clearance of scFv from the blood pool and normal tissues has been shown to be much more rapid than that seen with intact IgG, F(ab′)₂, or Fab fragments (64, 65), offering the possibility of earlier imaging and a reduction of the radiation absorbed dose to normal tissues in a therapeutic setting. Second, autoradiographic studies have shown that scFv can penetrate into a tumor much more rapidly than intact mAbs and larger fragments (71). This is important for RIT applications because of the potential for increasing the homogeneity of radiation dose deposition within tumors.

scFv constructs have been made using a variety of mAbs to both complex polypeptide antigens and small-molecular-weight haptens. The scFv fragments have been shown to retain the antigen-binding affinity of the

monovalent Fab fragment in most cases. However, some antigen–intact antibody interactions involve both antigen-binding sites of the immunoglobulin, either for binding to a molecule with more than one antigenic determinant or for bridging the two separate cell surface molecules. There are reports indicating a decrease in the binding affinity of the scFv fragments as compared to the whole antibodies (72, 73). Intact antibodies are polyvalent molecules that provide a significant increase in the functional affinity (avidity) due to the simultaneous binding to two or more target antigens. Thus, multivalency is an effective means for increasing the functional affinity of an antibody fragment. The simplest approaches to production of multivalent scFvs are based on the spontaneous formation of noncovalent dimers (Fig. 5.3) such as 50 kDa diabodies (74) or trimers such as triabodies, trimeric constructs having no additional linker sequence between the V_L and V_H chains (75, 76). A number of investigators have reported that, for certain scFv fragments, a degree of dimerization or even multimerization can spontaneously occur (77, 78). Such multimeric

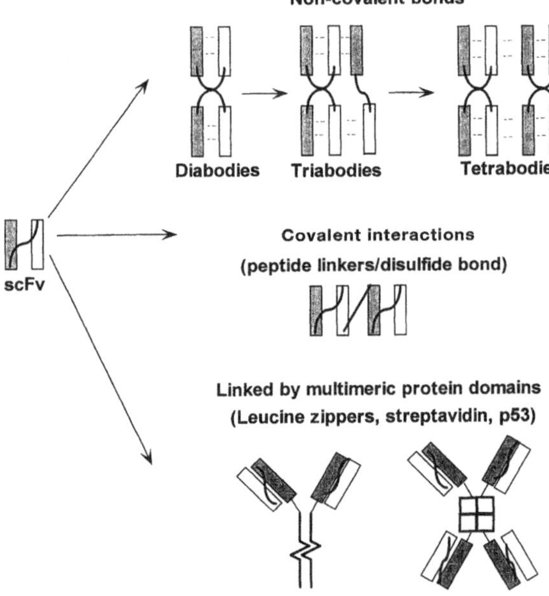

Fig. 5.3   Recombinant monovalent and multivalent single-chain Fvs of tumor-specific antibodies generated for effective tumor targeting. ScFvs are comprised of variable regions of heavy and light chains connected by an artificial linker. ScFvs can associate to form multimers by noncovalent interactions (74–76); covalent interactions such as disulfide bonds (90) and peptide linkers (81, 155); and multimeric protein domains such as helix bundles (84), zipper sequences (156, 157), protein A (158), etc.

molecules were thought to be dependent on the primary sequence of the V_L and V_H regions and on the length of the linker. Molecular modeling (74) and the determination of the crystal structure of a dimeric scFv (79) have shown that the V_L and V_H domains can come apart and associate with a second scFv molecule, creating one molecule containing two V_L/V_H assemblies. The formation of dimer from the monomer seems to depend upon a concentration-dependent equilibrium (80). Pluckthun and Pack (67) reported that the formation of dimers is related to the order of the variable chain domains, with the V_H–linker–V_L order forming predominantly monomers, whereas dimers are formed in the V_L–linker–V_H construct. The reasoning behind this report lies with the interpretation of the crystal structural data and the angle of rotation about the pseudo-twofold axis (parallel to the interface). Another unique approach for generating a covalent stable dimer of scFv involves the addition of a flexible helical structure linker (Fig. 5.3) at the C-terminus of the scFv fragment (81, 82). Furthermore, a tetravalent scFv was formed by a noncovalent association of the covalent dimer sc(Fv)$_2$. The (sc(Fv)$_2$)$_2$ with four potentially active antigen binding sites showed improved *in vitro* binding properties as compared to divalent sc(Fv)$_2$. (sc(Fv)$_2$)$_2$ showed a binding constant (K_A) 1.02×10^8 M^{-1} that was similar to that of IgG CC49 (1.14×10^8 M^{-1}) and was fourfold higher than that of its divalent scFv (sc(Fv)$_2$, 2.75×10^7 M^{-1}).

Covalent heterodimeric scFv molecules have also been generated. These constructs are made using two different binding Fv regions that are linked by a peptide linker (83). Stable divalent and multivalent scFvs have been constructed by fusion to amphipathic helix (84), transcriptional factor p53 (85), and core streptavidin (86). The C-terminal fragment of C4-binding plasma protein has also been used for the multimerization of scFvs (87). Recently, bispecific tetravalent antibodies have been made by fusing scFvs to the C-terminus (C_H3–scFv) or to the hinge region (hinge–scFv) of an antibody of a different specificity (88). Alt *et al.* (89) developed a bispecific tetravalent construct by combining diabodies (Db) with the Fc (scDb–Fc) or C_H3 (scDb–C_H3) region of the human immunoglobulin γ1 chain. Another approach has been to introduce a cysteine at the C-terminus of the scFv, which can be used to covalently link two scFvs together via a site-specific dimerization. Adams *et al.* (90) prepared a divalent-scFv with the specificity of anti-erb-2 monoclonal antibody 741F8 using cysteine residues at the carboxy terminal. A greater tumor localization is seen with the divalent scFv as compared to monovalent scFv, suggesting that the increased avidity of the dimer is a factor of its tumor retention.

We have constructed monovalent, divalent, and tetravalent scFv constructs of mAb CC49 and have characterized them for *in vitro* binding characteristics and *in vivo* tumor targeting and therapy. Pharmacokinetic analysis of blood clearance studies showed the elimination half-lives for (sc(Fv)$_2$)$_2$, sc(Fv)$_2$, scFv, and IgG to be 170, 50, 10, and 330 minutes, respectively (81, 82, 91). The CC49 Fab′ generated enzymatically from the parent murine mAb had a blood clearance that was faster than that of the noncovalent (scFv)$_2$ with half of the activity cleared from the serum of 30 and 50 minutes, respectively (91). Compared to sc(Fv)$_2$, (sc(Fv)$_2$)$_2$ has a threefold increase in the circulating half-life. Biodistribution studies showed that the percentage of injected dose accumulated pen gram of LS-174T colon carcinoma xenografts was 21.3 ± 1.3 % i.d./g for radioiodinated (sc(Fv)$_2$)$_2$, 9.8 ± 1.3 % i.d./g for sc(Fv)$_2$, and 17.3 ± 1.1 % i.d./g for IgG (Fig. 5.4) at 6 hours postadministration. This increased persistence of the tetramer in the blood allows increased uptake by the tumor. The blood half-life for CC49 IgG was twice as long as that for sc(Fv)$_2$)$_2$, explaining the higher levels of nonspecific organs. Whole-body clearance studies showed that the blood clearance of radiolabeled antibody constructs was indeed due to the removal of the radionuclide from the body and not to the accumulation in some specific organ or extravascular space. At 24 hours, the tetravalent scFv exhibited a tumor:blood ratio that was about 15-fold higher than that of IgG and 1.5-fold higher than that of sc(Fv)$_2$ (Fig. 5.4). Similarly, (sc(Fv)$_2$)$_2$, demonstrated a higher RI than sc(Fv)$_2$ and intact IgG in all the other organs tested with the exception of liver, which could be the possible site for the elimination of tetravalent scFv as also evidenced by the lower kidney uptake of (sc(Fv)$_2$)$_2$ (Table 5.6).

King *et al.* (92) found that the di-Fab′ and tri-Fab′ molecules accumulated to relatively high levels in the tumor when compared to IgG, with high tumor:blood ratios. However, chemically cross-linked scFv molecules demonstrated rapid clearance from the circulation, giving rise to only relatively low levels of activity accumulated at the tumor.

Recently, the therapeutic potential of CC49 (scFv)$_2$ was examined in RIT studies in athymic mice bearing established small-cell human colon carcinoma (LS-174T) xenografts (93). The group of mice treated with the lowest dose of ^{131}I-(scFv)$_2$ (500 μCi) showed statis-

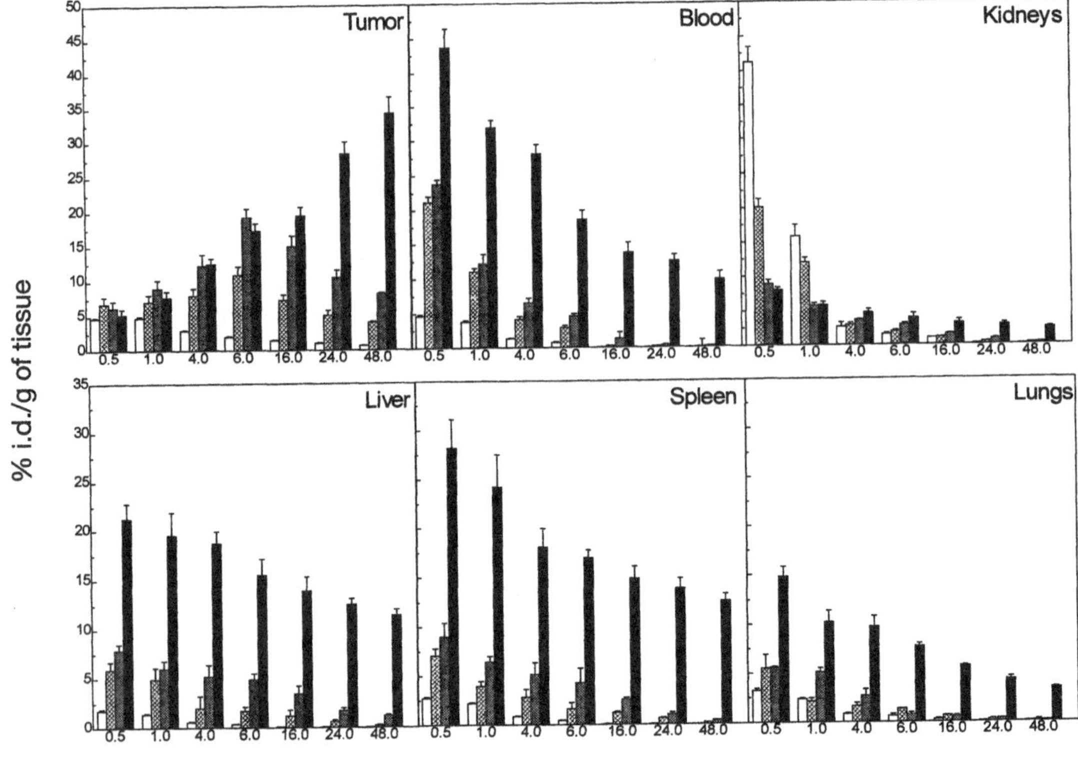

Fig. 5.4 Biodistribution of radioiodinated scFv (open histograms), sc(Fv)$_2$ (crossed histograms), (sc(Fv)$_2$)$_2$ (gray), and CC49 IgG (black) in groups of six athymic mice bearing LS-174T human colon carcinoma xenografts. The results are the per cent injected dose/gram of tissue ± SD (% i.d./g ± SD); n = 6 mice.

Table 5.6 Comparative biodistribution studies of CC49 IgG and various scFv fragments (radiolocalization index) at 24 hours after administration

Tissue	Radiolocalization index (RI)*			
	CC49 IgG	scFv	sc(Fv)$_2$	(sc(Fv)$_2$)$_2$
Blood	2.1	23.2	24.1	33.9
Kidneys	9.7	7.3	12.3	13.5
Liver	2.3	16.6	8.1	3.9
Lungs	6.5	16.6	24.1	40.5
Spleen	2.6	19.3	8.2	10.4

* Iodinated CC49 and various scFvs were injected into athymic mice (6 per group) bearing LS-174T tumors. The mice were sacrificed at 24 h and the radiolocalization index (% i.d./g of tumor divided by % i.d./g of normal tissue) for each organ was determined as described by Colcher *et al.* (148) and Goel *et al.* (82).

tically significant prolonged survival when compared to controls ($p = 0.036$). At 15 days postadministration, the tumors were 37 per cent the size of control tumors in mice given 1500 μCi of labeled (scFv)$_2$ and 19 and 15 per cent the size of control tumors in animals given 250 and 500 μCi of labeled IgG, respectively. Comparisons of single and fractionated therapeutic regimes showed median survival as 20 ($p = 0.8262$) and 32 days ($p < 0.0001$), respectively, for sc(Fv)$_2$ (Fig. 5.5). The median survival for the control group was 20 days. Furthermore, tetravalent scFv showed statistically significant prolonged survival with both single and fractionated administrations with media survival of 26 ($p = 0.0003$) and 47 days ($p < 0.0001$), respectively (Fig. 5.5).

Although advances in DNA recombinant technology have provided a variety of antigen-binding proteins showing high tumor:normal ratio, the absolute amount of radioactivity delivered by them is generally low due to fast clearance. Directly labeled scFvs usually provide high RI values at the cost of low tumor uptake. In a clinical trial with five patients, the scFv monomer was found to be safe and showed rapid clearance allowing same-day imaging (61). However, the absolute amount

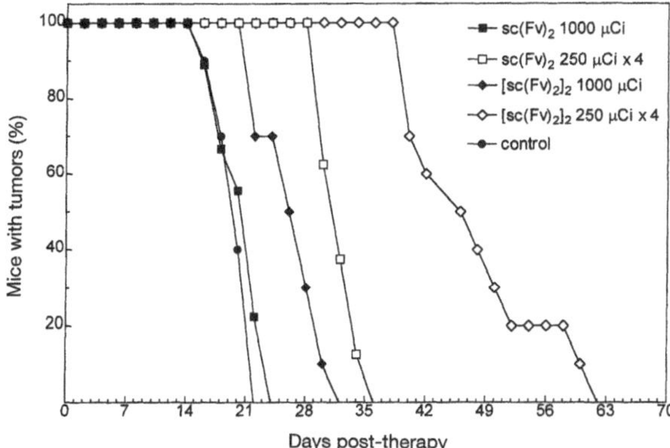

Fig. 5.5 Survival analysis of athymic mice bearing LS-174T human colon carcinoma xenografts versus time after a single administration of 1000 μCi of (black square) sc(Fv)₂ or (black diamond) (sc(Fv)₂)₂ or four injections of 250 μCi each at days 0, 1, 2, and 3 or (white square) sc(Fv)₂ or (white diamond) (sc(Fv)₂)₂. (Black circle) The control group was injected with phosphate-buffered saline (PBS), pH 7.4. The survival fraction of each group (n = 10) was evaluated. Mice were sacrificed when tumors exceeded 10 per cent of the total body weight, tumor ulceration was detected, or the animals lost ≥ 20 per cent of their original body weight.

uptake in the tumor was < 0.0005–0l0025 % i.d./g and was not of therapeutic benefit. Recently, Mayer *et al.* (62) used an scFv construct (MFE-23-his) directed against CEA in 34 patients for radioimmunoguided surgery (RIGS), with an 84 per cent accuracy between the tumor localization of antibody-targeted radionuclide and histological examination.

Optimization of radioimmunotherapy

Encouraging results are being obtained from clinical and preclinical trials in RIT using novel antibodies, radioisotopes, and genetically engineered antibody fragments. To overcome the low uptake of radioactivity by tumors and to increase tumor:normal tissue ratio, a variety of approaches including the upregulation of antigen expression by biological modifiers, increase of blood flow and vascular permeability by hyperthermia (94), vasoactive cytokines (95), radiosensitizers, and radioprotectors are being investigated.

In a novel pretargeting approach, the mAb is modified so that the radiolabel can bind to the antibody in the subsequent step. The modified mAb (antibody–conjugate) should have the properties of the same specificity and affinity for the tumor cells as the parent antibody if it is not internalized and stays on tumor cells enough (slow dissociation rate) to allow the unbound antibody to be cleared before administration of the radioisotope–hapten. The antibody–conjugate is first administered and allowed to localize in the tumor and undergo clearance from blood and normal tissues. Radiolabel–hapten is then injected to allow binding with the pretargeted antibody and acts to concentrate radiation in the tumor. The optimal timing of administration of the radioisotope for pretargeted RIT is when the tumor:normal tissue ratio of unlabeled antibody is at the peak level. In theory, the pretargeting approach has the potential to increase achievable tumor doses and improve the tumor:normal tissue ratio. Using a pretargeting approach, a 100 per cent cure (10/10) in mice bearing human colon or small cell lung and 80 per cent (8/10) in mice with human breast cancer xenografts was obtained without significant toxicity (96).

Pretargeting strategies use either an avidin–biotin system (97) or bispecific antibodies (98). In the avidin–biotin system, biotinylated or streptavidin (avidin)-conjugated mAb is used as an antibody–conjugate. Streptavidin or biotin is labeled for the carriage of radionuclides. The advantage of this approach is that biotin has high affinity (dissociation constant, $K_d = 10^{-15}$ M) for avidin and can clear rapidly (small molecular weight) from the whole body. The application of this approach is currently limited by the immunogenicity of avidin and strepavidin. Bispecific or bifunctional antibodies have two different antigen-binding sites, one for the TAA and the other for the radioactive hapten. This approach, using humanized or human antibodies, could be useful due to the limited immunogenicity of these constructs.

Conclusions and future trends

MAbs directed against tumor-associated antigens have been conjugated to various radioisotopes. Radiolabeled mAb-based targeted therapy, RIT, is a modality that can deliver radiation to tumor cells at levels significantly higher (up to 50 times) than to the normal tissue. In RIT, the emission properties of the therapeutic radionuclide are or equal importance to the targeting antibody and the characteristics of the targeted tumor and antigen. Several radioimmunoconjugates have shown impressive preclinical results and encouraging responses in patients. However, murine mAbs have several inherent limitations that have hampered their successful routine clinical application. Methods of improving the therapeutic index (tumor:normal tissue ratio) are needed for the development of more effective RIT for solid tumors. Several modifications have improved the efficacy of radioimmunoconjugates. Immunogenicity has been reduced by the chimerization and humanization of murine mAbs. The ability to engineer antibody molecules has now advanced to the stage where one can realistically envision creating pharmacologically useful targeting agents with desired functions. With the advance of combinatorial expression libraries and the power to develop antibodies that can then be mutagenized to imitate affinity maturation, it will certainly be possible in the near future to combine specificity, affinity, avidity, and stability in a construct that contains the minimal antigen-binding site. These recombinant antibodies appear to be promising vehicles for future innovative radiolabeled therapy of solid tumors. A variety of novel approaches for improving the efficacy of RIT are available including the development of new targeting molecules (genetically engineered antibodies), improved labeling chemistry, the development of additional radionuclides, dose fractionation, local administration, pretargeting, the use of biological response modifiers, and gene transfer techniques that upregulate expression of TAAs. Finally, combined modalities of RIT, chemotherapy, and gene therapy can synergize the therapeutic efficacy in cancer patients.

References

1. Köhler G. Milstein C. Continuous cultures of fused cells secreting antibody of predefined specificity. Nature 1975, **256**, 495–7.
2. Chester KA, Hawkins RE. Clinical issues in antibody design. Trends Biotechnol 1995, **13**, 294–300.
3. Vaughan TJ, Osbourn JK, Tempest PR. Human antibodies by design. Nat Biotechnol 1998, **16**, 535–9.
4. Cairns J. The evolution of cancer research. Cancer Cells 1989, **1**, 1–8.
5. Urban JL, Schreiber H. Tumor antigens. Annu Rev Immunol 1992, **10**, 617–44.
6. Behr TM, Goldenberg DM, Becker WS. Radioimmunotherapy of solid tumors: a review 'of mice and men'. Hybridoma 1997, **16**, 101–7.
7. DeNardo SJ, Kroger LA, DeNardo GL. A new era for radiolabeled antibodies in cancer? Curr Opin Immunol 1999, **11**, 563–9.
8. Crippa F, Bolis G, Seregni E, et al. Single-dose intraperitoneal radioimmunotherapy with the murine monoclonal antibody I-131 MOv18: clinical results in patients with minimal residual disease of ovarian cancer. Eur J Cancer 1995, **5**, 686–90.
9. Juweid M, Sharkey RM, Behr T, et al. Radioimmunotherapy of medullary thyroid cancer with iodine-131-labeled anti-CEA antibodies. J Nucl Med 1996, **37**, 905–11.
10. Reilly RM, Sandhu J, Alvarez-Diez TM, et al. Problems of delivery of monoclonal antibodies. Pharmaceutical and pharmacokinetic solutions. Clin Pharmacokinet 1995, **28**, 126–42.
11. Esteban JM, Colcher D, Sugarbaker P, et al. Quantitative and qualitative aspect of radiolocalization in colon cancer patients of intravenously administered MAb B72.3. Int J Cancer 1987, **39**, 50–9.
12. Gendler SJ. Burchell JM, Duhig T, et al. Cloning of partial cDNA encoding differentiation and tumor-associated mucin glycoproteins expressed by human mammary epithelium. Proc Natl Acad Sci, USA 1987, **84**, 6060–4.
13. Gendler SJ, Cohen EP, Craston A, et al. The locus of the polymorphic epithelial mucin (PEM) tumour antigen on chromosome 1q21 shows a high frequency of alteration in primary human breast tumours. Int J Cancer 1990, **45**, 431–5.
14. Metzgar RS, Hollingsworth MA, Kaufman B. In: The pancreas biology, pathology, and diseases, Vol. 2. ed. VLW Go and EP Dimagno. Raven Press, New York, 1993, 351–67.
15. Ohuchi N, Thor A, Nose M, et al. Tumor-associated glycoprotein (TAG-72) detected in adenocarcinomas and benign lesions of the stomach. Int J Cancer 1986, **38**, 643–50.
16. Thor A, Gorstein F, Ohuchi N, et al. Tumor-associated glycoprotein (TAG-72) in ovarian carcinomas defined by monoclonal antibody B72.3. J Natl Cancer Inst 1986, **76**, 995–1006.
17. Tempero M, Takasaki H, Uchida E, et al. Co-expression of CA 19-9, DU-PAN-2, CA 125, and TAG-72 in pancreatic adenocarcinoma. Am J Surg Pathol 1989, **13**, 89–95.
18. Wynant GE, Murphy GP, Horoszewicz JS, et al. Immunoscintigraphy of prostatic cancer: preliminary results with 111In-labeled monoclonal antibody 7E11-C5.3 (CYT-356). Prostate 1991, **18**, 229–41.
19. Gottlinger HG, Funke I, Johnson JP, et al. The epithelial cell surface antigen 17-1A, a target for antibody-mediated tumor therapy: its biochemical nature, tissue distribution and recognition by different monoclonal antibodies. Int J Cancer 1986, **38**, 47–53.
20. Willingham MC, Fitz-Gerald DJ, Pastan I. *Pseudomonas* exotoxin coupled to a monoclonal antibody against ovarian cancer inhibits the growth of human ovarian cancer cells in a mouse model. Proc Natl Acad Sci, USA 1987, **84**, 2474–8.
21. Breitz HB, Fisher DR, Weiden PL, et al. Dosimetry of rhenium-186-labeled monoclonal antibodies: methods, prediction from technetium-99m-labeled antibodies and results of phase I trials (see comments). J Nucl Med 1993, **34**, 908–17.
22. Barendswaard EC, Scott AM, Divgi CR, et al. Rapid and specific targeting of monoclonal antibody A33 to a colon cancer xenograft in nude mice. Int J Oncol 1998, **12**, 45–53.
23. Bhargava KK, Acharya SA. Labeling of monoclonal antibodies with radionuclides. Sem Nucl Med 1989, **19**, 187–201.

24. Mausner LF, Srivastava SC. Selection of radionuclides for radioimmunotherapy. Med Phys 1993, **20**, 503–9.

25. Meares CF, Moi MK, Diril H, *et al.* Macrocyclic chelates of radiometals for diagnosis and therapy. Br J Cancer Suppl 1990, **10**, 21–6.

26. Gansow OA, Brechbiel MW, Mirzadeh S, *et al.* Chelates and antibodies: current methods and new directions. Cancer Treat Res 1990, **51**, 153–71.

27. Li M, Meares CF. Synthesis, metal chelate stability studies, and enzyme digestion of a peptide-linked DOTA derivative and its corresponding radio-labeled immunoconjugates. Bioconjug Chem 1993, **4**, 275–83.

28. DeNardo GL, Kroger LA, Meares CF, *et al.* Comparison of 1,4,7,10-tetraazacyclododecane-N,N′, N″,N‴-tetraacetic acid (DOTA)-peptide-ChL6, a novel immunoconjugate with catabolizable linker, to 2-iminothiolane-2-[*p*-(bromoacetamido)benzyl]-DOTA-ChL6 in breast cancer xenografts. Clin Cancer Res 1998, **4**, 2483–90.

29. Elkind, MM. DNA damage and cell killing. Cause and effect? Cancer 1985, **56**, 2351–63.

30. Uckun FM, Gillis S, Souza L, *et al.* Effects of recombinant growth factors on radiation survival of human bone marrow progenitor cells. Int J Radiat Oncol Biol Phys 1989, **16**, 415–35.

31. Haimovitz-Friedman A, Falcone DJ, Eldor A, *et al.* Activation of platelet heparitinase by tumor cell-derived factors. Blood 1991, **78**, 789–96.

32. Chae HP, Jarvis LJ, Uckun FM. Role of tyrosine phosphorylation in radiation-induced activation of c-jun protooncogene in human lymphohematopoietic precursor cells. Cancer Res 1993, **53**, 447–51.

33. Kastan MB, Zhan Q, el-Deiry WS, *et al.* A mammalian cell cycle checkpoint pathway utilizing p53 and GADD45 is defective in ataxia–telangiectasia. Cell 1992, **71**, 587–97.

34. Muschel RJ, Zhang HB, Iliakis G, *et al.* Cyclin B expression in HeLa cells during the G2 block induced by ionizing radiation. Cancer Res 1991, **51**, 5113–17.

35. Tempero M, Colcher D. Radiolabeled monoclonal antibodies: therapy of solid tumors. Encyclopedia of Cancer 1997, **III**, 1448–58.

36. Knox SJ. Radioimmunotherapy of the non-Hodgkin's lymphomas. Sem Radiat Oncol 1995, **5**, 331–41.

37. Liu SY, Press OW. The potential for immunoconjugates in lymphoma therapy. Hematol Oncol Clin N Am 1997, **11**, 987–1006.

38. McLaughlin P, Grillo-Lopez AJ, Link BK, *et al.* Rituximab chimeric anti-CD20 monoclonal antibody therapy for relapsed indolent lymphoma: half of patients respond to a four-dose treatment program. J Clin Oncol 1998, **16**, 2825–33.

39. Press OW, Eary JF, Appelbaum FR, *et al.* Phase II trial of 131I-B1 (anti-CD20) antibody therapy with autologous stem cell transplantation for relapsed B cell lymphomas. Lancet 1995, **346**, 336–40.

40. Juweid ME, Stadtmauer E, Hajjar G, *et al.* Pharmacokinetics, dosimetry, and initial therapeutic results with 131I- and (111)In-/90Y-labeled humanized LL2 anti-CD22 monoclonal antibody in patients with relapsed, refractory non-Hodgkin's lymphoma. Clin Cancer Res 1999, **5**, 3292s–303s.

41. Foon KA. Biological response modifiers: the new immunotherapy [published erratum appears in Cancer Res 1990, 50 (1), 212]. Cancer Res 1989, **49**, 1621–39.

42. Jain RK. Transport of molecules across tumor vasculature. Cancer Metastasis Rev 1987, **6**, 559–93.

43. Milenic DE, Esteban JM, Colcher D. Comparison of methods for the generation of immunoreactive fragments of monoclonal antibody (B72.3) reactive with human carcinomas. J Immunol Methods 1989, **120**, 71–83.

44. Khazaeli MB, Conry RM, LoBuglio AF. Human immune response to monoclonal antibodies. J Immunother 1994, **15**, 42–52.

45. Milenic DE, Detrick B, Reynolds JC, *et al.* Characterization of primate antibody responses to administered murine monoclonal immunoglobulin. Int J Biol Markers 1990, **5**, 177–87.

46. DeNardo GL, O'Donnell RT, Kroger LA, *et al.* Strategies for developing effective radioimmunotherapy for solid tumors. Clin Cancer Res 1999, **5**, 3219s–23s.

47. Schlom J, Molinolo A, Simpson JF, *et al.* Advantage of dose fractionation in monoclonal antibody-targeted radioimmunotherapy. J Natl Cancer Inst 1990, **82**, 763–71.

48. Meredith RF, Khazaeli MB, Liu T, *et al.* Dose fractionation of radiolabeled antibodies in patients with metastatic colon cancer. J Nucl Med 1992, **33**, 1648–53.

49. Buchsbaum D, Khazaeli MB, Liu T, *et al.* Fractionated radioimmunotherapy of human colon carcinoma zenografts with 131I-labeled monoclonal antibody CC49. Cancer Res 1995, **55**, 5881s–7s.

50. Morrison SL. Transfectomas provide novel chimeric antibodies. Science 1985, **229**, 1202–17.

51. Shin SU. Chimeric antibody: potential applications for drug delivery and immunotherapy. Biotherapy 1991, **3**, 43–53.

52. Gilles SD. Wesolowski JS. Antigen binding and biological activities of engineered mutant chimeric antibodies with human tumor specificities. Hum Antibodies Hybridomas 1990, **1**, 47–54.

53. Mueller BM, Romerdahl CA, Gilles SD, *et al.* Enhancement of antibody-dependent cytotoxicity with a chimeric anti-GD2 antibody. J Immunol 1990, **144**, 1382–6.

54. Slavin-Chiorini DC, Horan Hand PH, Kashmiri SV, *et al.* Biologic properties of a CH2 domain-deleted recombinant immunoglobulin. Int J Cancer 1993, **53**, 97–103.

55. Slavin-Chiorini DC, Kashmiri SV, Schlom J, *et al.* Biological properties of chimeric domain-deleted anti-carcinoma immunoglobulins. Cancer Res 1995, **55**, 5957s–67s.

56. Chester KA, Robson L, Keep PA, *et al.* Production and tumour-binding characterization of a chimeric anti-CEA Fab expressed in *Escherichia coli*. Int J Cancer 1994, **57**, 67–72.

57. Wright A, Morrison SL. Effect of altered CH2-associated carbohydrate structure on the functional properties and *in vivo* fate of chimeric mouse–human immunoglobulin G1. J Exp Med 1994, **180**, 1087–96.

58. Tao MH, Canfield SM, Morrison SL. The differential ability of human IgG1 and IgG4 to activate complement is determined by the COOH-terminal sequence of the C_H2 domain. J Exp Med 1991, **173**, 1025–8.

59. Hand PH, Calvo B, Milenic D Comparative biological properties of a recombinant chimeric anti-carcinoma mAb and a recombinant aglycosylated variant. Cancer Immunol Immunother 1992, **35**, 165–74.

60. Denardo SJ, Richman CM, Goldstein DS, *et al.* Yttrium-90/indium-111-DOTA-peptide-chimeric L6: pharmacokinetic, dosimetry and initial results in patients with incurable breast cancer. Anticancer Res 1997, **17**, 1735–44.

61. Larson SM, EL-Shirbiny AM, Divgi CR, *et al.* Single chain antigen binding protein (scFv CC49): first human studies in colorectal carcinoma metastatic to liver. Cancer 1997, **80**, 2458–68.

62. Mayer A, Tsiompanou E, O'Malley D, *et al.* Radioimmunoguided surgery in colorectal cancer using a genetically engineered anti-CEA single-chain Fv antibody (In Process Citation). Clin Cancer Res 2000, **6**, 1711–19.

63. Skerra A, Pluckthun A. Assembly of a functional immunoglobulin Fv fragment in *Escherichia coli.* Science 1988, **240**, 1038–41.

64. Riechmann L, Foote J, Winter G. Expression of an antibody Fv fragment in myeloma cells. J Mol Biol 1988, **203**, 825–8.

65. Skerra A. Bacterial expression of immunoglobulin fragments. Curr Opin Immunol 1993, **5**, 256–62.

66. Pluckthun A. *Escherichia coli* producing recombinant antibodies. Bioprocess Technol 1994, **19**, 233–52.

67. Pluckthun A, Pack P. New protein engineering approaches to multivalent and bispecific antibody fragments. Immunotechnology 1997, **3**, 83–105.

68. Glockshuber R, Malia M. Pfitzinger I, *et al.* A comparison of strategies to stabilize immunoglobulin Fv-fragments. Biochemistry 1990, **29**, 1362–7.

69. Huston JS, Levinson D, Mudgett-Hunter M, *et al.* Protein engineering of antibody binding sites: recovery of specific activity in an anti-digoxin single-chain Fv analogue produced in *Escherichia coli.* Proc Natl Acad Sci, USA 1988, **85**, 5879–83.

70. Bird RE, Hardman KD, Jacobson JW, *et al.* Single-chain antigen-binding proteins [published erratum appears in Science 1989, **244** (4903), 409]. Science 1988, **242**, 423–6.

71. Yokota T, Milenic DE, Whitlow M, *et al.* Rapid tumor penetration of a single-chain Fv and comparison with other immunoglobulin forms. Cancer Res 1992, **52**, 3402–8.

72. Condra JH, Sardana W, Tomassini JE, *et al.* Bacterial expression of antibody fragments that block human rhinovirus infection of cultured cells. J Biol Chem 1990, **265**, 2292–5.

73. Milenic DE, Yokota T, Filpula DR, *et al.* Construction, binding properties, metabolism, and tumor targeting of a single-chain Fv derived from the pancarcinoma monoclonal antibody CC49. Cancer Res 1991, **51**, 6363–71.

74. Holliger P, Prospero T, Winter G. 'Diabodies': small bivalent and bispecific antibody fragments. Proc Natl Acad Sci, USA 1993, **90**, 6444–8.

75. Iliades P, Kortt AA, Hudson PJ. Triabodies: single chain Fv fragments without a linker form trivalent trimers. FEBS Lett 1997, **409**, 437–41.

76. Le Gall F, Kipriyanov SM, Moldenhauer G, Little M. Di-, tri- and tetrameric single chain Fv antibody fragments against human CD19: effect of valency on cell binding. FEBS Lett 1999, **453**, 164–8.

77. Griffiths AD, Malmqvist M, Marks JD, *et al.* Human anti-self antibodies with high specificity from phage display libraries. Embo J 1993, **12**, 725–34.

78. Wu AM, Chen W, Raubitschek A, *et al.* Tumor localization of anti-CEA single-chain Fvs: improved targeting by non-covalent dimers. Immunotechnology 1996, **2**, 21–36.

79. Perisic O, Webb PA, Holliger P, *et al.* Crystal structure of a diabody, a bivalent antibody fragment. Structure 1994, **2**, 1217–26.

80. Kortt AA, Malby RL, Caldwell JB, *et al.* Recombinant anti-sialidase single-chain variable fragment antibody. Characterization, formation of dimer and higher-molecular-mass multimers and the solution of the crystal structure of the single-chain variable fragment/sialidase complex. Eur J Biochem 1994, **221**, 151–7.

81. Beresford GW, Pavlinkova G, Booth BJ, *et al.* Binding characteristics and tumor targeting of a covalently linked divalent CC49 single-chain antibody. Int J Cancer 1999, **81**, 911–17.

82. Goel A, Beresford GW, Colcher D, *et al.* Divalent forms of CC49 single-chain antibody constructs in *Pichia pastoris*: expression, purification, and characterization. J Biochem (Tokyo) 2000, **127**, 829–36.

83. Cao Y, Suresh MR. Bispecific antibodies as novel bioconjugates. Bioconjug Chem 1998, **9**, 635–44.

84. Pack P, Muller K, Zahn R, *et al.* Tetravalent miniantibodies with high avidity assembling in *Escherichia coli.* J Mol Biol 1995, **246**, 28–34.

85. Rheinnecker M, Hardt C, Ilag LL, *et al.* Multivalent antibody fragments with high functional affinity for a tumor-associated carbohydrate antigen. J Immunol 1996, **157**, 2989–97.

86. Dubel S, Breitling F, Kontermann R, *et al.* Bifunctional and multimeric complexes of streptavidin fused to single chain antibodies (scFv). J Immunol Methods 1995, **178**, 201–9.

87. Libyh MT, Goossens D, Oudin S, *et al.* A recombinant human scFv anti-Rh(D) antibody with multiple valences using a C-terminal fragment of C4-binding protein. Blood 1997, **90**, 3978–83.

88. Coloma MJ, Morrison SL. Design and production of novel tetravalent bispecific antibodies [see comments]. Nat Biotechnol 1997, **15**, 159–63.

89. Alt M, Muller R, Kontermann RE. Novel tetravalent and bispecific IgG-like antibody molecules combining single-chain diabodies with the immunoglobulin gamma 1 Fc or C_H3 region. FEBS Lett 1999, **454**, 90–4.

90. Adams GP, McCartney JE, Tai MS, *et al.* Highly specific *in vivo* tumor targeting by monovalent and divalent forms of 741F8 anti-c-erbB-2 single-chair Fv. Cancer Res 1993, **53**, 4026–34.

91. Pavlinkova G, Beresford GW, Booth BJ, *et al.* Pharmacokinetics and biodistribution of engineered single-chain antibody constructs of MAb CC49 in colon carcinoma xenografts. J Nucl Med 1999, **40**, 1536–46.

92. King DJ, Turner A, Farnsworth AP, *et al.* Improved tumor targeting with chemically cross-linked recombi-

nant antibody fragments. Cancer Res 1994, **54**, 6176–85.

93. Pavlinkova G, Booth BJ, Batra SK, *et al.* Radioimmunotherapy of human colon cancer xenografts using a dimeric single-chain Fv antibody construct. Clin Cancer Res 1999, **5**, 2613–19.

94. Cope DA, Dewhirst MW, Friedman HS, *et al.* Enhanced delivery of a monoclonal antibody F(ab′)2 fragment to subcutaneous human glioma xenografts using local hyperthermia. Cancer Res 1990, **50**, 1803–9.

95. DeNardo GL, Lamborn KR, DeNardo SJ, *et al.* Use of response surface statistical designs to detect effects of biologic response modifiers such as IL-2. Biotechnol Ther 1994, **5**, 15–26.

96. Axworthy DB, Reno JM, Hylarides MD, *et al.* Cure of human carcinoma xenografts by a single dose of pretargeted yttrium-90 with negligible toxicity. Proc Natl Acad Sci, USA 2000, **97**, 1802–7.

97. Sakahara H, Saga T. Avidin–biotin system for delivery of diagnostic agents. Advan Drug Deliv Rev 1999, **37**, 89–101.

98. Segal DM, Weiner GJ, Weiner LM. Bispecific antibodies in cancer therapy. Curr Opin Immunol 1999, **11**, 558–62.

99. Press OW, Eary JF, Appelbaum FR, *et al.* Radiolabeled-antibody therapy B-cell lymphoma with autologous bone marrow support (see comments). New Engl J Med 1993, **329**, 1219–24.

100. Kaminski MS, Zasadny KR, Francis IR, *et al.* Radioimmunotherapy of B-cell lymphoma with [131I]anti-B1 (anti-CD20) antibody. New Engl J Med 1993, **329**, 459–65.

101. Kaminski MS, Zasadny KR, Francis IR, *et al.* Iodine-131-anti-B1 radioimmunotherapy for B-cell lymphoma. J Clin Oncol 1996, **14**, 1974–81.

102. Knox SJ, Goris ML, Trisler K, *et al.* Yttrium-90-labeled anti-CD20 monoclonal antibody therapy of recurrent B-cell lymphoma. Clin Cancer Res 1996, **2**, 457–70.

103. Breitz HB, Fisher DR, Goris ML, *et al.* Radiation absorbed dose estimation for 90Y-DOTA-biotin with pretargeted NR-LU-10/streptavidin [In Process Citation]. Cancer Biother Radiopharm 1999, **14**, 381–95.

104. Czuczman MS, Straus DJ, Divgi Cr, *et al.* Phase I dose-escalation trial of iodine 131-labeled monoclonal antibody OKB7 in patients with non-Hodgkin's lymphoma. J Clin Oncol 1993, **11**, 202–9.

105. Goldenberg DM, Horowitz JA, Sharkey RM, *et al.* Targeting, dosimetry, and radioimmunotherapy of B-cell lymphomas with iodine-131-labeled LL2 monoclonal antibody (see comments). J Clin Oncol 1991, **9**, 548–64.

106. Press OW, Eary JF, Badger CC, *et al.* Treatment of refractory non-Hodgkin's lymphoma with radiolabeled MB-1 (anti-CD37) antibody. J Clin Oncol 1989, **7**, 1027–38.

107. Kaminski MS, Fig LM, Zasadny KR, *et al.* Imaging, dosimetry, and radioimmunotherapy with iodine 131-labeled anti-CD37 antibody in B-cell lymphoma. J Clin Oncol 1992, **10**, 1696–711.

108. DeNardo GL, DeNardo SJ, Lamborn KR, *et al.* Low-dose, fractionated radioimmunotherapy for B-cell malignancies using 131I-Lym-1 antibody [In Process Citation]. Cancer Biother Radiopharm 1998, **13**, 239–54.

109. DeNardo GL, DeNardo SJ, Goldstein DS, *et al.* Maximum-tolerated dose, toxicity, and efficacy of (131)I-Lym-1 antibody for fractionated radioimmunotherapy of non-Hodgkin's lymphoma. J Clin Oncol 1998, **16**, 3246–56.

110. Lenhard Jr RE, Order SE, Spunberg JJ, *et al.* Isotopic immunoglobulin: a new systemic therapy for advanced Hodgkin's disease. J Clin Oncol 1985, **3**, 1296–300.

111. Vriesendorp HM, Herpst JM, Leichner PK, *et al.* Polyclonal 90Yttrium labeled antiferritin for refractory Hodgkin's disease. Int J Radiat Oncol Biol Phys 1989, **17**, 815–21.

112. Jurcic JG, Caron PC, Miller WH, *et al.* Sequential targeted therapy for relapsed acute promyelocytic leukemia with all-trans retinoic acid and anti-CD33 monoclonal antibody M195. Leukemia 1995, **9**, 244–8.

113. Jurcic JG, Caron PC, Nikula TK, *et al.* Radiolabeled anti-CD33 monoclonal antibody M195 for myeloid leukemias. Cancer Res 1995, **55**, 5908s–10s.

114. Schrier DM, Stemmer SM, Johnson T, *et al.* High-dose 90Y Mx-diethylene-triaminepentaacetic acid (DTPA)-BrE-3 and autologous hematopoietic stem cell support (AHSCS) for the treatment of advanced breast cancer: a phase I trial. Cancer Res 1995, **55**, 5921s–5924s.

115. DeNardo SJ, Kramer EL, O'Donnell RT, *et al.* Radioimmunotherapy for breast cancer using indium-111/yttrium-90 BrE-3: results of a phase I clinical trial. J Nucl Med 1997, **38**, 1180–5.

116. Richman CM, DeNardo SJ, O'Donnell RT, *et al.* Dosimetry-based therapy in metastatic breast cancer patients using 90Y monoclonal antibody 170H.82 with autologous stem cell support and cyclosporin A. Clin Cancer Res 1999, **5**, 3243s–8s.

117. Welt S, Divgi CR, Scott AM, *et al.* Antibody targeting in metastatic colon cancer: a phase I study of monoclonal antibody F19 against a cell-surface protein of reactive tumor stromal fibroblasts. J Clin Oncol 1994, **12**, 1193–203.

118. Murray JL, Macey DJ, Kasi LP, *et al.* Phase II radioimmunotherapy trial with 131I-CC49 in colorectal cancer. Cancer 1994, **73**, 1057–66.

119. Meredith RF, Partridge EE, Alvarez RD, *et al.* Intraperitoneal radioimmunotherapy of ovarian cancer with lutetium-177-CC49. J Nucl Med 1996, **37**, 1491–6.

120. Welt S, Scott AM, Divgi CR, *et al.* Phase I/II study of iodine 125-labeled monoclonal antibody A33 in patients with advanced colon cancer. J Clin Oncol 1996, **14**, 1787–97.

121. Knox SJ, Goris ML, Tempero M, *et al.* Phase II trial of yttrium-90-DOTA-biotin pretargeted by NR-LU-10 antibody/streptavidin in patients with metastatic colon cancer. Clin Cancer Res 2000, **6**, 406–14.

122. Pai-Scherf LH, Carrasquillo JA, Paik C, *et al.* Imaging and phase I study of 111In- and 90Y-labeled anti-Lewis Y monoclonal antibody B3 (In Process Citation). Clin Cancer Res 2000, **6**, 1720–30.

123. Zeng ZC, Tang ZY, Liu KD, *et al.* Improved long-term survival for unresectable hepatocellular carcinoma

(HCC) with a combination of surgery and intrahepatic arterial infusion of 131I-anti-HCC mAb. Phase I/II clinical trials. J Cancer Res Clin Oncol 1998, **124**, 275–80.

124. Cheung NK, Kushner BH, Yeh SD, *et al.* 3F8 monoclonal antibody treatment of patients with stage 4 neuroblastoma: a phase II study. Int J Oncol 1998, **12**, 1299–306.

125. Bigner DD, Brown MT, Friedman AH, *et al.* Iodine-131-labeled antitenascin monoclonal antibody 81C6 treatment of patients with recurrent malignant gliomas: phase I trial results. J Clin Oncol 1998, **16**, 2202–12.

126. Akabani G, Cokgor I, Coleman RE, *et al.* Dosimetry and dose-response relationships in newly diagnosed patients with malignant gliomas treated with iodine-131-labeled anti-tenascin monoclonal antibody 81C6 therapy. Int J Radiat Oncol Biol Phys 2000, **46**, 947–58.

127. Brown MT, Coleman RE, Friedman AH, *et al.* Intrathecal 131I-labeled antitenascin monoclonal antibody 81C6 treatment of patients with leptomeningeal neoplasms or primary brain tumor resection cavities with subarachnoid communication: phase I trial results. Clin Cancer Res 1996, **2**, 963–72.

128. Meredith RF, Khazaeli MB, Plott WE, *et al.* Phase II study of dual 131I-labeled monoclonal antibody therapy with interferon in patients with metastatic colorectal cancer. Clin Cancer Res 1996, **2**, 1811–18.

129. Alvarez RD, Partridge EE, Khazaeli MB, *et al.* Intraperitoneal radioimmunotherapy of ovarian cancer with 177Lu-CC49: a phase I/II study. Gynecol Oncol 1997, **65**, 94–101.

130. Nicholson S, Gooden CS, Hird V, *et al.* Radioimmunotherapy after chemotherapy compared to chemotherapy alone in the treatment of advanced ovarian cancer: a matched analysis. Oncol Rep 1998, **5**, 223–6.

131. Rosenblum MG, Verschraegen CF, Murray JL, *et al.* Phase I study of 90Y-labeled B72.3 intraperitoneal administration in patients with ovarian cancer: effect of dose and EDTA coadministration on pharmacokinetics and toxicity. Clin Cancer Res 1999, **5**, 953–61.

132. Meredith RF, Khazaeli MB, Macey DJ, *et al.* Phase II study of interferon-enhanced 131I-labeled high affinity CC49 monoclonal antibody therapy in patients with metastatic prostate cancer. Clin Cancer Res 1999, **5**, 3254s–8s.

133. Divgi CR, Bander NH, Scott AM, *et al.* Phase I/II radioimmunotherapy trial with iodine-131-labeled monoclonal antibody G250 in metastatic renal cell carcinoma. Clin Cancer Res 1998, **4**, 2729–39.

134. Lane DM, Eagle KF, Begent RH, *et al.* Radioimmunotherapy of metastatic colorectal tumours with iodine-131-labelled antibody to carcinoembryonic antigen: phase I/II study with comparative biodistribution of intact and F(ab')₂ antibodies. Br J Cancer 1994, **70**, 521–5.

135. Bigner DD, Brown M, Coleman RE, *et al.* Phase I studies of treatment of malignant gliomas and neoplastic meningitis with 131I-radiolabeled monoclonal antibodies anti-tenascin 81C6 and anti-chondroitin proteoglycan sulfate Me1-14 F (ab')₂—a preliminary report. J Neurooncol 1995, **24**, 109–22.

136. Juweid ME, Hajjar G, Stein R, *et al.* Initial experience with high-dose radioimmunotherapy of metastatic medullary thyroid cancer using 131I-MN-14 F(ab')₂ anti-carcinoembryonic antigen MAb and AHSCR [see comments]. J Nucl Med 2000, **41**, 93–103.

137. Denardo SJ, O'Grady LF, Richman CM, *et al.* Radioimmunotherapy for advanced breast cancer using I-131-ChL6 antibody. Anticancer Res 1997, **17**, 1745–51.

138. Wong JY, Somlo G, Odom-Maryon T, *et al.* Initial clinical experience evaluating yttrium-90-chimeric T84.66 anticarcinoembryonic antigen antibody and autologous hematopoietic stem cell support in patients with carcinoembryonic antigen-producing metastatic breast cancer. Clin Cancer Res 1999, **5**, 3224s–31s.

139. Meredith RF, Khazaeli MB, Plott WE, *et al.* Phase I trial of iodine-131-chimeric B72.3 (human IgG4) in metastatic colorectal cancer [see comments]. J Nucl Med 1992, **33**, 23–9.

140. Weiden PL, Breitz HB, Seiler CA, *et al.* Rhenium-186-labeled chimeric antibody NR-LU-13: pharmacokinetics, biodistribution and immunogenicity relative to murine analog NR-LU-10. J Nucl Med 1993, **34**, 2111–19.

141. Wong JY, Chu DZ, Yamauchi D, *et al.* Dose escalation trial of indium-111-labeled anti-carcinoembryonic antigen chimeric monoclonal antibody (chimeric T84.66) in presurgical colorectal cancer patients. J Nucl Med 1998, **39**, 2097–104.

142. Juweid M, Swayne LC, Sharkey RM, *et al.* Prospects of radioimmunotherapy in epithelial ovarian cancer: results with iodine-131-labeled murine and humanized MN-14 anti-carcinoembryonic antigen monoclonal antibodies. Gynecol Oncol 1997, **67**, 259–71.

143. Molthoff CF, Prinssen HM, Kenemans P, *et al.* Escalating protein doses of chimeric monoclonal antibody MOv18 immunoglobulin G in ovarian carcinoma patients: a phase I study. Cancer 1997, **80**, 2712–20.

144. Buijs WC, Tibben JG, Boerman OC, *et al.* Dosimetric analysis of chimeric monoclonal antibody cMOv18IgG in ovarian carcinoma patients after intraperitoneal and intravenous administration. Eur J Nucl Med 1998, **25**, 1552–61.

145. Steffens MG, Boerman OC, de Mulder PH, *et al.* Phase I radioimmunotherapy of metastatic renal cell carcinoma with 131I-labeled chimeric monoclonal antibody G250. Clin Cancer Res 1999, **5**, 3268s–74s.

146. Kossman SE, Scheinberg DA, Jurcic JG, *et al.* A phase I trial of humanized monoclonal antibody HuM195 (anti-CD33) with lose-dose interleukin 2 in acute myelogenous leukemia. Clin Cancer Res 1999, **5**, 2748–55.

147. Sgouros G, Ballangrud AM, Jurcic JG, *et al.* Pharmacokinetics and dosimetry of an alpha-particle emitter labeled antibody: 213Bi-HuM195 (anti-CD33) in patients with leukemia. J Nucl Med 1999, **40**, 1935–46.

148. Colcher D, Goel A, Pavlinkova G, *et al.* Effects of genetic engineering on the pharmacokinetics of antibodies. Quart J Nucl Med 1999, **43**, 132–9.

149. Wolff EA, Esselstyn J, Maloney G, *et al.* Human monoclonal antibody homodimers. Effect of valency on *in vitro* and *in vivo* antibacterial activity. J Immunol 1992, **148**, 2469–74.

150. Casey JL, King DJ, Chaplin LC, *et al.* Preparation, characterisation and tumour targeting of cross-linked divalent and trivalent anti-tumour Fab' fragments. Br J Cancer 1996, **74**, 1397–405.

151. Kashmiri SV, Shu L, Padlan EA, *et al.* Generation, characterization, and *in vivo* studies of humanized anticarcinoma antibody CC49. Hybridoma 1995, **14**, 461–73.

152. Hutzell P, Kashmiri S, Colcher D, *et al.* Generation and characterization of a recombinant/chimeric B72.3 (human gamma 1). Cancer Res 1991, **51**, 181–9.

153. Lee HS, Shu L, De Pascalis R, *et al.* Generation and characterization of a novel single-gene-encoded single-chain immunoglobulin molecule with antigen binding activity and effector functions. Mol Immunol 1999, **36**, 61–71.

154. Hu S, Shively L, Raubitschek A, *et al.* Minibody: a novel engineered anti-carcinoembryonic antigen antibody fragment (single-chain Fv-C_H3) which exhibits rapid, high-level targeting of xenografts. Cancer Res 1996, **56**, 3055–61.

155. Kurucz I, Titus JA, Jost CR, *et al.* Retargeting of CTL by an efficiently refolded bispecific single-chain Fv dimer produced in bacteria. J Immunol 1995, **154**, 4576–82.

156. Kostelny SA, Cole MS, Tso JY. Formation of a bispecific antibody by the use of leucine zippers. J Immunol 1992, **148**, 1547–53.

157. Pack P, Pluckthun A. Miniantibodies: use of amphipathic helices to produce functional, flexibly linked dimeric FV fragments with high avidity in *Escherichia coli*. Biochemistry 1992, **31**, 1579–84.

158. Ito W, Kurosawa Y. Development of an artificial antibody system with multiple valency using an Fv fragment fused to a fragment of protein A. J Biol Chem 1993, **268**, 20668–75.

6 | *Combined external beam radiotherapy and radioimmunotherapy*

David Raben and Donald J. Buchsbaum

Introduction

Clinical experience and success with radioimmunotherapy (RIT) utilizing radiolabeled monoclonal antibodies (mAbs) has evolved rapidly over the last decade, facilitating recent investigations into the feasibility of combining RIT with external beam radiation therapy (EBRT) to improve therapeutic outcome for patients with both hematological and solid malignancies. RIT is a form of systemic radiotherapy in which there is preferential tumor uptake due to the binding of radiolabeled antibody to tumor-associated antigens or receptors, but there is also nonspecific distribution that results in a normal tissue and whole-body radiation dose deposition that limits the quantity of radiolabeled mAb that can be administered. RIT has potential advantages over alternative systemic treatments due to its tumor specificity. It may have a secondary role in the treatment of local disease in combination with surgery or EBRT. RIT results in continuous dose delivery at a low dose rate that is exponentially decreasing, compared to high-dose-rate EBRT. The use of RIT in clinical trials has resulted in impressive response rates and durable complete remissions in patients with B-cell lymphomas (1–6). Excellent outcomes have been reported with the use of high-dose RIT in combination with bone marrow or stem cell transplantation (7–9). In some institutions, RIT has replaced total body irradiation (TBI) as part of the preparatory regimen for bone marrow transplants in patients with B-cell lymphomas (7). The clinical efficacy of RIT for treatment of solid tumors has been undermined by their lower radiosensitivity compared to B-cell lymphoma, limitations from bone marrow suppression, low uptake of radiolabeled antibody, and the restricted diffusion capacity of antibodies into large tumors, which results in an inadequate radiation-absorbed dose delivered to the tumor. However, these same limitations have led to insights into improved delivery and targeting of either intact antibodies, antibody fragments, or peptides for treatment of solid tumors.

A strategy to enhance therapeutic efficacy is to combine therapeutic modalities, such as EBRT and chemotherapy, in an effort to produce synergistic or additive effects. An increase in tumor control rate might be achieved with combined therapies of EBRT and RIT as compared to EBRT alone, since these therapies have different normal tissue toxicities and RIT may be effective against local, locally disseminated, or metastatic disease. The concept is that a combined radiation treatment, not unlike implant brachytherapy and EBRT, may improve the therapeutic outcome. Thus, RIT could be considered as a boost to conventional EBRT for elimination of minimal residual disease. One major difference between RIT and EBRT is that radiolabeled antibodies have a heterogeneous distribution in most tumors and thus a heterogeneous dose deposition throughout the tumor (10, 11). Furthermore, the radiation dose rate in RIT is relatively low, so that a given radiation dose may be less efficient in producing cell kill than a similar dose given by EBRT, due to increased repair of DNA double-strand breaks with the low-dose-rate radiation(12). However, normal tissue toxicity might decrease more than the tumor response at the low dose rates delivered by RIT (13, 14). Regional or systemic RIT, whose primary toxicity is hemopoietic suppression, in combination with EBRT might result in an increase in local and metastatic tumor control, without a reduction in the EBRT dose due to their differences in normal tissue toxicity. There have been some preclinical and clinical studies that have combined RIT with EBRT. The objective of this chapter is to introduce the concept of combination treatment with EBRT and RIT, to discuss the results obtained in preclinical animal model studies and clinical trials, and to put into perspective the potential for this approach in clinical cancer treatment.

External beam radiotherapy

Since the earliest therapeutic applications of X-rays in the late 1800s, important technical advances in the delivery of EBRT have resulted in improved therapeutic outcome in a variety of malignancies. The ability to clearly visualize the tumor and its relationship with surrounding normal tissue through the use of computerized tomography (CT) and magnetic resonance imaging (MRI) have greatly enhanced the precision with which EBRT is rendered. Three-dimensional reconstruction of a patient's external and internal contours enables the radiation oncologist to see the intended tumor target through a beam's eye view, and treatment-planning computers allow for rapid dose calculations and assessment of the optimal treatment plan (Fig. 6.1). Modern treatment machines are equipped with multileaf collimators, large numbers of individually controlled leaves that are moved into the radiation beam to block out normal tissue and assist in conforming the radiation beam around the tumor. Intensity-modulated radiation therapy (IMRT) is accomplished using dynamic multileaf collimators that are moved into and out of the treatment field. Thus, the intensity of the radiation is modified in specific areas during the actual treatment. The advantage of IMRT is its ability to conform the beam around irregularly shaped tumors thus sparing more normal tissue. An example of this would be the treatment of prostate cancer. The prostate lies in close proximity to the rectum. IMRT can assist in directing the beam to curve around the anterior wall of the rectum and thus enable the radiation oncologist to prescribe higher total doses to the prostate gland without fear of causing increased toxicity to the rectum.

Advances in radiobiology have led to altered fractionation schemes that have generally followed one or a combination of two patterns.

1. Hyperfractionation is a strategy whereby multiple fractions per day are given, with a reduction of the dose per fraction by approximately 40 to 50 per cent. The total dose is, therefore, increased approximately 10 to 15 per cent over conventional radiation therapy, and the overall treatment time generally remains about the same. The

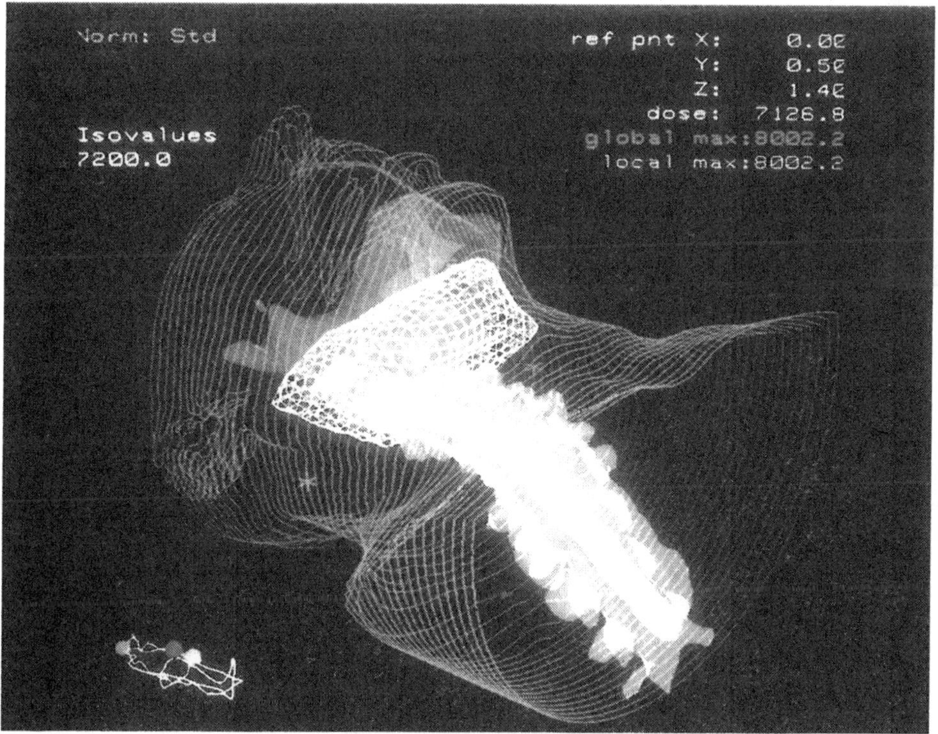

Fig. 6.1 Example of three-dimensional reconstruction of patient with locally advanced squamous cell cancer of the oropharynx. Conformal isodose curve to prescribed dose of 72 Gy surrounds the target volume. (See also 'Plates' section.)

rationale for this alteration in dose per fraction is based on the hypothesis that improved sublethal repair of late-responding tissue occurs, allowing higher total doses of radiation to be given to the tumor. It is also hypothesized that hyperfractionation takes advantage of cell cycle redistribution, improving chances of interfering with cancer cells during radiation-sensitive parts of the cell cycle.

2. Accelerated fractionation attempts to reduce the overall treatment time by delivering multiple fractions per day but only reducing the dose per fraction by approximately 20 to 30 per cent. The intent is to limit tumor cell proliferation.

One approach combines continuous hyperfractionated accelerated radiotherapy (CHART). A recent British multicenter randomized trial compared conventional fractionated radiotherapy (60 Gy in 30 fractions over 6 weeks) to CHART (54 Gy in 36 fractions for 12 days). The trial accrued 563 patients and revealed a significant overall survival advantage for the CHART approach. This was primarily seen in patients with squamous cell histology (15). The advantages of this approach include not only short treatment time with minimal treatment breaks, which is more convenient for the patient, but also potentially decreased cost for the patient. Retrospective and prospective randomized studies have reported superior local control and survival outcomes with the use of altered fractionation regimens over once-daily treatments (16–18).

Although great strides have been made with the use of EBRT in the treatment of solid and hemopoietic malignancies, there remains considerable room for improvement in regards to local/regional control rates. Tumors of the central nervous system continue to represent a therapeutic challenge. Gliomas respond modestly to EBRT doses in the range of 60 Gy. Brachytherapy or radiosurgical boosts appear to provide some increase in local control and survival but their applications are limited to patients whose tumors are surgically accessible, or to patients with small tumor dimensions encompassable by stereotactic beams. RIT in conjunction with EBRT might augment the effects of EBRT. Cancers of the head/neck and lung are difficult to treat with EBRT due to important surrounding structures including major salivary glands, optic structures, esophagus, and spinal cord. Local control rates in lung cancer after EBRT, as measured by bronchoscopic biopsies, are less than 20 per cent (19). Tumors, such as neuroblastomas, have a high propensity for systemic spread and require newer strategies in conjunction with EBRT and chemotherapy to improve outcomes. Hepatomas can be difficult to treat because of the sensitivity of the liver to high doses of EBRT. These are examples of malignancies where the investigation of RIT in conjunction with EBRT might prove to be fruitful. Perhaps, the disadvantages of each strategy would be overcome by the other's advantages and thus improve the therapeutic gain.

Radioimmunotherapy

Antibodies

The development of radiolabeled antibodies that bind to tumor-associated antigens for RIT of cancer has been reviewed elsewhere (20–25). Although mouse mAbs have been the most widely used for RIT studies, the problems related to bone marrow suppression and immunogenicity have resulted in antibody modifications. One approach has been enzymatic cleavage of intact antibodies to form $F(ab')_2$ and Fab fragments, or the use of genetic engineering to produce single-chain antibody (scFv) or diabody molecules and heavy-chain deletions (for example, $\Delta C_H 2$ fragments) (26–30). Genetically engineered humanized antibody constructs (mouse–human chimeric, complementarity-determining region (CDR)-grafted, minibodies) have been produced with longer effective half-lives that may produce a higher tumor uptake and radiation-absorbed dose in tumor (5, 31, 32). These molecules are often less immunogenic, which may allow for repeated dosing.

Determinants of RIT effects and approaches to improve the therapeutic ratio

The therapeutic ratio of RIT depends on the amount of radiation-absorbed dose deposited in tumors versus that in normal tissues. There are a number of pathological and physiological factors that affect the efficacy of RIT (33–38). These may result in poor delivery of radiolabeled antibody to tumor resulting in an unsatisfactory therapeutic ratio. A more favorable biodistribution is desirable with higher concentrations of radiolabeled mAb in tumor than in normal organs.

The biodistribution of intravenously (IV) administered radiolabeled mAbs has been unfavorable in lymphoma patients with splenomegaly or large tumor burdens, resulting in similar localization of antibody in normal organs and tumor (7, 39, 40). Predosing with unlabeled antibody before injection of radiolabeled mAb has improved the biodistribution and pharmacokinetics of radiolabeled antibody (7, 41–43). Improvements in biodistribution of radiolabeled mAb following predosing of unlabeled mAb are due to decreased binding to normal B cells in lymphoid tissue and decreased binding to Fc receptors within the reticuloendothelial system as a result of the binding of the preadministered unlabeled antibody.

In addition to predosing, other areas of research have been pursued for the purpose of improving the therapeutic ratio (22, 44). In addition to the genetic engineering of humanized antibody constructs, other modifications include: (1) more stable bifunctional chelating agents; (2) pretargeting strategies; (3) hyperthermia, external beam radiation, and physiological manipulations that may increase tumor blood flow and vascular permeability; (4) adjuvant use of radiosensitizers or radioprotectors, growth factors, and cytokines; and (5) integration with gene therapy in a manner that may amplify tumor targeting or produce radiosensitization. Another very promising approach is local/regional delivery of the radiolabeled mAb as described in the next section.

Through efforts in experimental animal studies, the feasibility of direct intralesional administration of radiolabeled antibodies or peptides has been demonstrated. This has resulted in significantly higher tumor radioactivity deposition compared to normal tissue uptake. Human head and neck squamous cell carcinomas are generally radiosensitive. However, there are limitations with regard to the total tumor dose that one can deliver because of the significant radiation-absorbed dose to surrounding normal tissues resulting in severe late toxicity. In this regard, recent preclinical studies with nude mice bearing subcutaneous head and neck squamous cell carcinoma xenografts have demonstrated the advantage of local intralesional injections of antibodies labeled with the pure high-energy beta emitter yttrium-90 (^{90}Y) compared to IV injection. Intralesional delivery of ^{90}Y-labeled IgM resulted in a significantly higher radiation-absorbed dose within the tumor volume with decreased normal tissue absorbed dose in comparison to IV delivered radiolabeled antibody (45). Similar strategies have been applied to the intratumoral injections of radiolabeled peptides into human cancer xenografts. RC-160, a somatostatin analog, was labeled with rhenium-188 (^{188}Re, medium energy beta and photon emitter) and used to treat human prostate adenocarcinoma xenografts via direct intralesional

injections. A significant decrease in tumor volume and increased survival were noted with prolonged retention of the radionuclide in the tumor. Importantly, minimal radioactivity was demonstrated in normal tissues such as the spleen, bone, and lungs. In this study, multiple intratumoral administrations of ^{188}Re-labeled RC-160 were employed in providing information for potential therapeutic applications used alone or in combination with EBRT (46).

The main potential benefit of RIT may be for disseminated tumor deposits. For larger tumors, RIT is likely to be suboptimal, as a result of low tumor uptake or heterogeneous intratumor distribution (47). However, a potential benefit of combining RIT and EBRT is the possible reduction of dosimetric nonuniformity in large tumors.

An approach to overcome the nonuniform tumor uptake of radiolabeled mAbs as well as hemopoietic toxicity is through the use of pretargeting strategies in which an unlabeled bifunctional mAb that binds to a tumor-associated antigen and a hapten is administered IV (48). At a later time, when the blood concentration of the bifunctional mAb is low, a radiolabeled low-molecular-weight hapten is injected IV which binds to the preadministered unlabeled mAb localized in the tumor and clears the circulation rapidly through the kidneys, thus producing a low radiation absorbed dose in other normal tissues. This promising approach is in clinical trials (49–51).

Comparisons of RIT and EBRT in preclinical in vivo studies

Prior to combining RIT and EBRT it was important to provide quantitative comparisons of the efficacy of both radiotherapeutic approaches. A comparison of radiolabeled antibody therapy and EBRT in the treatment of human glioma xenografts (52) demonstrated the need for delivery of a threefold greater total dose of ^{90}Y-labeled antibodies to achieve tumor regrowth delays similar to those in multifraction EBRT treatments. This was thought to be due to a large fractionation effect from EBRT, suggesting that the ineffectiveness of radiolabeled antibody in this system was caused by a large dose-rate effect of the low-dose-rate RIT (52). This is similar to findings by Buchsbaum *et al.* using a human colon cancer xenograft model wherein three times the amount of RIT dose with mAb labeled with ^{131}I (medium energy beta and photon emitter) was needed to produce growth delays similar to those with single-fraction EBRT (53). The relative effectiveness per unit dose delivered by ^{131}I-labeled A33 mAb reactive with colon cancers was about one-third of that produced by fractionated EBRT as measured by tumor xenograft regrowth delay (54). However, several investigators reported greater antitumor responses in other tumor types following RIT than for EBRT (55, 56). Certainly, a multitude of factors, including tumor size, hypoxia, radiosensitivity, dose-rate, heterogeneity of intratumor distribution of radiolabeled mAb, etc., would affect responses to RIT or EBRT. Moreover, single-fraction EBRT may also be an inappropriate therapy to compare to RIT especially in hypoxic conditions and is less relevant in a clinical setting. Buras *et al.* (57) compared RIT and EBRT in a nude mouse model containing subcutaneous human colon cancer xenografts. Here, RIT was delivered through intraperitoneal injections of ^{90}Y-labeled anti-carcinoembryonic antigen (anti-CEA) mAb. The radiosensitive human colon cancer line (LS174T) and a more radioresistant human colon cancer line (WiDr) were evaluated for response to RIT in comparison to single-fraction EBRT by serial measurements of size. RIT produced tumor growth delay similar to that of single-fraction EBRT for the LS174T xenografts based on radiation absorbed dose estimates; in contrast RIT was less effective in comparison to single-fraction EBRT for the WiDr xenografts. Conclusions drawn from these studies suggest that RIT can produce biological responses similar to those for EBRT in tumor cell lines that may have a diminished capacity for DNA repair. Explanations for the diminished response seen with RIT in the WiDr line include increased DNA repair capacity in comparison to the LS174T human colon cancer cell line, decreased CEA expression, and possible differences in ^{90}Y distribution within these tumor xenografts (57). Review of conflicting data from other groups in regard to the greater or lesser efficacy of RIT in comparison to either single- or multi-fraction EBRT also suggests a relationship to the different capacities of the tumor cell lines to repair DNA damage, tumor growth rate, cell cycle redistribution, reoxygenation, and uptake of radiolabeled antibody (58).

Combining RIT and EBRT in vitro and in vivo: preclinical studies

With the understanding from the studies described above that RIT has a range of effectiveness based on the DNA repair capacities of various cancer cell lines, it has been demonstrated that by combining RIT with EBRT one could potentially modulate the radiosensitivities of the different cancer cell lines through low-dose-rate and high-dose-rate radiation exposure. Combined high-dose-rate and continuous low-dose-rate irradiation has been evaluated both *in vitro* and *in vivo* in human malignant glioma cell lines (59). Increased cytotoxicity was noted with human U251 glioma cells exposed to media containing tritiated water yielding a dose-rate of 0.03 Gy/hour in combination with fractionated high-dose-rate treatments in comparison to low-dose-rate or high-dose-rate radiation treatments alone. More importantly, *in vivo* experiments with U251 glioma subcutaneous xenografts in nude mice demonstrated that, when high-dose-rate EBRT was combined with either ^{125}I seed brachytherapy at a dose-rate of 0.05 Gy/hour or whole-body continuous low-dose-rate (0.03 Gy/hour) radiation, prolongation of regrowth delay occurred in contrast to either of these modalities delivered alone. Linear quadratic modeling revealed an increase in the beta coefficient of the linear quadratic model for cell killing *in vitro* (59). These preclinical experiments have provided promising results, suggesting that, in select situations, RIT combined with EBRT might improve the therapeutic outcome.

Exploring this concept further, Bender *et al.* (60) demonstrated enhanced cytotoxicity of human glioma cells *in vitro* when treated with ^{125}I-labeled mAb 425 specific for human epidermal growth factor receptor (EGFR) in combination with EBRT. The sequential treatment with EBRT followed by ^{125}I-labeled 425 mAb showed additive effects on cell survival. Interestingly, the greatest effect was seen when the antibody was added at day 2 after EBRT in contrast to no effect when 425 mAb was added 4 or 7 days after radiation. EBRT appeared to increase surface binding of 425 mAb 3–5-fold as compared to untreated cells perhaps due to an increase in EGFR expression (61). Additionally, internalization of ^{125}I-labeled 425 mAb was enhanced in a dose-dependent fashion on the human glioma cell lines tested (U87-MG, A1207) with increasing EBRT doses. Mechanisms behind the additive effects seen with the addition of RIT after EBRT were thought to be a result of the conversion of potentially lethal damage into lethal damage as a result of the internalization of ^{125}I-labeled 425 mAb and delivery of ^{125}I (Auger high linear energy transfer electron emitter) to the nucleus (62). When the interval between the delivery of EBRT and exposure to radiolabeled mAb was too long, the added effects decreased significantly leading to speculation that this was due to DNA repair. Moreover, EBRT induced a mitotic block that resulted in a dose-dependent increase in cell volume. A reduction in cell cycling might promote enhanced ability of ^{125}I-labeled 425 mAb to induce lethal damage. Thus, although the treatments were not concurrent, this data is certainly encouraging in that, the closer these two treatment modalities were to one another, the more enhanced was cytotoxic effect noted. It might have been interesting to evaluate the level of apoptosis as an additional mechanism for enhanced cytotoxicity in this study. The results support the potential adjuvant use of RIT in the treatment of glioma (63). Bone marrow suppression for the combination treatment was similar to that with RIT alone.

The effects of sequential RIT and fractionated EBRT have been assessed in human colon cancer xenografts as summarized in Table 6.1. Buchegger *et al.* (64) administered ^{131}I-labeled anti-CEA F(ab′)$_2$ fragments in two doses of 1.5 mCi via the tail vein in nude mice bearing two human colon cancer xenografts (Co112 and LS174T). The first injection was administered on the last day of radiation therapy followed by a second injection 4 days later. The results were compared to those in animals treated with radiolabeled antibody fragments alone or EBRT alone. EBRT doses were either 16 or 25 Gy in five fractions over 5 days (Table 6.1). Biodistribution studies were performed in animals injected with ^{131}I-labeled anti-CEA F(ab′)$_2$ compared to control groups receiving ^{125}I-labeled control F(ab′)$_2$. An uptake of 11 per cent injected dose/gram of tumor (% i.d./g) was measured in Co112 xenografts, which increased to 16% i.d./g after 16 Gy of EBRT. This slightly enhanced tumor uptake of radiolabeled anti-CEA antibody was noted only when low amounts of antibody were injected. For LS174T xenografts, uptake into tumors was reported as 10.6% i.d./g when low amounts of antibody were injected. Tumor uptake was reduced to 5.5% i.d./g when larger amounts of antibody fragments were employed. Uptake

was not increased when tumors were pretreated with 25 Gy EBRT. In the Co112 tumor xenografts, transient regression of tumor was noted in all mice treated with EBRT doses of radiation up to 50 Gy. In experiments combining radiation therapy with RIT, an additive therapeutic effect was noted through increased tumor regrowth delay and local control (64). Significant long-term remissions were noted in several experiments with Co112 xenografts when EBRT and RIT were combined. The number of long-term tumor remissions increased with increasing EBRT dose. Results were significantly better than for EBRT alone, RIT alone, or EBRT combined with radiolabeled control antibodies. No mice bearing Co112 tumors were locally controlled with a 32-Gy EBRT dose alone, while 32 Gy of EBRT combined with RIT produced 100 per cent complete regressions. The combined treatment of LS174T tumors with 25-Gy EBRT and RIT also showed a tumor regrowth delay significantly longer than with EBRT or RIT alone or EBRT followed by RIT. One limitation of this study is that both EBRT and RIT were administered in high doses per fraction. Skin toxicity was noted after EBRT and hematological toxicity, as expected, coupled with some early weight loss was noted after RIT. Local skin toxicity was only noted with total doses above 25 Gy of fractionated EBRT. No additional skin toxicity was noted with the combination of EBRT and RIT as compared to RIT alone at the varying dose levels studied. Thus, adding RIT may allow one to reduce the EBRT dose by 10–20 per cent without a loss of tumor control thereby increasing the therapeutic gain. By reducing the dose of RIT the therapeutic gain could be increased further by the reduction of acute and late side-effects. Alternatively, the combination of RIT and EBRT might allow an increase of the tumor radiation absorbed dose while maintaining acceptable normal tissue toxicity.

The timing effects of RIT combined with EBRT were assessed in athymic nude mice bearing Co112 human colon carcinoma xenografts (65). EBRT (30 Gy,

Table 6.1 Preclinical studies combining EBRT and RIT

Tumor model	Radiolabeled mAb	RIT dose	EBRT dose	EBRT/RIT sequencing	Ref.
Colon (Co112, LS174T)	^{131}I-anti-CEA F(ab′)$_2$	1.5 mCi + 1.5 mCi	16 or 25 Gy (5 fractions/5 days)	EBRT → RIT	64
Colon (Co112)	^{131}I-anti-CEA	0.3 mCi × 3 (weekly)	30 Gy (10 fractions/12 days)	RIT → EBRT RIT + EBRT EBRT → RIT*	65
Colon (LS174T liver metastases)	^{131}I-anti-CEA	0.15 mCi × 2 (2.5 days)	30 Gy (15 fractions/17 days)	EBRT → RIT → EBRT → RIT	66

* Immediately or after 2 weeks.

10 fractions over 12 days) was combined with thrice weekly IV injections of 200 μCi ^{131}I-labeled anti-CEA mAbs in four different treatment schedules (Table 6.1). RIT was given either prior to, concurrently with, immediately after, or 2 weeks after EBRT. The longest tumor growth inhibition, and the smallest tumor volumes, were observed in mice treated by concurrent administration of EBRT and RIT, which was a substantially greater effect than for EBRT or RIT alone, or the other treatment combinations. EBRT immediately followed by RIT produced the smallest tumor volumes among the sequential therapy schedules. The toxicity of all combined regimens was minimal. Thus, RIT can produce a good antitumor effect when given concurrently with EBRT. RIT could also provide the advantages of potentially treating micrometastatic disease in distant sites.

The combination of RIT and fractionated radiotherapy could also be utilized as a therapeutic strategy in patients with metastatic cancer. A significant percentage of patients with colorectal cancer will develop liver metastasis as the first site of local/regional failure. With multiple liver metastases, treatment options are limited generally to either IV or intraarterial therapy. Vogel *et al.* (66) evaluated the utility of combining RIT and fractionated EBRT to nude mice bearing human colon cancer engrafted liver metastases. This was based on previous work showing that concomitant administration of EBRT and RIT resulted in the longest delays of tumor regrowth in comparison to sequential EBRT and RIT (67). The CEA-expressing human colon cancer line LS174T was used for engraftment into the spleens of nude mice, which subsequently resulted in liver metastases. In this regard, EBRT and RIT were given simultaneously over a 17-day period with treatment beginning 2 weeks after engraftment. Five fractions of 2 Gy of EBRT were delivered over a 2.5 day period and then the first dose of RIT consisting of 150 μCi ^{131}I-labeled anti-CEA mAb was administered by tail vein injection (Table 6.1). Another 10 Gy of EBRT at five fractions over 5 days was then started on day 6 followed by an additional injection of 150 μCi ^{131}I-labeled anti-CEA mAb. An additional 10 Gy of radiation was delivered in five fractions starting at day 13. The EBRT was focused on the liver. Increased survival was seen in 5 of 11 mice after the combined therapy. The majority of the mice (8 of 10) had died at 60 days in the untreated control group. Importantly the majority of mice treated with RIT or EBRT alone were dead at 79 days. Combined treatment resulted in a cure rate of 45 per cent, which was a statistically significant

improvement in comparison to RIT or EBRT alone. The greatest survival increase was seen in mice treated 1 week after engraftment. In contrast, RIT initiated 2 weeks after engraftment revealed a survival increase compared to that in untreated controls, but the number of long-term survivors was similar to background. No survival increase was seen in mice treated 3 weeks after engraftment. An expected improvement in survival in these studies occurred in animals with smaller tumor nodules in comparison to mice with larger tumors. This was thought to be due to nonhomogeneous antibody distribution and hypoxia in the larger tumors. Hematological toxicity was noted in mice receiving RIT alone or combined with EBRT. Weight loss was also noted in mice treated with RIT with recovery at approximately 2 weeks. Skin toxicity with EBRT was noted in the dose range of 40–70 Gy (grade I/II). Toxicity usually appeared 2 months after treatment initiation. Several mice died from late toxicity 3 months after receiving 50–70 Gy of EBRT with noted development of ascites at autopsy.

This animal study was important for several reasons, including the fact that a clinically relevant fractionated dose of EBRT was employed. Unfortunately, a significant portion of the abdomen was exposed to radiation that certainly would enhance late toxicity. In the clinic a more conformal radiation therapy approach to the liver with significant sparing of surrounding normal organs would be desirable in an effort to reduce both organ and bone marrow toxicity if patients were to be treated in combination with RIT. Additionally, RIT was shown to cure a high percentage of mice that would have otherwise died of liver metastases (> 60 per cent).

The combination of EBRT and RIT may produce enhanced toxicity in selected situations. Wang *et al.*(68) observed temporary veno-occlusive disease in 3 of 3 beagle dogs treated with 30 Gy to the whole liver, delivered in 2 Gy fractions over 3 weeks. Reversible bone marrow toxicity was noted after 2 injections of 18.5 MBq per kg body weight ^{90}Y-labeled ZCE025 anti-CEA mAb in 3 of 3 dogs tested. The antibody injections were administered 1 week apart. When 3 dogs were treated with EBRT followed by RIT added during the last 2 weeks of EBRT, significant radiation hepatitis developed, starting at approximately 35 days after the end of treatment. Two dogs required euthanasia secondary to terminal liver failure at approximately day 90 after treatment. Radiolabeled ZCE025 previously demonstrated high liver uptake from serial scans with gamma camera imaging. Combination of liver radiation and RIT did cause enhanced changes in lymphocyte and platelet levels. The estimated combined dose of EBRT and RIT in this series of experiments was 36 Gy, resulting in lethal radiation hepatitis in 2/3 dogs receiving this combined treatment. This is a dose that is in a range that has resulted in the development of radiation hepatitis in humans. This might not be representative of what might occur in human clinical trials with the use of antibodies that have improved targeting to either tumor metastases or primary tumors of the liver. Smaller antibody fragments or radiolabeled peptides might provide more rapid elimination and better diffusion into tumor thus reducing the amount of normal liver exposed to radiation. One could certainly consider reducing the volume of liver exposed to EBRT using conformal techniques as well as reducing the dose of EBRT when combining it either sequentially or concurrently with RIT.

Dose–response relationship and radiosensitivity to RIT

It is more difficult to establish a radiation dose–response relationship for clinical RIT than for EBRT since the dose calculations are subject to more uncertainty, the radiation absorbed dose is usually much more heterogeneous, and the probability for cure depends on the regions receiving the least dose which may be underdosed (69). There are also several physiological and biological factors such as oxygenation status and proliferation rate that are usually not included in the dose calculations (47, 70, 71). Possible methods to reduce the heterogeneity in dose deposition include the use of combined modality therapy, fractionated RIT, or RIT and fractionated EBRT as discussed below (71). Other approaches include the use of smaller targeting molecules such as radiolabeled antibody fragments or radiolabeled haptens, and radionuclides with higher energies and emission ranges such as ^{90}Y and ^{188}Re (47).

The extended survival of some lymphoma patients treated with low-dose RIT or high-dose RIT and bone marrow transplantation after failing conventional therapies is encouraging (7–9). Tumor doses have ranged from approximately 18.5–200 cGy/mCi in patients with non-Hodgkin's lymphoma with variable relationship between tumor response and estimated tumor dose (72). The greater success in treating lymphomas than other solid tumors is probably related to

their greater radiosensitivity, and susceptibility to low-dose-rate radiation and antibody-induced apoptosis. These factors may explain in part the relatively high response rate at relatively low tumor doses that has been observed.

High-dose RIT for patients with gastrointestinal tumors has resulted in substantially fewer objective responses than achieved in patients with lymphomas and no complete remissions (73). Local/regional rather than IV administration of radiolabeled antibodies allows higher radiation absorbed doses to be delivered without excess toxicity. Central nervous system (CNS) malignancies, which are often relatively resistant to EBRT, have shown responses to RIT, but the doses delivered are generally higher than those tolerated with EBRT (69).

The results of intraperitoneal (IP) RIT for ovarian cancer suggest both a radionuclide dose and tumor size dependence. Patients receiving less than 50 mCi ^{131}I-2G3 mAb progressed, whereas 75 per cent of those given ≥ 50 mCi experienced palliation of ascites (74). It has been reported that, the smaller the size of tumor masses, the better the response to IP RIT (75, 76). No objective responses were noted among patients with tumors ≥ 2 cm whereas 9/16 patients with smaller measurable nodules and 50 per cent of patients with microscopic disease responded to therapy.

It has been reported that the CC49 anti-TAG-72 antibody labeled with lutetium-177 (^{177}Lu, medium energy beta and photon emitter) and administered IP resulted in higher radiation absorbed doses and greater efficacy for ovarian cancer than when the antibody was labeled with ^{131}I or ^{90}Y and injected IV for prostate, lung, breast, and gastrointestinal malignancies (73, 77, 78). The greater radiosensitivity of ovarian cancer compared to that of other adenocarcinomas is also suggested by other RIT studies where IV ^{131}I-MN-14 therapy resulted in objective responses in ovarian cancer patients, but not in patients with other CEA-reactive tumors (79, 80).

A considerable amount of effort has been put into radiobiological modeling to explore combination RIT and EBRT strategies for treatment of disseminated malignancies with different radiosensitivity and patterns of metastatic spread. One of these strategies has focused on delivering radiolabeled antibodies in conjunction with TBI followed by bone marrow rescue (81, 82). External beam TBI would be used to treat tumor cells that escape RIT. These modeling studies have suggested that RIT and TBI would be superior to either component used alone and would predict for a high tumor curability in the treatment of disseminated solid malignancies. The dose of TBI is dependent on tumor radiosensitivity with TBI dose increasing as the radiosensitivity decreases. The optimal dose of radionuclide administered would depend on the tumor radiosensitivity, the amount of microscopic disease present, and the uptake of the targeted molecules as well as the TBI dose. Localized EBRT might also be required if a tumor mass ≥ 1 cm is present. Mathematical modeling assumed uniformity of radionuclide distribution within each tumor. This is unlikely to be the case clinically; however, combination EBRT and RIT strategies may counteract the heterogeneity problems that RIT alone would encounter.

RIT effects on normal tissues

Normal organ dose tolerances for RIT are not well defined but appear to be higher than the $TD_{5/5}$ for fractionated EBRT (69). Therefore, most organs should be less sensitive to the lower-dose-rate irradiation from RIT than to high-dose-rate EBRT. The dose-limiting toxicity for systemic and IP RIT not followed by bone marrow transplantation has been bone marrow suppression. In high-dose RIT studies, cardiopulmonary (40) and hepatic (83–85) toxicity have become dose-limiting when the limitations of hematological toxicity are overcome by using bone marrow or peripheral blood stem cell transplantation. The late toxicity that has been observed after high-dose systemic RIT with ^{131}I-labeled antibodies (40) has been abnormal thyroid function.

Clinical applications of combination RIT and EBRT

There are several published studies in which combination treatment with EBRT and RIT has been used, as discussed below. These include CNS tumors, neuroblastoma, head and neck cancer, and hepatoma. Other potential cancers for combination EBRT and RIT include localized pancreatic cancer and lung cancer (Fig. 6.2), or metastatic prostate cancer and breast cancer.

CNS tumors

Several antibodies, radionuclides, and routes of administration have been tested in the RIT of CNS disease.

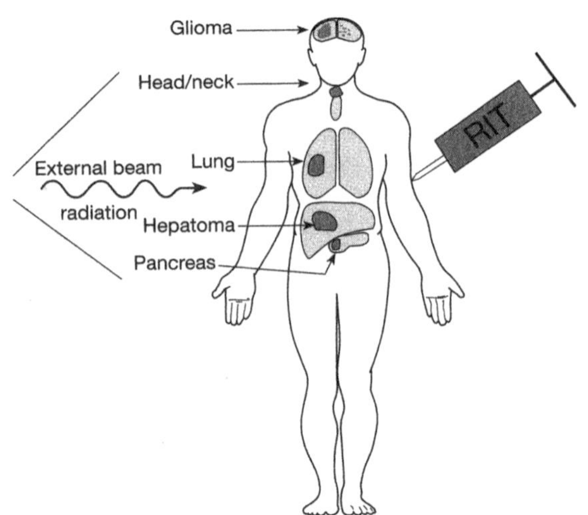

Fig. 6.2 Examples of current treatment sites (glioma, head/neck, hepatoma) and potential treatment sites (pancreas, lung) for combination EBRT and RIT.

These studies are summarized in Table 6.2. Brady *et al.*(63) reported a prolongation of overall survival in patients with glioma treated with surgery, EBRT, and RIT with ^{125}I-labeled mAb 425, which binds to EGFR, compared to surgery and EBRT only (Table 6.2). EBRT is known to break down the blood–brain barrier in brain tumors in patients (86) and thus might increase mAb accumulation after systemic injection. Riva *et al.* (87) used direct intralesional injections of anti-tenascin ^{131}I-labeled mAbs BC-2 and BC-4 intracranially in patients with malignant gliomas. A significant portion of these patients were treated in the recurrent setting after failing previous combinations of surgery and EBRT. Multiple courses of intralesional injections of ^{131}I-labeled mAbs in patients with glioma were delivered with modest adverse affects and a very favorable median survival of 23 months with a response rate of 52 per cent (87). Follow-up studies in a similar patient population incorporated ^{90}Y-labeled BC-4 in an effort to improve radiation penetration into the tumor or tumor cavity; the maximum tolerated dose was 25 mCi (88). The most favorable outcomes were observed in cases with small tumor burden. Thus, this study demonstrated the potential benefits of direct local/regional injections of radiolabeled mAbs as an adjuvant treatment in the clinic. The hypothesis is that the radiolabeled mAbs will bind to the microscopic infiltrates of tumor cells that have spread from the detectable tumor mass into normal brain, which cannot be eradicated by surgery or EBRT. Concurrent or sequential RIT with EBRT may result in increased

Table 6.2   Clinical studies combining EBRT and RIT

No. patients	Radiolabeled antibody	RIT dose	EBRT dose	EBRT/RIT sequencing	Ref.
Disease: glioma					
25	^{125}I-mAb 425	35–90 mCi/infusion/IV (total dose range, 40–224 mCi)	Mean dose, 61 Gy	EBRT → (4–6 wks) → RIT	63
20	^{90}Y-mAb BC-4 Anti-tenascin	5–30 mCI intralesional; mean dose to tumor cavity: 3200 cGy/mCi	Not stated	Surgery → EBRT Recurrence ⇻ Surgery → RIT	88
105	^{131}I-mAb BC-2, BC-4 Anti-tenascin	Mean dose: 54 mCI/ intralesional	55–65 Gy	(a) Surgery → EBRT → RIT (b) Surgery → EBRT → Recurrence ⇻ Surgery → RIT	87
Disease: neuroblastoma					
5	^{131}I-MIBG	5.2 Gy absorbed tumor dose/IV	TBI: 12.6 Gy, 23.4 Gy; EBRT*	Chemotherapy → Surgery → TBI → RIT → EBRT*	89
Disease: head/neck (tonsil)					
1	Biotinylated anti-CEA + avidin + ^{90}Y-DOTA–biotin + ^{111}In-DOTA–biotin	2.59 GBq [90]Y + 74 MBq ^{111}In-DOTA–biotin/IV	70 Gy	EBRT → RIT	91
Disease: hepatoma					
105[†]	^{131}I-antiferritin	(a) Single-dose escalation (30–150 mCi/mCi)/IV	21 Gy (3 Gy 4×/wk) to whole liver	(a) RTOG 79-28: EBRT + adriamycin/5FU → monthly adriamycin/5FU → single-dose RIT	92
		(b) 30 mCi on day 0; mCi on day 5; total dose: ~ 200 mCi/IV	20 21 Gy (3 Gy 4×/wk) to whole liver	(b) RTOG 83-01: adriamycin/5FU → 4 cycles of RIT (polyclonal)	
		(c) Same as (b)/IV	21 Gy (3 Gy 4×/wk) to whole liver	(c) RTOG 83-11: EBRT + adriamycin/5FU → 4 cycles of RIT (polyclonal)[‡]	

* EBRT in one patient only (1.8 Gy twice daily).
[†] Total in three sequential studies.
[‡] Higher doses of adriamycin used; RIT doses modified if grade 3/4 hematological toxicity occurred.

tumor radiation absorbed dose with relative sparing of surrounding normal brain.

Pediatric malignancies

Neuroblastomas are radiosensitive tumors and thus provide an optimal setting in which to study combination RIT and TBI, as this tumor tends to gravitate to bone and bone marrow. Amin *et al.* (82) provided a modeling of different combined RIT and TBI schedules that would produce the same effect on normal tissue, assuming an 'α/β ratio' of 3 Gy for late responding normal tissues. From this modeling data, optimal combination schedules for tumor groups with varying radiosensitivities have been derived with increasing TBI dose required as the tumor becomes more radioresistant. Tumor uptake levels in which the 90 and 50 per cent cure probabilities are obtainable were provided suggesting that small differences in tumor uptake levels

impact significantly on cure probabilities. Difficulties in optimizing the various combinations of RIT and TBI become even more complex when considering a scenario of disseminated metastatic cancers with different tumor sizes. Amin *et al.* (89) provided elegant theoretical data for optimum combination strategies for different tumor sizes with differing intrinsic radiosensitivities. It was suggested that, for tumors with given radiosensitivities, the probabilities of tumor cure are dependent on the proportions of TBI and radionuclide therapy used and that it is variable when metastatic patterns are different for tumors with similar radiosensitivities. For a patient with a radiosensitive tumor with distribution 3 (in fig. 7 of reference 89), TBI would be required with an increased emphasis on targeted RIT for optimal outcome. This is in contrast to a patient with a more radioresistant tumor with a similar metastatic distribution pattern who would require a higher dose delivered from the TBI regimen than from RIT.

Combination RIT and TBI has recently been translated into the clinic in a pilot study of children suffering from stage IV neuroblastoma. Patients were treated with ^{131}I-labeled meta-iodobenzyl guanidine (^{131}I-MIBG), which exhibits uptake in most neuroblastomas, with a quantity designed to give a whole-body absorbed radiation dose of approximately 2 Gy administered on day 0 (Table 6.2). Scintigraphy was performed to determine the accumulation of ^{131}I-MIBG in the body. Ten days later, a chemoablative regimen was delivered, followed by TBI on days 12–15 at 1.8 Gy fractions for a maximum dose of 12.6 Gy delivered in a twice-daily fashion over 4 days. Patients then underwent bone marrow transplantation, either autologous or allogeneic. Localized EBRT was given to a patient who had a residual tumor mass. The study indicated that the treatment was well tolerated with no toxic deaths. The primary toxicity was, as expected, hematological. All patients suffered from infective complications as well as severe mucosal reactions. One patient experienced graft versus host disease following an allogeneic bone marrow transplant. Three patients at the time of this report were alive and disease-free at 9, 14, and 15 months after treatment. Two patients subsequently relapsed and died after remissions of 10 and 14 months. Conclusions drawn from these studies and extrapolated to additional radiobiological modeling have confirmed earlier conclusions that wide dissemination of micrometastases necessitates that TBI remain as the primary component of treatment but that control of radiosensitive tumors would be augmented with an increased contribution by RIT. The approach of using ^{131}I-MIBG in combination with TBI and local radiotherapy as well as ablative chemotherapy was found to be feasible.

Head and neck tumors

Maraveyas *et al.* (90) elegantly reconstructed a larynx phantom to be used as a representative anatomical structure of the head and neck in an effort to begin evaluating concurrent combinations of EBRT and RIT. To generate data for this phantom model, patients were injected with ^{125}I-labeled human milk fat globulin 1 (HMFG-1) mAb, an antibody that reacts strongly with both human adenocarcinomas and squamous cell carcinomas. Injections were given prior to patients undergoing surgical resection of the larynx. Tumors, as well as normal tissue including skin, muscle, fat, cartilage, and lymph nodes, were evaluated for antibody uptake. Three-dimensional information on the weights of the larynx and cartilage obtained from the surgical specimens was used to obtain dosimetric data pertaining to the major tissues that constitute the larynx.

The point of this endeavor was to determine whether one could safely administer RIT at the same time as EBRT to reduce the total EBRT dose without a loss in local tumor control. Tumor/normal antibody uptake ratios in this study were greater than 5:1 with the tumor/mucosa ratio of approximately 2.5:1 secondary to cross-reactivity of the antibody with surrounding mucosa on the larynx. Considerations regarding the most effective way of combining EBRT and RIT include the dose rate of each radioimmunoconjugate, as well as the effective half-lives of the radioconjugates in order to determine the adjustment of EBRT dose required for each patient. Additional considerations would include the type of fractionation pattern used with EBRT. Modifications to EBRT become more complicated if one considers which fractions of EBRT would require alterations. Would the EBRT fractions that fall within two effective half-lives of the radioimmunoconjugate be the fractions requiring modification? It may be that relatively little dose adjustment is required with EBRT due to the fact that the surrounding normal mucosa including the mandible and parotid glands will receive minimal radiation dose from RIT.

A case report evaluating the effects of combined EBRT and pretargeted RIT in a patient with advanced oropharyngeal cancer has been recently published (91). This case study involved a 73-year-old man diagnosed with a T4N3M0 squamous cell carcinoma of the right tonsil. The tumor was excised along with a functional right neck dissection and myocutaneous flap reconstruction. The patient had gross disease remaining in the right lower cervical chain and residual tumor in the right tonsillar fossa infiltrating into the oropharyngeal wall, extending to the superclavicular fossa creating a fistula. The patient in the postoperative setting had received concomitant chemotherapy and radiation therapy. The total radiation dose was 70 Gy in 2 Gy daily fractions delivered 5 days a week. A persistent mass was noted at the end of the therapy in the right tonsillar region. After immunohistochemistry indicated uptake by both anti-CEA and B72.3 mAbs, this man was injected with 10 mg biotinylated anti-CEA and 20 mg of biotinylated B72.3 anti-TAG-72 antibody (Table 6.2). Thirty-six hours later, 30 mg of avidin was injected followed by 50 mg of streptavidin. Eighteen hours later, ^{90}Y-labeled 1,4,7,10-tetraazacyclododecane-N,N',N'',N''' tetraacetic acid (^{90}Y-DOTA)–biotin was injected IV. The preparation was spiked with 74 MBq of ^{111}In-DOTA–biotin (0.05 mg). Biodistribution scintigraphic studies revealed maximum uptake within the tumor observed 1 hour after administration, at a level of 0.55 ± 0.06 per cent injected dose. At 16 hours, the uptake was 0.35 ± 0.04 per cent injected dose. Dosimetric calculations revealed 13.4 MBq delivered to the tumor in contrast to 1.5, 3.8, and 0.7 cGy/37 MBq to the liver, kidney, and bone marrow, respectively. Thus it was calculated that the tumor had received a dose of 10 Gy.

There was no significant toxicity reported from this RIT administration and, 17 months after RIT, the patient was alive and disease-free by clinical examination and radiographic evaluation. Although the EBRT and RIT treatments were not delivered concurrently, this provides exciting preliminary clinical data that suggests that using RIT as a boost with EBRT is feasible and might significantly impact on local/regional tumor control in patients with head and neck cancer. Additionally, this case demonstrated no significant increase in mucosal toxicity, which is one of the limiting factors in using EBRT. Clearly, one cannot derive significant conclusions from this case study as the authors did not provide definitive evidence through biopsy that the cancer was progressing prior to the administration of RIT. Residual abnormality on CT scan after definitive EBRT is not uncommon in cancers of the head and neck and may simply represent fibrosis.

Hepatoma

Combined RIT, EBRT, and chemotherapy has been used for therapy of hepatoma, with some impressive tumor regressions (92). The Radiation Therapy Oncology Group (RTOG) has studied the use of sequential EBRT and RIT. One hundred-five patients with hepatoma were treated with ^{131}I-antiferritin. The initial pilot study, RTOG 79-28, combined EBRT in 300 cGy fractions to a total dose of 2100 cGy to the entire liver concurrently with doxorubicin and 5-fluorouracil (5FU) as induction therapy (Table 6.2). Patients then received monthly doxorubicin and 5FU at 60 and 500 mg/m^2, respectively, followed by ^{131}I-antiferritin, in a single-dose escalation study of 30, 50, 100, and 150 mCi. The next protocol, RTOG 83-01, deleted the intermediate cycles of chemotherapy; ^{131}I-antiferritin employed in each fraction was derived from different animal species. Based on the tumor saturation data from the first protocol a dose of 30 mCi on day 0 and 20 mCi on day 5, ^{131}I-antiferritin was administered for four cycles with rotating antibodies from animals including rabbit, pig, monkey, and bovine.

Important findings emerged from these studies combining sequential EBRT and RIT. These include the following.

- Enhanced uptake of targeted RIT in the tumor with the use of EBRT resulted in improved antibody targeting.
- Toxicities were not significantly amplified because of the use of EBRT prior to RIT.
- Thrombocytopenia was the major toxicity noted with the use of ^{131}I-antiferritin and was more severe with doses greater than or equal to 100 mCi or when combined concurrently with chemotherapy.

No fatalities occurred that were thought to be treatment-related. The survival in 46 alpha fetoprotein-positive (AFP$^+$) patients was 5 months and for 59 AFP$^-$ patients was 7 months, which improved to 10.5 months when patients with metastasis and/or failure of previous treatments were deleted. A subsequent randomized prospective phase III trial (RTOG 83-19) compared a radiolabeled antibody to full-dose chemotherapy with similar survivals noted (93).

Breast and prostate cancers

Carabasi *et al.* (94) have conducted phase I studies for high-performance status patients with hormone-resistant metastatic prostate cancer or metastatic breast cancer. ^{131}I-CC49 mAb (100–150 mCi/m^2) was followed by 1320 cGy TBI and autologous stem cell reinfusion. Breast cancer patients also received thiotepa (5 mg/kg 2 days after TBI). Three prostate cancer patients and nine breast cancer patients were treated. Prostate cancer patients had objective evidence of response including normalization of prostate-specific antigen (PSA) and/or radiographic response. All survived > 9 months with good quality of life, and without need for additional therapy for > 5 months. Two breast cancer patients had a partial response by radiographic criteria. This combined-modality therapy with high-dose RIT and TBI for metastatic solid tumors was well tolerated and resulted in higher objective response rates than usually obtained with non-myeloablative RIT studies of adenocarcinomas.

Conclusions

Significant advances have been made in improving tumor targeting through humanization of antibodies and use of smaller radiolabeled molecules. Significant advances in EBRT techniques include the development of three-dimensional conformal strategies, and investigators have now begun to set some foundations in the clinic for combining the two strategies. A significant amount of work remains in regard to optimizing combination treatment. In the preliminary data presented in this review, both preclinical and clinical, it is clear that important strides have been made in developing newer treatment strategies for patients with solid and hemopoietic malignancies by combining EBRT and RIT. The main advantages for combining RIT and EBRT are to both improve local control of various tumors by providing a boost with RIT to enhance dose deposition to the tumor and also to spare a greater percentage of normal tissue. This would potentially allow one to reduce the EBRT dose without compromising the therapeutic gain. RIT may also provide enhanced distant control as well. The use of sequential or concurrent EBRT and RIT warrants further investigation to determine optimal dosing and scheduling patterns for the two modalities and opens the door for exciting new clinical trials in the future.

References

1. Kaminski MS, Zasadny KR, Francis IR, *et al*. Iodine-131-anti-B1 radioimmunotherapy for B-cell lymphoma. J Clin Oncol 1996, **14**, 1974–81.
2. Knox SJ, Goris ML, Trisler K, *et al*. Yttrium-90-labeled anti-CD20 monoclonal antibody therapy of recurrent B-cell lymphoma. Clin Cancer Res 1996, **2**, 457–70.
3. Lamborn KR, DeNardo GL, DeNardo SJ, *et al*. Treatment-related parameters predicting efficacy of Lym-1 radioimmunotherapy in patients with B-lymphocytic malignancies. Clin Cancer Res 1997, **3**, 1253–60.
4. Wahl RL, Zasadny KR, MacFarlane D, *et al*. Iodine-131 anti-B1 antibody for B-cell lymphoma: an update on the Michigan phase I experience. J Nucl Med 1998, **39** (suppl.), 21S–7S.
5. Juweid ME, Stadtmauer E, Hajjar G, *et al*. Pharmacokinetics, dosimetry, and initial therapeutic results with ^{131}I- and ^{111}In-/^{90}Y-labeled humanized LL2 anti-CD22 monoclonal antibody in patients with relapsed, refractory non-Hodgkin's lymphoma. Clin Cancer Res 1999, **5** (suppl.), 3292s–303s.
6. Wiseman GA, White CA, Witzig TE, *et al*. Radioimmunotherapy of relapsed non-Hodgkin's lymphoma with Zevalin, a ^{90}Y-labeled anti-CD20 monoclonal antibody. Clin Cancer Res 1999, **5** (suppl.), 3281s–6s.
7. Press OW, Eary JF, Appelbaum FR, *et al*. Radiolabeled-antibody therapy of B-cell lymphoma with autologous bone marrow support. New Engl J Med 1993, **329**, 1219–24.
8. Press OW, Eary JF, Appelbaum FR, *et al*. Phase II trial of ^{131}I-B1 (anti-CD20) antibody therapy with autologous stem cell transplantation for relapsed B cell lymphomas. Lancet 1995, **346**, 336–40.
9. Liu SY, Eary JF, Petersdorf SH, *et al*. Follow-up of relapsed B-cell lymphoma patients treated with iodine-131-labeled anti-CD20 antibody and autologous stem-cell rescue. J Clin Oncol 1998, **16**, 3270–8.
10. Humm JL. Dosimetric aspects of radiolabeled antibodies for tumor therapy. J Nucl Med 1986, **27**, 1490–7.
11. Buchsbaum DJ, Wessels BW. Introduction: radiolabeled antibody tumor dosimetry. Med Phys 1993, **20**, 499–501.
12. Fowler JF. Radiobiological aspects of low dose rates in radioimmunotherapy. Int J Radiat Oncol Biol Phys 1990, **18**, 1261–9.
13. Moulder JE, Fish BL, Wilson JF. Tumor and normal tissue tolerance for fractionated low-dose-rate radiotherapy. Int J Radiat Oncol Biol Phys 1990, **19**, 341–8.
14. Williams JR, Zhang YG, Dillehay LE. Sensitization processes in human tumor cells during protracted irradiation: possible exploitation in the clinic. Int J Radiat Oncol Biol Phys 1992, **24**, 699–704.
15. Saunders M, Dische S, Barrett A, *et al*. Continuous hyperfractionated accelerated radiotherapy (CHART) versus conventional radiotherapy in non-small-cell lung cancer: a randomised multicentre trial. CHART Steering Committee. Lancet 1997, **350**, 161–5.
16. Horiot JC, LeFur R, N'Guyen T, *et al*. Hyperfractionation versus conventional fractionation in oropharyngeal carcinoma: final analysis of a randomized trial of the EORTC cooperative group of radiotherapy. Radiother Oncol 1992, **25**, 231–41.
17. Datta NR, Choudhrly AD, Gupta S, *et al*. Twice a day versus once a day radiation therapy in head and neck cancer. Int J Radiat Oncol Biol Phys 1989, **17**, 132–3.
18. Pinto LH, Canary PCV, Araujo CMM, *et al*. Prospective randomized trial comparing hyperfractionated versus conventional radiotherapy in stages III and IV oropharyngeal carcinoma. Int J Radiat Oncol Biol Phys 1991, **21**, 557–62.
19. Le Chevalier T, Arriagada R, Quoix E, *et al*. Radiotherapy alone versus combined chemotherapy and radiotherapy in unresectable non-small cell lung carcinoma. Lung Cancer 1994, **10** (suppl. 1), S239–S44.
20. Goldenberg DM. New developments in monoclonal antibodies for cancer detection and therapy. CA Cancer J Clin 1994, **44**, 43–64.
21. Larson SM, Divgi CR, Scott A, *et al*. Current status of radioimmunotherapy. Nucl Med Biol 1994, **21**, 785–92.
22. Buchsbaum DJ. Experimental radioimmunotherapy and methods to increase therapeutic efficacy. In: Cancer therapy with radiolabeled antibodies (ed. DM Goldenberg). CRC Press, Boca Raton, 1995, 115–40.
23. Meredith RF, Buchsbaum DJ. Radioimmunotherapy of Solid Tumors. In: Nuclear medicine (ed. RE Henkin, MA

Boles, GJ Dillehay, JR Halama, *et al.*) Mosby-Year Book, Inc, St. Louis, 1996, 601–8.

24. Wilder RB, DeNardo GL, DeNardo SJ. Radioimmunotherapy: recent results and future directions. J Clin Oncol 1996, **14**, 1383–400.

25. Meredith RF, LoBuglio AF. Recent progress in radioimmunotherapy for cancer. Oncology 1997, **11**, 979–87.

26. Buchegger F, Pelegrin A, Delaloye B, *et al.* Iodine-131-labeled MAb F(ab')₂ fragments are more efficient and less toxic than intact anti-CEA antibodies in radioimmunotherapy of large human colon carcinoma grafted in nude mice. J Nucl Med 1990, **31**, 1035–44.

27. Yokota T, Milenic DE, Whitlow M, *et al.* Rapid tumor penetration of a single-chain Fv and comparison with other immunoglobulin forms. Cancer Res 1992, **52**, 3402–8.

28. Slavin-Chiorini DC, Kashmiri SVS, Lee H-S, *et al.* A CDR-grafted (humanized) domain deleted antitumor antibody. Cancer Biother Radiopharm 1997, **12**, 305–16.

29. Behr TM, Memtsoudis S, Sharkey RM, *et al.* Experimental studies on the role of antibody fragments in cancer radio-immunotherapy: influence of radiation dose and dose rate on toxicity and anti-tumor efficacy. Int J Cancer 1998, **77**, 787–95.

30. Shan D, Press OW, Tsu TT, *et al.* Characterization of scFv-Ig constructs generated from the anti-CD20 mAb 1F5 using linker peptides of varying lengths. J Immunol 1999, **162**, 6589–95.

31. Riechmann L, Clark M, Waldmann H, *et al.* Reshaping human antibodies for therapy. Nature 1988, **332**, 323–7.

32. James K. Human monoclonal antibodies and engineered antibodies in the management of cancer. Sem Cancer Biol 1990, **1**, 243–53.

33. Sands H, Jones PL. Physiology of monoclonal antibody accretion by tumors. In: Cancer imaging with radiolabeled antibodies (ed. DM Goldenberg). Kluwer Publishers, Boston, 1990, 97–122.

34. Schlom J, Horan Hand P, Greiner JW, *et al.* Innovations that influence the pharmacology of monoclonal antibody guided tumor targeting. Cancer Res (suppl.) 1990, **50**, 820s–7s.

35. Jain RK. Vascular and interstitial barriers to delivery of therapeutic agents in tumors. Cancer Metastasis Rev 1990, **9**, 253–66.

36. van Osdol W, Fujimori K, Weinstein JN. An analysis of monoclonal antibody distribution in microscopic tumor nodules: consequences of a 'binding site barrier'. Cancer Res 1991, **51**, 4776–84.

37. Baxter LT, Yuan F, Jain RK. Pharmacokinetic analysis of the perivascular distribution of bifunctional antibodies and haptens: comparison with experimental data. Cancer Res 1992, **52**, 5838–44.

38. Neuwelt EA, Barnett PA, Hellstrom KE, *et al.* Effect of blood–brain barrier disruption on intact and fragmented monoclonal antibody localization in intracerebral lung carcinoma xenografts. J Nucl Med 1994, **35**, 1831–41.

39. Press OW, Eary JF, Appelbaum FR, *et al.* Radiolabeled antibody therapy of lymphomas. In: Biologic therapy of cancer, Vol. 4 (ed. VT DeVita, S Hellman, and SA Rosenberg). Lippincott Healthcare Publications, Philadelphia, 1994, 1–13.

40. Press OW, Eary JF, Appelbaum FR, *et al.* Treatment of relapsed B cell lymphomas with high dose radioimmunotherapy and bone marrow transplantation. In: Cancer therapy with radiolabeled antibodies (ed. DM Goldenberg). CRC Press, Boca Raton, 1995, 229–37.

41. Bunn PA, Jr, Carrasquillo JA, Keenan AM, *et al.* Imaging of T-cell lymphoma by radiolabelled monoclonal antibody. Lancet 1984, **2**, 1219–21.

42. Kaminski MS, Zasadny KR, Frances IR, *et al.* Radioimmunotherapy of B-cell lymphoma with [¹³¹I]anti-B1 (anti-CD20) antibody. New Engl J Med 1993, **329**, 459–65.

43. Knox SJ, Goris ML, Trisler K, *et al.* ⁹⁰Y-labeled anti-CD20 monoclonal antibody therapy of recurrent B cell lymphoma. Clin Cancer Res 1996, **2**, 457–70.

44. Knox SJ. Overview of studies on experimental radioimmunotherapy. Cancer Res 1995, **55** (suppl.), 5832s–6s.

45. Borchardt PE, Quadri SM, Freedman RS, *et al.* Intralesional radiolabeled human monoclonal IgM in human tumor xenografts. Radiother Oncol 1997, **44**, 283–93.

46. Zamora PO, Gulhke S, Bender H, *et al.* Experimental radiotherapy of receptor-positive human prostate adenocarcinoma with ¹⁸⁸Re-RC-160, a directly-radiolabeled somatostatin analogue. Int J Cancer 1996, **65**, 214–20.

47. O'Donoghue JA. Implications of nonuniform tumor doses for radioimmunotherapy. J Nucl Med 1999, **40**, 1337–41.

48. Goodwin DA, Meares CF. Pretargeting: general principles; October 10–12, 1996. Cancer 1997, **80** (suppl.), 2675–80.

49. Barbet J, Kraeber-Bodéré F, Vuillez J-P, *et al.* Pretargeting with the affinity enhancement system for radioimmunotherapy. Cancer Biother Radiopharm 1999, **14**, 153–66.

50. Cremonesi M, Ferrari M, Chinol M, *et al.* Three-step radioimmunotherapy with yttrium-90 biotin: dosimetry and pharmacokinetics in cancer patients. Eur J Nucl Med 1999, **26**, 110–20.

51. Vuillez J-P, Kraeber-Bodéré F, Moro D, *et al.* Radioimmunotherapy of small cell lung carcinoma with the two-step method using a bispecific anti-carcinoembryonic antigen/anti-diethylenetriaminepentaacetic acid (DTPA) antibody and iodine-131 di-DTPA hapten: results of a phase I/II trial. Clin Cancer Res 1999, **5** (suppl.), 3259s–67s.

52. Williams JA, Edwards JA, Dillehay LE. Quantitative comparison of radiolabeled antibody therapy and external beam radiotherapy in the treatment of human glioma xenografts. Int J Radiat Oncol Biol Phys 1992, **24**, 111–17.

53. Buchsbaum DJ, Ten Haken RK, Heidorn DB, *et al.* A comparison of ¹³¹I-labeled monoclonal antibody 17–1A treatment to external beam irradiation on the growth of LS174T human colon carcinoma xenografts. Int J Radiat Oncol Biol Phys 1990, **18**, 1033–41.

54. Barendswaard EC, O'Donoghue JA, Larson SM, *et al.* ¹³¹I radioimmunotherapy and fractionated external beam radiotherapy: comparative effectiveness in a human tumor xenograft. J Nucl Med 1999, **40**, 1764–8.

55. Wessels BW, Vessella RL, Palme DF, *et al.* Radiobiological comparison of external beam irradiation

and radioimmunotherapy in renal cell carcinoma xenografts. Int J Radiat Oncol Biol Phys 1989, **17**, 1257–63.

56. Knox SJ, Levy R, Miller RA, *et al.* Determinants of the antitumor effect of radiolabeled monoclonal antibodies. Cancer Res 1990, **50**, 4935–40.

57. Buras RR, Wong JYC, Kuhn JA, *et al.* Comparison of radioimmunotherapy and external beam radiotherapy in colon cancer xenografts. Int J Radiat Oncol Biol Phys 1993, **25**, 473–9.

58. Ning S, Trisler K, Wessels BW, *et al.* Radiobiologic studies of radioimmunotherapy and external beam radiotherapy *in vitro* and *in vivo* in human renal cell carcinoma xenografts. Cancer 1997, **80**, 2519–28.

59. Williams JA, Williams JR, Yuan X, *et al.* Protracted exposure radiosensitization of experimental human malignant glioma. Radiat Oncol Invest 1998, **6**, 255–63.

60. Bender H, Emrich JG, Eshelman J, *et al.* External beam radiation enhances antibody mediated radiocytotoxicity in human glioma cells *in vitro*. Anticancer Res 1997, **17**, 1797–802.

61. Peter RU, Beetz A, Ried C, *et al.* Increased expression of the epidermal growth factor receptor in human epidermal keratinocytes after exposure to ionizing radiation. Radiat Res 1993, **136**, 65–70.

62. Sastry KS. Biological effects of the Auger emitter iodine-125: a review. Report no. 1 of AAPM Nuclear Medicine Task Group No. 6. Med Phys 1992, **19**, 1361–70.

63. Brady LW, Miyamoto C, Woo DV, *et al.* Malignant astrocytomas treated with iodine-125 labeled monoclonal antibody 425 against epidermal growth factor receptor: a phase II trial. Int J Radiat Oncol Biol Phys 1991, **22**, 225–30.

64. Buchegger F, Rojas A, Delaloye AB, *et al.* Combined radioimmunotherapy and radiotherapy of human colon carcinoma grafted in nude mice. Cancer Res 1995, **55**, 83–9.

65. Sun L-Q, Vogel C-A, Mirimanoff R-O, *et al.* Timing effects of combined radioimmunotherapy and radiotherapy on a human solid tumor in nude mice. Cancer Res 1997, **57**, 1312–19.

66. Vogel C-A, Galmiche MC, Buchegger F. Radioimmunotherapy and fractionated radiotherapy of human colon cancer liver metastases in nude mice. Cancer Res 1997, **57**, 447–53.

67. Sharkey RM, Weadock KS, Natale A, *et al.* Successful radioimmunotherapy for lung metastasis of human colonic cancer in nude mice. J Natl Cancer Inst 1991, **83**, 627–32.

68. Wang S, Quadri SM, Tang X-Z, *et al.* Liver toxicity induced by combined external-beam irradiation and radioimmunoglobulin therapy. Radiat Res 1995, **141**, 294–302.

69. Meredith RF, Buchsbaum DJ, Knox SJ. Radioimmunotherapy. In: Clinical radiation oncology, (ed. L Gunderson and J Tepper). Churchill Livingston, Edinburgh, 2000, p. 283–98.

70. Roberson PL, Buchsbaum DJ. Reconciliation of tumor dose response to external beam radiotherapy *versus* radioimmunotherapy with ^{131}iodine-labeled antibody for a colon cancer model. Cancer Res 1995, **55** (suppl.), 5811s–16s.

71. O'Donoghue JA. Dosimetric aspects of radioimmunotherapy. Tumor Targeting 1998, **3**, 105–11.

72. Siegel JA, Goldenberg DM, Badger CC. Radioimmunotherapy dose estimation in patients with B-cell lymphoma. Med Phys 1993, **20** (suppl.), 579–82.

73. Tempero M, Leichner P, Dalrymple G, *et al.* High-dose therapy with iodine-131-labeled monoclonal antibody CC49 in patients with gastrointestinal cancers: a phase I trial. J Clin Oncol 1997, **15**, 1518–28.

74. Buckman R, De Angelis C, Shaw P, *et al.* Intraperitoneal therapy of malignant ascites associated with carcinoma of ovary and breast using radioiodinated monoclonal antibody 2G3. Gynecol Oncol 1992, **47**, 102–9.

75. Epenetos AA, Munro AJ, Stewart S, *et al.* Antibody-guided irradiation of advanced ovarian cancer with intraperitoneally administered radiolabeled monoclonal antibodies. J Clin Oncol 1987, **5**, 1890–9.

76. Stewart JSW, Hird V, Snook D, *et al.* Intraperitoneal radioimmunotherapy for ovarian cancer: pharmacokinetics, toxicity, and efficacy of I-131 labeled monoclonal antibodies. Int J Radiat Oncol Biol Phys 1989, **16**, 405–13.

77. Murray JL. Radioimmunotherapy of colorectal cancer. In: Cancer therapy with radiolabeled antibodies (ed. DM Goldenberg). CRC Press, Inc, Boca Raton, 1995, 173–88.

78. Meredith RF, Khazaeli MB, Carabasi MH, *et al.* Radioimmunotherapy of prostate cancer. In: Therapy of malignancies with radioconjugate monoclonal antibodies: present possibilities and future perspectives (ed. P Riva). Harwood Academic Publisher, 1997.

79. Juweid M, Sharkey RM, Swayne LC, *et al.* Phase I dose-escalation trial of ^{131}I-labeled MN-14 anti-carcinoembryonic antigen (CEA) monoclonal antibody in patients with epithelial ovarian cancer. Tumor Targeting 1996, **2**, 189.

80. Juweid M, Sharkey RM, Alavi A, *et al.* Regression of advanced refractory ovarian cancer treated with iodine-131-labeled anti-CEA monoclonal antibody. J Nucl Med 1997, **38**, 257–60.

81. O'Donoghue JA. Optimal scheduling of biologically targeted radiotherapy and total body irradiation with bone marrow rescue for the treatment of systemic malignant disease. Int J Radiat Oncol Biol Phys 1991, **21**, 1587–94.

82. Amin AE, Wheldon TE, O'Donoghue JA, *et al.* Radiobiological modeling of combined targeted ^{131}I therapy and total body irradiation for treatment of disseminated tumors of differing radiosensitivity. Int J Radiat Oncol Biol Phys 1993, **27**, 323–30.

83. Vriesendorp HM, Quadri SM, Stinson RL, *et al.* Selection of reagents for human radioimmunotherapy. Int J Radiat Oncol Biol Phys 1991, **22**, 37–45.

84. Vriesendorp HM, Shao Y, Blum JE, *et al.* Fractionated intravenous administration of ^{90}Y-labeled B72.3 GYK-DTPA immunoconjugate in beagle dogs. Nucl Med Biol 1993, **20**, 571–8.

85. Leichner PK, Akabani G, Colcher D, *et al.* Patient-specific dosimetry of indium-111 and yttrium-90-labeled monoclonal antibody CC49. J Nucl Med 1997, **38**, 512–16.

86. Quin DX, Zheng R, Tang L, *et al.* Influence of radiation on the blood–brain barrier and optimum time of

chemotherapy. Int J Radiat Oncol Biol Phys 1990, **19**, 1507–10.

87. Riva P, Franceschi G, Arista A, *et al.* Local application of radiolabeled monoclonal antibodies in the treatment of high grade malignant gliomas: a six-year clinical experience. Cancer 1997, **80**, 2733–42.

88. Riva P, Franceschi G, Frattarelli M. Loco-regional radioimmunotherapy of high-grade malignant gliomas using specific monoclonal antibodies labeled with ^{90}Y: a phase I study. Clin Cancer Res 1999, **5** (suppl.), 3275s–80s.

89. Amin AE, Wheldon TE, O'Donoghue JA, *et al.* Optimum combination of targeted ^{131}I and total body irradiation for treatment of disseminated cancer. Int J Radiat Oncol Biol Phys 1995, **32**, 713–21.

90. Maraveyas A, Myers M, Stafford N, *et al.* Radiolabeled antibody combined with external radiotherapy for the treatment of head and neck cancer: reconstruction of a theoretical phantom of the larynx for radiation dose calculation to local tissues. Cancer Res 1995, **55**, 1020–7.

91. Paganelli G, Orecchia R, Jereczek-Fossa B, *et al.* Combined treatment of advanced oropharyngeal cancer with external radiotherapy and three-step radioimmunotherapy. Eur J Nucl Med 1998, **25**, 1336–9.

92. Order SE, Sleeper AM, Stillwagon GB, *et al.* Radiolabeled antibodies: results and potential in cancer therapy. Cancer Res 1990, **50**, 1011s–13s.

93. Order SE, Stillwagon GB, Klein JL, *et al.* Iodine 131 antiferritin, a new treatment modality in hepatoma: a Radiation Therapy Oncology Group study. J Clin Oncol 1985, **3**, 1573–82.

94. Carabasi M, Meredith R, Khazaeli MB, *et al.* Combined modality radiation using radioimmunotherapy and external beam radiation (TBI) for breast and prostate cancer. Cancer Biother Radiopharm 1999, **14** (suppl.), 318.

Section III

7

Genetic immunotherapy for cancer

Hardev S. Pandha

Introduction

Remarkable recent insights into the molecular biology of cancer development and progression have allowed us to contemplate new molecular and genetic approaches to augment current anticancer therapies such as chemotherapy and radiotherapy. The key developments include techniques to identify tumor-associated antigens; insights into the mechanisms of antigen recognition, processing, and presentation to T cells; and the technology termed gene therapy—that is, the transfer of genes into cells in order to replace, correct, or modify function in a wide range of benign diseases as well as cancer. The limitations to success for immunotherapy involving genetic manipulation will be the same as those for other gene therapy strategies. These include the lack of efficient delivery systems, problems in sustaining gene expression, as well as host immune reactions to foreign gene products. One particular frustration has been an inability to target cellular compartments or tumor-associated factors with a high degree of specificity. The plethora of human gene therapy trials commenced worldwide was perceived as premature, but have shown that biological responses to gene transfer are possible without toxicity. They have also highlighted the need for renewed emphasis on the basic science behind gene therapy—particularly the three intertwined fields of tumor immunology, vectorology, and cell biology.

Currently, immunotherapy has a small but defined role in the conventional treatment of certain malignancies. This consists mainly of the use of monoclonal antibodies, exogenous systemic recombinant cytokines, or intratumoral injection of infective agents such as bacille Calmette–Guérin (BCG). In contrast to prophylactic vaccines against infectious agents, in which the generation of neutralizing humoral immunity is the most important feature, the major focus in cancer vaccine development has been on the generation of antigen-specific T-cell responses. The use of immunotherapy has been limited by lack of specificity, limited efficacy, and serious systemic toxicity. The explosion in interest in gene therapy over the last decade has coincided with major advances in the understanding of the molecular basis of humoral and cellular immune responses, recognition of tumor-associated antigens, and the identification and culture of potent antigen-presenting cells (APCs). Advances in gene transfer techniques have been crucial in this evolution and have provided opportunities for introducing immunostimulatory genes into tumor or immune effector cells, with the aim of boosting immune responses and causing the selective destruction of tumor cells. At the same time, there have also been important insights into the intricate and ingenious mechanisms by which cancers may evade immune destruction, and some of these may provide realistic targets for future cancer immunotherapy.

T-cell immunotherapy

In the last century William Coley observed that tumor regression could be induced by stimulating the immune system with bacterial toxins (1). Since then the goal of tumor immunologists has been to activate tumor-specific immune responses capable of recognizing and eradicating metastatic tumor deposits. Early attempts at achieving this used crude vaccines consisting of allogeneic or autologous tumor cells, or infective agents such as BCG. These approaches shared the limitation of poor specificity while still stimulating a wide spectrum of immune responses to tumor-associated antigens presumed to be present. The occurrence of isolated spontaneous tumor regressions, the presence of mononuclear infiltrates in certain tumors, and response to exogenous cytokines and adoptive transfer of cytokine genes into tumor cells kept alive hopes that immune intervention may be effective in some patients. Some of the immune mechanisms involved in antitumor immune responses have now been elucidated, and T cells have been shown to play a critical role (2). Human T cells that accumulate within the mass of a tumor have been shown to specifically lyse autologous tumor cells *in vitro*. T cells may secrete numerous cytokines and proliferate in response to stimulation with autologous tumor cells (3). T cells with antitumor activity can be grown to large numbers *in vitro*, and transferred adoptively to treat large tumor burdens in human patients (4). Finally, tumor antigens recognized by cytotoxic T lymphocytes (CTLs) have been identified and provide further compelling evidence that a T-cell immune response can occur against an autologous tumor. Advances in understanding the molecular basis of immune recognition of tumor antigens, effector cell function, and the complex interactions with co-stimulatory molecules and professional APCs have finally led to genetic approaches to immunotherapy.

Immune surveillance

Cancer vaccines are therapeutic and involve attempts to activate immune responses against antigens in the tumor to which the immune system has already been exposed. Tumors are considered immunogenic if they induce resistance to a secondary challenge of the same tumor following immunization of syngeneic animals through expression of specific determinants (that is, tumor-associated transplantation antigens). Some tumors clearly express tumor antigens that are recognized by components of the immune system (5). However, it is unclear why spontaneously occurring tumors expressing neoantigens such as point mutations in oncogenes are poorly or even non-immunogenic (6). A number of mechanisms for this non-responsiveness have been proposed including the loss of expression of major histocompatibility complex (MHC) class I molecules, antigen loss tumor variants, downregulation of antigen processing in the proteosome, and expression of local inhibitory molecules such as transforming growth factor and Fas ligand. More fundamentally, recent studies indicate that, when the immune system encounters a new antigen (in the periphery), the outcome is not necessarily activation and the induction

of memory T cells. Firstly, the state of tolerance may be a result of ignorance, anergy, or T-cell deletion. The outcome of antigen encounter depends on the context of antigen presentation to the immune system. The outcome of tissue destruction or inflammation that occurs during bacterial or viral infection is usually activation. This contrasts with the endogenous expression of antigen, in the absence of the danger signals accompanying tissue destruction and inflammation, where tolerance results. Secondly, T-cell responses are dependent on co-stimulatory signals present at the time of antigen recognition. In response to certain cytokines, APCs express co-stimulatory molecules such as the B7 family that promote T-cell activation. In the absence of B7 expression, engagement of the T-cell receptor may lead to ignorance, anergy, or apoptosis of the antigen-specific T cell. It appears therefore that tumors are poor stimulators of the immune system and may be capable of inducing tolerance. Cancer vaccines must break down this tolerance or activate a population of T cells that escaped the tolerance by virtue of their low affinity for antigens expressed by the tumor, termed subdominant epitopes.

We now recognize that one of the key goals of cancer vaccines is to target the immunizing antigen to bone-marrow-derived APCs. Antigen may be presented as whole cell, protein, or peptide exogenous to the APC (Fig. 7.1). Tumor antigens are endocytosed, processed, and presented on the surface of the APC to CD4+ T cells in association with MHC class II molecules. Antigen may enter the endogenous processing route by viral infection or deliberately by a number of gene transfer methods. Processed antigen is then presented to CD8+ T cells in association with MHC class I molecules. Exogenous peptide antigen may enter the MHC class I processing machinery by 'cross-priming' or target APCs directly by loading empty MHC molecules on the surface of the APC, bypassing the normal processing machinery. Ultimately, the factors that determine whether the immune system is activated are the density of peptide/MHC complexes on the APC cell surface and the expression of co-stimulatory molecules.

Th1/Th2 paradigm

CD4+ T helper cells (Th cells) can be subdivided into three subsets, Th0, Th1, and Th2. All three fulfil important immunoregulatory functions by secreting

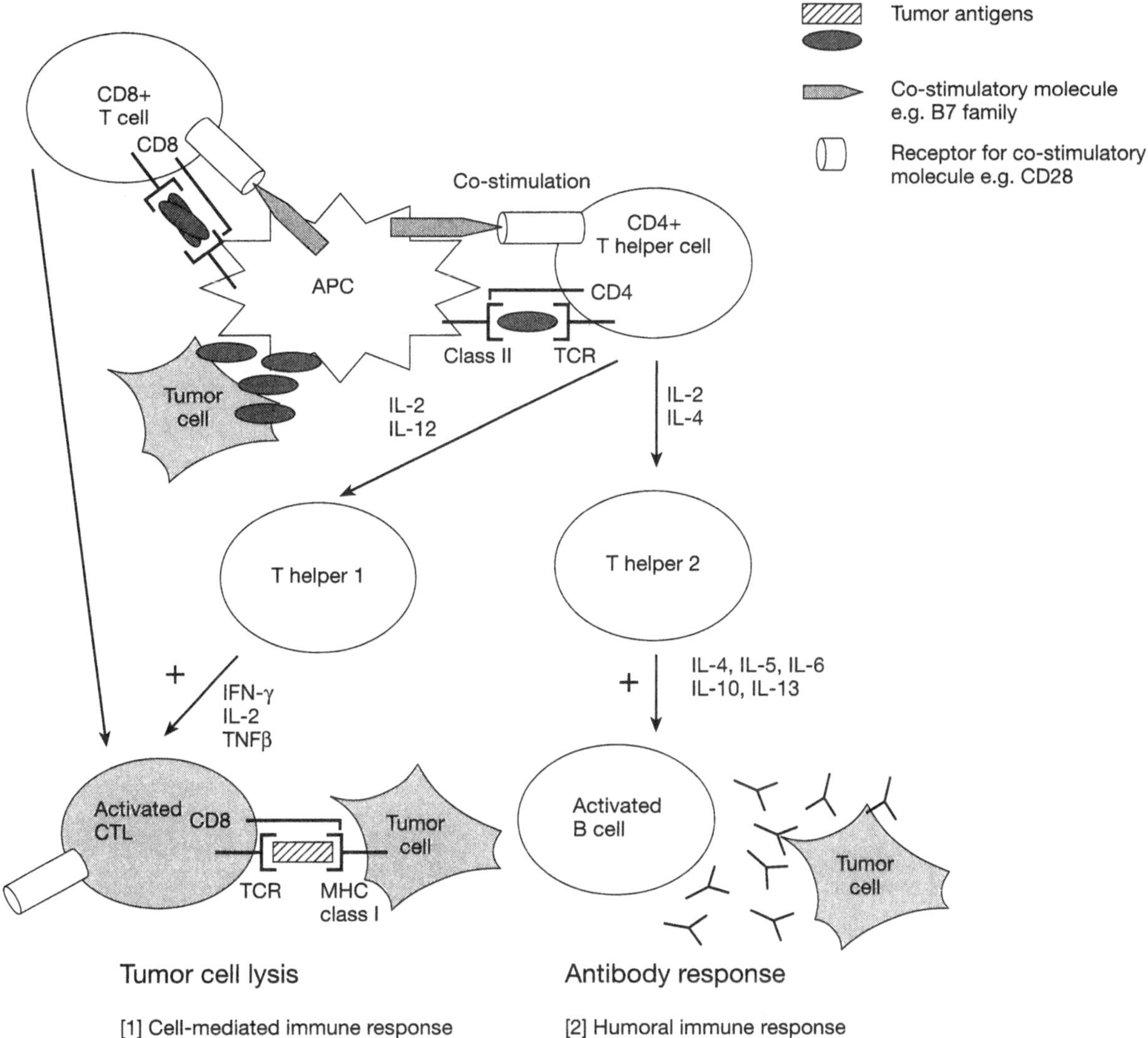

Fig. 7.1 Immune responses to tumor antigens. Activation of pre-cytotoxic CD8[+] T cells depends on recognition by the T-cell receptor (TCR) of a specific epitope presented by an MHC class I molecule on the tumor cell. Cytokines secreted by CD4[+] cells directly influence T helper differentiation and provide further stimulatory signals for pre-cytotoxic CD8[+] T cells. Alternatively, tumor antigens are taken up by APCs that are able to activate T helper cells or prime pre-cytotoxic CD8[+] T cells.

cytokines with autocrine and paracrine effects. Differentiation into an individual subset depends on the local cytokine environment, the nature of the antigenic challenge, and the influences of co-stimulation. This clonal restriction is a useful functional classification, which appears less absolute for human CD4[+] cells than for mice. Th1 cells enhance cytotoxicity and cell-mediated inflammatory responses against, for example tumor cells, by producing interleukin 2 (IL-2), interferon γ (IFN-γ), and lymphotoxin. In contrast, Th2 cells promote B-cell responses and secrete interleukins, IL-4, IL-5, IL-6, IL-9, IL-10, and IL-13, which may also cause destruction of tumor cells by sensitizing tumor cells to macrophage attack. Cells producing cytokines typical of both groups have been designated Th0. The eventual fate of the bipotent CD4[+] cell to differentiate into mutually antagonistic Th1 or Th2 is influenced by local cytokine production from macrophages and dendritic cells (IL-12), natural killer (NK) cells (IFN-γ), or basophiles (IL-4). A Th1 response is stimulated by IFN-γ (which suppresses Th2) and IL-12, while IL-4 favors a Th2 response (and suppresses Th1) (7, 8). Current strategies have focused on polarizing immune responses towards Th1 and cellular toxicity, using specific methods of gene delivery such as DNA vaccination or delivering Th1-type cytokines.

Immune adjuvants

Recent vaccine studies have highlighted the importance of immunological adjuvants such as KLH (keyhole limpet hemocyanin), QS1 (a saponin derivative), and granulocyte–macrophage colony-stimulating factor (GM-CSF). There is no standard adjuvant for immunizing humans to peptides. Studies in rats established that GM-CSF is a potent adjuvant for the generation of immune responses to rat neu peptide. The peptide-based vaccine using GM-CSF was most effective in rats when injected intradermally (ID) versus subcutaneously (SC) presumably because of the role of ID GM-CSF as a chemoattractant and growth and differentiation factor for dermal dendritic cells (DCs) (9). GM-CSF has been shown to be a powerful adjuvant in a number of studies of peptide vaccines including the elicitation of a strong delayed-type hypersensitivity (DTH) response.

Mechanisms of resistance

Tumors may effectively evade the immune system by several mechanisms, which are not only confined to tumor cells, but may also be related to impaired function of immune responses in a tumor-bearing host. Some of these defects may be overcome at least partially by restoration of immunoregulatory gene expression. There may be loss of expression of MHC class I antigens or defects in antigen processing such as transporter-associated protein (TAP) (10, 11). Outgrowth of antigen-negative clones of tumor cells may result as a lack of T-cell recognition. As indicated earlier, tumor cells do not express co-stimulatory molecules and may lose expression of adhesion molecules. The Fas system is a major cytolytic pathway used by CTLs to kill target cells and is also a key element in elimination of activated T cells during downregulation of the immune response. Fas-mediated cell suicide is one of the basic mechanisms of apoptosis. Immune cells expressing Fas receptor (FasR) after binding the cell expressing Fas ligand (FasL) undergo apoptotic cell death. Most cells

of the immune system express FasR and/or FasL. Functional FasL expression has been detected in tumor cells. It has been postulated that FasL-positive tumor cells may 'kill' sensitive (Fas-positive) CD4+ and CD8+ T lymphocytes (12). Tumor cells may secrete immuno-inhibitory factors into the local environment such as IL-10, transforming growth factor beta (TGFβ), prostaglandin E2, inhibitory neuropeptides. Factors such as vascular endothelial growth factor (VEGF) have an inhibitory effect on APCs (13). New insights into the molecular recognition of immune responses have identified inhibitory pathways of T-cell activation that may be amenable to blockade. One of the most promising of these is blockade of the CTL antigen 4 (CTLA4) inhibitory pathway. CTLA4 binds B7 with 10-fold higher affinity than its natural ligand CD28. CTLA4 binding inhibits CD28 T-cell activation and cytokine induction (14). However, complete loss of CTLA4 as observed in CTLA4 knock-out mice results in a severe lymphoproliferative disorder and organ destruction, exemplifying the need for transient, reversible blocking strategies only (15). This has been achieved in part by the use of an anti-CTLA4 antibody, which has been shown to enhance vaccine efficacy in a mouse model.

Tumor antigens

An important approach in cancer immunotherapy has been to identify tumor-specific or tumor-associated antigens that are recognized by cyotoxic T cells. Techniques applied to define tumor-derived peptides presented to CTL have included screening recombinant DNA libraries with CTL, analysing peptides eluted from MHC complexes expressed on tumor cells, and serological identification of antigens by recombinant expression cloning (SEREX).

The MHC class I allele-specific peptide size and sequence requirements are known as the peptide-binding motifs and are of enormous importance to the peptide repertoire presented at the cell surface. For several MHC class I alleles, specific motifs have now been determined and, on the basis of these, candidate CTL epitopes have been predicted with some success (16). Self-proteins expressed by melanoma cells, such as melanocyte differentiation antigens gp100, MAGE, and MART-1, have been found to be immunogenic in humans who have had melanoma. Self-proteins known to be involved in malignant

Table 7.1 Examples of human tumor antigens recognized by CTLs

Tumor antigen element	Restriction	Peptide epitope
Melanoma-derived antigens		
Shared antigens		
MAGE-1	HLA-A1	EADPTGHSY
MAGE-3	HLA-A2	FLWGPRALV
BAGE	HLA-Cw16	AARAVFLAL
GAGE	HLA-Cw6	YRPRPRRY
Melanocyte-specific antigens		
Tyrosinase	HLA-A2	YMNGTMSQV
MART-1/ Melan A	HLA-A2	AAGIGILTV
gp100	HLA-A2	LLDGTATLRL
Mutated antigens		
CDK4	HLA-A2	ACDPHSGHFV
β-catenin	HLA-A24	SYLDSGIHF
Non-melanoma antigens		
ERBB2	HLA-A2	ELVSEFSRM
MUC-1	Unrestricted	PPAGHVTSAPDTRPAPGSTA
KRAS	HLA-A31	MTEYKLVVVGASGVGKSALTIQ

transformation, such as ERBB2 and c-myc, have also been found to stimulate an immune response in patients whose cancers express those proteins.

As Table 7.1 shows, a large variety of peptide epitopes for CD8$^+$ T cells have been demonstrated in both animal and human cancers as potential targets for *in vitro* CTL activity. Several of these can be present on the same tumor cells and some have high, or even absolute tumor specificity. Although an antigenic protein may contain multiple motif-fitting peptides, CTL responses are directed against a very limited number of 'immunodominant' epitopes (17). Where tumors express a truly cancer-specific oncoprotein due to point mutations such as for mutant RAS and p53, immune responses are not necessarily solely directed at the areas of mutation but may also be directed against the non-mutated or 'self'-epitopes. For model antigens such as OVA, there appears to be a hierarchy among class I binding peptides; potential epitopes may be dominant, subdominant, or cryptic (as they are presented at levels too low to elicit CTL responses) (18). However, responses to subdominant peptide epitopes have been demonstrated after primary CTL elicitation by a dominant epitope (19). Subdominant epitopes have also been described in melanoma-expressing gp100 antigen. In cancer patients, peptides may bind their MHC class 1 restriction element with relatively weaker affinities than epitopes recognized, for example, in acute viral infections. Some of the CTL reactivities directed against the highest MHC class I-binding epitopes may be inacti-

vated by thymic education of peripheral tolerance and, paradoxically, dominant tumor epitopes may be, in fact, relatively low-affinity binders.

Gene transfer vectors—gene delivery

The addition, substitution, or ablation of DNA sequences may be achieved by any of the following.

- Injection of naked DNA into skeletal muscle by simple needle and syringe.
- DNA transfer by liposomes (delivered by the intravascular, intratracheal, intraperitoneal, or intracolonic routes).
- DNA coated on the surface of gold pellets which are air-propelled into the epidermis (the 'gene gun').
- Biological vehicles (vectors) such as viruses and bacteria. Viruses are genetically engineered not to replicate once inside the host. They are currently the most efficient means of gene transfer. Individual features of viral vectors are compared in Table 7.2.

Other techniques involve fusion of whole cells or viral envelopes, electroporation, microinjection, or chemical precipitation of DNA into cells.

Table 7.2 Viral vectors used for gene transfer

Retrovirus	Adenovirus	Adeno-associated virus	Herpes virus
Advantages			
Small genome	High viral titers	Small genome	High viral titers
Stable co-linear integration	Stable integration	Integrates into chromosome 19	
Efficient gene transfer	Highly efficient gene transfer	Efficient gene transfer	Highly efficient gene transfer
Nontoxic to host	Nontoxic to host Can infect non-dividing cells	Nonpathogenic in humans Can infect non-dividing cells	Neural tropism Can infect non-dividing cells
Biology well understood			
Disadvantages			
Requires actively dividing cells	Transient expression	Not well studied	Large genome
Small DNA sequences only carried	Small DNA sequences only carried	Small DNA sequences only carried	Lytic virus
Low titer, transient expression			
Random integration			
Insertional mutagenesis			

The efficiency of transfer of therapeutic DNA required (dictated by the nature of the genetic defect) influences the choice of vector. For example, for gene replacement, high-efficiency viral vectors are desirable, whereas short-term gene expression to prime an immune response or sensitize cells to radiotherapy may be achieved by liposomal delivery.

Some of the above strategies can be achieved *ex vivo* by transfer of a therapeutic gene into isolated cancer or noncancer cells, which are then re-implanted into the host. Others require delivery and expression of genes to target cancer cells *in vivo* (at much lower efficiency than *ex vivo* transfer) by exploiting transcriptional differences of specific genes between cancer and normal cells. The efficiency of gene transfer also varies greatly according to cell type targeted (low in neural and hemopoietic cells, high in myocytes, fibroblasts, and hepatocytes, and variable among different tumors).

Genetically modified tumor vaccines have been used in the context of phase I/II clinical trials. The various strategies are summarized in Table 7.3. The approaches using cytokine-gene-modified tumor cells, polynucleotide vaccination, and dendritic cell therapies are discussed in detail.

Table 7.3 Clinical trials with genetically modified tumor vaccines

	Strategy*		Providing propagation signal to tumor microenvironment
	Presentation of tumor antigen		
	Direct	Indirect	
Cell type	Autologous or/and allogeneic tumor cells	DCs, fibroblasts	Fibroblasts, TIL
Gene type	TA, cytokines (IL-2; IFN-γ; GM-CS; IL-4, -7, -12; TNF; IL-6/sIL-6R; co-stimulatory molecules (B-7.1); HLA molecules (HLA-B7); beta-2 m	TA alone or with cytokines (e.g. Th1 type cytokines: IL-2, IL-12, IFNα)	Cytokines (IL-2, IL-4, IL-12, TNF)
Gene delivery system	*Ex vivo* (retroviral, nonviral-lipid), *In vivo* (nonviral-lipid, adenoviral)	*Ex vivo* (nonviral retroviral) *In vivo* (pox virus)	*Ex vivo* (retroviral)

* TA, Tumor antigen; TIL, tumor-infiltrating lymphocyte.

Cytokine-modified tumor cells as vaccines

Despite the success so far in identifying cancer-associated antigens and CTL epitopes, we currently have little insight into the most important tumor rejection antigens for the majority of human cancers. Most cancer vaccine strategies therefore use tumor cells themselves as a source of antigen. This, in turn, relies on their capacity to induce stronger immunity against tumor-specific or tumor-selective antigens than against ubiquitously expressed self-antigens within the tumor. Genetically modified cell vaccines are an alternative approach to traditional cell vaccines, which comprised syngeneic tumor cell lysates or irradiated whole cells often admixed with microbial adjuvants. The revolution in gene transfer technology using high-efficiency viral transfer systems has resulted in tumor-cells stably expressing cytokine genes. Originally, Lindenmann and Klein showed that vaccination with influenza virus–infected tumor cell lysates generated enhanced systemic immune responses following challenge with the original tumor(20). In mouse models, a wide variety of tumor cell types have been genetically engineered to secrete IL-2, IL-4, tumor necrosis factor alpha (TNFα), interferon, or GM-CSF, in order to make them more immunogenic. Mice are treated with irradiated cytokine-secreting tumors. These animals then develop protective immunity against subsequent tumor challenge. This protective immunity includes induction of antitumor CTLs. In the case of cytokines such as IL-2, the injection of IL-2 secreting cells into the patient should lead to high local release and avoid system side-effects associated with treatment with recombinant IL-2, as well as inducing CTL responses. This approach has reached a phase I clinical trial where antitumor DTH responses and CTLs were induced with no evidence of systemic toxicity (21). GM-CSF is the most potent stimulator of a systemic antitumor response when transduced into autologous tumor cells (22). The potency of GM-CSF in modulating an antitumor response has been attributed to its role as an important growth and differentiation factor for DCs at the vaccination site (23). The use of GM-CSF in this way has extended to human trials of renal cell carcinoma and malignant melanoma (24). The limitation on autologous cytokine secretion is the technical effort required to prepare autologous vaccine. Each preparation requires the expansion of tumor explant into a homogenous culture, followed by gene transfer, cell selection, cell expansion, assays for GM-CSF secretion level, and irradiation before the vaccine can be used (25). The yield of cytokine from *in vitro* cell expansion may be unreliable and too low to elicit an immune response. These limitations may be circumvented by using a universal vaccine that is readily available and has a predetermined and effective level of cytokine expression. GM-CSF-transduced allogeneic cell lines have been evaluated for this purpose. The feasibility of this approach has been supported by the findings that host APCs, rather than the tumor vaccine cells themselves, present the tumor-specific antigens and prime the host T cells through a process called cross-priming. Allogeneic delivery does not reduce antitumor protection by paracrine GM-CSF. Rather, the allogeneic immune response in the host seems to enhance the specific antitumor response (26). Most of the current studies using allogeneic tumor-cell based-vaccines utilize tumor-specific and not antigen-specific vaccines.

The distinct advantage of this approach is a dramatic reduction in systemic toxicity. This is best seen in

Table 7.4 Clinical trials with genetically modified tumor vaccines

Tumor	Gene transferred	No. of patients
Melanoma	IL-2, GM-CSF, IL-6/slL-6R, IL-7, IL-12, IFNγ, TNF, B-7.1, HLA-B7/β-2m, MART-1, gp-100	620
Renal cell cancer	IL-2, 1L-7, GM-CSF, TNF, IL-4, HLA-B7/β-2 m	145
Colorectal carcinoma	IL-2, TNF, B-7, 1, HLA-B7/β-2m, CEA	80
Breast cancer	IL-2, B-7, 1, TNF, HLA-B7/β-2m, MUC1, CEA, BRCA-1	72
Ovarian cancer	B-7, 1/1L-12, BRCA-1, CEA, HLA-A2, HLA-B13, H2K	65
Prostate cancer, non-small-cell lung cancer, malignant gliomas, neuroblastomas, head and neck cancer, mesothelioma, cervical carcinoma, lymphomas	IL-2, IFN-γ, IL-4, IL-12, HLA-B7/β-2m, GM-CSF, IFN-β, PSA, BRCA-1, HPV	82

cytokine gene transfer where sustained local release of cytokines produces local inflammation without systemic effects or toxicity, even when a large number of transduced tumor cells are used. To date, the most effective cytokine gene in terms of antitumor efficacy in animal models has been GM-CSF (22). The enhanced effect of paracrine GM-CSF in multiple tumor vaccine models relates specifically to its role in promoting local DC differentiation at the vaccination site (23, 27). DCs are felt to be the primary cells necessary for activating naive T cells; their role in priming the immune response is now considered central. The phase I clinical trials shown in Table 7.4 have shown promise in terms of efficacy but may be prohibitively expensive for routine application. Alternative approaches that maintain the immunological activity of paracrine cytokine elaboration include the use of transduced allogeneic tumor cells, based on the assumption that some tumor rejection antigens are shared rather than unique, and that the host APCs rather than the tumor vaccine cells themselves present tumor antigen and prime T cells through cross-priming (28, 29). Furthermore, it is clear that tumor antigens are presented to the immune system by the patient's own bone-marrow-derived APCs rather than the vaccinating tumor itself, so that tissue compatibility for allogeneic vaccination is not required.

Antigen-specific cancer vaccines

Peptide vaccines

Activation of immune responses against selected defined immunodominant tumor antigens has theoretical advantages in terms of control in targeting immune responses. As indicated earlier, a wide range of tumor-associated antigens have been identified but these are rarely cancer-specific. Initial approaches included the use of peptide vaccines using synthetic peptide sequences presented by common human leukocyte antigen (HLA) alleles. The first reported successful protective CTL response from peptide vaccination was for cytomegalovirus (CMV) and Sendai virus mixed with Freund's incomplete adjuvant (30). Almost all peptide-based vaccines have so far used MHC class I-restricted antigenic peptides. Through cross-priming, both MHC class I and class II responses by T-cell profile have resulted as well as documented evidence of protection against syngeneic tumor challenge. This relies on

loading empty MHC molecules specifically on APCs *in vivo*. Peptide loading of other immune cells not expressing co-stimulatory molecules may paradoxically lead to immune tolerance as a number of studies have shown. A number of phase I clinical trials in malignant melanoma have been completed with encouraging results. However, the few clinical responses observed did not correlate with immunological read-out assays such as CTL responses (31, 32).

Polynucleotide (DNA) vaccination

The models for the development of anticancer polynucleotide vaccines have been based on observations that protective antiviral immunity can be induced following genetic immunization with plasmid DNA encoding viral antigens. It was shown that CTLs could be generated against epitopes from influenza virus nucleoprotein, and that these cells provided cross-strain protection in a mouse model (33). Furthermore, DNA immunization was superior to traditional influenza vaccine and immunogenicity by this method was induced by very low doses (10 μg) of plasmid DNA injection.

The DNA transfer into tissue by injection is followed by uptake of plasmid molecules into the cytoplasm and subsequently into the cell nucleus. They are then translated into functional proteins, processed into peptides, and presented by MHC molecules to naive T cells. Importantly, specific T-cell-mediated immunity may be stimulated by vaccine-transfected APCs without prior knowledge of responder MHC haplotypes or relevant MHC class I- or class II-restricted peptide epitopes (Fig. 7.2). Several genes encoding relevant antigens can be applied simultaneously, including genes encoding immunostimulatory cytokines such as GM-CSF, IL-2, and IL-12, which have been shown to direct the nature of the resulting immune response and to augment the efficacy of the vaccine (34–36). The advantages of DNA over protein and peptide vaccines include ease of production and storage, lower cost, low risk of insertional mutagenesis, prolonged antigen expression, induction of antibody, both CD8[+] CTL responses and CD4[+] responses, and Th1 cytokines. DNA vaccination has successfully induced both humoral and cellular immune responses to reporter genes (37), tumor-associated antigens such as carcinoembryonic antigen (CEA)(38) and MUC-1 (39), as well as to viral antigens such as influenza (33) and parasites (40), and has shown efficacy in terms of protection against tumor or

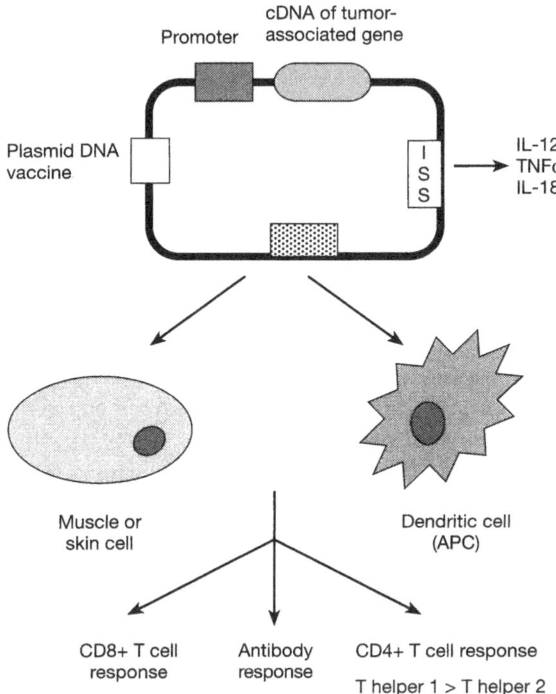

Fig. 7.2 DNA vaccination leads to activation of cellular and humoral immunity. The DNA vaccine comprises a transcriptional unit of cDNA sequence driven by the cytomegalovirus promoter/enhancer. Immunostimulatory sequences (ISS) in the DNA backbone stimulate cytokine release. Expression of transgene in muscle or skin cells, and possibly dendritic cells, leads to the induction of cellular and humoral immune responses.

infectious agent challenge. An important feature of plasmid DNA is the presence of unmethylated CpG motifs that have Th1 activity (41). In nature, the immunostimulatory activity of bacterial DNA is likely to help mobilize immune responses against invading microbes. In vaccine plasmids, these same sequences may serve to mobilize the immune response against the DNA-expressed immunogen. In the unmethylated form, CpG motifs stimulate monocytes and macrophages to secrete Th1 cytokines, including IL-12 and TNFα, and to recruit further immune cells such as NK cells (42).

Dendritic cells in targeted immunotherapy

DCs have emerged as the most potent professional APCs known. Since their discovery 25 years ago, a number of technological advances have resulted in the ability to culture large numbers of DCs *in vitro*, and thereby allow their basic biology to be studied. Progress in this field has fortunately coincided with new insights into the antigens that tumor cells commonly express and, in particular, identification of specific T-cell epitopes for some of these antigens (43). DC-based tumor vaccines have already been translated into clinical trials and in some cases resulted in significant antitumor responses. These encouraging early results also point to the exigency for modification of DC-based vaccines before they become a commonly used modality for the treatment of cancer. DCs are distinguished by their dendritic or veiled morphology and high expression of MHC class I and class II as well as co-stimulatory and adhesion molecules involved in T-cell activation such as B7.1 and B7.2 (44). Although there is no single marker defining DC populations, DCs express unique genes such as one encoding a T-cell-specific chemokine rendering DCs' unique prowess in initiating T-cell responses. DCs reside in the spleen and lymph nodes and comprise less than 1 per cent of the circulating white cell population. They may also arise from cells such as epidermal Langerhans cells or monocytes. DCs can be generated *in vitro* from bone-marrow-derived CD34+ hemopoietic progenitor cells or CD14+ adherent monocytes under specific culture conditions in the presence of GM-CSF and IL-4 (45). This results in 'immature DCs', which have marked phagocytic and endocytic activity but limited ability to present antigen. DC maturation, when cells develop enhanced T-cell activation and migratory capacity, is inducible *in vitro* by using TNFα, lipopolysaccharide, a monocyte-conditioning medium, or a number of other cytokines. Genetic modification of DCs has involved the transfer of genes encoding cytokines or tumor-associated antigens and the creation of DC–tumor-cell fusions.

Gene transfer into dendritic cells

This technology has been established since we have been able to grow DCs in large numbers. There have been comparisons of various methods of gene transfer to DCs. These have included DNA/liposomal transfer, electroporation, CaPO4 co-precipitation, and the use of recombinant adenoviral and retroviral vectors (46, 47). The physical methods result in low-efficiency transfer, while viral methods of transfer are the most efficient. Recombinant adenoviral vectors encoding reporter, cytokine, or tumor-associated genes have been the most efficient vectors. Studies have shown that, just as in control transfections of cell lines, gene expression in DCs was a linear function of multiplicity of infection (MOI). At MOIs of 100:1 and above, transduction efficiencies of up to 95 per cent have been observed, and functionally important levels of cytokine production have been achieved (48).

Dendritic cells and cancer therapies

DCs may not be able to capture and process antigens from malignant cells *in vivo* because of tumor-secreted factors such as IL-10 and vascular endothelial growth factor, which inhibit DC differentiation and antigen-presenting function (13). The use of DCs as immunological adjuvants has followed after successful cytokine-stimulated expansion of autologous DCs *in vitro*, which have been pulsed with antigenic peptide or transduced with genes encoding tumor antigen, and re-infused to induce T-cell responses. This would bypass the proposed obstacle, that is, that tumor antigens do not access DCs *in vivo*. In cancer patients, the antigen-presenting efficacy of pooled mature peripheral DCs has been shown to be inferior compared to that of DCs generated from peripheral blood precursors using a range of cytokines (49). Strategies using such immunocompetent DCs should ensure the presentation of high levels of immunostimulatory signal, which may not normally be provided by most tumor cells.

Nonspecific protein fractions

It is not clear which of the recently identified tumor-specific or tumor-associated antigens is the best choice to mount an effective antitumor response *in vivo*. This was highlighted by the fact that some HLA-A2 patients who develop malignant melanoma have detectable circulating CTL populations, which are not necessarily directed at melanoma antigens, Mart-1, tyrosinase, gp100, or MAGE-3 (50). Alternative approaches to overcome these limitations include the use of unfractionated tumor peptides or tumor proteins as a source of tumor antigen. The drawbacks of this approach are poor efficacy of vaccines due to low concentration of putative antigens in the protein frac-

tions, the requirement for large amounts of tumor from patients to prepare proteins for DC pulsing, and the possibility of vaccination with unfractionated tumor proteins inducing autoimmune responses against self-antigens (51).

Early reports include data on mice immunization with semi-purified DCs pulsed with tumor protein extracts, or with DCs purified from lymph nodes draining the tumor (52). DCs pulsed with such peptides/proteins and used as vaccines were capable of inducing protective immunity against tumor challenge (53), and reducing the growth of subcutaneously established, weakly immunogenic tumors (54). The immunogenicity of peptide-pulsed DCs appears to be directly correlated to the ability of the vaccine to prime *in vivo* splenic antitumor CTLs (55).

Specific peptides

Difficulties in defining truly tumor-specific antigens have limited the potential of DCs in immunotherapy and created so much interest in using unfractionated proteins. However, there are a number of examples where a tumor-associated peptide-pulsed DC strategy has had *in vitro* and *in vivo* efficacy. These include DCs pulsed with peptide CTL epitopes derived from missense mutation at codon 234 of p53 on established murine sarcomas (56); melanoma-associated MZ2-E nonapeptide (encoded by the MAGE-1 gene) (57) and gp100 antigen (58); and HPV type 16 peptide (59) tumor-specific idiotype protein in B-cell lymphoma (60); and oncogenic RAS (61).

Tumor antigen RNA

The limitation in the number of defined tumor antigens has recently highlighted the potential of using mRNA isolated from tumor extracts. The rationale has been that mRNA can be amplified from very small numbers of cells, and tumor-specific RNA can be enriched by subtractive hybridization with RNA from normal tissue to increase the concentration of the tumor-specific antigens present and hence the potency of the vaccine. More importantly, this would reduce the concentration of non-tumor-specific antigens or possibly self-antigens lessening the potential for autoimmunity. There is evidence that antigen mRNA transfer using liposomal vectors and intramuscular or intradermal injections has elicited cellular immune responses to influenza nucleoprotein (62) and CEA (63). DCs lipofected with unfractionated tumor-derived RNA have successfully resulted in the induction of antigen-specific CTLs and protection against syngeneic tumor challenge. The effect was abrogated by treatment with antigen-specific antisense oligodeoxynucleotides (64).

Tumor antigen gene transduction of dendritic cells for immunotherapy

In addition to methods described earlier, it is clear that *in vivo* priming of DCs is possible by cutaneous intradermal injection with naked DNA (65). This results in transfection of skin-derived dendritic cells, which localize to draining lymph nodes and result in potent antigen-specific CTL-mediated protective immunity. Intramuscular delivery of naked DNA-transduced DCs also results in enhanced protective immunity associated with an increased Th1 CD4$^+$ T-cell response, but, notably, this is a specific function of DCs as similarly transfected macrophages lack immunogenicity even though plasmid expression occurs *in vitro* (66).

DCs lipofected with plasmid DNA encoding the antigens glycoprotein B or immediate–early protein IPC27 of herpes simplex virus (HSV) were used to stimulate enriched populations of naive T cells *in vitro*. Antigen-specific CD8$^+$ CTLs that reacted both with specific protein-expressing targets and with syngeneic targets infected with HSV could be demonstrated (67).

Transfection of murine IL-12 gene into murine DCs using retrovirus or lipofection has also resulted in enhanced antitumor-, antigen-specific CTL responses. Adenovirus-mediated transduction of DCs with DF3/MUC-1 tumor-associated antigen results in significant immunogenicity in terms of eliciting CTL responses specific for the transgene, potency in a mixed leukocyte reaction (MLR), and protection against syngeneic tumor challenge. The nature of the T-cell response was further defined to be both CD4$^+$ and CD8$^+$, as determined by antibody blocking to these subsets.

Dendritic cells, immunotolerance, and T-cell apoptosis

DCs comprise less that 1 per cent of peripheral leukocytes and are found in trace (< 0.5 per cent) amounts in tumors such as melanoma using the CD83 marker (68). There are few data on the functional properties of these tumor-associated DCs and, despite their presence, no marked antitumoral response appears to be induced by these cells. A comparison of functions of DCs obtained from syngeneic progressive versus nonprogressive metastases has been possible (69). Compared to cells isolated from nonprogressive lesions, DCs derived from progressive lesions have been shown to be less potent inducers of an allogeneic MLR, have reduced surface CD86 expression, and induce anergy in CD3-stimulated T cells, possibly by high levels of IL-10 secreted locally in tumor tissue. In this way, tumor-associated factors may be able to convert the APC function of DCs from immunogenicity to tolerance induction against tumor tissue.

DCs exhibit immunoregulatory (including tolerogenic) properties *in vivo* and *in vitro*, partly through the ability to subvert T-cell responses (70). DCs have a central role in thymic deletion (central tolerance) and are able to induce peripheral T-cell unresponsiveness *in vivo* (71). In the context of tissue transplantation, donor-derived DCs can be seen in the tissues of long-surviving (therefore spontaneously tolerant) organ allograft recipients, and propagated from their bone marrow (72). There is evidence that DCs present peptides from apoptotic (and not necessarily necrotic) cells. Accordingly DCs may be able to present self-antigens, derived from normal turnover of somatic cells, to T cells and thus induce tolerance to self-proteins that have no access to the thymus (73). A recent report has shown that B7 and FasL molecules expressed on DCs play counterregulatory roles in determining T-cell survival and proliferation, and that DCs may be capable of inducing T-cell apoptosis in the absence of co-stimulation (74). FasL expression on lymphoid DCs has been linked to the ability of DCs to induce low levels of apoptosis in activated T cells (not seen in DCs from FasL-deficient mice). This effect is enhanced by CTLA4Ig, implicating CD28 co-stimulation in the prevention of T cell death mediated by FasL-dependent or -independent mechanisms.

Clinical studies using dendritic cells for immunotherapy

Idiotype protein-pulsed DCs for lymphoma

DCs pulsed with either naturally processed or synthetic peptides have already been used as immunostimulants in humans, and recent studies have used idiotype protein loaded on to DCs with some success in treating lymphoma (60). In mice, this type of immunization had previously resulted in the eradication of established tumors (75). The tumor antigen pulsed on to DCs was the monoclonal surface immunoglobulin (idiotype protein) present in each patient's lymphoma. Infusions of between 2 and 32 million pulsed DCs plus subcutaneous boosts of idiotypic protein with KLH adjuvant resulted in measurable antitumor cellular responses. This was absent prior to immunization, appeared after one or two vaccinations, and was specific for the autologous tumor idiotype protein. Meaningful clinical responses were seen in two patients. As with autologous cell vaccines, this approach involves the laborious task of identifying and purifying idiotypic protein for each individual patient.

Melanoma peptide-pulsed DCs

Early trials consisting of peptide vaccines using antigens, such as gp100, MART-1, tyrosinase, MAGE-1, or MAGE-3, rarely produced clinical responses despite impressive *in vitro* CTL killing (76). In a recent study, an immunodominant peptide of gp100 with a single anchor residue and an intermediate affinity for HLA-A2 was modified to endow it with dual anchor residues and enhanced CTL-generating activity *in vitro*. Vaccination with the modified peptide plus high-dose IL-2 induced T-cell and clinical responses in 91 and 42 per cent of patients, respectively. Remarkably, the sites of tumor regression included liver and brain, which is rarely seen with conventional therapies. The addition of exogenous IL-2 was essential and reduced the frequency of T-cell response without affecting the clinical response (31). A further clinical trial used melanoma peptide-loaded DCs as therapeutic vaccines. This involved the use of numerous melanoma-associated peptides or crude tumor lysates co-cultured with the patients' own DCs, which were then injected directly into lymph nodes to favor efficient entry into the immune system. The highly immunogenic adjuvant KLH was included in the culture to recruit CD4+ T cells and promote the maturation of a memory CTL response. Tumor regressions occurred in 5 of 16 patients. Notably, two of the six responders were given crude lysate-pulsed cells, allowing this approach to be considered for other cancers. All patients had evidence of antigen-specific skin test reactivity (77).

Future developments in dendritic-cell-based immunotherapy

DCs are physiological carriers of antigen and appear to be well tolerated when re-infused into patients. Their sensitivity to culture medium conditions may indicate that we have yet to optimize their yield and immunopotency for clinical use. The use of allogeneic DCs rather than relying on an individual patient's *ex vivo* culture for autologous cells would greatly advance progress and reduce costs. These allogeneic DCs should share some HLA alleles with the recipient to allow T-cell recognition of antigen. Alleles at the HLA locus are extremely polymorphic but only partial matching of HLA between donor DC and recipient may be necessary. Certain class I and class II alleles are common in the population (HLA-A2 in 30 per cent of the population) so only a limited number of HLA haplotypes may need to be included.

This approach has already been tested. *In vitro* challenge of allogeneic DCs derived from peripheral blood of healthy individuals stimulated human immuodeficiency virus (HIV)-specific T cells from the peripheral blood of HIV-infected individuals. Modification of DC maturation may also be achieved by transfer of genes encoding cytokines. There is increasing interest in IL-12, a multifunctional cytokine secreted by DCs upon their interaction with CD4+ T helper lymphocytes through ligation of the co-stimulatory molecule CD40. IL-12 is crucial for the development of Th1-type cell-mediated immune responses as discussed earlier. Genes encoding the whole tumor antigen protein can be processed endogenously and overcome the problem of MHC restriction applicable to peptide antigen pulsing of DCs where recognition will only occur if the patient expresses an appropriate MHC allele (78). CD40 ligand (CD40L) is expressed mainly by a small number of activated circulating CD4+ T cells. CD40L exerts a broad range of humoral and cellular immune responses The CD40L receptor is present on professional APCs such as DCs. The CD40L–CD40R interaction upregulates the expression of co-stimulatory molecules such as B7.1 and B7.2 on these cells. These molecules together with specific MHC/peptide antigen interaction with the T-cell receptor help provide the necessary signals for T-cell activation. APC activation by CD40L increases the APCs' production of IL-12 (and IFN-γ), which helps to polarize the immune response to a Th1 phenotype and enhance NK activity. A recent study has shown that expression of CD40L in neuroblastoma cells by retroviral transfection resulted in effective antitumor response even though only 1.4 per cent of cells expressed the transgene (79).

Conclusion

The last decade has seen an unprecedented investment of research hours and human resources in the field of cancer vaccinology. Many advances have only been possible due to new insights into the molecular immunology of cancer, identification of tumor-associated antigens, and gene transfer technology. However, this enthusiasm has been tempered by the lack of efficacy of any vaccine therapy in clinical trials completed so far. This, in turn, has led to a new appreciation of mechanisms of tumor tolerance and evasion from immune recognition. Data from animal models of genetic vaccination is extremely encouraging and reiterates the challenge of extending experimental success to provide effective treatment for patients.

References

1. Coley W. The treatment of malignant tumors by repeated inoculations of erysipelas with a report of 10 original cases. Am J Med Sci 1893, **105**, 487–490.
2. Rosenberg SA. Adoptive immunotherapy of cancer using lymphokine activated killer cells and recombinant interleukin-2. Important Adv Oncol 1986, 55–91.
3. Barth A, Hoon DS, Foshag LJ, Nizze JA, Famatiga E, Okun E, Morton DL. Polyvalent melanoma cell vaccine induces delayed-type hypersensitivity and *in vitro* cellular immune response. Cancer Res 1994, **54**, 3342–5.
4. Rosenberg SA, Packard BS, Aebersold PM, Solomon D, Topalian SL, Toy ST, Simon P, Lotze MT, Yang JC, Seipp CA, *et al.* Use of lymphocytes and interleukin-2 in the immunotherapy of patients with metastatic melanoma. A preliminary report [see comments]. New Engl J Med 1988, **319**, 1676–80.
5. Boon T, Cerottini J-C, Van den Eynde B, van der Bruggen P, Van Pel A. Tumor antigens recognised by lymphocytes. Annu Rev Immunol 1994, **12**, 337–65.
6. Pardoll D, Carrera A. Thymic selection. Curr Opin Immunol 1992, **4**, 162–5.
7. Mosmann TR, Sad S. The expanding universe of T-cell subsets: Th1, Th2 and more. Immunol Today 1996, **17**, 138–46.
8. Paul WE, Seder RA. Lymphocyte responses and cytokines. Cell 1994, **76**, 241–51.
9. Cox JC, Coulter AR. Adjuvants—a classification and review of their modes of action. Vaccine 1997, **15**, 248–56.
10. Kaklamanis L, Leek R, Koukourakis M, Gatter KC, Harris AL. Loss of transporter in antigen processing 1. Transport protein and major histocompatibility complex class I molecules in metastatic versus primary breast cancer. Cancer Res 1995, **55**, 5191–4.
11. Korkolopoulou P, Kaklamanis L, Pezzella F, Harris AL, Gatter KC. Loss of antigen-presenting molecules (MHC class I and TAP-1) in lung cancer. Br J Cancer 1996, **73**, 148–53.
12. Strand S, Hofmann WJ, Hug H, Muller M, Otto G, Strand D, Mariani SM, Stremmel W, Krammer PH, Galle PR. Lymphocyte apoptosis induced by CD95 (APO-1/Fas) ligand-expressing tumor cells—a mechanism of immune evasion? [see comments]. Nat Med 1996, **2**, 1361–6.
13. Gabrilovich DI, Chen HL, Girgis KR, Cunningham HT, Meny GM, Nadaf S, Kavanaugh D, Carbone DP. Production of vascular endothelial growth factor by human tumors inhibits the functional maturation of dendritic cells [published erratum appears in Nat Med 1996, 2 (11), 1267]. Nat Med 1996, **2**, 1096–103.
14. Krummel MF, Sullivan TJ, Allison JP. Superantigen responses and co-stimulation: CD28 and CTLA-4 have opposing effects on T cell expansion *in vitro* and *in vivo*. Int Immunol 1996, **8**, 519–23.
15. Waterhouse P, Penninger JM, Timms E, Wakeham A, Shahinian A, Lee KP, Thompson CB, Griesser H, Mak TW. Lymphoproliferative disorders with early lethality in mice deficient in Ctla-4. Science 1995, **270**, 985–8.
16. Sijts EJAM, Leupers CJM, Mengede EAM, Loenen WAM, van den Elsen PJ, Melief CJM. Cloning of the MCF1233 murine leukemia virus and identification of sequences involved in viral tropism, oncogenicity and T cell epitope formation. Virus Res 1994, **34**, 339–49.
17. Barber LD, Parham P. The essence of epitopes. J Exp Med 1994, **180**, 1191–4.
18. Oukka M, Riche N, Kosmatopoulos K. A nonimmunodominant nucleoprotein-derived peptide is presented by influenza A virus-infected H-2b cells. J Immunol 1994, **152**, 4843–51.
19. van der Most RG, Sette A, Oseroff C, Alexander J, Murali-Krishna K, Lau LL, Southwood S, Sidney J, Chesnut RW, Matloubian M, Ahmed R. Analysis of cytotoxic T cell responses to dominant and subdominant epitopes during acute and chronic lymphocytic choriomeningitis virus infection. J Immunol 1996, **157**, 5543–54.
20. Lindenmann J, Klein PA. Viral oncolysis: increased immunogenicity of host cell antigen associated with influenza virus. J Exp Med 1967, **126**, 93–108.

21. Palmer K, Moore J, Everard M, Harris JD, Rodgers S, Rees RC, Murray AK, Mascari R, Kirkwood J, Riches PG, Fisher C, Thomas JM, Harries M, Johnston SR, Collins MK, Gore ME. Gene therapy with autologous, interleukin 2-secreting tumor cells in patients with malignant melanoma. Hum Gene Ther 1999, **10**, 1261–8.

22. Dranoff G, Jaffee E, Lazenby A, Golumbek P, Levitsky H, Brose K, Jackson V, Hamada H, Pardoll D, Mulligan RC. Vaccination with irradiated tumor cells engineered to secrete murine granulocyte–macrophage colony-stimulating factor stimulates potent, specific, and long-lasting anti-tumor immunity. Proc Natl Acad Sci, USA 1993, **90**, 3539–43.

23. Steinman RM. The dendritic cell system and its role in immunogenicity. Annu Rev Immunol 1991, **9**, 271–96.

24. Simons JW, Jaffee EM, Weber CE, Levitsky HI, Nelson WG, Carducci MA, Lazenby AJ, Cohen LK, Finn CC, Clift SM, Hauda KM, Beck LA, Leiferman KM, Owens AH, Jr, Piantadosi S, Dranoff G, Mulligan RC, Pardoll DM, Marshall FF. Bioactivity of autologous irradiated renal cell carcinoma vaccines generated by *ex vivo* granulocyte–macrophage colony-stimulating factor gene transfer. Cancer Res 1997, **57**, 1537–46.

25. Jaffee EM, Pardoll DM. Considerations for the clinical development of cytokine gene-transduced tumor cell vaccines. Methods 1997, **12**, 143–53.

26. Toes RE, Blom RJ, van der Voort E, Offringa R, Melief CJ, Kast WM. Protective antitumor immunity induced by immunization with completely allogeneic tumor cells. Cancer Res 1996, **56**, 3782–7.

27. Huang AYC, Golumbek P, Ahmadzadeh M, Jaffee E, Pardoll D, Levitsky H. Role of bone marrow-derived cells in presenting MHC class I-restricted tumor antigens. Science 1994, **264**, 961–5.

28. Huang AY, Golumbek P, Ahmadzadeh M, Jaffee E, Pardoll D, Levitsky H. Bone marrow-derived cells present MHC class I-restricted tumor antigens in priming of antitumor immune responses. Ciba Found Symp 1994, **187**, 229–40.

29. Huang AYC, Bruce AT, Pardoll DM, Levitsky HI. *In vivo* cross-priming of MHC class I-restricted antigens requires the TAP transporter. Immunity 1996, **4**, 349–55.

30. Schulz M, Zinkernagel RM, Hengartner H. Peptide-induced antiviral protection by cytotoxic T cells. Proc Natl Acad Sci, USA 1991, **88**, 991–3.

31. Rosenberg SA, Yang JC, Schwartzentruber DJ, Hwu P, Marincola FM, Topalian SL, Restifo NP, Dudley ME, Schwarz SL, Spiess PJ, Wunderlich JR, Parkhurst MR, Kawakami Y, Seipp CA, Einhorn JH, White DE. Immunologic and therapeutic evaluation of a synthetic peptide vaccine for the treatment of patients with metastatic melanoma [see comments]. Nat Med 1998, **4**, 321–7.

32. Parkhurst MR, Salgaller ML, Southwood S, Robbins PF, Sette A, Rosenberg SA, Kawakami Y. Improved induction of melanoma-reactive CTL with peptides from the melanoma antigen gp100 modified at HLA-A*0201-binding residues. J Immunol 1996, **157**, 2539–48.

33. Ulmer JB, Donnelly JJ, Parker SE, Rhodes GH, Felgner PL, Dwarki VJ, Gromkowski SH, Deck RR, DeWitt CM, Friedman A, Hawe LA, Leander KR, Martinez D, Perry HC, Shiver JW, Montgomery DL, Liu MA. Heterologous protection against influenza by injection of DNA encoding a viral protein. Science 1993, **259**, 1745–9.

34. Davis HL, Mancini M, Michel ML, Whalen RG. DNA-mediated immunization to hepatitis B surface antigen: longevity of primary response and effect of boost. Vaccine 1996, **14**, 910–15.

35. Trinchieri G. Recognition of major histocompatibility complex class I antigens by natural killer cells. J Exp Med 1994, **180**, 417–21.

36. Syrengelas AD, Chen TT, Levy R. DNA immunization induces protective immunity against B-cell lymphoma. Nat Med 1996, **2**, 1038–41.

37. Forg P, von Hoegen P, Dalemans W, Schirrmacher V. Superiority of the ear pinna over muscle tissue as site for DNA vaccination. Gene Ther 1998, **5**, 789–97.

38. Conry RM, LoBuglio AF, Loechel F, Moore SE, Sumerel LA, Barlow DL, Curiel DT. A carcinoembryonic antigen polynucleotide vaccine has *in vivo* antitumor activity. Gene Ther 1995, **2**, 59–65.

39. Graham RA, Burchell JM, Beverley P, Taylor-Papadimitriou J. Intramuscular immunisation with MUC1 cDNA can protect C57 mice challenged with MUC1-expressing syngeneic mouse tumor cells. Int J Cancer 1996, **65**, 664–70.

40. Sedegah M, Hedstrom R, Hobart P, Hoffman SL. Protection against malaria by immunization with plasmid DNA encoding circumsporozoite protein. Proc Natl Acad Sci, USA 1994, **91**, 9866–70.

41. Krieg AM, Yi AK, Schorr J, Davis HL. The role of CpG dinucleotides in DNA vaccines. Trends Microbiol 1998, **6**, 23–7.

42. Klinman DM, Yamshchikov G, Ishigatsubo Y. Contribution of CpG motifs to the immunogenicity of DNA vaccines. J Immunol 1997, **158**, 3635–9.

43. Banchereau J, Steinman RM. Dendritic cells and the control of immunity. Nature 1998, **392**, 245–52.

44. Bender A, Sapp M, Schuler G, Steinman RM, Bhardwaj N. Improved methods for the generation of dendritic cells from nonproliferating progenitors in human blood. J Immunol Methods 1996, **196**, 121–35.

45. Talmor M, Mirza A, Turley S, Mellman I, Hoffman LA, Steinman RM. Generation or large numbers of immature and mature dendritic cells from rat bone marrow cultures. Eur J Immunol 1998, **28**, 811–17.

46. Arthur JF, Butterfield LH, Roth MD, Bui LA, Kiertscher SM, Lau R, Dubinett S, Glaspy J, McBride WH, Economou JS. A comparison of gene transfer methods in human dendritic cells. Cancer Gene Ther 1997, **4**, 17–25.

47. Alijagic S, Moller P, Artuc M, Jurgovsky K, Czarnetzki BM, Schadendorf D. Dendritic cells generated from peripheral blood transfected with human tyrosinase induce specific T cell activation. Eur J Immunol 1995, **25**, 3100–7.

48. Gong J, Chen L, Chen D, Kashiwaba M, Manome Y, Tanaka T, Kufe D. Induction of antigen-specific antitu-

mor immunity with adenovirus-transduced dendritic cells. Gene Ther 1997, **4**, 1023–8.

49. Gabrilovich DI, Corak J, Ciernik IF, Kavanaugh D, Carbone DP. Decreased antigen presentation by dendritic cells in patients with breast cancer. Clin Cancer Res 1997, **3**, 483–90.

50. Anichini A, Mortarini R, Maccalli C, Squarcina P, Fleischhauer K, Mascheroni L, Parmiani G. Cytotoxic T cells directed to tumor antigens not expressed on normal melanocytes dominate HLA-A2.1-restricted immune repertoire to melanoma. J Immunol 1996, **156**, 208–17.

51. Houghton AN. Cancer antigens: immune recognition of self and altered self [comment]. J Exp Med 1994, **180**, 1–4.

52. Gyure LA, Barfoot R, Denham S, Hall JG. Immunity to a syngeneic sarcoma induced in rats by dendritic lymph cells exposed to the tumor either *in vivo* or *in vitro*. Br J Cancer 1987, **55**, 17–20.

53. Grabbe S, Bruvers S, Gallo RL, Knisely TL, Nazareno R, Granstein RD. Tumor antigen presentation by murine epidermal cells. J Immunol 1991, **146**, 3656–61.

54. Zitvogel L, Mayordomo JI, Tjandrawan T, DeLeo AB, Clarke MR, Lotze MT, Storkus WJ. Therapy of murine tumors with tumor peptide-pulsed dendritic cells: dependence on T cells, B7 costimulation, and T helper cell 1-associated cytokines [see comments]. J Exp Med 1996, **183**, 87–97.

55. Celluzzi CM, Mayordomo JI, Storkus WJ, Lotze MT, Falo LD, Jr. Peptide-pulsed dendritic cells induce antigen-specific CTL-mediated protective tumor immunity [see comments]. J Exp Med 1996, **183**, 283–7.

56. Mayordomo JI, Loftus DJ, Sakamoto H, De Cesare CM, Appasamy PM, Lotze MT, Storkus WJ, Appella E, DeLeo AB. Therapy of murine tumors with p53 wild-type and mutant sequence peptide-based vaccines. J Exp Med 1996, **183**, 1357–65.

57. Mukherji B, Chakraborty NG. Immunobiology and immunotherapy of melanoma [see comments]. Curr Opin Oncol 1995, **7**, 175–84.

58. Tsai V, Southwood S, Sidney J, Sakaguchi K, Kawakami Y, Appella E, Sette A, Celis E. Identification of subdominant CTL epitopes of the GP100 melanoma-associated tumor antigen by primary *in vitro* immunization with peptide-pulsed dendritic cells. J Immunol 1997, **158**, 1796–802.

59. Ossevoort MA, Feltkamp MC, van Veen KJ, Melief CJ, Kast WM. Dendritic cells as carriers for a cytotoxic T-lymphocyte epitope-based peptide vaccine in protection against a human papillomavirus type 16-induced tumor. J Immunother Emphasis Tumor Immunol 1995, **18**, 86–94.

60. Hsu FJ, Benike C, Fagnoni F, Liles TM, Czerwinski D, Taidi B, Engleman EG, Levy R. Vaccination of patients with B-cell lymphoma using autologous antigen-pulsed dendritic cells. Nat Med 1996, **2**, 52–8.

61. Gjertsen MK, Bakka A, Breivik J, Saeterdal I, Gedde-Dahl T, 3rd, Stokke KT, Solheim BG, Egge TS, Soreide O, Thorsby E, Gaudernack G. *Ex vivo* ras peptide vaccination in patients with advanced pancreatic cancer: results of a phase I/II study. Int J Cancer 1996, **65**, 450–3.

62. Martinon F, Krishnan S, Lenzen G, Magne R, Gomard E, Guillet JG, Levy JP, Meulien P. Induction of virus-specific cytotoxic T lymphocytes *in vivo* by liposome-entrapped mRNA. Eur J Immunol 1993, **23**, 1719–22.

63. Conry RM, LoBuglio AF, Wright M, Sumerel L, Pike MJ, Johanning F, Benjamin R, Lu D, Curiel DT. Characterization of a messenger RNA polynucleotide vaccine vector. Cancer Res 1995, **55**, 1397–400.

64. Boczkowski D, Nair SK, Snyder D, Gilboa E. Dendritic cells pulsed with RNA are potent antigen-presenting cells *in vitro* and *in vivo*. J Exp Med 1996, **184**, 465–72.

65. Condon C, Watkins SC, Celluzzi CM, Thompson K, Falo LD. DNA-based immunization by *in vivo* transfection of dendritic cells. Nat Med 1996, **2**, 1122–8.

66. Manickan E, Kanangat S, Rouse RJ, Yu Z, Rouse BT. Enhancement of immune response to naked DNA vaccine by immunization with transfected dendritic cells. J Leuk Biol 1997, **61**, 125–32.

67. Rouse RJ, Nair SK, Lydy SL, Bowen JC, Rouse BT. Induction *in vitro* of primary cytotoxic T-lymphocyte responses with DNA encoding herpes simplex virus proteins. J Virol 1994, **68**, 5685–9.

68. Zhou LJ, Tedder TF. Human blood dendritic cells selectively express CD83, a member of the immunoglobulin superfamily. J Immunol 1995, **154**, 3821–35.

69. Enk AH, Jonuleit H, Saloga J, Knop J. Dendritic cells as mediators of tumor-induced tolerance in metastatic melanoma. Int J Cancer 1997, **73**, 309–16.

70. Finkelman FD, Lees A, Birnbaum R, Gause WC, Morris SC. Dendritic cells can present antigen *in vivo* in a tolerogenic or immunogenic fashion. J Immunol 1996, **157**, 1406–14.

71. Khoury SJ, Gallon L, Chen W, Betres K, Russell ME, Hancock WW, Carpenter CB, Sayegh MH, Weiner HL. Mechanisms of acquired thymic tolerance in experimental autoimmune encephalomyelitis: thymic dendritic-enriched cells induce specific peripheral T cell unresponsiveness *in vivo*. J Exp Med 1995, **182**, 357–66.

72. Starzl TE, Demetris AJ, Murase N, Trucco M, Thomson AW, Rao AS. The changing immunology of organ transplantation. Hosp Pract (Off Ed) 1995, **30**, 31–4, 37–42.

73. Albert ML, Sauter B, Bhardwaj N. Dendritic cells acquire antigen from apoptotic cells and induce class I-restricted CTLs. Nature 1998, **392**, 86–9.

74. Lu L, Qian S, Hershberger PA, Rudert WA, Lynch DH, Thomson AW. Fas ligand (CD95L) and B7 expression on dendritic cells provide counter-regulatory signals for T cell survival and proliferation. J Immunol 1997, **158**, 5676–84.

75. Mayordomo JI, Zorina T, Storkus WI, Zitvogel L, Celluzi C, Falo LD, Melief CJ, Ildstad ST, Kast WM, Deleo AB, Lotze MT. Bone marrow-derived dendritic cells pulsed with synthetic tumor peptides elicit protective and therapeutic antitumor immunity. Nat Med 1995, **1**, 1297–302.

76. Jaeger E, Bernhard H, Romero P, Ringhoffer M, Arand M, Karbach J, Ilsemann C, Hagedorn M, Knuth A.

Generation of cytotoxic T-cell responses with synthetic melanoma-associated peptides *in vivo*: implications for tumor vaccines with melanoma-associated antigens. Int J Cancer 1996, **66**, 162–9.

77. Nestle FO, Alijagic S, Gilliet M, Sun Y, Grabbe S, Dummer R, Burg G, Schadendorf D. Vaccination of melanoma patients with peptide- or tumor lysate-pulsed dendritic cells [see comments]. Nat Med 1998, **4**, 328–32.

78. Storkus WJ, Wei M, Cresswell P, Dawson JR. Class I-like CD1A-C do not protect target cells from NK-mediated cytolysis. Cell Immunol 1996, **167**, 154–6.

79. Grossmann ME, Brown MP, Brenner MK. Antitumor responses induced by transgenic expression of CD40 ligand. Hum Gene Ther 1997, **8**, 1935–43.

8

Targeting of cancer gene therapy

Kevin J. Harrington and Richard G. Vile

Introduction

Cancer gene therapy (CGT) involves the delivery of genetic material to malignant (or normal) human cells with a therapeutic intent. This new field of study has emerged from our rapidly expanding understanding of the molecular biology of cancer and represents an exciting means of designing rational new targeted-treatment strategies. The key components of an effective CGT approach are the therapeutic gene that is to be introduced into a cell, the vehicle that delivers it to the cell and mediates its entry, and the means by which its expression is controlled to maximize efficacy and limit toxicity (Fig. 8.1). Each of these individual pieces of the jigsaw represents an extremely active area of research. The initial studies focused largely on the identification of therapeutic genes with the ability to kill cancer cells *in vitro* and *in vivo*. This search yielded (and continues to yield) a large number of candidate genes with various mechanisms of action. More recently, attention has shifted towards controling the expression of these genes in target tissues and limiting their potential toxicity in normal tissues (reviewed in reference 1). The development of viral and nonviral vectors that are capable of delivering therapeutic genes efficiently to tumor cells has identified an increasing

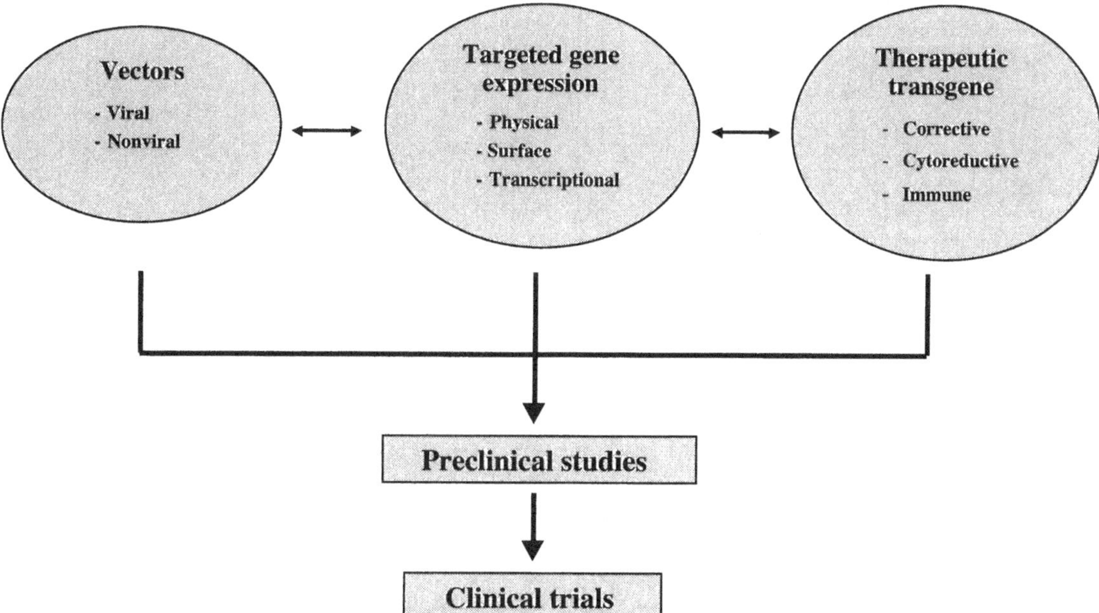

Fig. 8.1 Key components of a gene therapy system. The aim of current research is to develop systemically administered vectors that can be used to deliver potent therapeutic transgenes that can be precisely controled such that their effects are manifest only in target tissues. Careful development and subsequent integration of each of these components will pave the way for future preclinical and clinical trials.

number of candidates, which are undergoing intensive analysis (2). In this chapter, the key background to CGT will be presented and an attempt will be made to focus on those aspects of the subject that offer the prospect of novel, clinically applicable targeted-therapy strategies.

Development of vectors for CGT

In recent years it has become clear that the issue of vector development will determine the success or failure of CGT. Efforts to identify effective therapeutic transgenes and the means of ensuring their selective expression in target tissues will come to nothing unless they can be delivered to a substantial fraction of clonogenic cells (3, 4). Until now, preclinical and clinical studies have largely relied on direct intratumoral injection or infusion, but this technique has limited relevance to clinical situations, such as disseminated metastatic disease, in which systemic delivery will be required. Immunomodulatory gene therapy is an exception to this rule in that the purpose of treatment is to use locoregional gene delivery to prime a systemic immune response that will be capable of dealing with both local and distant metastatic cancer (5). Vectors for CGT can be considered under the broad headings of viral and nonviral systems.

Viral vectors

During infection of a cell, viruses use specific entry mechanisms and subvert the biosynthetic machinery of the infected cell to secure expression of their genes in order to allow viral replication and release. While these properties make viruses extremely attractive as vectors for CGT, they are also responsible for their pathogenicity. Therefore, the challenge of developing viral vectors for CGT lies in harnessing the targeting efficiency of viruses while abrogating their ability to cause infection and disease. The most commonly used means of achieving these objectives has been by modification of the viral genome. Genetic sequences required for viral binding, entry, and gene delivery can be retained, while those that mediate viral replication and pathogenicity are removed. Such changes leave 'space' in the viral genome that may be replaced with exogenous therapeutic genes. Genetically engineered viral vectors theoretically retain the cellular tropism of the wild-type virus and deliver the transgene to the malignant cell

population without being propagated as an ongoing infection. Additional attempts have been made to modify the tropism of wild-type viruses and re-target them specifically to cancer cells. Such attempts have focused on replacing those viral components that mediate cell binding and internalization with re-engineered receptors that recognize cancer-associated antigens (6–9).

Many viral vectors are under development, each with its own potential strengths and weaknesses. Most work has focused on retroviruses (RV), adenoviruses (AV), herpes simplex viruses (HSV), adeno-associated viruses (AAV), and pox viruses (PV), although other viruses that are under investigation include reovirus (10), Newcastle disease virus (11), alphaviruses (12), and vesicular stomatitis virus (13). However, a detailed discussion of all of the viruses that are currently under active development is beyond the scope of this chapter, which will be restricted to RV, AV, HSV, AAV, and PV.

Retroviral vectors

RV are single-stranded diploid RNA viruses, the basic structure of which is illustrated in Fig. 8.2. C-type RV, based on the Moloney murine leukemia virus (MoMLV), have been investigated most intensively (14). RV have a complex life cycle (15). They enter cells by binding of surface envelope proteins (encoded by the *env* gene) to specific cellular receptors. Upon entry to the cell, the viral enzyme reverse transcriptase (encoded by the *pol* gene) transcribes a double-stranded DNA copy of the viral genome. This DNA sequence is able to enter the nucleus of dividing cells (because the nuclear membrane has broken down) and integrate at random sites into the genome of the host under the action of the viral integrase enzyme (encoded by the *pol* gene). This step accounts for a significant potential advantage of RV vectors, namely, that of stable integration and expression of genes, although this is of limited relevance in strategies aiming to kill the targeted cell. In the case of wild-type RV, gene expression results in viral replication, assembly, and packaging with subsequent propagation of the viral infection. Clearly, if RV-targeted CGT caused an ongoing RV infection, this would have serious safety implications. Therefore, RV used for CGT protocols have been manipulated to render them replication-deficient. This is accomplished by producing RV from so-called

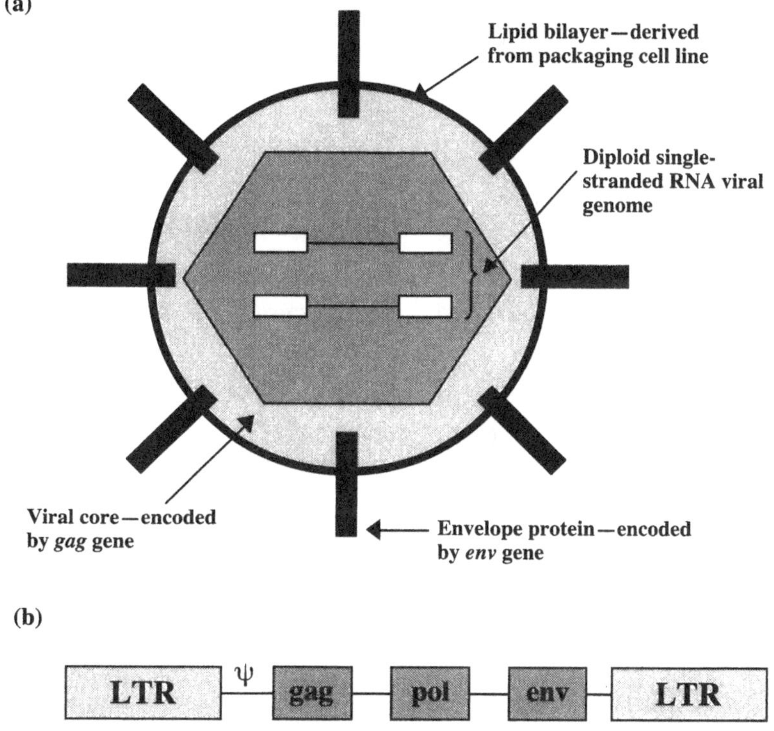

Fig 8.2 Diagrammatic representation of the morphological and genetic structure of a typical retrovirus: (a) Morphology. RV are single-stranded diploid RNA viruses that have a liped bilayer membrane surrounding the viral core. Envelope proteins mediate cell entry through interactions with specific cellular receptors (b) Genome. The RV genome consists of a packaging sequence (ψ and 3 genes (gag, pol, and env). The RV gag, pol, and env genes can be deleted and replaced by therapeutic transgenes. The resulting viral particles derived from producer cell lines are infectious and can secure expression of the transgenes they contain but are not capable of directing further viral replication. LTR, Long terminal repeat, important in replication and transcriptional control; ψ, sequence that mediates viral packaging and release from infected cells. Gag encodes the viral core proteins, pal encodes the reverse transcriplase enzyme, and env encodes the viral protein.

packaging cell lines which have been engineered stably to express the RV *gag, pol,* and *env* genes from plasmids lacking the packaging sequence (Ψ).

Delivery of the therapeutic gene in a construct containing the RV long terminal repeats (LTR) and Ψ into such a packaging cell line permits assembly, packaging, and release of infectious but non-replicative RV that can be harvested from the supernatant and concentrated. In recent years it has been appreciated that RV have a number of potential disadvantages as vectors for CGT: (1) RV packaging cell lines yield relatively low titers (10^7 infectious units/ml); (2) the RV genome is small, which limits the size of the therapeutic gene constructs that RV can carry to approximately 8000 base pairs (8 kb); (3) random integration into the host genome may disrupt cellular genes (insertional mutagenesis); and (4) RV-mediated gene delivery is only successful in dividing cells since RV constructs lack the

ability to pass the intact nuclear membrane. The lentiviruses (a subtype of RV) may represent a powerful alternative to C-type RV. Lentiviruses such as human, simian, and feline immunodeficiency viruses (HIV, SIV, and FIV, respectively) can infect nondividing cells (16) and integrate in the same way as other RV. Clearly, the development of lentiviral vectors will need special emphasis on the safety aspects of the viral constructs, in view of the serious nature of the clinical syndromes caused by these agents.

Adenoviral vectors

AV are non-enveloped, protein-encapsidated viruses that contain a genome composed of double-stranded DNA (Fig. 8.3). The viral capsid is made of an icosahedral mosaic of 240 hexones and 12 pen tone bases from which protrude antennae-like fibers terminating

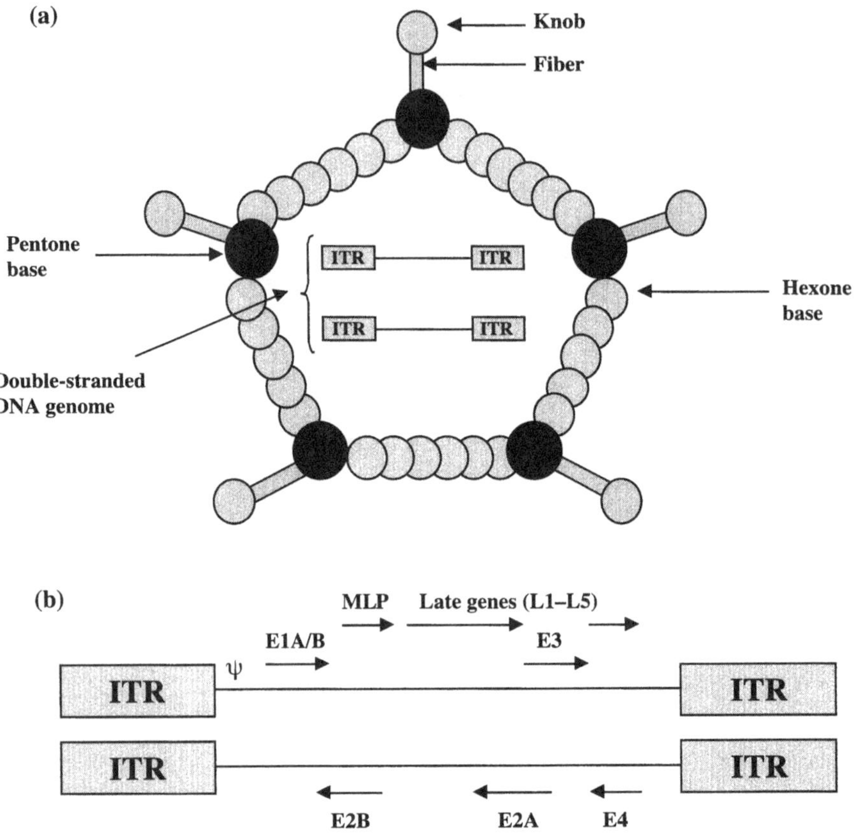

Fig. 8.3　Diagrammatic representation of the morphological and genetic structure of a typical adenovirus. (a) Morphology. AV are double-stranded DNA viruses composed of non-enveloped icosahedral proteins capsids (hexones and pentones) that bind to the CAR receptor through the knob domain of the fiber. (b) Genome. The AV genes are divided into early (E) and late (L) genes. Deletion of the E1 genes renders AV replication-defective. Further deletion of other early genes (E2, E3, and E4) serves the function of reducing the risk of emergence of replication-competent AV and makes additional space for packaging of therapeutic transgenes. In recent years there has been increasing interest in the development of conditionally replication-competent AV in which the E1 gene is restored under the control of a tissue/tumor-specific promoter. ITR, Inverted terminal repeat, important in transcriptional control; ψ, packaging signal; E1A/B, encode proteins involved in regulation of transcription of viral genes; E2A/B, encode proteins involved in viral replication; E3, involved in preventing cytolysis by T lymphocytes and cytokines; E4, involved in DNA replication; MLP, major late promoter, which directs transcription of the late genes; L1–L5, late genes that encode structured element of the virus.

in a knob protein that mediates binding of the virus to the cellular coxsackie and adenovirus receptor (CAR) (17). After CAR binding, viral internalization occurs by interaction of viral argininq–glycine–aspartate (RGD) sequences with cellular $\alpha_v\beta_3$ and $\alpha_v\beta_5$ integrins. The virus escapes from endosomes and, once in the cytoplasm, disassembles and translocates to the nucleus under the influence of nuclear localising signals within the capsid proteins. Upon entry to the nucleus, viral gene expression can begin. It has been reported recently that CAR expression is downregulated in a number of tumor types (18) This phenomenon may have important implications for the use of AV vectors in CGT and increases the potential importance of work aiming to alter the natural tropism of these viruses (6–8).

More than 40 AV serotypes, subdivided into six groups (groups A to F), have been identified. Viruses from group C (serotypes 2 and 5, Ad2 and Ad5) have been most extensively evaluated as candidates for gene delivery (19). However, up to 70 per cent of the population have circulating neutralizing anti-Ad2 and anti-Ad5 antibodies that accelerate viral clearance after the first administration. Furthermore, the immunogenicity of AV precludes repeated dosing with the same serotype, even in patients who have previously not been exposed.

Administering replicating AV to patients with cancer is potentially dangerous. In an attempt to improve the safety profile of AV vectors, replication-defective AV (RDAV) have been generated by deleting the El gene that is essential for viral gene transcription. Further levels of control have been added by deleting other early genes (E2, E3, and E4). More recently, the whole AV coding sequence has been removed to form minimal-sequence or 'gutless' AV (19). Such viruses, which have a residual inverted terminal repeat (ITR) sequence and the packaging signal, have enormous capacity to carry therapeutic genes but must be grown in producer cell lines in the presence of helper viruses, which are unable to package themselves but which can supply all the necessary viral gene functions to facilitate packaging of infectious) RDAV containing the therapeutic transgene. RDAV have a number of potential advantages over RV as vectors for CGT: (1) they can be produced in high titers (10^{10}–10^{11} infectious units/ml); (2) they can infect nondividing cells (due to the presence of viral nuclear localizing signals); (3) gene expression occurs without integration into the host genome, which removes the risk of insertional mutagenesis; and (4) gutless AV offer the chance to develop vectors with vastly expanded capacity for therapeutic transgenes.

In recent years, there has been a move towards the investigation of replication–competent AV (RCAV) for CGT (20). Two general approaches have been described: (1) the generation of AV with genetic defects that prevent their replication in normal cells but which permit their replication in malignant cells (21–24); and (2) the generation of AV with essential portions of the viral genome under transcriptional regulation which endows them with specificity for tumor cells (25–28). The most widely studied RCAV is the ONYX-015 (dl1520) virus (21). This virus contains a deletion in the E1B 55 kDa gene, the product of which is responsible for binding and inactivating cellular p53. Therefore, this ElB-deleted virus theoretically replicates preferentially in p53-deficient tumor cells as compared to normal p53 wild-type cells (although this matter is not as clear-cut as originally described). This agent has been shown to have activity against tumors in mice (29, 30) and appears to enhance the effect of both cytotoxic chemotherapy and radiotherapy in preclinical studies (31, 32]. ONYX-015 has entered phase I/II studies in head and neck, colorectal, pancreatic, and ovarian cancers where it has been shown to yield tumor responses both alone and in combination with cisplatin chemotherapy (33–35).

Herpes simplex viral vectors

HSV are large viruses with a linear double-stranded DNA genome of approximately 150 kb that encodes over 70 proteins (36). Entry into cells is mediated by binding of the viral gB and gD glycoproteins to heparan sulfate residues on the cell surface. HSV are human pathogens that establish latent infections (a matter that carries limited therapeutic significance but which poses safety concerns for CGT applications). HSV can be rendered replication-defective by inactivating key immediate early genes (ICPO, ICP4, ICP22, and ICP27) that are essential for subsequent expression of other viral genes. In addition, deletion or disruption of key viral genes can yield oncolytic HSV with preferential toxicity for tumor, as opposed to normal, cells. Furthermore, since many HSV genes can be deleted without compromising the ability to produce viral, vectors, HSV vectors can contain large DNA sequences comprising multiple genes and their regulatory elements. In this regard, there has been much interest in so-called HSV amplicon vectors that contain multiple repetitions of partial HSV sequence consisting of an origin of replication and a cleavage/packaging sequence (37). Such vectors retain their ability to infect cells, are non-replicative, and have enormous packaging capacity. Their use potentially circumvents the cytotoxicity and immune activation associated with viral gene expression. However, in the context of CGT such considerations have limited significance and these vectors are more likely to be of use in the treatment of nonmalignant conditions.

In the setting of CGT, thus far, most attention has focused on the creation of oncolytic HSV vectors. It has been shown that HSV mutants defective in HSV thymidine kinase (HSVtk) replicate preferentially in mitotic cells (38) although the use of such viruses presents a potential problem in that they are resistant to the use of ganciclovir as a means of aborting a productive infection. Other HSV mutants with defects in the ICP6 (hrR3) or ICP34.5 (HSV-1716) or both (G207) genes lyse dividing tumor cells without causing significant toxicity in normal cells, have antitumor activity in animal models and have entered clinical trials in patients (39–45). In an alternative approach, an HSV with a deletion in the glycoprotein H gene has been shown to be able to infect, replicate in, and kill cells but is incapable of cellular exit and subsequent propagation of the infection. This agent has been called HSV-DISC (disabled infectious single cycle) and has been shown to have activity against colorectal cancer cells *in vitro* and *in vivo* (46).

Adeno-associated viral vectors

AAV are single-stranded DNA viruses composed of non-enveloped icosahedral protein capsids. They are native, non-pathogenic human viruses that require co-infection with another 'helper' virus (adenovirus or herpesvirus) in order to replicate (47). In the absence of helper virus, AAV infection of a cell leads to latency in which the viral genome persists either in an integrated form or as episomal DNA. AAV vectors have a number of potential advantages over RV and AV vectors. They are capable of infecting nondividing cells and are stably integrated/maintained in the host genome, although this issue is of lesser importance in CGT where transient expression of cytotoxic genes should be sufficient to achieve a therapeutic effect. An additional benefit is that, in contrast to RV, the risk of insertional mutagenesis is reduced since integration occurs preferentially at a site-dependent locus on chromosome 19. However, in AAV vectors for CGT this characteristic integration is lost due to deletion of rep proteins (in an attempt to reduce the risk of the emergence of replication competent AAV). However, AAV also have a number of potential drawbacks as vectors for CGT. They have limited packaging capacity (approximately 5 kb) and gene expression may be slow to reach its peak. Production requires the use of helper viruses which means that preparations for pre-clinical and clinical use may be contaminated with these entities.

Pox virus vectors

PV, which include vaccinia and canarypox (ALVAC,) are double-stranded DNA viruses. PV that contain a defective thymidine kinase gene have been shown to replicate preferentially in tumor cells and a number of studies have demonstrated levels of gene expression up to 188 000-fold greater in tumor compared with normal tissue after regional or systemic administration (48–50). Direct intraprostatic administration of a PV vector in association with various solid state vehicles (gelatin matrix, suture material) has been reported in a murine model. This form of delivery resulted in durable gene expression and enhanced activity (51). In addition, persistent gene expression was demonstrated in patients with mesothelioma who received multiple injections of PV vectors over a period of 3 months despite the development of an antibody response (52). Initial therapeutic studies with PV vectors have focused on their ability to deliver immunostimulatory cytokine genes (see below) (53, 54). Such studies have led to phase I clinical trials in patients with melanoma and adenocarcinomas (55–58).

Nonviral vectors

Naked DNA

Physical injection of a complementary DNA (cDNA) sequence into a tumor is the simplest and most direct form of CGT (59). In this approach, a circular piece of DNA (plasmid or naked DNA) containing the therapeutic transgene and promoter/enhancer elements to drive transcription is taken into cells after injection by undefined mechanisms and translocated to the nucleus where it may be expressed transiently, from an episomal location, or stably, if integration into the host genome occurs. This process of functional gene transfer into cells is known as transfection or transduction. Intratumoral injection of naked DNA has been shown to be feasible in a number of tumor types (59), although it results in rapid clearance from the tumor (60). This process can be retarded by complexing the DNA with macromolecules (see below). However, a limitation of the process is the fact that these complexes do not diffuse far from the injection site and are unlikely to transduce many cells. At present, for reasons that remain obscure, skeletal muscle is most efficiently transduced by injection of naked DNA. Therefore, for the foreseeable future, this approach is likely to be of use only in situations in which synthesis and release of a protein into the circulation will be of therapeutic benefit (61). Examples of this sort of therapeutic approach in the treatment of cancer include the delivery of anti-angiogenic proteins (endostatin, angiostatin) (62) or specific antigens during vaccination strategies (63) (see below).

DNA-coated gold particles

The efficiency of transduction of tumor cells *in vivo* can be increased by administering the DNA in a form in which it is adsorbed onto gold particles and injected under pressure using a 'gene gun' (64). This process has also been termed biolistic transformation (65). The precise mechanism by which this procedure improves DNA delivery to cells is presently unknown. Responses have been seen in animal tumor models following intratumoral gene gun delivery of therapeutic cytokine genes (66).

Lipoplexes

Liposomes composed of phospholipid bilayer membranes can encapsulate a range of substances including DNA (67). Preparations of lipids and DNA form complexes (lipoplexes) that can transfect cells both *in vitro* and *in vivo* (68–71). Lipid-mediated gene delivery has the following potential advantages over viral systems: (1) the ability to transfect various cell types without interacting with specific receptors; (2) lack of significant immunogenicity, which allows repeated administration; (3) the ability to deliver large DNA sequences; (4) ease of production. However, they are not without their potential drawbacks, which can be summarised as follows: (1) relatively low transduction efficiency; (2) only transient expression of DNA; (3) release of plasmid DNA from the lipoplex can mediate inflammatory and/or immune reactions; (4) lipid components in lipoplexes may have distinct normal-tissue toxicity profiles (72).

Many lipid formulations have been described, with different abilities to deliver DNA to cells. Although many of these agents are highly effective *in vitro*, they may run into serious problems after *in vivo* administration. Standard liposomal preparations are cleared from the circulation promptly after intravenous injection, mainly by the lungs, reticuloendothelial system, and the heart, and lack the ability to achieve effective targeting of tumors after systemic administration. As a consequence, their use has been largely restricted to intralesional injection. The development of polyethylene glycol (PEG)-derivatized (PEGylated) liposomes has been shown to increase the circulation half-life of liposomes after intravenous administration and enhances their ability to localize to tumors (67). Unfortunately, the coating of PEG on PEGylated liposomes significantly reduces their ability to interact with the cell membrane and impairs their ability to deliver DNA. The pharmacokinetics, biodistribution, and fusogenicity of liposomes can be varied by altering the composition of the lipid membrane. In particular, incorporation of certain cationic lipids (for example DMRIE, DOSPA, and DOTAP) along with neutral or helper co-lipids (cholesterol or DOPE) in liposomes has been shown to increase markedly their ability to fuse with cell membranes and deliver their contents into cells. Phase I/II trials have confirmed the ability of these agents to deliver genes to human tumors *in vivo* (73, 74). Further development of both conventional and PEGylated liposomes represents an extremely active area of research, which is likely to result in the creation of improved therapeutic vectors in the future.

Polymer–DNA complexes

Many nonlipid polycationic polymers (poly-L-lysine, polyethylenimine, polyglucosamines, peptoids) form complexes with DNA (polyplexes) and enhance its delivery to cells (71, 75–78). Poly-L-lysine–DNA complexes are rapidly removed from the circulation, probably due to interactions with serum proteins (79). Polyethylenimine has been shown to protect complexed DNA from degradation and promotes its release from cellular endosomes and its subsequent transportation to the nucleus (75, 76). Recently, it has been shown that PEGylated polyethylenimine polymers have reduced interactions with serum proteins, extended circulation half-life and the ability to deliver genes to tumors without significant toxicity (80). Goldman *et al.* (1997) (77) have shown that polyglucosamine-based gene delivery into intracranial tumors can yield levels of expression comparable with those of viral systems. These vectors elicit a minimal immunological response and have limited toxicity *in vivo*.

Regulation of the expression of therapeutic genes

The clinical utility of a CGT approach will be dependent on its therapeutic index–the chance of a beneficial outcome compared to the risk of a serious adverse event (1). Therefore, in order to maximize the therapeutic index, the expression of therapeutic genes should be restricted exclusively to the tissue of interest. This is especially relevant to the delivery of genes with direct toxic actions since even low-level expression in normal tissues might cause severe toxicity. A number of levels of control can be built into CGT systems. Delivery of the therapeutic gene to the target tissue can be controlled either by means of direct local injection or infusion (physical targeting) or through tumor-specific ligand/receptor interactions (physiological or surface targeting). However, no matter how 'specific' such targeting appears, there will always be some gene delivery to local and distant normal tissues. An additional safeguard can be incorporated into the system by controlling gene expression very tightly at the transcriptional level, and a number of strategies have been proposed to exploit this mechanism. The process by which a gene is transcribed into mRNA and then translated into a cellular protein is complex and subject to multiple levels of control. Regulation of transcription is the key initiating event in this process and is mediated by the interaction between enhancer/promoter elements in the DNA and specific proteins (transcription factors) which bind to them. A highly simplified schematic representation of this process is shown in Fig. 8.4. For the purposes of this discussion, the term 'promoter' will be used to refer to any construct containing combinations of promoter and enhancer elements and these will be described briefly under the following headings: (1) tissue-specific promoters; (2) tumor-specific promoters; (3) inducible promoters; and (4) customized promoters.

Tissue-specific promoters

With few exceptions, each cell in the body contains a complete copy of the human genome. Despite this fact, cells from different body tissues that are genotypically homogeneous can be phenotypically heterogeneous by virtue of differences in their individual patterns of gene expression. This process is largely regulated at the tran-

scriptional level. Certain tissues make proteins that are, more or less, specific to that tissue (for example, tyrosinase in melanocytes, prostate-specific antigen (PSA) in prostate cells (81–108). The promoters that control these genes have been called tissue-specific promoters (TSP). In the context of CGT, an ideal TSP should have the following characteristics: (1) its activity should be reliably restricted to a single tissue type; (2) the normal tissue (in which it will also be active) should be expendable, replaceable, or located far from the site of gene delivery/expression. Thus, a CGT strategy using a TSP driving a gene that ablates melanocytes, prostate, or thyroid tissue may be clinically acceptable, whereas a similar approach which causes appreciable toxicity to liver or neuronal tissues would be unacceptable. A number of TSP that are under development for CGT approaches are detailed in Table 8.1.

Tumor-specific promoters

The dividing line between tissue- and tumor-specific promoters is not entirely clear. For the purposes of this discussion, a distinction is made on the basis that certain promoters are either silent or active at very low background levels in normal tissues but highly active in

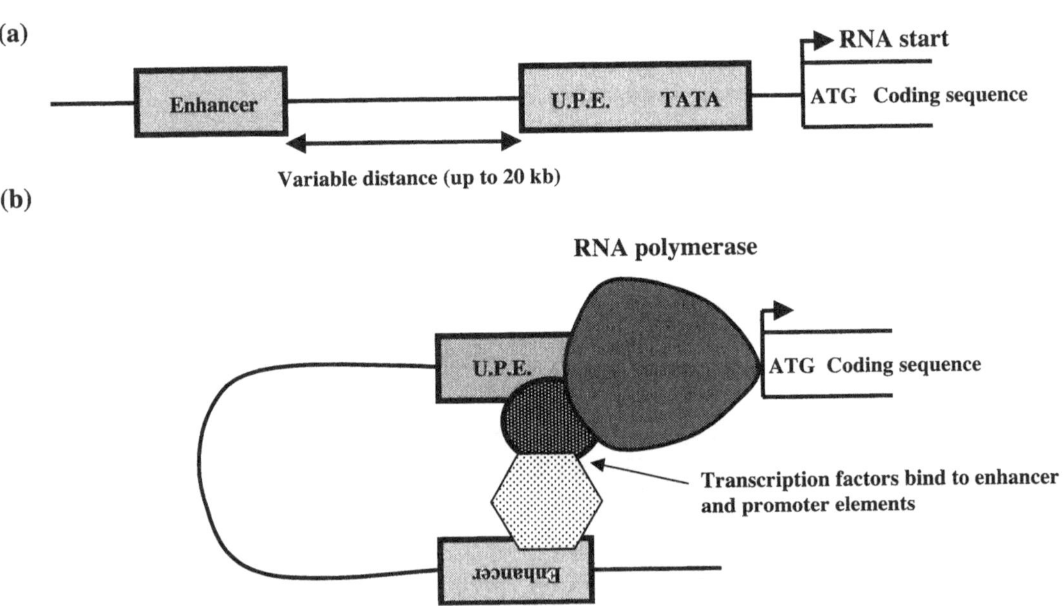

Fig. 8.4   Diagrammatic representation of the basic transcriptional control elements involved in regulating gene expression. (a) The coding sequence of a gene that begins at the first ATG is controlled by a proximal upstream promoter element (U.P.E) and a distal enhancer. The U.P.E contains a TATA-box sequence that acts as a binding site for the TATA factor. (b) Binding of regulatory proteins (transcription factors) to the enhancer and promoter regions regulates their interaction and co-ordinates the assembly of the transcriptional machinery and subsequent mRNA synthesis by RNA polymerase (adapted from reference 1).

Table 8.1　Tissue-specific promoters currently under development for cancer gene therapy strategies*

Tissue	Promoter	Vector	Transgene	Reference	Notes
Prostate	PSA/probasin/MMTV	AV	LacZ	81	Intraprostatic injections of AV vectors expressing β-galactosidase from three different promoters resulted in tight tissue-specific expression of the transgene (81). Subsequent AV-delivered suicide gene strategies have demonstrated effective *in vitro* and *in vivo* cell killing (82, 83, 86, 88). Plasmid delivery of the NIS transgene has been shown to confer on prostate cancer cells the ability to concentrate radioiodine and render them susceptible to therapeutic radioisotopes *in vitro* and *in vivo* (84, 85). Tissue-specific plasmid delivery of wild-type p53 has been shown to cause increased apoptosis *in vitro* (87)
	PSA	AV	HSVtk/PNP	82	
	PSA	AV	HSVtk	83	
	PSA	Plasmid	NIS	84, 85	
	PSA	AV	Nitroreductase	86	
	PSA	Plasmid	p53	87	
	Osteocalcin	AV	HSVtk	88	
Melanocyte	Tyrosinase/TRP1	Plasmid/RV	LacZ	89	Plasmid- and RV-delivered tyrosinase-driven constructs have shown tissue-specific gene expression *in vitro* and *in vivo* (89, 90). Delivery of cytokine genes in this fashion reduced tumorigenicity of murine melanoma *in vivo* (90). Suicide gene strategies have been shown to be effective in these models (91, 93, 94) which may prime systemic immune responses (91)
	Tyrosinase	Plasmid	IL-2, IL-4, M-CSF	90	
	Tyrosinase	RV	HSVtk	91	
	Tyrosinase	RV	IL-2	92	
	Tyrosinase	RV	CDase	93	
	Tyrosinase	Plasmid	PNP	94	
Glia	GFAP	HSV	LacZ	95	Astrocyte-specific expression of β-galactosidase has been demonstrated *in vitro* and *in vivo* with GFAP-driven HSV vectors (95). *In vitro* cytotoxicity has been has been reported with HSVtk and FasL transgenes (96, 97). MBP-driven reporter (99) and therapeutic (100) genes showed tissue specificity in glioma cell lines
	GFAP	Plasmid	HSVtk	96	
	GFAP/NSE	AV	FasL	97	
	Nestin	AV	LacZ	98	
	MBP	RV	LacZ/HSVtk	99, 100	
Osteoblast	Osteocalcin	AV	HSVtk	101	AV vector delivery of HSVtk therapeutic transgene under osteocalcin promoter control resulted in selective cytotoxycity in osteosarcoma cell lines *in vitro* and tumor regression *in vivo* (101). Combination of this gene therapy with methotrexate yielded an additive effect without exacerbating toxicity (102). Intravenous injection of AV with reporter and therapeutic genes showed tumor-specific expression and therapeutic efficacy in a lung metastasis model (103)
	Osteocalcin	AV	HSVtk	102	
	Osteocalcin	AV	LacZ/HSVtk	103	
Liver	Albumin/hAAT	AV	HAAT	104	RV vector delivery of hAAT reporter gene yielded strong tissue specific expression for up to 40 weeks *in vivo* (90). Albumin promoter-driven expression of viral ICP4 gene rendered mutant HSV (G92A) replication competent in albumin-expressing hepatoma cells but not in non-hepatoma cells (105, 106)
	Albumin	HSV	LacZ/ICP4	105, 106	
Thyroid	Thyroglobulin	RV	HSVtk	107	*In vitro* cytotoxicity assays demonstrated thyroglobulin expression status-dependent cell killing by transduction of RV vector encoding HSVtk. Significant growth inhibition, but not complete tumor eradication was seen in subcutaneous tumor xenografts (107). In a subsequent study, the use of a Cre-loxP system was shown to increase transcriptional activity by approximately 10-fold (108)
	Thyroglobulin		HSVtk	108	

* TRP1, tyrosinase-related protein-1; PSA, prostate-specific antigen; MMTV, murine mammary tumor virus; hAAT, human alpha-1-antitrypsin; GFAP, glial fibrillary acid protein; NSE, neuron-specific enolase; MBP, myelin basic protein; RV, retrovirus; AV, adenovirus; HSV, herpes simplex virus; lacZ, *E. coli* β-galactosidase gene; IL-2, interleukin 2; IL-4, interleukin 4; M-CSF, macrophage colony stimulating factor; HSVtk, herpes simplex virus thymidine kinase; CDase, cytosine deaminase; PNP, purine nucleoside phosphorylase; NIS, sodium iodide symporter; FasL, Fas ligand.

tumors. A number of so-called tumor-specific promoters can be included within this heterogeneous group.

1.   Promoters that are specific for the malignant process but that show no particular tissue specificity—so-called 'cancer-specific promoters'. Examples include the telomerase (109, 110), plastin (111, 112), and hexokinase II (113) promoters.

2.   Promoters of genes that encode oncofetal antigens and that have well-defined patterns of tissue specificity – so-called 'tumor-type specific promoters'. Examples include the promoters that control the expression of carcinoembryonic antigen (CEA) and alpha fetoprotein (AFP) (114–137) (see Table 8.2).

3.   Promoters responsive to pathophysiological conditions that predominate in tumor areas. Examples include promoters of genes that are responsive to hypoxia (phosphoglycerate kinase 1, erythropoietin, and vascular endothelial growth factor) (138, 139) or multidrug resistance (MDR-1) (140).

4.   Promoters that are specific to the vascular endothelium of tumor blood vessels. Examples include the E-selectin (141, 142) and endoglin (143) promoters.

Inducible promoters

The use of tissue- and tumor-specific promoters presents two main problems that may be difficult to overcome. The first is the relative weakness of existing promoters such that they direct only low-level transcription of transgenes. The second is the lack of true restriction of gene expression to the target tissue — a feature that is usually called 'leakiness'. The use of systems in which transgene transcription is controlled by administration of inducing or repressing agents that mediate their effects by modulating the binding of transcription factors to so-called inducible promoters represents a potential solution. These systems have been called 'gene switches' and may be particularly relevant for the temporal control of gene expression.

A number of agents, including drugs, radiation, and heat, can be used to control gene switches. The requirements of an optimal drug-inducible system can be defined as follows; the transcription factor should bind a DNA sequence that is not recognized by endogenous mammalian transcription factors and the inducing drug should be a small, nontoxic, orally bioavailable, cell-permeable molecule capable of reversibly modulating the activity of the transcription factor (144). Radiation and heat have an additional advantage in that their delivery can be controlled very accurately both spatially and temporally. Ideally, in the absence (or presence) of the modulating agent, the background transcription from the exogenous gene should be very low. However, on addition (or withdrawal) of the agent, induction ratios should be high with a wide dose–response range to meet the need for therapeutic requirements. Examples of drug-inducible systems include the use of tetracycline to suppress (tet-off) (145) or induce (tet-on) gene expression) (146), mifepristone (RU486) (147), ecdysone systems (148), and rapamycin (149). As yet, there have been few applications of drug-inducible systems in preclinical or clinical CGT approaches but it is likely that appropriate applications will be identified. In the realm of radioinducible promoters, most work has been performed with the Egr-1 (ziff/268) promoter which contains specific CArG (CC[A/T]$_6$(GG) motifs (150, 151) Delivery of genes under the control of heat-sensitive promoters followed by local hyperthermia represents an interesting means of physically regulating gene expression (152) Heat-inducible expression of green fluorescent protein (GFP) was reported from a glioma cell line engineered to express GFP stably under the control of the heat shock protein 70 (hsp70) minimal promoter (153).

Customized promoters

The perceived limitations of the natural promoter systems described above have fuelled the search for means of improving available wild-type sequences to derive so-called customized or designer promoters (154). The simplest of these strategies involves the attempt to identify mutant promoters with increased ability to drive transcription but with preserved tissue/tumor specificity (155, 156). Thus far, this approach has resulted in little benefit. More benefit has accrued from attempts to generate minimal enhancer/promoter sequences that retain the characteristics of the wild-type elements. Such studies involve generating a range of deletion and amplification mutants of the enhancer/promoter sequence driving a convenient reporter gene such as lacZ or chloramphenicol acetyltransferase (CAT). The DNA sequences that are derived from these studies are invariably smaller than the wild-type sequence, a feature that is of considerable significance to the issue

Table 8.2 Cancer-specific promoters currently under development for cancer gene therapy*

Tumor	Promoter	Vector	Transgene	Reference	Notes
Hepatoma	AFP	RV	HSVtk	114	Cell-specific expression of beta-galactosidase in AFP-positive cell lines (115, 117, 118). Cytotoxicity in AFP[+], but not AFP[-] cells *in vitro* (117, 118) and *in vivo* (116, 118) using both HSVtk and CDase systems. *In vitro* and *in vivo* activity against AFP and ALB expressing hepatoma tumor cell lines (119, 120). AFP-targeted expression of a retroviral ecotropic receptor has been used to facilitate subsequent targeted delivery of a RV HSVtk system (121)
	AFP	AV	LacZ/HSVtk	115–117	
	AFP	AV	LacZ/CD	118	
	AFP/ALB	AAV	HSVtk	119, 120	
	AFP	AV	MCAT/HSVtk	121	
Breast	c-erbB2	RV	CDase	122	c-erbB2 promoter-driven CD expression caused 5FC-induced cell death in c-erbB2[+] (but not c-erbB2[-]) breast cancer cells *in vitro* (122). Tumor-specific expression of GRPr driven by both c-erbB2 and Muc1 promoters resulted in receptor-mediated binding of 125I-labeled bombesin, which may have the potential to improve cancer radioimmunotherapy (123). RV vectors with HSVtk under the control of a chimeric Muc1/c-erbB2 promoter were selectively toxic to Muc1[+] cells *in vitro* (124). In addition, Muc1 and ALA/BLG were shown to be capable of driving breast-specific expression of β-galactosidase both *in vitro* and *in vivo*. Tumor-specific cytotoxicity *in vivo* was also seen with the HSVtk therapeutic transgene (125, 126)
	c-erbB2	AV	GRPr	123	
	Mucl/c-erbB2	RV	HSVtk	124	
	Muc1 (DF3)	AV	LacZ/HSVtk	125	
	Muc1 (DF3)	AV	GRPr	123	
	ALA/BLG	AV	LacZ/HSVtk	126	
Colorectal	CEA	AV	HSVtk	127	The activity of the CEA promoter has generally been shown to be weak *in vitro* and *in vivo*. However, suicide gene therapy using CEA-promoter-driven constructs caused less hepatotoxicity than equivalent CMV-promoter-driven constructs (127). Adenoviral vectors containing HSVtk (127, 128) and CDase (129) transgenes have been shown to have tissue-specific cytotoxicity *in vitro* and *in vivo*.
	CEA	AV	HSVtk	128	
	CEA	RV	CDase	129	
Pancreas	Amylase	AV	LacZ	130	AV-delivered β-galactosidase expression restricted to pancreatic tissue in neonatal and adult mice (130). Tumor-specific expression of GRPr driven by both c-erbB2 promoters resulted in receptor-mediated binding of 125I-labeled bombesin (123)
	c-erbB2	AV	GRPr	123	
Stomach	CEA	AV	LacZ/HSVtk	131, 132	β-galactosidase expression restricted to CEA[+] cells (131) with selective cytotoxicity of suicide gene therapy (131–133). *In vivo* delivery of a CD suicide gene resulted in tumor growth delay and improved survival (134)
	CEA	AV	LacZ/CD	133, 134	
Ovary	Muc1 (DF3)	AV	LacZ/BAX	135	Tumor-specific expression of β-galactosidase and pro-apoptotic BAX gene. *In vitro* and *in vivo* antitumor effect demonstrated through induction of apoptosis
Cervix	SLP1	Plasmid	HSVtk	136	*In vitro* cytotoxicity of SLP1[+] but not SLP[-], cell lines *in vitro*
Lung	CEA	Plasmid	HSVtk	137	*In vitro* and *in vivo* selective cell kill of CEA[+] lung cancer cells

* CEA, carcinoembryonic antigen; AFP, alpha-fetoprotein; ALB, albumin; ALA, alpha-lactalbumin; BLG, beta-lactoglobin; SLP1, secretory leukoprotease inhibitor; AV, adenovirus; RV, retrovirus; AAV, adeno-associated virus; HSVtk, herpes simplex virus thymidine kinase, CDase, cytosine deaminase; lacZ, *E. coli* β-galactosidase gene, MCAT, mouse cationic amino acid transporter-1; GRPr, gastrin-releasing peptide receptor.

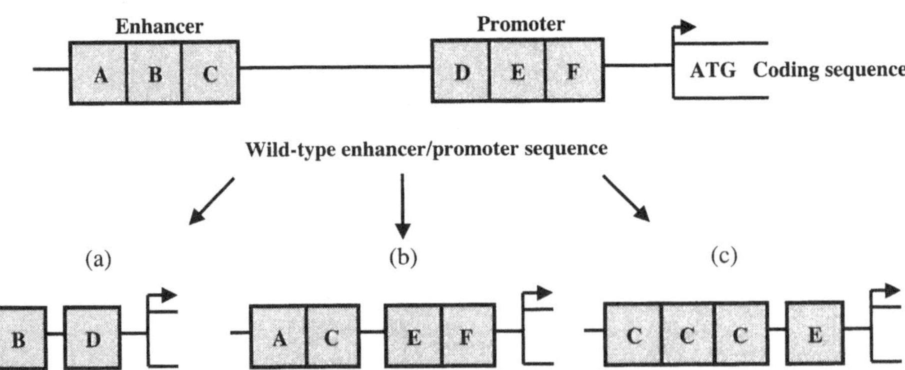

Fig. 8.5   Diagrammatic representation of the potential for building novel modular enhancer/promoter elements. Minimal sequences required for activity and specificity can be identified and combined to produce abbreviated sequences. Strong positively acting fragments can be included and negatively acting elements excluded. Multiple copies of particular sequences that confer activity and/or specificity can be used. (a) Single small modular sequences of the enhancer (B) and promoter (D) are combined. (b) Multiple small modules of the enhancer (A and C) and promoter (E and F) are combined. (c) Repeats of particularly active elements of the enhancer (C) have been used to improve activity and/or specificity of the minimal promoter sequence (E).

of generating viral vectors. Such studies have identified the crucial transcriptional control sequences for a number of genes and have led to the construction of a number of new smaller modular versions of previously identified promoters. Figure 8.5 illustrates this approach in a rather simplified form. Essentially, key positive and negative regulatory elements have been dissected out and the positive elements are recombined in novel shorter sequences with preserved, or even enhanced, activity. The elements that contribute to promoter activity or specificity can be multimerized to improve the effect (154), as has been shown for the CEA and PSA promoters (86, 157, 158). Another strategy involves the construction of chimeric promoters composed of regulatory elements from different promoters with the same tissue specificity. This tactic seeks to exploit the advantages of each of these promoters and to tighten the tissue specificity. This has been done with the AFP and albumin promoters with some success in a hepatoma model (119, 120) Alternatively, TSP have been used to drive the expression of exogenous bacterial or viral transcription factors, which can subsequently transactivate constructs containing therapeutic genes downstream of the appropriate DNA binding sites (159). It is likely that further developments will occur rapidly in this exciting arena (reviewed in Reference 154).

Strategies in cancer gene therapy

It is now widely accepted that the pathogenesis of cancer is a multistep process that involves the sequen-

tial accumulation of separate genetic defects (160). Indeed, the occurrence of the initial defects can destabilize the genome of the cancer cell such that further defects are increasingly more likely to accumulate. A diagrammatic, but far from complete, representation of some of the key cell/tissue functions that are involved in this process is shown in Fig. 8.6. Mutations of tumor suppressor genes and oncogenes give cells a growth or survival advantage over their neighbors and such changes frequently occur early in the process of malignant transformation (161). These changes often involve making the cell independent of the normal requirements for growth factors or allowing them to ignore antigrowth signals. As a tumor increases in size and begins to invade surrounding tissues, it accumulates mutations that allow it to recruit its own blood supply (162) and to loosen contacts with neighbouring cells (163). Further changes may be associated with downregulation of the expression of cellular markers (major histocompatibility complex (MHC) and tumor-associated antigen (TAA) molecules) that may allow the tumor to evade immunosurveillance (164). The process of tumor metastasis is complex and involves many steps including degradation of the extracellular matrix, cellular motility/migration, recruitment of new lymphatic vessels and expression of receptors for chemokines that may allow 'homing' to specific tissues (165–167). The development of disease that is refractory to treatment may occur as a result of overexpression of certain genes that reduce accumulation of cytotoxic chemotherapy (for example, P-glycoprotein/MDR1, MRP) or increase the ability of the cells to

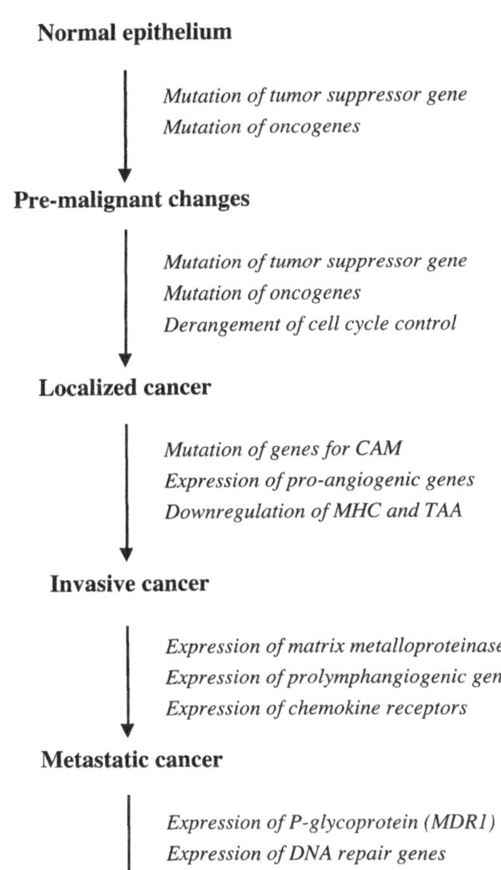

Fig. 8.6 Diagrammatic representation of the possible sequence of accumulation of genetic changes involved in the pathogenesis of the common cancers. This schema represents a hypothetical scenario by which a series of mutations may transform a normal epithelial cell into an aggressive, treatment-resistant metastatic cancer cell. The central themes of this progression are: (1) growth factor-independent cell growth; (2) immortalization; (3) circumvention of normal apoptotic signaling pathways; (4) recruitment of a secure blood supply; (5) local tissue invasion and spread (5) CAM, Cell adhesion molecule; MHC, major histocompatibility complex; TAA, tumor-associated antigen.

repair DNA damage (168, 169). Such is the pace of research that there is no doubt that further studies will identify other genes involved in the development, progression, spread, and refractoriness to treatment of the common cancers. Each of these abnormalities distinguishes a tumor cell from a normal cell and represents a possible target for genetic therapy.

For the purpose of this discussion, CGT strategies will be grouped as follows: (1) corrective gene therapy, which aims to restore normal function of a deleted or mutated gene (usually a tumor suppressor gene) or to counteract the effect of a mutated oncogene; (2) cytoreductive gene therapy, in which delivery of an exogenous gene results in cancer cell death either by metabolism of a prodrug to a toxic agent (suicide gene therapy), induction of apoptosis, anti-angiogenic activity, or enhanced localization of therapeutic radioisotopes; and (3) immunomodulatory gene therapy in which gene delivery to tumor or normal tissue enhances the ability of the immune system to mount an effective cytotoxic response.

Corrective gene therapy

In general terms, mutations of tumor suppressor genes and oncogenes enhance the growth potential and clonogenicity of malignant cells. Therefore, efforts to correct aberrations in the function of such genes have been seen as an appropriate approach to the treatment of cancer. The resulting strategies can take two forms: (1) attempts to restore to normal the function of a mutated or deleted cellular tumor suppressor gene; and (2) attempts to abolish the growth-promoting effects of oncogenes. The success of each of these approaches rests with the ability to deliver the therapeutic gene to every tumor cell and for its activity to be sufficient to reverse the malignant phenotype and/or to allow the action of the normal cellular machinery to trigger cell death either alone or in response to another cytotoxic treatment (radiotherapy or chemotherapy). The fact that cancer cells frequently have multiple mutations in a number of pathways may mean that correction of the function of a single mutated gene may not be sufficient to achieve a therapeutic effect, even if the problem of efficient gene delivery is solved. Therefore, it is likely that future approaches will involve targeting groups of genes simultaneously, in an analogous fashion to the use of multiagent chemotherapy regimens.

Restoration of normal tumor suppressor gene function

A variety of different tumor suppressor genes have been shown to be mutated in many common cancers. The complex interplay of a number of these factors in the pathogenesis of cancer is represented schematically in Fig. 8.7.

p53

p53, the 'guardian of the genome', is a nuclear phosphoprotein that plays a central part in many processes that protect the cell against genotoxic stress (170; see

                    Targeted therapy for cancer

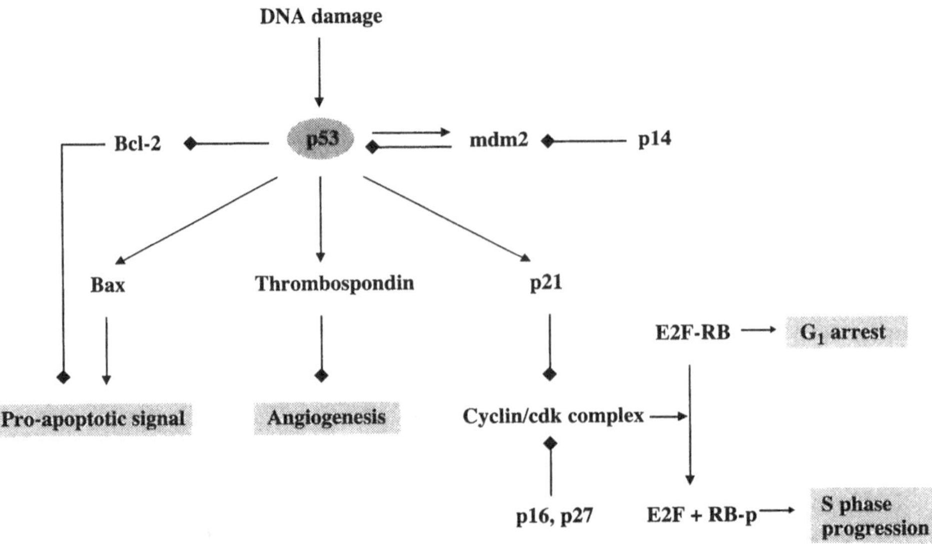

Fig. 8.7 Schematic representation of the role of p53 in mediating the cellular response to DNA damage. Arrows indicate a positive interaction (for example, p53 induces p21 expression) and diamonds indicate a negative interaction (for example, p53 reduces the level of Bcl-2). Following DNA damage, rapid induction of p53 leads to G_1 cell cycle arrest mediated through induction of p21, which, in concert with the cyclin-dependent kinase inhibitors p16 and p27, inhibits the activity of cyclin/cdk complexs. The activity of these complexes is required to release the transcription factor E2F from its inactive association with RB, an effect that is mediated by phosphorylation of RB to RB-phosphate (RB-p). Free E2F is able to promote transition across the G_1-S boundary. If the level of DNA damage exceeds the repair capacity of the cell, p53 signals a switch in the balance of anti-apoptotic (Bcl-2 and proapoptotic (Bax) molecules within the cell such that the cell is commited to apoptosis. Cellular levels of p53 protein are normally controlled by a negative feedback loop involving mdm2. Therefore, induction of p53 expression induces mdm2, which degrades the p53 protein and limits its activity. The level of mdm2 expressed is, in turn, negatively controlled by the expression of p14. Mutations in p53, p21, p16, p27, p14, Bcl-2, and mdm2 have all been documented in the common cancers, attesting to their central role in controling the response to DNA damage and cell cycle progression. As such, they are likely to be key targets for future gene therapy initiatives.

also Fig. 8.7). In cells that have sustained DNA damage, normal wild-type p53 protein mediates a G_1/S cell cycle arrest that allows time for DNA repair. However, if the damage exceeds the repair capacity of the cell, p53 acts to push the cell into the apoptotic pathway (l71). In contrast, cells with p53 mutations fail to undergo cell-cycle arrest or apoptosis in response to DNA damage and proceed through the cell cycle in the presence of unrepaired DNA damage that, if non-lethal, is passed on to daughter cells. In addition to these well-described functions, induction of p53 expression is associated with suppression of the growth-stimulating effects of certain oncogenes (c-myc, fibroblast growth factor (FGF)) and inhibition of angiogenesis through induction of the anti-angiogenic factor, thrombospondin-1 (l72).

Mutations of p53 have been reported in a wide variety of tumor types including the common epithelial tumors such as lung, breast, colorectal, prostate, zpancreatic, bladder, esophageal, and head and neck (173–181). Furthermore, there is abundant evidence that expression of mutant p53 is associated with a poor prognosis for most tumor types that have been reported (182–188). Preclinical studies have demonstrated decreased growth of cancer cells *in vitro* and *in vivo* after delivery of wild-type p53 by adenoviral (AV) (189–198), retroviral (RV) (l99, 200), and cationic liposomal vectors (201, 202). In addition, and perhaps most relevantly for clinical applications, liposome- and viral-mediated delivery of p53 has been shown to sensitize cancer cells to the effects of genotoxic agents such as radiotherapy (203–206) and chemotherapy (207–210) *in vitro* and *in vivo*. As a result of these positive preclinical data, p53 has been the subject of a number of preliminary phase I clinical trials (Table 8.3) (2ll–216). Most of the studies reported thus far have involved patients with lung cancer. Roth *et al.* (211) treated nine patients with relapsed non-small cell lung cancer (NSCLC) with an RV vector expressing wild-type p53. The therapy was very well tolerated and no significant treatment-related toxicity was documented. Following treatment, vector-specific p53 sequences were detected in posttreatment biopsies by

Table 8.3 Phase I clinical trials of corrective gene therapy: the reported studies involved either restitution of a mutated tumor suppressor gene or assessment of marker gene transfer efficiency*

Tumor	No. of patients	Transgene	Vector	Route	Outcomes	Ref.
NSCLC	9	p53	RV	IT	Single injection of 5×10^8 cfu delivered endobronchially (4 pts), percutaneously to chest wall (4 pts), and percutaneously to adrenal gland (1 pt). Gene expression confirmed in 3 injected tumors by PCR. Posttreatment biopsy confirmed increased apoptosis and 3 pts showed local PR. No treatment-related toxicity. No RCR isolated	211
NSCLC	6	lacZ	RDAV	IT	Two cohorts of 3 pts each received either 10^7 or 10^8 pfu by endobronchial injection. Tumor and peritumoral biopsies were performed at 8 days, 1, 2, and 3 months. Tumor expression of β-galactosidase was detected in 3 pts on day 8 biopsy. β-galactosidase was detected in blood on day 1, in sputum up to day 13, and in bronchial washings up to day 90 after injection. Minimal toxicity (including bleeding in the injection site)	212
Ovarian	12	BRCA1	RV	IP	Dose escalation study to 10^8 viral particles by four daily IP infusions every 4 weeks for up to 4 months. Acute sterile peritonitis in 3 pts which resolved spontaneously. Plasma and peritoneal antibodies to the RV envelope protein were detected only in patients treated at the highest does levels. Tumor reduction in 3 pts and SD in 8 pts	255
NSCLC	15	p53	RDAV	IT	Dose escalation study of 10^7–10^{10} pfu. Successful gene transfer documented by RT-PCR in 6 pts treated with the higher viral doses. Disease stabilization in 4 of 6 pts with documented gene transfer. No response in distant disease. No significant toxicity (maximal grade I/II fever/coryza)	213
NSCLC	28	p53	RDAV	IT	Dose-escalation study of 107–10 pfu delivered by CT-guided (23 pts) or bronchoscopic (5 pts) injection. Up to 6 injections at monthly intervals. Adenoviral DNA detected by PCR in 18 of 21 pts who underwent posttreatment biopsy. Vector-specific p53 mRNA detected by RT-PCR in 12 of 26 evaluable pts. No significant toxicity. Therapeutic effect evaluable in 25 pts: PR 2 pts; SD 16 pts; PD 7 pts	214
SCCHN	15	p53	RDAV	IT	Dose-escalation study of 10^6–10^{11} pfu administered thrice weekly for 2 weeks as pre-, intra-, or postoperative treatment. Toxicity mainly seen at higher doses—fever in 6 pts, erythema in 3 pts	215
Ovarian	6	BRCA1	RV	IP	Daily injections through IP catheter of 4 days every 4 weeks for 3 cycles. Toxicity restricted to fever, peritonitis, and pleural effusion. No vector detectable in peritoneal fluid at 24 hours. No responses. Trial discontinued early because of poor vector stability and lack of objective responses	256
NSCLC	12	p53	RDAV	IT	Dose escalation study of 10^6–10^{11} pfu delivered by bronchoscopic injection every 4 weeks in pts with airway obstruction Treatment-related toxicity was minimal. Improvement of airway obstruction in 6 pts. PR in 3 pts	216

* cfu, Colony-forming units; CT, computerized tomography; IP, intraperitoneal; lacZ, gene encoding the bacterial enzyme β-galactosidase; mRNA, messenger RNA; NSCLC, non-small cell lung cancer; PCR, polymerase chain reaction; PD, progressive disease; pfu, plaque-forming units; PR, partial response; pt, patient; RCR, replication-competent retrovirus; RDAV, replication-deficient adenovirus; RT-PCR, reverse transcriptase polymerase chain reaction; RV, retrovirus; SCCHN, squamous cell cancer of the head and neck; SD, stable disease.

polymerase chain reaction (PCR) and *in situ* hybridization and there was evidence of increased cancer cell apoptosis. There were tumor regressions in three patients, including two patients in whom no viable tumor was detected at repeat biopsy. In a similar trial, 15 patients with lung cancer received p53 gene therapy using a RDAV delivered by endobronchial or percutaneous intratumoral injection without significant toxicity. Successful gene transfer was confirmed in 6 patients, of whom 4 showed evidence of disease stabilization on follow-up (213). In a larger study, Swisher *et al.* (214) treated 28 patients with treatment-refractory NSCLC with repeated escalating doses of an RDAV encoding p53. Gene transfer was confirmed in the tumors of nearly 50 per cent of the patients and this was most efficient with higher viral titers. As with previous studies, there was no significant toxicity associated with the treatment. The majority of the patients had stabilization of their local disease and 2 patients achieved a partial response.

These promising preliminary data have spawned a number of follow-up trials in different tumor types, the results of which should be available in the near future. Although these studies have demonstrated that replacement of normal p53 function can yield tumor responses, even in patients with advanced and/or metastatic disease, it is likely that clinical application of this approach will involve integration of p53 gene therapy with radiotherapy and/or cytotoxic chemotherapy (203–210). As yet, no clinical trials of this strategy have been reported.

Cell cycle control genes

The processes governing entry to, transit through, and exit from the cell cycle are very tightly controlled in normal eukaryotic cells (217). However orderly control of cell cycle progression is frequently grossly deranged in cancer cells. As detailed in Fig. 8.7, the transition across the G_1 checkpoint into S phase (the phase in which DNA synthesis occurs) is a critical component of normal cell cycle control. This process is regulated by three important tumor suppressor gene families, the Rb pocket proteins (218–220) and the Cip/Kip (p21, p27) and Ink4 (pl6 and pl4) cyclin-dependent kinase inhibitors (220–223). In normal cells, DNA damage leads to induction of expression of these genes and subsequent cell cycle arrest in G_0/G_1. However, mutations in cyclin-dependent kinase inhibitors, which are negative regulators of cell-cycle progression, confer on cells a growth advantage. Aberrant expression of Rb and cyclin-dependent kinase inhibitors has been confirmed in a wide range of tumor types (224–227) and has been shown to correlate with disease outcome in a number of different tumor types (reviewed in reference 222).

Such findings confirm the importance of this group of genes in the development, progression, and response to treatment of a range of common cancers and justifies the investigation of gene therapy approaches directed towards restoring their expression. Preclinical *in vitro* and *in vivo* studies have demonstrated that restitution of normal expression of Rb (228-230), p21 (231–237), p27 (238–24l), pl6 (242–252), and pl4 (253) by a variety of vectors can result in reduced tumor growth in a number of different model systems. These studies have confirmed that the therapeutic effect is mediated through arrest of cell cycle progression and proliferation and an increase in tumor cell apoptosis. It is anticipated that clinical trials using viral delivery of these genes will be reported in the near future.

Other tumor suppressor genes

A number of other tumor suppressor genes (for example, BRCA1, promyelocytic-leukemia (PML), deleted in colorectal cancer (DCC), and mutated in multiple advanced cancers 1/phosphatase and tensin homolog (MMAC1/PTEN) genes) have been identified. As yet, few have been investigated as candidates for CGT. Mutations of BRCA1 have been shown to be associated with susceptibility to breast and ovarian cancer (254). Phase I and II clinical trials have been conducted using intraperitoneal injections of a RV vector to deliver BRCA1 to patients with ovarian cancer (Table 8.3) (255, 256). Conflicting results were obtained with three responses in the phase I trial (255) but no responses in the phase II trial, which was abandoned prematurely (256). Subsequent analysis revealed very poor stability of the viral vector *in vivo*, possibly due to complement-mediated viral lysis. The PML gene has been shown to mediate a G_1 cell-cycle arrest and promote apoptosis *in vitro* (257). Delivery of AV vectors containing the PML gene caused reduced breast and prostate cancer growth *in vitro* and reduced tumorigenicity *in vivo*. Furthermore, direct injection into prostate cancer xenograft tumors in mice resulted in significant tumor regressions (258). The PTEN gene is mutated in a number of cancer types. Adenoviral delivery of this gene has been shown to yield *in vitro* and *in vivo* effects against glioma and endometrial and ovarian cancers (259–261).

Suppression of oncogene function

Mutations may also directly activate cellular oncogenes that give tumors a growth advantage or the ability to circumvent normal apoptotic signaling pathways. Examples of oncogenes that are frequently mutated in cancers are ras, myc, erbB2, and bc1-2 (reviewed in reference 161). CGT strategies can be designed to negate the activating function of these mutated genes by targeting the transcriptional/translational machinery of the cell with the aim of preventing the cell from making functional oncogenic proteins (see Fig. 8.8). Transcription involves partial uncoiling of the double-stranded DNA helix into its two complementary strands. The antisense strand functions as a template used by DNA-dependent RNA polymerase to generate a sense messenger RNA (mRNA) copy. This mRNA is subsequently edited (spliced) to remove noncoding regions (introns), exported from the nucleus, and translated at the ribosome to yield the encoded protein product. Therapeutic strategies can be designed to interfere with transcription or prevent the transcribed mRNA being translated into protein. Two main strategies have been proposed: (1) antisense oligonucleotides (AO) that can interfere with either transcription or translation; (2) catalytic ribozymes that interfere with translation.

Antisense oligonucleotides

AO are oligomers of 15–20 nucleotide bases. Naturally occurring phosphodiester DNA oligonucleotides have an extremely short half-life in both *in vitro* and *in vivo* systems as a result of degradation by exonucleases and endonucleases and are likely to have limited clinical utility (262). Therefore, attempts have been made to alter the pharmacokinetic profile of AO by increasing their biological half-life through manipulation of the oligonucleotide sugar–phosphate backbone to increase their resistance to nuclease-mediated destruction. Such modifications have included the generation of phosphorothioate, methylphosphonate, phosphoramide, and mixed-backbone oligonucleotides (263). As yet, the optimal formulation for AO remains to be defined but preliminary clinical studies have focused on the use of phosphorothioate backbones (see below).

The precise mechanism of action of AO remains to be determined definitively. In addition to their putative antisense effects, AO have been shown to mediate anti-angiogenic effects (264–266) and immune stimulation

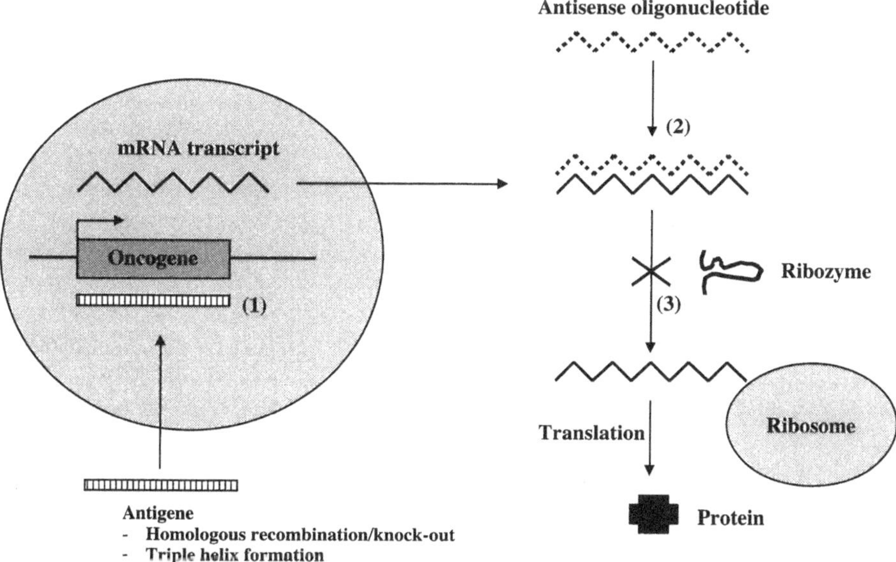

Fig. 8.8 Gene therapy approaches that target the cellular transcriptional/translational machinery. Three basic strategies have been developed. (1) The delivery of oligonucleotides that are complementary to the sequence of a targeted gene facilitates homologous recombination to 'knock-out' the gene the formation of a triple helix to prevent transcription or sequestration of the factors that are required to initiate transcription. (2) The delivery of antisense oligonucleotides that prevent translation of messenger RNA either by promoting degradation by RNases or by preventing a functional interaction with the ribosome. (3) The delivery of catalytic ribozymes that degrade specific target messenger RNA species and prevent their translation.

through the presence of so-called CpG motifs (267). However, the relative importance of these effects remains unclear and this discussion will be limited to the ability of AO to block cellular transcription and/or translation, an effect that can occur at a number of levels (Fig. 8.8). First, delivery of molecules that contain 5′ and 3′ sequences that are identical to a target gene can be used as a vehicle to mediate homologous recombination. This process involves replacing or 'knocking-out' all or part of a gene at cell division with a similar nonfunctional sequence (268). Although this elegant technology may appear attractive, it has not yet reached the stage of being applicable *in vivo*. In an alternative approach, a specific oligonucleotide DNA sequence can be used to form triple-stranded DNA sequences (triplexes) that can block transcription (263). This strategy has the obvious attraction of only needing to target two molecules within each cell but, thus far, it has been difficult to achieve reliably, even in *in vitro* systems. Similarly, the delivery of specific 'decoy' oligonucleotide sequences that are capable of sequestering cellular pools of transcription factors and preventing them from interacting with their endogenous DNA binding sites potentially represents an interesting approach (269). Although this strategy has not been tested in clinical studies of patients with cancer, it has demonstrated activity as a means of preventing restenosis in patients treated with coronary angioplasty (270).

The most well-known and best developed form of oncogene suppression involves the use of antisense molecules that can be used to target specific mRNA sequences and prevent their translation, either by promoting their destruction by cytoplasmic RNase H or by steric inhibition of translation (263). A number of *in vitro* and preclinical *in vivo* systems have been investigated. Delivery of AO against the c-myc, bcl-2, and ras oncogene families (or their downstream signaling pathways) have been shown to reduce the growth of various malignant tumors *in vitro* and *in vivo* both alone and in combination with cytotoxic chemotherapy (271–279).

On the basis of these promising data, a number of AO sequences have entered preliminary clinical trials and these are summarized in Table 8.4 (280–288). The primary goal of these studies has been to define the toxicity profile of AO treatment. Animal studies had suggested that complement activation and coagulopathy would be problematic and potentially dose-limiting. However, in practice, this has not been found to be the case. Indeed, many phase I studies have failed to define a maximum tolerated dose and toxicity has

been largely confined to inflammation at the local injection site (281, 287), fatigue (283, 285), fever (282, 283) and nausea/vomiting (282). Among the first reported studies, Bishop *et al.*(280) treated 16 patients with acute myeloblastic leukemia or myelodysplastic syndrome with a continuous 10-day intravenous infusion of a 20-base phosphorothioate AO complementary to p53 mRNA. This study demonstrated that the treatment was feasible and tolerable, although no responses were reported. Webb *et al.* (281) reported the therapeutic activity of an 18-base phosphorothioate AO against bcl-2 delivered as a 14-day subcutaneous infusion in 9 patients with relapsed non-Hodgkin's lymphoma. Toxicity was largely limited to local inflammation at the injection site. There was a single complete response to therapy and in two other patients there was a significant fall in the number of circulating lymphoma cells. In an updated report from the same group, 21 patients received the same AO with further dose escalation. Three patients showed evidence of disease response (1 complete and 2 minor responses) (287). In a separate study using a 20-base AO to protein kinase C-α, two patients with non-Hodgkin's lymphoma achieved complete responses (282). The same agent has also been shown to possess activity against ovarian cancer with objective responses in 3 of 4 treated patients (285).

Therefore, from the above studies, it can be concluded that AO therapy is safe and has yielded sporadic responses in patients with relapsed/advanced disease. However, it is very unlikely that it will have much impact as a single modality therapy. Instead, it is most likely to be of benefit combined with other standard therapies such as chemotherapy or radiotherapy. A number of preclinical studies have demonstrated the potential value of AO in this regard but, as yet, no clinical data are available (266, 274, 276, 278). Further studies of AO need to provide answers to important questions such as what are the most promising mRNA targets, the optimal oligonucleotide formulation(s), the most efficacious route(s) of administration, and treatment schedules. Finally, and perhaps most importantly, the issue of integrating AO into rational combination therapy strategies needs to be addressed.

Catalytic ribozymes

Ribozymes are RNA molecules with catalytic activity that enables them to degrade phosphodiester bonds in mRNA molecules without the aid of protein-based enzymes (263). Ribozymes bind to target mRNA molecules through specific base pairing and this means that

Table 8.4 Clinical trials of antisense oligonucleotide therapy of cancer*

Tumor	No. of patients	Sequence target	Route	Outcomes	Ref.
AML/MDS	16	p53 (20-mer)	IV infusion	Dose-escalation protocol from 0.05 mg/kg to 0.25 mg/kg per hour for 10 days. Plasma concentration and AUC were correlated linearly with dose. Intact AO was recovered from the urine. No responses	280
NHL	9	Bcl-2 (18-mer)	SC infusion	Dose-escalation protocol from 4.6 mg/m^2 to 73.6 mg/m^2 per day for 14 days. Toxicity limited mainly to local inflammation at the injection site. One CR, 3 SD, 5 PD. Significant reduction in circulating lymphocytes in 2 patients	281
Various	36	Protein kinase C α (20-mer)	IV infusion	Dose-escalation protocol from 0.15 mg/kg to 6.0 mg/kg three times per week for 3 weeks of a 4-week cycle. Moderate nausea/vomiting, fever, chills, and thrombocytopenia. No dose-limiting toxicity. Two CR in patients with NHL	282
Various	31	c-raf-1	IV infusion	Dose-escalation protocol from 0.15 mg/kg to 6.0 mg/kg three times per week for 3 weeks of a 4-week cycle. The AUC was correlated linearly with dose. Fever and fatigue were the main toxicities but the MTD was not determined. Two patients with SD had documented reductions in c-raf-1 expression in peripheral blood mononuclear cells	283,284
Various	21	Protein kinase C a (20-mer)	IV infusion	Dose-escalation protocol from 0.5 mg/kg to 3.0 mg/kg per day as continuous infusion for 3 weeks of a 4 week cycle. MTD was 5.0 mg/kg per day. Dose-limiting toxicity was fatigue and thrombocytopenia	285
Various	34	c-raf-1	IV infusion	Dose-escalation protocol from 0.5 mg/kg to 5.0 mg/kg per day as a continuous infusion for 3 weeks of a 4-week cycle. Minimal toxicity. SD in 2 pts; marker response in 1 pt with ovarian cancer	286
NHL	21	Bcl-2 (18-mer)	SC infusion	Dose-escalation protocol from 4.6 to 195.8 mg/m^2 per day. The MTD was 147.2 mg/ m^2 per day. Dose-limiting toxicities were thrombocytopenia, hypotension, fever, and asthenia. 1 CR, 2 MR, 9 SD, and 9 PD	287
Various	14	Type 1 Protein kinase A	IV infusion	Dose-escalation protocol from 2.5 mg/kg to 9 mg/kg. Pharmacokinetic parameters correlated linearly with dose. Mild fever and fatigue. No thrombocytopenia or complement activation. Stabilization of CEA level in one patient	288

* AML, Acute myeloblastic leukemia; AO, antisense oligonucleotide; AUC, area under the curve; CEA, carcinoembryonic antigen; CR, complete response; IV, intravenous; MDS, myelodysplastic syndrome; MR, minor response; MTD, maximum tolerated dose; NHL, non-Hodgkin's lymphoma; PD, progressive disease; SC, subcutaneous; SD, stable disease.

different ribozymes exhibit specificity for particular mRNA sequences, a matter of considerable importance for their potential clinical application. The most clearly defined molecules in this class are the hammerhead (HmR) and hairpin ribozymes (HpR), so-called because of their predicted molecular shapes. Both HmR and HpR demonstrate selective cleavage of certain specific RNA sequences, although this restriction is by no means absolute. The efficacy of a number of HmR that target bcl-2, ras, or c-erbB2 mRNA has been reported both *in vitro* (289–292) and *in vivo* in prostate, pancreatic, breast, and lung cancer models (289, 293–295). These agents delivered by various vectors have been shown to be able to reduce tumor cell growth *in vitro* and to yield responses in established tumors *in vivo*. A potential obstacle to the use of HmR *in vivo* is their requirement of a relatively high, non-physiological concentration of Mg^{2+} for optimal activity. However, although HpR are also dependent on the presence of metal ions, other molecules such as aminoglycoside antibiotics or endogenous cellular polyamines (for example, spermine) have been shown to support efficient catalytic activity at physiological ionic concentrations (296). Therefore, HpR would seem to have more likelihood of being clinically useful (263). Nonetheless, as yet, the use of ribozymes in CGT remains a theoretical possibility and there have been no clinical trials with this modality.

Cytoreductive gene therapy

The term cytoreductive gene therapy embraces approaches that aim to deliver genes that kill cells either directly or indirectly (by sensitizing them to the effects of drugs or radiation or by depriving them of their blood supply). A range of strategies can be considered under this heading, including gene-directed enzyme prodrug therapy (GDEPT) or 'suicide' gene therapy, genetic induction of apoptosis, anti-angiogenic gene therapy, and gene-directed radioisotopic therapy. A great deal of preclinical work has been completed and a number of promising genes have been identified, although, as yet, only GDEPT approaches have reached the stage of clinical trials.

GDEPT

GDEPT involves the delivery of a gene that encodes an enzyme that is able to convert a relatively innocuous prodrug to a toxic active agent within tumor cells. The strength of this approach lies in its potential to avoid the systemic toxicity and lack of tumor specificity associated with existing cytotoxic agents by ensuring that they are generated in high concentrations only at the tumor site, thus increasing their therapeutic index (297). The components of an idealized GDEPT system are as follows: (1) a gene that encodes an enzyme that catalyzes the conversion of a prodrug to a cytotoxic metabolite; (2) a mechanism of restricting gene expression to tumor tissue; (3) an enzyme that elicits only a minimal host immune response (although in the case of immunomodulatory gene therapy such an immune response may be beneficial); (4) a prodrug with minimal intrinsic cytotoxicity and well-established pharmacokinetics; (5) a toxic product that kills both cycling and non-cycling cells; (6) a toxic agent that is able to diffuse to adjacent tumor cells to cause a bystander effect (see Fig. 8.9).

A number of candidate suicide genes have undergone preliminary preclinical evaluation (298–310) (see Table 8.5). The two most widely studied examples of GDEPT are: (1) the herpes simplex virus thymidine kinase (HSVtk) and ganciclovir (GCV) system; (2) the *Escherichia coli* bacterial cytosine deaminase (CDase) and 5-fluorocytosine (5FC) system. Each of these systems has undergone extensive preclinical evaluation (reviewed in reference 311), and they have now entered clinical trials, the design and results of which are presented in Table 8.6 (88, 312–322). The majority of these studies have employed either RV or RDAV vectors to deliver a HSVtk transgene followed 7–14 days later by administration of the prodrug ganciclovir. The studies that have used RV vectors have involved direct intralesional or intracavitary instillation of murine cell lines (PA317 or M11) that produce and release RV *in situ* in patients with melanomas on brain or breast tumors. The endpoints of these studies have included evaluation of safety issues (such as the generation of replication-competent retroviruses) and documentation of toxicity (88, 312–322), *in situ* gene expression (312, 313, 315, 318), and responses (312–320, 322). In the studies reported to date, no replication-competent retroviruses have been detected and no patient has suffered an illness consistent with propagation of a retroviral infection. In general, toxicity has been mild and has been restricted to local inflammatory effects (314, 319, 322), fever (322), and the systemic toxicity of ganciclovir (313, 316). In direct contrast, the studies of RDAV have used direct intratumoral, intrapleural, or intraperitoneal administration of recombinant viral particles. All of these studies have been conducted as dose-escalation protocols with the

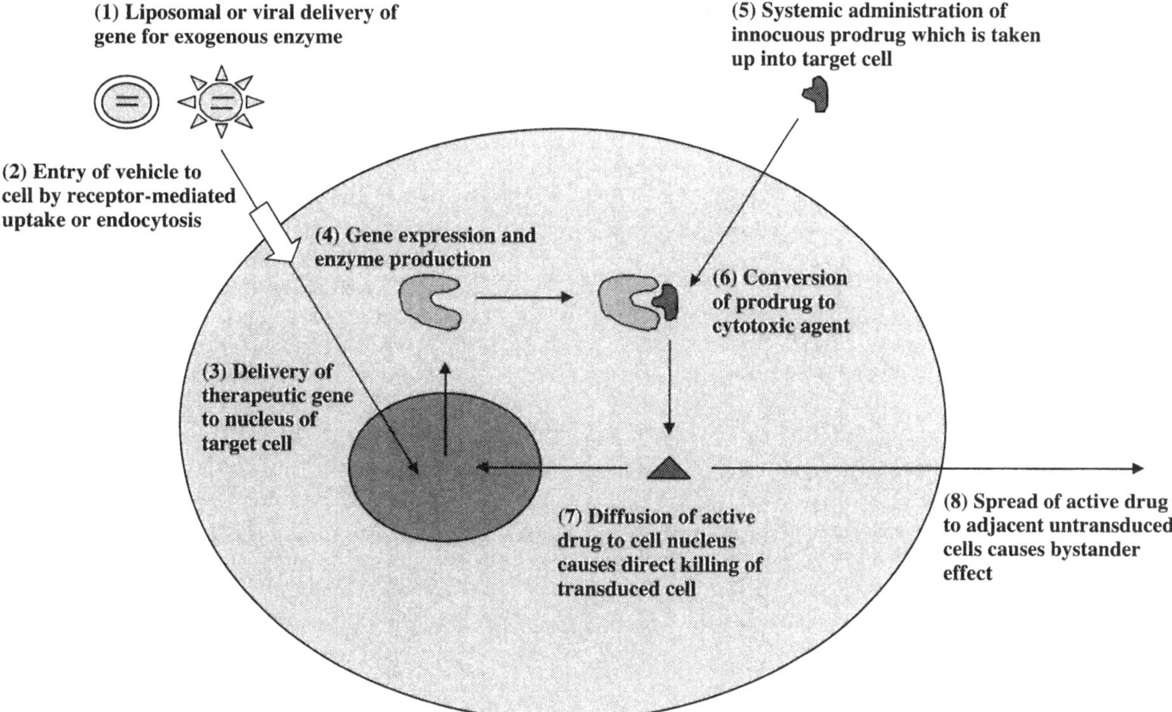

Fig. 8.9 Diagrammatic representation of the key components of gene-directed enzyme prodrug therapy (GDEPT).

aim of defining toxicological parameters. In most cases, toxicity has been mild and has involved fever, myelo-suppression, and deranged liver function (88, 313, 316, 320–322). The results of these initial studies are encouraging but, as yet, there has been little evidence of clinical benefit with either RV or RDAV vectors. It must be borne in mind, however, that they are essentially phase I studies that have employed GDEPT as a single agent in patients with aggressive, recurrent disease. In such situations, the reports of minor responses and disease stabilization can be seen as a promising start and have provided the necessary background for designing future trials.

Genetic induction of apoptosis

Apoptosis (programed cell death) is a carefully controlled process in which cells that have fulfilled their function or have sustained irreparable damage are disassembled from within and removed from a tissue (323). Under normal conditions, cells receive a regular supply of signals 'instructing' them not to die. Changes in the patterns of input of these signals are responsible for switching on the apoptotic machinery. There are two basic pathways that can direct a cell to undergo apoptosis: (1) positively-acting external signals mediated by binding of apoptosis-inducing ligands (for example, tumor necrosis factor (TNF), TNF-related apoptosis-inducing ligand (TRAIL), Fas ligand (FasL)) to their receptors (TNF receptor, Fas) on the cell surface (Fig. 8.10); (2) negatively acting signals in which reduced levels of growth factor support to the cell mediate changes in the intracellular balance of pro- and anti-apoptotic molecules that lead to release of cytochrome C from the mitochondria (Fig. 8.11). Each of these pathways converges in the activation of cellular enzymes called caspases (cytosolic aspartate-specific proteases) that degrade cellular proteins and commit the cell to self-destruction.

Derangement of normal apoptotic signaling pathways is a central component of malignant transformation (163). Therefore, dissection of the underlying molecular biology of apoptosis has opened up new prospects for gene therapy. Studies have addressed switching on apoptosis through both of the pathways described above. Signaling into tumor cells via specific apoptosis-inducing ligands has been reported for TNF (324), TRAIL (325), and FasL (326–331). Griffith

Table 8.5 Examples of GDEPT systems that are currently the subject of preclinical and clinical investigation (modified from ref. 298)

Enzyme	Prodrug	Active drug	Ref.
HSVtk	Ganciclovir	Ganciclovir triphosphate	299
Cytosine deaminase	5-fluorocytosine	5-fluorouracil	300
DT diaphorase	5-(aziridin-1-yl)-2,4-dinitrobenzamide (CB 1954)	5-(aziridin-1-yl)-4-hydroxylamino-2-nitrobenzamide	301
Nitroreductase	5-(aziridin-1-yl)-2,4-dinitrobenzamide (CB 1954)	5-(aziridin-1-yl)-4-hydroxylamino-2-nitrobenzamide	302
Guanine phosphoribosyl transferase	6-thioxanthine	6-thioxanthine monophosphate	303
Purine nucleoside phosphorylase	6-methyl-purine-2'-deoxynucleoside	6-methylpurine	304
Thymidine phosphorylase	5'-deoxy-5-fluorouridine	5-fluorouracil	305
Carboxylesterase	Irinotecan (CPT-11)	SN-38	306
Folylpolyglutamyl synthetase	Edatrexate	Edatrexate polyglutamate	307
Carboxypeptidase A1	Methotrexate-a-peptides	Methotrexate	308
Carboxypeptidase G2	Benzoic acid mustard glutamates	Benzoic acid mustards	309
Cytochrome P-450 (CYP2B1)	Cyclophosphamide, ifosfamide	Phosphoramide mustard	310

Table 8.6 Clinical trials of gene-directed enzyme prodrug therapy (GDEPT) for cancer*

Tumor	No. of patients	Transgene	Vector	Route	Outcomes	Ref.
Prostate	11	HSVtk	RDAV	IT	Dose escalation from 2.5×10^{10}–2.5×10^{10} pfu. HSVtk transgene under control of the osteocalcin promoter. Intralesional injections into local recurrence, nodal and bone metastases. Side-effects limited to flue-like illness and transient lymphopenia. No response data reported	88
Glioma, melanoma, breast	15	HSVtk	RV	IC	19 discrete tumors treated with intracerebral RV-producing murine PA317 packaging cell line. GCV commenced 7 days later. *In situ* gene expression demonstrated. Antitumor responses in 5 lesions	312
Mesothelioma	21	HSVtk	RDAV	IPL	Dose escalation from 10^9–10^{12} pfu. Gene expression documented in 11 of 20 evaluable pts. Toxicity fever in 20 pts; deranged LTF in 13 pts; decreased hemoglobin in 17 pts; leukopenia in 1 pt. No objectiv responses. SD in 3 pts	313
Glioma	12	HSVtk	RV	IC/IT	Tumors treated with intracerebral RV-producing murine M11 packaging cell line after debulking surgery. GCV commenced 7 days later for 2 weeks.No serious side-effects. PD in 4 pts at 4 months. Three-year survival in 1 pt	314
Melanoma	8	HSVtk	RV	IT	Tumors treated with intralesional RV-producing murine M11 packaging cell line for up to 3 courses. GCV commenced 7 days later for 2 weeks. Toxicity limited to local inflammation and fever. HSVtk expression seen in 3 pts who underwent biopsy. In 3 pts necrosis was seen in treated, but not untreated, tumor	315
Prostate	18	HSVtk	RDAV	IT	Dose escalation from 10^8–10^{11} infectious units. Mainly grade 1–2 toxicity except grade 3 hepatotoxicity and grade 4 thrombocytopenia in one pt. PSA feel by > 50% in 3 pts	316
Glioma	48	HSVtk	RV	IC/IT	resection of recurrent glioma followed by instillation of RV-producing murine PA317 packaging cell line into sides of resection cavity. GCV commenced 14 days later for 2 weeks. Toxicity mild. No recurrence in 4 pts at 12 months	317
Breast	12	E. coli CD	Plasmid	IT	Dose escalation study using intralesional plasmid cDNA containing CD transgene under control of the c-erbB2 promoter. Targeted gene expression documented in 11 of 12 pts. Minor responses in 4 pts. Minimal toxicity	318
Brain	12	HSVtk	RV	IC/IT	Intracavitary instillation of RV-producing murine PA317 packaging cell line after debulking surgery in 7 gliomas, 3 PNETs, and 2 ependymomas. Serious acute adverse reactions in 4 pts which resolved with conservative management. No RCR detected. PD in all pts	319
Glioma	13	HSVtk	RDAV	IT	Dose escalation from 2×10^9–2×10^{12} particles. Acute neurological toxicity (confusion, hyponatremia, seizures) in pts at highest dose. Death within 10 months in 10 pts. Post-mortem examination revealed cavitation and necrosis at injection site. Prolonged survival (29 months) in 1 pt	320
Ovary	10	HSVtk	RDAV	IP	Dose escalation from 2×10^{10}–2×10^{13} pfu instilled intraperitoneally after secondary debulking surgery of stage IIIc ovarian cancer. GCV and topotecan commenced 24 hours later. Toxicity limited to myelosuppression. No response data reported	321

Table 8.6 Continued

Tumor	No. of patients	Transgene	Vector	Route	Outcomes	Ref.
Glioma	14	HSVtk	RV or RDAV	IC/IT	Pts received intracerebral injections of either RV-producing murine PA317 packaging cell line (7 pts) or RDAV (7 pts). Toxicity limited to fever and increased seizure frequency in 2 pts. RV-treated tumors all progressed at 3 months. Three pts treated with RDAV had SD at 3 months. Mean survival times 7.4 and 15.0 months for RV- and RDAV-treated pts, respectively	322

* cDNA, complementary DNA; *E. coli*, CDase, cytosine deaminase derived from *Escherichia coli*; IC, intracerebral; IC/IT, intracavitary/intratumoral; IP, intraperitoneal; IPL, intrapleural; IT, intratumoral; GCV, ganciclovir; HSVtk, herpes simplex virus thymidine kinase; LFT, liver function tests; PD, progressive disease; pfu, plaque forming units; PNET, primitive neuroectodermal tumor; pt, patient; RCR, replication-competent retrovirus; RDAV, replication-deficient adenovirus; RV, retrovirus; SD, stable disease.

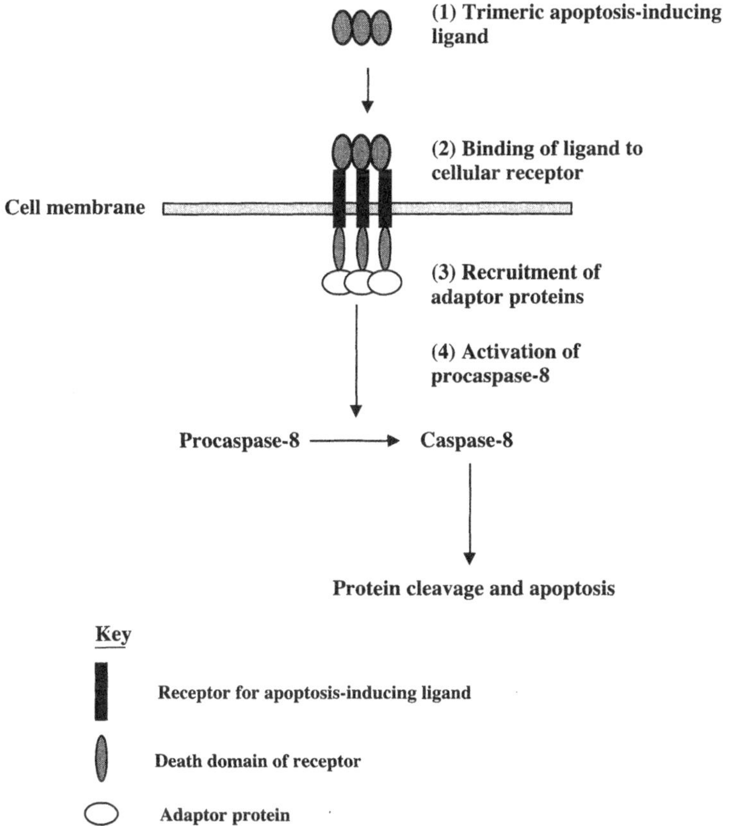

Fig. 8.10 Apoptosis signaling pathway. Binding of a positively acting apoptosis-inducing ligand to its cellular receptor leads to trimerization of the receptor and recruitment of activating adaptor proteins to the death domains of the receptor. The resulting protein complex is able to convert the inactive procaspase-8 into its active form, which degrades key cellular proteins and initiates the apoptotic cascade.

et al. (325) recently demonstrated that an AV vector directing expression of TRAIL was able to induce apoptosis through caspase activation in a variety of cancer cell lines *in vitro*. Much work has been done with FasL, which has been shown to be effective after direct viral delivery to cancer cells (326, 328–331) or after delivery by FasL-secreting myoblast cells (327). Significantly, this approach has been shown to be capable of inducing apoptosis in cell lines that were resistant to induction of apoptosis by conventional Fas-mediated pathways (agonist anti-Fas antibody or membrane-bound recombinant FasL) (331). Alternative approaches have involved the delivery of proapoptotic members of the Bcl-2 family, such as Bak (332) or Bax (333, 334), or active caspase molecules (335–338). Such approaches have been shown to be effective both *in vitro* and *in vivo*. As yet, no clinical studies of CGT using proapoptotic molecules have been reported. Clearly, as with all other approaches, tight control of

the expression of these genes will be necessary to guard against the risk of toxicity.

Anti-angiogenic gene therapy

The growth of a tumor beyond a diameter of 1–2 mm requires it to recruit its own blood supply through the process of angiogenesis (162, 163). This process is carefully regulated under normal physiological conditions by the interaction of pro-angiogenic (basic fibroblast growth factor (bFGF), vascular endothelial growth factor (VEGF), platelet-derived endothelial growth factor (PDGF)) and anti-angiogenic (angiostatin, endostatin, thrombospondin-1) factors. As a consequence, in health, angiogenesis is confined to the female reproductive cycle, pregnancy, and tissue healing (339). A central theme of cancer development and progression is the ability of tumors to circumvent these normal homeostatic mechanisms in order to promote the formation

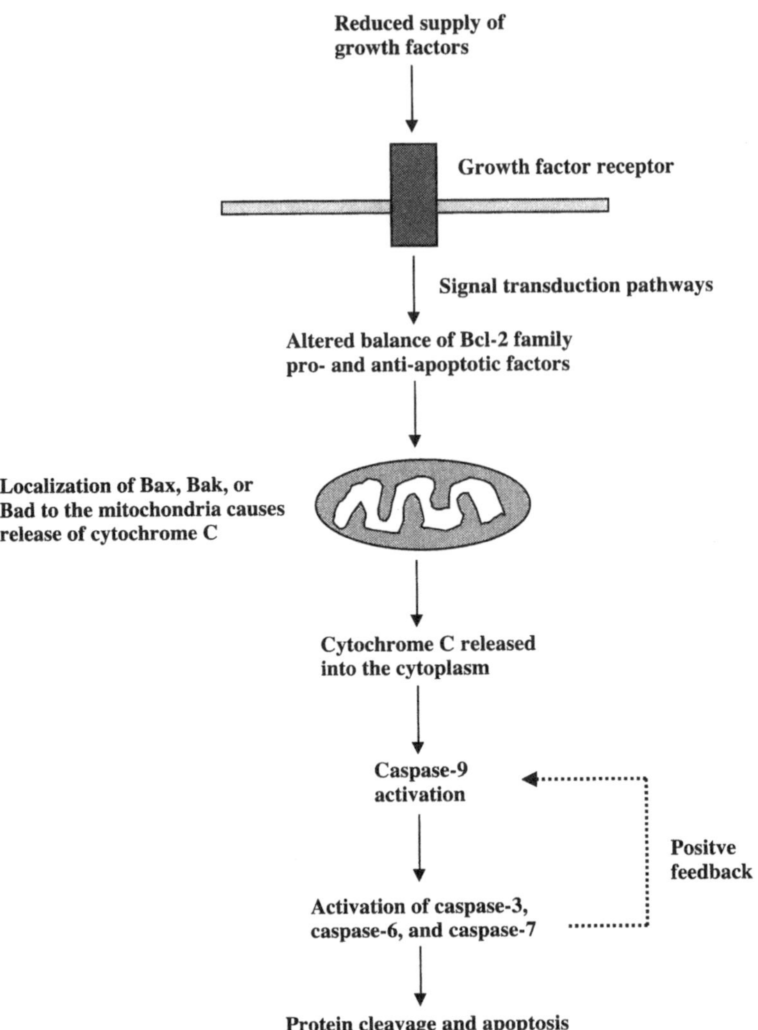

Fig. 8.11 Apoptosis signaling pathway. Alterations in the pattern of input of cellular growth factors lead to an altered balance of anti- and proapoptotic factors within the cell in favor of a proapoptotic state. Proapoptotic members of the Bcl-2 family of proteins localize to the mitochondria and cause membrane permeabilization and release of cytochrome C. The presence of this mitochondrial protein in the cytoplasm leads to activation of caspase-9 (and other downstream caspases) that are able to degrade cellular proteins and commit the cell to apoptosis.

of new blood vessels by upregulating expression of pro-angiogenic factors and downregulating expression of anti-angiogenic factors. Each of the essential steps in the process of angiogenesis (endothelial cell migration, proliferation, and maturation) represents a potential target for therapeutic intervention (340, 341). Furthermore, since this process is essentially restricted to tumor tissue, there exists the prospect of designing specific anti-angiogenic gene therapy strategies with minimal risk of toxic effects in normal tissues. An additional benefit accrues from the fact that endothelial cells, which are the targets of anti-angiogenic gene therapy, have not undergone malignant transformation. Therefore, they remain responsive to normal physiological controls and are unlikely to develop a resistant phenotype through the selection of mutant clones—a problem that is a feature of tumors. Furthermore, tumor endothelium-specific promoters have been identified and characterized and may be used to drive expression of therapeutic genes preferentially in the blood vessels that feed tumors (141, 142, 342). Destruction of tumor neovasculature may yield a very powerful bystander effect by killing all the cells that rely on a particular vessel to supply their oxygen and nutrient requirements.

Angiostatin and endostatin, which are angiogenesis inhibitors, have been shown to have very impressive therapeutic efficacy in tumor models in animals (343–346). As yet, there have been no published accounts of the activity of these agents in clinical studies. Because angiostatin and endostatin are proteins, their clinical use demands frequent parenteral administration. This requirement represents a serious potential barrier to clinical application of these promising agents. Delivery as plasmid DNA or by viral vectors offers the prospect of circumventing this problem by facilitating continuous endogenous production of the protein. Furthermore, because these agents are active after systemic administration, their expression from nontumor sites (for example, from muscle) may well be adequate for a therapeutic effect. Such considerations offer a means of overcoming the vexed issue of vector targeting to tumor tissue. It has been shown in mouse models that systemic administration of recombinant adenoviruses containing the endostatin gene yield serum levels sufficient to delay tumor engraftment (347, 348) reduce growth of established tumors (347, 349), and prevent the development of lung metastases (347). In another study, it was reported that a soluble form of the anti-angiogenic platelet factor-4 expressed from both RV and AV vectors delayed tumor progression after local injection in an intracerebral glioma model (350). In a different murine model, the ability of an AV vector expressing a secretable form of the amino-terminal fragment of urokinase to protect the liver from the development of metastases after injection of colon carcinoma cells was demonstrated (351).

In addition to direct delivery of anti-angiogenic genes, attention has been given to strategies involving the use of factors that block the action of pro-angiogenic factors. The activity of VEGF can be blocked by expressing a truncated, soluble form of the VEGF receptor (sFLT-1). This approach has the dual benefits of preventing VEGF from interacting with its functional receptor by sequestering it in the extracellular fluid while at the same time inactivating nascent VEGF receptors by forming nonfunctional intracellular heterodimers. Tumor cell lines stably transfected with sFLT-1 have been shown to grow more slowly as subcutaneous or direct intracranial implants and to have significantly reduced metastatic potential (352). A similar approach involving intratumoral delivery of an

AV vector expressing soluble Tie2 (an endothelium-specific receptor tyrosine kinase for the pro-angiogenic factor angiopoietin-1) resulted in delayed tumor progression by sequestration of angiopoietin-1. In addition, administration of this AV vector at the time of intravenous tumor inoculation or tumor excision decreased the incidence of subsequent lung metastases (353).

These studies suggest that anti-angiogenic gene therapy strategies may have a number of advantages over other CGT approaches. Therefore, the results of ongoing clinical studies using recombinant angiostatin and endostatin are eagerly awaited because they will give an indication of the potential benefits that might accrue from genetic delivery of anti-angiogenic therapy.

Genetic radioisotopic therapy

The efficacy of β-emitting radioisotopes in the treatment of certain tumor types has encouraged research into means of expanding the applicability of this therapy. Thus far, two genes that appear to have promise in this regard have been identified. Uptake of the radiolabelled catecholamine analog, ^{131}I-meta-iodobenzylguanidine (^{131}I-MIBG), into cells that express the norepinephrine (also called noradrenaline) transporter (NAT) forms the basis of treating pheochromocytoma, neuroblastoma, and carcinoid and medullary thyroid carcinoma in the clinic. It has been shown that NAT gene transfer can increase the localization and cytotoxicity of ^{131}I-MIBG in glioma and neuroblastoma cells *in vitro* (354, 355). As yet, no *in vivo* studies of this approach have been reported. An alternative strategy is based on the sodium iodide symporter (NIS)-mediated uptake of iodide into normal and malignant thyroid cells (reviewed in reference 356). Spitzweg *et al.* (84, 85) have reported NIS-mediated uptake of radioiodine in prostate cancer cells *in vitro* and have demonstrated that radioiodine can be used specifically to kill prostate cancer cells *in vitro* and xenograft tumors *in vivo*. NIS-expressing tumors accumulated 25–30 per cent of an intraperitoneal dose of radioiodine and retained it with a biological half-life of 45 hours. A single 111 MBq dose of a therapeutic ^{131}I resulted in an average tumor volume reduction of more than 90 per cent and complete tumor regression in up to 60 per cent of NIS-expressing tumors but not in the non-expressing controls. Boland *et al.* (357) expressed the rat NIS gene in a number of cell lines by adenovirus-mediated gene transfer and were able to demonstrate radioiodine uptake as well as a selective cytotoxic effect of trapped radioiodine *in vitro. In vivo* models using breast and cervix cancer cells demonstrated uptake to levels of 11 per cent of the injected radioiodine dose per gram of tumor tissue, although no therapeutic effect was reported. These studies demonstrate the potential of NIS gene transfer followed by radioiodine therapy as a novel cytoreductive gene therapy approach for nonthyroidal cancers, although no clinical data are available yet.

Immunomodulatory gene therapy

Many cancer cells display on their surfaces so-called tumor-associated antigens (TAA), which can be recognized by the humoral and cellular limbs of the immune system. Despite this fact, the immune system is rarely seen to mount a clinically meaningful antitumor response. Indeed, there is extensive evidence that the tumor is able to evade immune surveillance both by reducing its own immunogenicity and by inhibiting the ability of the immune system to mount an effective response against it (5). A number of mechanisms that appear to contribute to this phenomenon have been identified. Total or partial loss of expression of the MHC class I and co-stimulatory B7.1/B7.2 molecules has been documented in many cancer types and serves to reduce the efficiency of presentation of TAA to cytotoxic T lymphocytes (CTL) (see below). Mutations in the pathways regulating the transport and presentation of peptides on the surface of tumor cells may also shield them from detection by CTL. In addition, those CTL that infiltrate cancers may be killed by means of release of soluble FasL from the tumor cells, which themselves appear to be partially resistant to this important pathway of cell killing.

The identification of these aberrations in the immune system has fuelled interest in approaches aimed at delivering genes to enhance the immunogenicity of tumors and the immune responses mounted against them (5358). Enlisting the services of the immune system may have a number of benefits: (1) the inherent specificity of the immune response should limit the occurrence of normal tissue toxicity; (2) an immune response generated at one site should prime the immune system to react to disease deposits at other local and distant sites, yielding a potent bystander effect; (3) the system involves significant signal amplification such that a small immunogenic stimulus has the capacity to trigger a large response; (4) once established, antitumor immunity should persist through the generation of memory cells that should act to prevent disease recurrence.

The central components of an antitumor immune response are presented in a simplified form in Fig. 8.12. The essence of the process is the activation of specific CD8+CTL that are able to recognize TAA and kill cells that express them. A number of the steps required for this process are deranged locally and/or systemically in patients with cancer and are, therefore, suitable targets for immunomodulatory CGT. The means by which delivery of therapeutic genes could be used to generate or enhance the immune response against tumors can be summarized thus: (1) intratumoral delivery and expres-

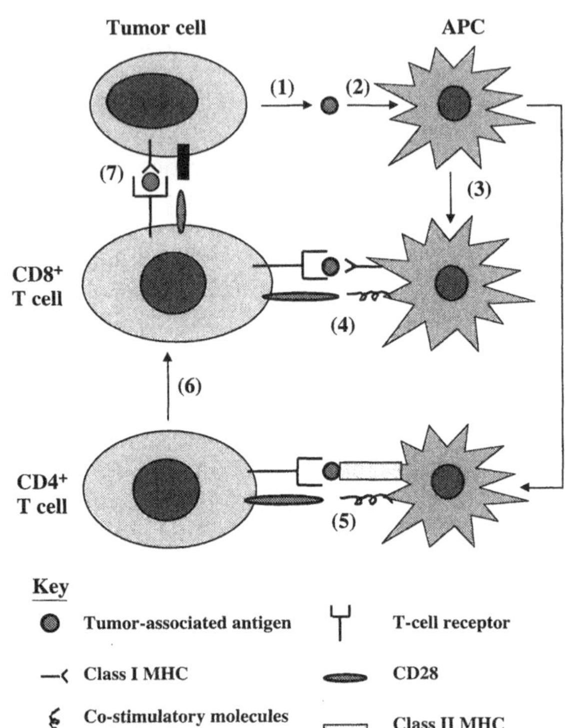

Fig. 8.12 A schematic representation of the key components of a cell-mediated specific antitumor response: (1) Tumor-associated antigen (TAA) is released from tumor cells either as part of a normal physiological process or in response to cytotoxic therapy. (2) The TAA is phagocytosed by an immature antigen-presenting cell (APC). (3) The process of exposure to and uptake of TAA causes maturation of the APC. (4) The APC processes the TAA and presents it in the context of MHC class I and B7.1/B7.2 co-stimulatory molecules to a CD8+ T cell that expresses the appropriate T-cell receptor. This interaction activates the CD8+ cytotoxic T cell (CTL). (5) The APC can also present the TAA to a CD4+ T cell in context of MHC class II and B7.1/B7.2 co-stimulatory molecules. This interaction activates the CD4+ cell. (6) The CD4+ T cell (T helper cell) secretes cytokines to stimulate the CD8+ T cell and help it to become a CTL. (7) The CTL kills tumor cells expressing the TAA in the context of MHC class I and appropriate co-stimulatory molecules.

sion of cytokine genes to increase trafficking of antigen-presenting cells (APC) and T cells into the tumor and to enhance their ability to mount an immune response (359); (2) intratumoral delivery of genes encoding co-stimulatory molecules, such as B7.1 and B7.2, with the goal of enhancing the ability of CTL to recognize, engage, and kill tumor cells (360); (3) intratumoral delivery of exogenous foreign immunogens (for example, allogeneic tumor cells or MHC molecules) to generate a local immune/inflammatory reaction that will increase the ability of APC to take up TAA (so-called cross-priming of an immune response) (361) (4) tumor cell killing by cytoreductive CGT (for example, GDEPT or genetic radioisotopic therapy) with subsequent release of TAA, which can be processed by APC and presented to immune effector cells in an environment that is perceived as 'dangerous' (91, 362); (5) intramuscular delivery of plasmid cDNA encoding cloned TAA leading to local uptake and expression by APC and subsequent presentation to immune effector cells (363).

In the arena of clinical development of immunomodulatory CGT, studies have focused on two particular approaches. The first involves attempts to deliver genes encoding MHC molecules or cytokines directly into tumor cells *in vivo*. The published data dealing with this approach are summarized in Table 8.7 (55, 73, 74, 364–371). A number of trials have examined the ability of a cationic liposome to deliver plasmid cDNA for the HLA-B7 molecule in association with β_2-microglobulin in patients with a variety of tumor types (73, 74, 364, 365, 367). The early phase I studies involved dose-escalation protocols using intratumoral injections of cDNA encapsulated in cationic liposomes. The treatment was very well tolerated and successful gene transfer was demonstrated by means of PCR of posttreatment tumor biopsy specimens. Stable disease and occasional partial responses were reported in patients with melanoma and head and neck and renal cancer (73, 74, 364, 367). Subsequently, a large phase II trial in 52 patients confirmed the activity of this agent, although no patient achieved a complete response. Delivery of cytokine genes (granulocyte–macrophage colony stimulating factor (GM-CSF), interferon-γ (IFN-γ), and interleukin-2 (IL-2)) has been accomplished using replication-deficient vaccinia, and retroviral and adenoviral vectors in patients with melanoma and breast, colonic, and pancreatic cancers (55, 368–370). Once again, these approaches have been shown to have good safety profiles and to be capable of transducing tumor cells *in vivo*. However, as with the studies involving cationic liposomal vehicles, there have been few objective responses, although a number of patients have experienced disease stabilization.

The second approach to clinical immunomodulatory gene therapy has involved using genetically modified normal or malignant cells as cancer vaccines. The published clinical studies are summarized in Table 8.8 (372–381). In most studies, the patient's own (autologous) tumor cells have been harvested, transduced with a therapeutic cytokine gene (GM-CSF, IFN-γ, IL-2, and IL-12), and re-injected (after irradiation to stop them forming 'metastatic' deposits). This strategy has been seen as most likely to yield a meaningful clinical response because the tumor cells are likely to display the relevant antigens necessary for inducing antitumor immunity. Studies of this type have been reported in patients with melanoma and glioma using *ex vivo* transduction of tumor cells with plasmid cDNA or RV vectors (372, 373, 376, 379, 380). In general, treatment has been very well tolerated with side-effects limited to local inflammatory changes and fever. Surrogate measures of antitumor immunity have included generation of delayed type hypersensitivity (DYH) reactions (373, 376), CTL (373), and intratumoral immune infiltrates (373, 379). Responses in these studies have largely been limited to disease stabilization, although occasional objective responses have been reported. Despite the obvious attraction of using autologous tumor cells, there are a number of technical problems inherent in this approach which are likely to limit its clinical utility. These problems include the need to harvest and grow each patient's tumor, transduce it *ex vivo*, assay the levels of gene transfer, and ensure that the whole procedure is conducted in accordance with guidelines laid down by regulatory bodies. A potential means of circumventing these problems is to use generic tumor cell lines that are derived either from other patients (allogeneic tumor cells) or from animals of a different species (xenogeneic cells). Each of these strategies has been subjected to phase I clinical evaluation (375, 377, 381). Again, these studies have yielded preliminary data demonstrating immune activation as evidenced by the generation of DTH responses (381), specific antibodies (377), and the occurrence of vitiligo in a patient with melanoma (375). However, response data have been limited to disease stabilization or, at best, mixed or partial responses.

Conclusions

As this review has demonstrated, gene therapy has been an extremely active field of research in the last 2

140

Table 8.7 Summary of clinical trials involving direct intratumoural delivery of major histocompatibility complex or cytokine genes for immunomodulatory cancer gene therapy. Studies have involved gene delivery by cationic liposomes or recombinant vaccinia, retroviral or adenoviral vectors.

Tumour	Pts	Transgene	Vector	Route	Outcomes	Ref
Melanoma	7	GM-CSF	Vaccinia	IT	Twice weekly injections for 6 weeks. Virally encoded GM-CSF detected at injection site for up to 8 months. Dense CD4, CD8 and eosinophil infiltrate. Minimal toxicity. 1 CR, 1 PR, 3 MR, 2PD.	[55]
Renal	15	HLA-B7/β_2MG	CL	IT	HLA-B7 expression demonstrated in 8 of 14 evaluable lesions. Toxicity $\leq$ Grade 2. SD in 12 of 15 patients during study. No objective responses.	[73]
Melanoma, Renal, Sarcoma	24 (Phase I) 52 (Phase II)	IL-2	CL	IT	Phase I study demonstrated minimal toxicity. Phase II study: PR in 2 of 17 renal, 1 of 18 melanoma and 0 of 17 sarcoma; SD in 2 of 17 renal, 3 of 18 melanoma, 6 of 17 sarcoma patients.	[74]
Melanoma	10	HLA-B7/β_2MG	CL	IT	Dose escalation study using 3 injections of cDNA. Gene transfer seen in 9 of 10 patients. Dense intratumoural lymphocytic infiltrate detected. One pt had a PR.	[364]
Colorectal	15	HLA-B7/β_2MG	CL	IT	Dose escalation study of IT injection of liver metastases. Plasmid DNA detected by PCR in biopsies from 14 of 15 patients. HLA-B7 protein detected evaluable samples. No serious toxicity. No response data reported.	[365]
NSCLC, Melanoma, Breast, Cervix, Ovary	19	HLA-A2, HLA-B 13, murine H-2K^k	CL	IT	Weekly IT injections. No toxicity. HLA-A2 induced 2 CR and 4 PR in 8 patients with cutaneous nodules from cervical and ovarian cancer. CR in axillary nodes in patient with non-small cell lung cancer.	[366]
Head and neck	9	HLA-B7/β_2MG	CL	IT	Two weekly injections ($\times$ 4). Histopathological evidence of weak HLA-B7 expression and increased apoptosis (TUNEL staining) in 2 patients. No treatment-related toxicity. 4 PR with stable disease for 12–72 weeks.	[367]
Melanoma, Breast	13	IFN-γ	RV	IT	Injections of RV vector encoding IFN-γ gene for 5 consecutive days (1.5 $\times$ 10^8 cfu total dose). Tumour resection 3 days after final injection. No RCR isolated. IFN-γ transduction seen in 3 of 10 tumours. No objective responses at distant sites.	[368]
Melanoma	17	IFN-γ	RV	IT	Daily IT injections for 5 days per treatment course. Increased anti-melanoma antibodies in 8 patients. Minimal toxicity. No RCR. SD in 1 of 9 pts treated with single course and in 8 of 8 treated with multiple courses.	[369]
Melanoma, Breast	23	IL-2	RDAV	IT	10^7–10^{10} pfu per injection. Anti-adenoviral antibodies detected in all patients pre-treatment and increased post-treatment. Toxicity limited to local inflammation and fever. SD in 6 patients (5 of 15 melanoma, 1 of 8 breast cancer).	[370]
Colon, Pancreas	6	IL-2	RDAV	IT	10^7–10^8 pfu per injection. Transient increase in serum IL-2 levels seen at days 10 and 14. No acute toxicity. No response data reported.	[371]

Table 8.8 Summary of Phase I clinical trials of cancer vaccine strategies using genetically modified cells.

Tumour	Pts	Transgene	Vehicle	Route	Outcomes	Ref
Melanoma	5	IFN-γ	Autologous tumour cells	sc	Autologous tumour cells were transduced *ex vivo* with a RV vector expressing IFN-γ. Expansion of the cells was attempted in 64 pts, successfully in only 12 pts. Five pts received sc injections of tumour cells expressing IFN-γ. SD in 3 pts, PD in 2 pts.	[372]
Melanoma	6	IL-12	Autologous tumour cells	sc	Autologous tumour cells were transduced with plasmid cDNA encoding IL-12 by direct gene gun injection. All pts received > 4 sc injections of these cells. Mild fever occurred in 2 pts. DTH response and increased CTL were seen in 2 pts. MR in 1 pt, SD in 3 pts. Responding pt had a heavy intratumoural infiltrate of CD4+ and CD8+ cells.	[373]
Colorectal	10	IL-2	Autologous fibroblasts	sc	Autologous fibroblasts from a skin biopsy transduced *ex vivo* with RV encoding IL-2 and mixed with autologous tumour cells. Pts received 10^7 autologous tumour cells plus IL-2-transduced fibroblasts in escalating doses to a minimum of 3 doses. Toxicity limited to fatigue and a flu-like syndrome. Positive DTH responses seen in 5 pts. One pt with SD, 9 with PD.	[374]
Various	9	IL-2	Xenogeneic Veto cells	IT	Monkey fibroblast (Vero) cells engineered to express human IL-2. Intra-tumoural injection of escalating doses of cells (5×10^5 to 5×10^7 cells) on three occasions. MR in 1 pt, SD in 4 pts. Development of vitiligo in one pt with melanoma.	[375]
Melanoma	12	IL-2	Autologous tumour cells	sc	Autologous tumour cells were transduced *ex vivo* with a RV vector expressing IL-2 and re-injected sc. Local reactions occurred at 11 of the 24 injection sites. Minor systemic reactions occurred after 6 injections. Antitumour DTH response was seen in 1 pt. No objective responses. SD in 3 pts.	[376]
Melanoma	12	IL-4	Allogeneic tumour cells	sc	Allogeneic tumour cells were transduced *ex vivo* with a RV vector expressing IL-4 and re-injected sc. Minor toxicity (Grade 1–2). Anti-alloantigen antibody responses in 2 of 11 assessable pts. Anti-autologous antigen antibody responses in 1 of 6 assessable pts. Two pts with MR.	[377]
Renal, colorectal, lymphoma	10	IL-2	CIK cells	ivi	CIK cells transduced *ex vivo* by electroporation to express IL-2. Following ivi, CIK cells were detected in the blood by PCR for 2 weeks. Systemic levels of IFN-γ, GM-CSF and TGF-β were elevated. CR in 1 pt with lymphoma.	[378]
Melanoma	5	GM-CSF	Autologous tumour cells	ID	Intradermal vaccination with autologous tumour cells that either had or had not been transduced *ex vivo* with RV expressing GM-CSF. Vaccination site and draining lymph nodes were removed at 7–10 days. Increased infiltration with dendritic cells noted at the GM-CSF primed sites and nodes. One pt had a CR.	[379]
Glioma	12	None	Autologous tumour cells	ID	Autologous tumour harvested, irradiated, mixed with GM-CSF and injected ID in to the thigh. The draining inguinal nodes were harvested and cultured *ex vivo* in the presence of IL-2. The resulting population of cells (71% CD4+) were re-infused iv. There was mild toxicity. PR in 4 pts, including 2 pts with glioblastoma multiforme.	[380]
Pancreas	14	GM-CSF	Allogeneic tumour cells	ID	Following pancreaticoduodenectomy, pts received 4 vaccinations with allogeneic pancreatic cancer cell lines (both GM-CSF expressing and non-expressing cells) at doses of $1 \times 10^7 - 5 \times 10^8$ cells. Three additional vaccinations administerred to 6 pts still in remission after adjuvant chemotherapy and radiotherapy. No dose-limiting toxicities occurred. DTH responses against autologous tumour cells detected in 3 pts who also had a prolonged disease-Free interval (> 2 years).	[381]

Key: cDNA – complementary DNA, CIK – cytokine-induced killer, CR – complete response, CTL – cytotoxic T-lymphocytes, DTH – delayed type hypersensitivity, GM-CSF – granulocyte-macrophage colony stimulating factor, ID – intradermal, IFN-γ – interferon γ, IL-2 – interleukin 2, IT – intratumoural, ivi – intravenous infusion, MR – mixed response ie complete or partial response in one site with progressive disease in another, PCR – polymerase chain reaction, PD – progressive disease, PR – partial response, pt – patient, RV – retrovirus, sc – subcutaneous, SD – stable disease, TGF-β – transforming growth factor β.

decades. Enormous effort has been devoted to elucidating the genetic mechanisms underlying malignant disease with a view to finding novel therapeutic targets. We now stand on the threshold of a period in which many of these new therapies will be subjected to rigorous clinical evaluation. When gene therapy was in its infancy, there was great optimism that such standard therapies as surgery, radiotherapy, and chemotherapy would eventually be rendered obsolete by the new science of molecular therapy. However, in the last 10 years, there has been a substantial reassessment of the situation. There is an increasing awareness that gene therapy is most likely to be introduced into clinical practice as an adjuvant treatment in conjunction with the currently used standard modalities. Indeed, the direction of current preclinical studies demonstrates that there is a strong trend towards using gene therapy to maximize the therapeutic benefit of radiotherapy and chemotherapy. The challenge for the next decade lies in identifying the most valuable gene therapy approaches and working out ways to integrate them into a diversified clinical armamentarium.

References

1. Harrington KJ, Linardakis E, Vile RG. Transcriptional control: an essential component of cancer gene therapy strategies? Adv Drug Deliv Rel 2000, 44, 167–84.
2. Vile RG, Russell SJ, Lemoine NR. Cancer gene therapy: hard lessons and new courses. Gene Ther 2000, 7, 2–8.
3. Verma IM, Somia N. Gene therapy—promises, problems and prospects. Nature 1997, 389, 239–42.
4. Peng KW, Vile RG. Vector development for cancer gene therapy. Tumor Targeting 1999, 4, 3–11.
5. Melcher A, Gough M, Todryk S, Vile R. Apoptosis or necrosis for tumour immunotherapy: what's in a name? J Mol Med 1999, 77, 824–33.
6. Krasnykh VN, Mikheeva GV, Douglas JT, Curiel DT. Generation of recombinant adenovirus vectors with modified fibers for altering viral tropism. J Virol 1996, 70, 6839–46.
7. Kasono K, Blackwell JL, Douglas JT, *et al.* Selective gene delivery to head and neck cancer cells via an integrin targeted adenoviral vector. Clin Cancer Res 1999, 5, 2571–9.
8. Wickham TJ. Targeting adenovirus. Gene Ther 2000, 7, 110–14.
9. Cosset FL, Russell SJ. Targeting retrovirus entry. Gene Ther 1996, 3, 946–56.
10. Coffey MC, Strong JE, Forsyth PA, Lee PW. Reovirus therapy of tumours with activated Ras pathway. Science 1998, 282, 1332–4.
11. Schirrmacher V, Haas C, Bonifer R, Ahlert T, Gerhards R, Ertel C. Human tumour cell modification by virus infection: an efficient and safe way to produce cancer vaccine with pleiotropic immune stimulatory properties when using Newcastle disease virus. Gene Ther 1999, 6, 63–73.
12. Wahlfors JJ, Zullo SA, Loimas S, Nelson DM, Morgan RA. Evaluation of recombinant alphaviruses as vectors in gene therapy. Gene Ther 2000, 7, 472–80.
13. Stojdl DF, Lichty B, Knowles S, *et al.* Exploiting tumour-specific defects in the interferon pathway with a previously unknown oncolytic virus. Nat Med 2000, 6, 821–5.
14. Miller AD. Retroviral vectors. Curr Top Microbiol Immunol 1992, 158, 1–24.
15. Vile RG, Russell SJ. Retroviruses as vectors. Br Med Bull 1995, 51, 12–30.
16. Naldini L, Blomer U, Gallay P, *et al. In vivo* gene delivery and stable transduction of nondividing cells by a lentiviral vector. Science 1996, 272, 263–7.
17. Zhang WW. Development and application of adenoviral vectors for gene therapy of cancer. Cancer Gene Ther 1999, 6, 113–38.
18. Curiel DT. Strategies to adapt adenoviral vectors for targeted delivery. Ann NY Acad Sci 1999, 886, 158–71.
19. Kochanek S. High-capacity adenoviral vectors for gene transfer and somatic gene therapy. Hum Gene Ther 1999, 10, 2451–9.
20. Curiel DT. The development of conditionally replicative adenoviruses for cancer therapy. Clin Cancer Res 20001, 6, 3395–9.
21. Bischoff JR, Kim DH, Williams A, *et al.* An adenovirus mutant that replicates selectively in p53-deficient human tumor cells. Science 1996, 274, 373–6.
22. Shinoura N, Yoshida Y, Tsunoda R, *et al.* Highly augmented cytopathic effect of a fiber-mutant E1B-defective adenovirus for gene therapy of gliomas. Cancer Res 1999, 59, 3411–16.
23. Wildner 0, Blaese RM, Morris JC. Therapy of colon cancer with oncolytic adenovirus is enhanced by the addition of herpes simplex virus-thymidine kinase. Cancer Res 1999, 59, 410–13.
24. Freytag SO, Rogulski KR, Paielli DL, Gilbert JD, Kim JH. A novel three-pronged approach to kill cancer cells selectively: concomitant viral, double suicide gene, and radiotherapy. Hum Gene Ther 1998, 9, 1323–33.
25. Rodriguez R, Schuur ER, Lim HY, Henderson GA, Simons JW, Henderson DR. Prostate attenuated replication competent adenovirus (ARCA) CN706: a selective-cytotoxic for prostate-specific antigen-positive prostate cancer cells. Cancer Res 1997, 57, 2559–63.
26. Yu DC, Sakamoto GT, Henderson DR. Identification of the transcriptional regulatory sequences of human kallikrein 2 and their use in the construction of calydon virus 764, an attenuated replication competent adenovirus for prostate cancer therapy. Cancer Res 1999, 59, 1498–504.
27. Yu DC, Chen Y, Seng M, Dilley J, Henderson DR. The addition of adenovirus type 5 region E3 enables calydon virus 787 to eliminate distant prostate tumour xenografts. Cancer Res 1999, 59, 4200–3.
28. Hallenbeck PL, Chang YN, Hay C, *et al.* A novel tumor-specific replication-restricted adenoviral vector

for gene therapy of hepatocellular carcinoma. Hum Gene Ther 1999, **10**, 1721–33.

29. Heise C, Sampson-Johannes A, Williams A, McCormick F, Von Hoff DD, Kirn DH. ONYX-015, an E1B gene-attenuated adenovirus, causes tumour-specific cytolysis and antitumoural efficacy that can be augmented by standard chemotherapeutic agents. Nat Med 1997, **3**, 639–45.

30. Heise CC, Williams AM, Xue S, Propst M, Kim DH. Intravenous administration of ONYX-015, a selectively replicating adenovirus, induces antitumoral efficacy. Cancer Res 1999, **59**, 2623–8.

31. You L, Yang CT, Jablons DM. ONYX-015 works synergistically with chemotherapy in lung cancer cell lines and primary cultures freshly made from lung cancer patients. Cancer Res 2000, **60**, 1009–13.

32. Rogulski KR, Freytag SO, Zhang K, *et al. In vivo* antitumor activity of ONYX-015 is influenced by p53 status and is augmented by radiotherapy. Cancer Res 2000, **60**, 1193–6.

33. Kirn D, Hermiston T, McCormick F. ONYX-015: clinical data are encouraging. Nat Med 1998, **4**, 1341–2.

34. Khuri FR, Nemunaitis J, Ganly I, *et al.* A controlled trial of intratumoral ONYX-015, a selectively-replicating adenovirus, in combination with cisplatin and 5-fluorouracil in patients with recurrent head and neck cancer. Nat Med 2000, **6**, 879–85.

35. Nemunaitis J, Ganly I, Khuri F, *et al.* Selective replication and oncolysis in p53 mutant tumors with ONYX-015, an ElB-55kD gene-deleted adenovirus, in patients with advanced head and neck cancer: a phase II trial. Cancer Res 2000, **60**, 6359–66.

36. Fink DJ, Glorioso JC. Engineering herpes simplex virus vectors for gene transfer to neurons. Nat Med 1997, **3**, 357–9.

37. Sena-Esteves M, Saeki Y, Fraefel C, Breakefield XO. HSV-1 amplicon vector-simplicity and versatility. Mol. Ther 2000, **2**, 9–15.

38. Martuza RL, Malick A, Markert JM, Ruffner KL, Coen DM. Experimental therapy of human glioma by means of a genetically engineered virus mutant. Science 1991, **252**, 854–6.

39. Boviatsis EJ, Scharf JM, Chase M, *et al.* Antitumor activity and reporter gene transfer into rat brain neoplasms inoculated with herpes simplex virus vectors defective in thymidine kinase or ribonucleotide reductase. Gene Ther 1994, **1**, 323–31.

40. Yoon SS, Nakamura H, Carroll NM, Bode BP, Chiocca EA, Tanabe KK. An oncolytic herpes simplex virus type 1 selectively destroys diffuse liver metastases from colon carcinoma. FASEB J 2000, **14**, 301–11.

41. Chiocca EA, Smith ER. Oncolytic viruses as novel anticancer agents: turning one scourge against another. Expert Opin Investig Drugs 2000, **9**, 311–27.

42. Rampling R, Cruickshank G, Papanastassiou V, *et al.* Toxicity evaluation of replication-competent herpes simplex virus (ICP 34.5 null mutant 1716) in patients with recurrent malignant glioma. Gene Ther 2000, **7**, 859–66.

43. Mineta T, Rabkin SD, Yazaki T, Hunter WD, Martuza RL. Attenuated multi-mutated herpes simplex virus-1 for the treatment of malignant gliomas. Nat Med 1995, **1**, 938–43.

44. Oyama M, Ohigashi T, Hoshi M, *et al.* Intravesical and intravenous therapy of human bladder cancer by the herpes vector G207. Hum Gene Ther 2000, **11**, 1683–93.

45. Walker JR, McGeagh KG, Sundaresan P, Jorgensen TJ, Rabkin SD, Martuza RL. Local and systemic therapy of human prostate adenocarcinoma with the conditionally replicating herpes simplex virus vector G207. Hum Gene Ther 1999, **10**, 2237–43.

46. Todryk S, McLean C, Ali S, *et al.* Disabled infectious single-cycle herpes simplex virus as an oncolytic vector for immunotherapy of colorectal cancer. Hum Gene Ther 1999, **10**, 2757–68.

47. Flotte TR, Carter B.J. Adeno-associated viral vectors. In: Gene therapy technologies, applications and regulations (ed. A Meager). John Wiley and Sons, Chichester, 1999.

48. Gnant MF, Noll LA, Irvine KR, *et al.* Tumor-specific gene delivery using recombinant vaccinia virus in a rabbit model of liver metastases. J Natl Cancer Inst 1999, **91**, 174–50.

49. Gnant MF, Puhlmann M, Alexander HR Jr, Bartlett DL. Systemic administration of a recombinant vaccinia virus expressing the cytosine deaminase gene and subsequent treatment with 5-fluorocytosine leads to tumor-specific gene expression and prolongation of survival in mice. Cancer Res 1999, 59, 3396–403.

50. Puhlmann M, Brown CK, Gnant M, *et al.* Vaccinia as a vector for tumor-directed gene therapy: biodistribution of a thymidine kinase-deleted mutant. Cancer Gene Ther 2000, **7**, 66–73.

51. Siemens DR, Austin JC, Hedican SP, Tartaglia J, Ratliff TL. Viral vector delivery in solid-state vehicles: gene expression in a murine prostate cancer model. J Natl Cancer Inst 2000, **92**, 403–12.

52. Mukherjee S, Haenel T, Himbeck R, *et al.* Replication-restricted vaccinia as a cytokine gene therapy vector in cancer: persistent transgene expression despite antibody generation. Cancer Gene Ther 200Q, **7**, 663–70.

53. Qin H, Chatterjee SK. Cancer gene therapy using tumor cells infected with recombinant vaccinia virus expressing GM-CSF. Hum Gene Ther 1996, **7**, 1853–60.

54. Kawakita M, Rao GS, Ritchey JK, *et al.* Effect of canarypox virus (ALVAC)-mediated cytokine expression on murine prostate tumor growth. J Natl Cancer Inst 1997, **89**, 428–36.

55. Mastrangelo MJ, Maguire HC Jr, Eisenlohr LC, *et al.* Intratumoral recombinant GM-CSF-encoding virus as gene therapy in patients with cutaneous melanoma. Cancer Gene Ther 1999, **6**, 409–22.

56. Marshall JL, Hawkins MJ, Tsang KY, *et al.* Phase I study in cancer patients of a replication-defective avipox recombinant vaccine that expresses human carcinoembryonic antigen. J Clin Oncol 1999, **17**, 332–7.

57. von Mehren M, Arlen P, Tsang KY, *et al.* Pilot study of a dual gene recombinant avipox vaccine containing both carcinoembryonic antigen (CEA) and B7.1 transgenes in patients with recurrent CEA-expressing adenocarcinomas. Clin Cancer Res 2000, **6**, 2219–28.

58. Eder JP, Kantoff PW, Roper K, *et al*. A phase I trial of a recombinant vaccinia viru's expressing prostate-specific antigen in advanced prostate cancer. Clin Cancer Res 2000, **6**, 1632–8.

59. Yang JP, Huang L. Direct gene transfer to mouse melanoma by intratumour injection of free DNA. Gene Ther 1996, **3**, 542–8.

60. Nomura T, Nakajima S, Kawabata K, *et al*. Intratumoural pharmacokinetics and *in vivo* gene expression of naked plasmid DNA and its cationic liposome complexes after direct gene transfer. Cancer Res 1997, **57**, 2681–6.

61. Coe S, Harron M, Winslet M, Goldspink G. The use of skeletal muscle to express genes for the treatment of cancer. Adv Exp Med Biol 2000, **465**, 95–111.

62. Blezinger P, Wang J, Gondo M, *et al*. Systemic inhibition of tumor growth and tumor metastases by intramuscular administration of the endostatin gene. Nat Biotechnol 1991, **17**, 343–8.

63. Schreurs MW, de Boer AJ, Figdor CG, Adema GJ. Genetic vaccination against the melanocyte lineage-specific antigen gplOO induces cytotoxic T lymphocyte-mediated tumour protection. Cancer Res 1998, **58**, 2509–14.

64. Fynan EF, Webster RG, Fuller DH *et al*. DNA vaccines: protective immunizations by parenteral, mucosal, and gene-gun inoculations. Proc Natl Acad Sci, USA 1993, **90**, 11478–82.

65. Hui KM, Chia TF. Eradication of tumour growth via biolistic transformation with aliogeneic MHC genes. Gene Ther 1997, **4**, 762–7.

66. Sun WH, Burkholder JK, Sun J, *et al*. *In vivo* cytokine gene transfer by gene gun reduces tumour growth in mice. Proc Natl Acad Sci, USA 1995, **92**, 2889–93.

67. Lasic DD, Vallner JJ, Working PK. Sterically stabilised liposomes in cancer therapy and gene delivery. Curr Opin Mol Ther 1999, **1**, 177–85.

68. Feigner PL, Gadek TR, Holm M, *et al*. Lipofection: a highly efficient, lipid-mediated DNA-transfection procedure. Proc Natl Acad Sci, USA 1987, **84**, 7413–17.

69. Hug P, Sleight RG. Liposomes for the transformation of eukaryotic cells. Biochim Biophys Acta 1991, **1097**, 1–17.

70. Zhu N, Liggitt D, Liu Y, Debs R. Systemic gene expression after intravenous DNA delivery into adult mice. Science 1993, **261**, 209–11.

71. Li S, Huang L. *In vivo* gene transfer via intravenous administration of cationic lipid–protamine–DNA (LPD) complexes. Gene Ther 1997, **4**, 891–900.

72. Clark PR, Hersh EM. Cationic lipid-mediated gene transfer-Current concepts. Curr Opin Mol Ther 1999, **1**, 158–76.

73. Rini BI, Selk LM, Vogelzang NJ. Phase I study of direct intralesional gene transfer of HLA-B7 into metastatic renal carcinoma lesions. Clin Cancer Res 1999, **5**, 2766–72.

74. Galanis E, Hersh EM, Stopeck AT, *et al*. Immunotherapy of advanced malignancy direct gene transfer of an interleukin-2 DNA/DMRIE/DOPE lipid complex: phase I/II experience. J Clin Oncol 1999, **17**, 3313–23.

75. Boussif O, Lezoualc'h F, Zanta MA, *et al*. A versatile vector for gene and oligonucleotide transfer into cells in culture and *in vivo*: polyethylenimine. Proc Natl Acad Sci, USA 1995, **92**, 7297–301.

76. Godbey WT, Wu KK, Mikos AG. Poly(ethylenimine) and its role in gene delivery. J controlled Release 1999, **60**, 149–60.

77. Goldman CK, Soroceanu L, Smith N, *et al*. *In vitro* and *in vivo* gene delivery mediated by a synthetic polycationic amino polymer. Nat Biotechnol 1997, **15**, 462–6.

78. Murphy JE, Uno T, Hamer JD, *et al*. A combinatorial approach to the discovery of efficient cationic peptoid reagents for gene delivery. Proc Natl Acad Sci, USA 1998, **95**, 1517–22.

79. Dash PR, Read ML, Barrett LB, Wolfert MA, Seymour LW. Factors affecting blood clearance and *in vivo* distribution of polyelectrolyte complexes for gene delivery. Gene Ther 1999, **6**, 643–50.

80. Oris M. Brunner S, Schuller S, *et al*. PEGylated DNA/transferrin-PEI complexes: reduced interaction with blood components, extended circulation in blood and potential for systemic gene delivery. Gene Ther 1999, **6**, 595–605.

81. Steiner MS, Zhang Y. Carraher J. Lu Y. *In vivo* expression of prostate-specific adenoviral vectors in a canine model. Cancer Gene Ther 1999, **6**, 456–64.

82. Martiniello-Wilks R, Garcia-Aragon J, Daja MM, *et al*. *In vivo* gene therapy for prostate cancer: preclinical evaluation of two different enzyme-directed prodrug therapy systems delivered by identical adenovirus vectors. Hum Gene Ther 1998, **9**, 1617–26.

83. Gotoh A, Ko SC, Shirakawa T, *et al*. Development of prostate-specific antigen promoter-based gene therapy for androgen-independent human prostate cancer. J Urol l998, **160**, 220–9.

84. Spitzweg C, Zhang S, Bergert ER, *et al*. Prostate-specific antigen (PSA) promoter-driven androgen-inducible expression of sodium iodide symporter in prostate cancer cell lines. Cancer Res 1999, **59**, 2136–41.

85. Spitzweg C, 0'Connor MK, Bergert ER, Tindall DJ, Young CY, Morris JC. Treatment of prostate cancer by radioiodine therapy after tissue-specific expression of the sodium iodide symporter. Cancer Res 2000, **60**, 6526–30.

86. Latham JP, Searle PF, Mautner V, James ND. Prostate-specific antigen promoter/enhancer driven gene therapy for prostate cancer: construction and testing of a tissue-specific adenovirus vector. Cancer Res 2000, **60**, 334–41.

87. Lee SE, Jin RJ, Lee SG, Yoon SJ, *et al*. Development of a new plasmid vector with PSA-promoter and enhancer expressing tissue-specificity in prostate carcinoma cell lines. Anticancer Res 2000, **20**, 417–22.

88. Koeneman KS, Kao C, Ko SC, *et al*. Osteocalcin-directed gene therapy for prostate-cancer bone metastasis. World J Urol 2000, **18**, 102–10.

89. Vile RG, Hart IR. Use of tissue-specific expression of the herpes simplex virus thyrrudine kinase gene to inhibit growth of established murine melanomas following direct intratumoral injection of DNA. Cancer Res 1993, **53**, 3860–4.

90. Vile RG, Hart IR. Targeting of cytokine gene expression to malignant melanoma cells using tissue specific promoter sequences. Ann Oncol 1994, **5** (suppl. 4), 59–65

91. Vile RG, Nelson JA, Castleden S, Chong H, Hart IR. Systemic gene therapy of immune melanoma using

tissue specific expression of the HSVtk gene involves an immune component. Cancer Res 1994, **54**, 6228–34.

92. Vile RG, Diaz RM, Miller N, Mitchell S, Tuszyanski A, Russell SJ. Tissue-specific gene expression from Mo-MLV retroviral vectors with hybrid LTRs containing the murine tyrosinase enhancer/promoter. Virology 1995, **214**, 307–13.

93. Cao G, Zhang X, He X, Chen Q, Qi Z. A safe, effective *in vivo* gene therapy for melanoma using tyrosinase promoter-driven cytosine deaminase gene. *In Vivo* 1999, **13**, 181–7.

94. Park BJ, Brown CK, Hu Y, *et al.* Augmentation of melanoma-specific gene expression using a tandem melanocyte-specific enhancer results in increased cytotoxicity of the purine nucleoside phosphorylase gene in melanoma. Hum Gene Ther 1999, **10**, 889–98.

95. McKie EA, Graham DI, Brown SM. Selective astrocytic transgene expression *in vitro* and *in vivo* from the GFAP promoter in a HSV RL1 null mutant vector—potential glioblastoma targeting. Gene Ther 1998, **5**, 440–50.

96. Vandier D, Rixe 0, Brenner M, Gouyette A, Besnard F. Selective killing of glioma cell lines using an astrocyte-specific expression of the herpes simplex virus-thymidine kinase gene. Cancer Res 1998, **58**, 4577–80.

97. Morelli AE, Larregina AT, Smith-Arica J, *et al.* Neuronal and glial cell type-specific promoters within adenovirus recombinants restrict the expression of the apoptosis-inducing molecule Fas ligand to predetermined brain cell types, and abolish peripheral liver toxicity. J Gen Virol 1999, **80**, 571–83.

98. Kurihara H, Zama A, Tamura M, Takeda J, Sasaki T, Takeuchi T. Glioma/glioblastoma-specific adenoviral gene expression using the nestin gene regulator. Gene Ther 2000, **7**, 686–93.

99. Miyao Y, Shimizu K, Moriuchi S, Yamada M, Nakahira K, Nakajima K, Nakao J, Kuriyama S, Tsujii T, Mikoshiba K. Selective expression of foreign genes in glioma cells: use of the mouse myelin basic protein gene promoter to direct toxic gene expression. J Neurosci Res 1993, **36**, 472–9.

100. Miyao Y, Shimizu K, Tamura M, *et al.* Usefulness of a mouse myelin basic protein promoter for gene therapy of malignant glioma: myelin basic protein promoter is strongly active in human malignant glioma cells. Jpn J Cancer Res 1997, **88**, 678–86.

101. Ko SC, Cheon J, Kao C, Gotoh A, *et al.* Osteocalcin promoter-based toxic gene therapy for the treatment of osteosarcoma in experimental models. Cancer Res 1996, **56**, 4614–19.

102. Cheon J, Ko SC, Gardner TA, *et al.* Chemogene therapy: osteocalcin promoter-based suicide gene therapy in combination with methotrexate in a murine osteosarcoma model. Cancer Gene Ther 1997, **4**, 359–65.

103. Shirakawa T, Ko SC, Gardner TA, *et al. In vivo* suppression of osteosarcoma pulmonary metastasis with intravenous osteocalcin promoter-based toxic gene therapy. Cancer Gene Ther 1998, **5**, 274–80.

104. Hafenrichter DG, Ponder KP, Rettinger SD, *et al.* Liver-directed gene therapy evaluation of liver specific promoter elements. J Surg Res 1994, **56**, 510–17.

105. Miyatake S, Iyer A, Martuza RL, Rabkin SD. Transcriptional targeting of herpes simplex virus for cell specific replication. J Virol 1997, **71**, 5124–32.

106. Miyatake SI, Tani S, Feigenbaum F, *et al.* Hepatoma-specific antitumor activity of an albumin enhancer/promoter regulated herpes simplex virus *in vivo*. Gene Ther 1999, **6**, 564–72.

107. Braiden V, Nagayama Y, Iitaka M, Namba H, Niwa M, Yamashita S. Retro virus-mediated suicide gene/prodrug therapy targeting thyroid carcinoma using a thyroid-specific promoter. Endocrinology 1998, **139**, 3996–9.

108. Nagayama Y, Nishihara E, Iitaka M, Namba H, Yamashita S, Niwa M. Enhanced efficacy of transcriptionally targeted suicide gene/prodrug therapy for thyroid carcinoma with the Cre-1oxP system. Cancer Res 1999, **59**, 3049–52.

109. Gu J, Kagawa S, Takakura M, *et al.* Tumor-specific transgene expression from the human telomerase reverse transcriptase promoter enables targeting of the therapeutic effects of the Bax gene to cancers. Cancer Res 2000, **60**, 5359–64.

110. Koga S, Hirohata S, Kondo Y, *et al.* A novel telomerase-specific gene therapy: gene transfer of caspase-8 utilizing the human telomerase catalytic subunit gene promoter. Hum Gene Ther 2000, **11**, 1397–406.

111. Lin CS, Chen ZP, Park T, Ghosh K, Leavitt J. Characterization of the human L-plastin gene promoter in normal and neoplastic cells. J Biol Chem 1993, **268**, 2793–801.

112. Chung I, Schwartz PE, Crystal RG, Pizzorno G, Leavitt J, Deisseroth AB. Use L-plastin promoter to develop an adenoviral system that confers transgene expression in ovarian cancer cells but not in normal mesothelial cells. Cancer Gene 1999, **6**, 99–106.

113. Katabi MM, Chan HL, Karp SE, Batist G. Hexokinase type II: a novel tumor-specific promoter for gene-targeted therapy differentially expressed and regulated in human cancer cells. Hum Gene Ther 1999, **10**, 155–64.

114. Ido A, Nakata K, Kato Y, *et al.* Gene therapy for hepatoma cells using a retrovirus vector carrying herpes simplex virus thymidine kinase gene under the control of human alpha-fetoprotein gene promoter. Cancer Res 1995, **55**, 3105–9.

115. Arbuthnot PB, Bralet MP, Le Jossic C, *et al. In vitro* and *in vivo* hepatoma cell-specific expression of a gene transferred with an adenoviral vector. Hum Gene Ther 1996, **7**, 1503–14.

116. Kaneko S, Hallenbeck P, Kotani T, *et al.* Adenovirus-mediated gene therapy of hepatocellular carcinoma using cancer-specific gene expression. Cancer Res 1995, **55**, 5283–7.

117. Kanai F, Shiratori Y, Yoshida Y, *et al.* Gene therapy for alpha-fetoprotein-producing human hepatoma cells by adenovirus-mediated transfer of the herpes simplex virus thymidine kinase gene. Hepatology 1996, **23**, 1359–68.

118. Kanai F, Lan KH, Shiratori Y, *et al. In vivo* gene therapy for alpha-fetoprotein-producing hepatocellular carcinoma by adenovirus-mediated transfer of cytosine deaminase gene. Cancer Res 1997, **57**, 461–5.

119. Su H, Chang JC, Xu SM, Kan YW. Selective killing of AFP-positive hepatocellular carcinoma cells by adeno-associated virus transfer of the herpes simplex virus thymidine kinase gene. Hum Gene Ther 1996, **7**, 463–70.

120. Su H, Lu R, Chang JC, Kan YW. Tissue-specific expression of herpes simplex virus thymidine kinase gene delivered by adeno-associated virus inhibits the growth of human hepatocellular carcinoma in athymic mice. Proc Natl Acad Sci, USA 1997, **94**, 13891–6.

121. Uto H, Ido A, Hori T, *et al*. Hepatoma-specific gene therapy through retrovirus-mediated and targeted gene transfer using an adenovirus carrying the ecotropic receptor gene. Biochem Biophys Res Commun 1999, **265**, 550–5.

122. Harri JD, Gutierrez AA, Hurst HC, Sikora K, Lemoine NR. Gene therapy for cancer using tumour-specific prodrug activation. Gene Ther 1994, **1**, 170–5.

123. Stackhouse MA, Buchsbaum DJ, Kancharia SR, *et al*. Specific membrane receptor gene expression targeted with radiolabeled peptide employing the erbB-2 and DF3 promoter elements in adenoviral vectors. Cancer Gene Ther 1999, **6**, 209–19.

124. Ring CJ, Blouin P, Martin LA, Hurst HC, Lemoine NR. Use of transcriptional regulatory elements of the MUC1 and ERBB2 genes to drive tumour-selective expression of a prodrug activating enzyme. Gene Ther 1997, **4**, 1045–52.

125. Chen L, Chen D, Manome Y, Dong Y, Fine HA, Kufe DW. Breast cancer selective gene expression and therapy mediated by recombinant adenoviruses containing the DF3/MUC1 promoter. J Clin Invest 1995, **96**, 2775–82.

126. Anderson LM, Swaminathan S, Zackon I, Tajuddin AK, Thimmapaya B, Weitzman SA. Adenovirus-mediated tissue-targeted expression of the HSVtk gene for the treatment of breast cancer. Gene Ther 1999, **6**, 854–64.

127. Brand K, Loser P, Arnold W, Bartels T, Strauss M. Tumor cell-specific transgene expression prevents liver toxicity of the adeno-HSVtk/GCV approach. Gene Ther 1998, **5**, 1363–71.

128. Kijima T, Osaki T, Nishino K, *et al*. Application of the Cre recombinase/loxP system further enhances antitumor effects in cell type-specific gene therapy against carcmoembryonic antigen-producing cancer. Cancer Res 1999, **59**, 4906–11.

129. Cao G, Kuriyama S, Gao J, *et al*. Effective and safe gene therapy for colorectal carcinoma using the cytosine deaminase gene directed by the carcinoembryonic antigen promoter. Gene Ther 1999, **6**, 83–90.

130. Dematteo RP, McClane SJ, Fisher K, *et al*. Engineering tissue-specific expression of a recombinant adenovirus: selective transgene transcription in the pancreas using the amylase promoter. J Surg Res 1997, **72**, 155–61.

131. Tanaka T, Kanai F, Okabe S, *et al*. Adenovirus-mediated prodrug gene therapy for carcinoembryonic antigen-producing human gastric carcinoma cells *in vitro*. Cancer Res 1996, **56**, 1341–5.

132. Tanaka T, Kanai F, Lan KH, *et al*. Adenovirus-mediated gene therapy of gastric carcinoma using cancer-specific gene expression *in vivo*. Biochem Biophys Res Commun 1997, **231**, 775–9.

133. Lan KH, Kanai F, Shiratori Y, *et al*. Tumor-specific gene expression in carcinoembryonic antigen-producing gastric cancer cells using adenovirus vectors. Gastroenterology 1996, **111**, 1241–51.

134. Lan KH, Kanai F, Shiratori Y, *et al*. *In vivo* selective gene expression and therapy mediated by adenoviral vectors for human carcinoembryonic antigen-producing gastric carcinoma. Cancer Res 1997, **57**, 4279–84.

135. Tai YT, Strobel T, Kufe D, Cannistra SA. *In vivo* cytotoxicity of ovarian cancer cells through tumor-selective expression of the BAX gene. Cancer Res 1999, **59**, 2121–6.

136. Robertson MW 3rd, Wang M, Siegal GP, *et al*. Use of a tissue-specific promoter for targeted expression of the herpes simplex virus thymidine kinase gene in cervical carcinoma cells. Cancer Gene Ther 1998, **5**, 331–6.

137. Osaki T, Tanio Y, Tachibana I, *et al*. Gene therapy for carcinoembryonic antigen-producing human lung cancer cells by cell type-specific expression of herpes simplex virus thymidine kinase gene. Cancer Res 1994, **54**, 5258–61.

138. Dachs GU, Patterson AV, Firth JD, *et al*. Targeting gene expression to hypoxic tumor cells. Nat Med 1997, **3**, 515–20.

139. Binley K, Iqball S, Kingsman A, Kingsman S, Naylor S. An adenoviral vector regulated by hypoxia for the treatment of ischaemic disease and cancer. Gene Ther 1999, **6**, 1721–7.

140. Walther W, Wendt J, Stein U. Employment of the mdr1 promoter for the chemotherapy-inducible expression of therapeutic genes in cancer gene therapy. Gene Ther 1997, **4**, 544–52.

141. Jaggar RT, Chan HY, Harris AL, Bicknell R. Endothelial cell-specific expression of tumor necrosis factor-alpha from the KDR or E-selectin promoters following retroviral delivery. Hum Gene Ther 1997, **8**, 2239–47.

142. Walton T, Wang JL, Ribas A, Barsky SH, Economou J, Nguyen M. Endothelium-specific expression of an E-selectin promoter recombinant adenoviral vector. Anticancer Res 1998, **18**, 1357–60.

143. Graulich W, Nettelbeck DM, Fischer D, Kissel T, Muller R. Cell type specificity of the human endoglin promoter. Gene 1999, **227**, 55–62.

144. Clackson T. Controlling mammalian gene expression with small molecules. Curr Opin Chem Biol 1998, **1**, 210–18.

145. Gossen M, Bujard H. Tight control of gene expression in mammalian cells by tetracycline-responsive promoters. Proc Natl Acad Sci, USA 1992, **89**, 5547–51.

146. Gossen M, Freundlieb S, Bender G, Muller G, Hillen W, Bujard H. Transcriptional activation by tetracyclines in mammalian cells. Science 1995, **268**, 1766–9.

147. Burcin MM, Schiedner G, Kochanek S, Tsai SY, O'Malley BW, Adenovirus-mediated regulable target gene expression *in vivo*. Proc Natl Acad Sci, USA 1999, **96**, 355–60.

148. No D, Yao TP, Evans RM. Ecdysone-inducible gene expression in mammalian cells and transgenic mice. Proc Natl Acad Sci, USA 1996, **93**, 3346–51.

149. Rivera VM, Clackson T, Natesan S, *et al.* A humanized system for pharmacologic control of gene expression. Nat Med 1996, **2**, 1028–32.

150. Weichselbaum RR, Hallahan D, Fuks Z, Kufe D. Radiation induction of immediate early genes: effectors of the radiation-stress response. Int J Radiat Oncol Biol Phys 1994, **30**, 229–34.

151. Hallahan DE, Mauceri HJ, Seung LP, *et al.* Spatial and temporal control of gene therapy using ionizing radiation. Nat Med 1995, **1**, 786–91.

152. Gerner EW, Hersh EM, Pennington M, *et al.* Heat-inducible vectors for use in gene therapy. Int J Hyperthermia 2000, **16**, 171–81.

153. Vekris A, Maurange C, Moonen C, *et al.* Control of transgene expression using local hyperthermia in combination with a heat-sensitive promoter. J Gene Med 2000, **2**, 89–96.

154. Nettelbeck DM, Jerome V, Muller R. Gene therapy: designer promoters for tumour targeting. Trends Genet 2000, **16**, 174–81.

155. Stein U, Walther W, Shoemaker RH. Vincristine induction of mutant and wild-type human multidrug-resistance promoters is cell-type-specific and dose-dependent. J Cancer Res Clin Oncol 1996, **122**, 275–82.

156. Ishikawa H, Nakata K, Mawatari F, *et al.* Utilization of variant-type of human alpha-fetoprotein promoter in gene therapy targeting for hepatocellular carcinoma. Gene Ther 1999, **6**, 465–70.

157. Richards CA, Austin EA, Huber BE. Transcriptional regulatory sequences of carcinoembryonic antigen: identification and use with cytosine deaminase for tumor-specific gene therapy. Hum Gene Ther 1995, **6**, 881–93.

158. Pang S, Dannull J, Kaboo R, *et al.* Identification of a positive regulatory element responsible for tissue-specific expression of prostate-specific antigen. Cancer Res 1997, **57**, 495–9.

159. Segawa T, Takebayashi H, Kakehi Y, Yoshida O, Narumiya S, Kakizuka A. Prostate-specific amplification of expanded polyglutamine expression: a novel approach for cancer gene therapy. Cancer Res 1998, **58**, 2282–7.

160. Vogelstein B, Fearon ER. Hamilton SR, *et al.* Genetic alterations during colorectal-tumor development. New Engl J Med 1988, **319**, 525–32.

161. Teich NM. Oncogenes and cancer. In: Introduction to the cellular and molecular biology of cancer, 2nd edn (ed. LM Franks and NM Teich). Oxford Medical Publications, Oxford, 1991, **230**–68.

162. Hanahan D, Folkman J. Patterns and emerging mechanisms of the angiogenic switch during tumorigenesis. Cell 1996, **86**, 353–64.

163. Hanahan D, Weinberg RA. The hallmarks of cancer. Cell 2000, **100**, 57–70.

164. Smyth MJ, Godfrey DI, Trapani JA. A fresh look at tumor immunosurveillance and immunotherapy. Nat Immunol 2001, **2**, 293–9.

165. Meyer T, Hart IR. Mechanisms of tumour metastasis. Eur J Cancer 1998, **34**, 214–21.

166. Skobe M, Hawighorst T, Jackson DG, *et al.* Induction of tumor lymphangiogenesis by VEGF-C promotes breast cancer metastasis. Nat Med 2001, **7**, 192–8.

167. Muller A, Homey B, Soto H. *et al.* Involvement of chemokine receptors in breast cancer metastasis. Nature 2001, **410**, 50–6.

168. Kaye SB. Multidrug resistance: clinical relevance in solid tumours and strategies for circumvention. Curr Opin Oncol 1998, **10** (suppl. 1), S15–19.

169. Morgan WF, Mumane JP. A role for genomic instability in cellular radioresistance? Cancer Metastasis Rev 1995, **14**, 49–58.

170. Lane DP. Cancer, p53, guardian of the genome. Nature 1992, **358**, 15–16.

171. Schwartz D, Rotter V. p53-dependent cell cycle control: response to genotoxic stress. Semin Cancer Biol 1998, **8**, 325–36.

172. Dameron KM, Volpert OV, Tainsky MA, Bouck N. Control of angiogenesis in fibroblasts by p53 regulation of thrombospondin-1. Science 1994, **265**, 1582–4.

173. Takahashi T, Nau MM, Chiba I, *et al.* p53: a frequent target for genetic abnormalities in lung cancer. Science 1989, **246**, 491–4.

174. Prosser J, Thompson AM, Cranston G, Evans HJ. Evidence that p53 behaves as a tumour suppressor gene in sporadic breast tumours. Oncogene 1990, **5**, 1573–9.

175. Baker SJ, Fearon ER, Nigro JM, *et al.* Chromosome 17 deletions and p53 gene mutations in colorectal carcinomas. Science 1989, **244**, 217–21.

176. Chi SG, deVere White RW, Meyers FJ, *et al.* p53 in prostate cancer: frequent expressed transition mutations. J Natl Cancer Inst 1994, **86**, 926–33.

177. Ruggeri B, Zhang SY, Caamano J, DiRado M, Flynn SD, Klein-Szanto AJ. Human pancreatic carcinomas and cell lines reveal frequent and multiple alterations in the p53 and Rb-1 tumour-suppressor genes. Oncogene 1992, **7**, 1503–11.

178. Sidransky D, Von Eschenbach A, Tsai YC, *et al.* Identification of p53 gene mutations in bladder cancers and urine samples. Science 1991, **252**, 706–9.

179. Hollstein MC, Metcalf RA, Welsh JA, Montesano R, Harris CC. Frequent mutation of the p53 gene in human esophageal cancer. Proc Natl Acad Sci, USA 1990, **87**, 9958–61.

180. Brachman DG, Graves D, Yokes E, *et al.* Occurrence of p53 gene deletions and human papilloma virus infection in human head and neck cancer. Cancer Res 1992, **52**, 4832–6.

181. Sidransky D, Mikkelsen T, Schwechheimer K, Rosenblum ML, Cavanee W, Vogelstein B. Clonal expansion of p53 mutant cells is associated with brain tumour progression. Nature 1992, **355**, 846–7.

182. Remvikos Y, Tominaga O, Hammel P, *et al.* Increased p53 protein content of colorectal tumours correlates with poor survival. Br J Cancer 1992, **66**, 758–64.

183. Thor AD, Moore DH II, Edgerton SM, *et al.* Accumulation of p53 tumour suppressor gene protein: an independent marker of prognosis in breast cancers. J Natl Cancer Inst 1992, **84**, 845–55.

184. Koch WM, Brennan JA, Zahurak M, *et al.* p53 mutation and locoregional treatment failure in head and neck squamous cell carcinoma. J Natl Cancer Inst 1996, **88**, 1580–6.

185. Grignon DJ, Caplan R, Sarkar FH, *et al.* p53 status and prognosis of locally advanced prostatic adenocarci-

noma: a study based on RTOG 8610. J Natl Cancer Inst 1997, **89**, 158–65.

186. Eskelinen MJ, Haglund UH. Prognosis of human pancreatic adenocarcinoma: review of clinical and histopathological variables and possible uses of new molecular methods. Eur J Surg 1999, **165**, 292–306.

187. Mitsudomi T, Hamajima N, Ogawa M, Takahashi T. Prognostic significance of p53 alterations in patients with non-small cell lung cancer: a meta-analysis. Clin Cancer Res 2000, **6**, 4055–63.

188. Overgaard J, Yilmaz M, Guldberg P, Hansen LL, Alsner J. TP53 mutation is an independent prognostic marker for poor outcome in both node-negative and node-positive breast cancer. Acta Oncol 2000, **39**, 327–33.

189. Zhang WW, Fang X, Mazur W, *et al.* High-efficiency gene transfer and high-level expression of wild-type p53 in human lung cancer cells mediated by recombinant adenovirus. Cancer Gene Ther 1994, **1**, 5–13.

190. Liu TJ, Zhang WW, Taylor DL, Roth JA, Goepfert H, Clayman GL. Growth Suppression of human head and neck cancer cells by the introduction of a wild-type p53 gene via a recombinant adenovirus. Cancer Res 1994, **54**, 3662–7.

191. Eastham JA, Hall SJ, Sehgal I, *et al. In vivo* gene therapy with p53 or p21 adenovirus for prostate cancer. Cancer Res 1995, **55**, 5151–5.

192. Badie B, Drazan KE, Kramar MH, Shaked A, Black KL. Adenovirus-mediated p53 gene delivery inhibits 9L glioma growth in rats. Neurol Res 1995, **17**, 209–16.

193. Clayman GL, el-Naggar AK, Roth JA, *et al. In vivo* molecular therapy with p53 adenovirus for microscopic residual head and neck squamous carcinoma. Cancer Res 1995, **55**, 1–6.

194. Kock H, Harris MP, Anderson SC *et al.* Adenovirus-mediated p53 gene transfer Suppresses growth of human glioblastoma cells *in vitro* and *in vivo*. Int J Cancer 1996, **67**, 808–15.

195. Spitz FR, Nguyen D, Skibber JM, Cusack J, Roth JA, Cristiano RJ. *In vivo* adenovirus-mediated p53 tumour suppressor gene therapy for colorectal cancer. Anticancer Res 1996, **16**, 3415–22.

196. Ko SC, Gotoh A, Thalmann GN, *et al.* Molecular therapy with recombinant p53 adenovirus in an androgen-independent, metastatic human prostate cancer model. Hum Gene Ther 1996, **7**, 1683–91.

197. Seth P, Katayose D, Li Z, *et al.* A recombinant adenovirus expressing wild type p53 induces apoptosis in drug-resistant human breast cancer cells: a gene therapy approach for drug-resistant cancers. Cancer Gene Ther 1997, **4**, 383–90.

198. Bouvet M, Bold RJ, Lee J, *et al.* Adenovirus-mediated wild-type p53 tumour suppressor gene therapy induces apoptosis and suppresses growth of human pancreatic cancer. Ann Surg Oncol 1998, **5**, 681–8.

199. Fujiwara T, Cai DW, Georges RN, *et al.* Therapeutic effect of a retroviral wild-type p53 expression vector in an orthotopic lung cancer model. J Natl Cancer Inst 1994, **86**, 1458–62.

200. Hwang RF, Gordon EM, Anderson WF, Parekh D. Gene therapy for primary and metastatic pancreatic cancer with intraperitoneal retroviral vector bearing the wild-type p53 gene. Surgery 1998, **124**, 143–50.

201. Zou Y, Zong G, Ling YH, *et al.* Effective treatment of early endobronchial cancer with regional administration of liposome–p53 complexes. J Natl Cancer Inst 1998, **90**, 1130–7.

202. Lesoon-Wood LA, Kim WH, Kleinman HK, Weintraub BD, Mixson AJ. Systemic gene therapy with p53 reduces growth and metastases of a malignant human breast cancer in nude mice. Hum Gene Ther 1995, **6**, 395–405.

203. Spitz FR, Nguyen D, Skibber JM, Meyn RE, Cristiano RJ, Roth JA. Adenoviral-mediated wild-type p53 gene expression sensitizes colorectal cancer cells to ionizing radiation. Clin Cancer Res 1996, **2**, 1665–71.

204. Pirollo KF, Hao Z, Rait A, *et al.* p53 mediated sensitization of squamous cell carcinoma of the head and neck to radiotherapy. Oncogene 1997, **14**, 1735–46.

205. Badie B, Kramar MH, Lau R, Boothman DA, Economou JS, Black KL. Adenovirus-mediated p53 gene delivery potentiates the radiation-induced growth inhibition of experimental brain tumours. J Neurooncol 1998, **37**, 217–22.

206. Xu L, Pirollo KF, Tang WH, Rait A, Chang EH. Transferrin-liposome-mediated systemic p53 gene therapy in combination with radiation results in regression of human head and neck cancer xenografts. Hum Gene Ther 1999, **101**, 2941–52.

207. Nguyen DM, Spitz FR, Yen N, *et al.* Gene therapy for lung cancer: enhancement of tumour suppression by a combination of sequential systemic cisplatin and adenovirus-mediated p53 gene transfer. J Thorac Cardiovasc Surg 1996, **112**, 1372.

208. Osaki S, Nakanishi Y, Takayama K, *et al.* Alteration of drug chemosensitivity caused by the adenovirus-mediated transfer of the wild-type p53 gene in human lung cancer cells. Cancer Gene Ther 2000, **7**, 300.

209. Ogawa N, Fujiwara T, Kagawa S, *et al.* Novel combination therapy for human colon cancer with adenovirus-mediated wild-type p53 gene transfer and DNA-damaging chemotherapeutic agent. Int J Cancer 1997, **73**, 367–70.

210. Miyake H, Hara I, Hara S, Arakawa S, Kamidono S. Synergistic chemosensitization and inhibition of tumour growth and metastasis by adenovirus-mediated P53 gene transfer in human bladder cancer model. Urology 2000, **56**, 332–6.

211. Roth JA, Nguyen D, Lawrence DD, *et al.* Retro virus-mediated wild-type p53 gene transfer to tumors of patients with lung cancer. Nat Med 1996, **2**, 985–91.

212. Tursz T, Cesne AL, Baldeyrou P, *et al.* Phase I study of a recombinant adenovirus-mediated gene transfer in lung cancer patients. J Natl Cancer Inst 1996, **88**, 1857–63.

213. Schuler M, Rochlitz C, Horowitz JA, *et al.* A phase I study of adenovirus-mediated wild-type p53 gene transfer in patients with advanced non-small cell lung cancer. Hum Gene Ther 1998, **9**, 2075–82.

214. Swisher SG, Roth JA, Nemunaitis J, *et al.* Adenovirus-mediated p53 gene transfer in advanced non-small-cell lung cancer. J Natl Cancer Inst 1999, **91**, 763–71.

215. Clayman GL, Frank DK, Bruso PA, Goepfert H. Adenovirus-mediated wild-type p53 gene transfer as a surgical adjuvant in advanced head and neck cancers. Clin Cancer Res 1999, **5**, 1715–22.

216. Weill D, Mack M, Roth J, *et al.* Adenoviral-mediated p53 gene transfer to non-small cell lung cancer through endobronchial injection. Chest 2000, **118**, 966–70.

217. Nurse P. Regulation of the eukaryotic cell cycle. Eur J Cancer 1997, **33**, 1002–4.

218. Kaelin WG Jr. Alterations in G1/S cell-cycle control contributing to carcinogenesis. Ann NY Acad Sci 1997, **833**, 29–33.

219. Masciullo V, Khalili K, Giordano A. The Rb family of cell cycle regulatory factors: clinical implications. Int J Oncol 2000, **17**, 897–902.

220. Vidal A, Koff A. Cell-cycle inhibitors: three families united by a common cause. Gene 2000, **247**, 1–15.

221. Liggett WH Jr, Sidransky D. Role of the pl6 tumor suppressor gene in cancer. J Clin Oncol 1998, **16**, 1197–206.

222. Tsihlias J, Kapusta L, Slingerland J. The prognostic significance of altered cyclin-dependent kinase inhibitors in human cancer. Annu Rev Med 1999 50, 401–23.

223. Sherr CJ. The Pezcoller lecture: cancer cell cycles revisited. Cancer Res 2000, **60**, 3689–95.

224. Caldas C, Hahn SA, da Costa LT, *et al.* Frequent somatic mutations and homozygous deletions of the pl6 (MTS1) gene in pancreatic adenocarcinoma. Nat Genet 1994, **8**, 27–32.

225. Xiao S, Li D, Corson JM, Vijg J, Fletcher JA. Codeletion of pl5 and pl6 genes in primary non-small cell lung carcinoma. Cancer Res 1995, **55**, 2968–71.

226. Orlow I, Lacombe L, Hannon GJ, *et al.* Deletion of the pl6 and pl5 genes in human bladder tumors. J Natl Cancer Inst 1995, **87**, 1524–9.

227. Barbareschi M, Caffo 0, Doglioni C, *et al.* p21WAFl immunohistochemical expression in breast carcinoma: correlations with clinicopathological data, oestrogen receptor status, MIB1 expression, p53 gene and protein alterations and relapse-free survival. Br J Cancer 1996, **74**, 208–15.

228. Xu HJ, Zhou Y, Seigne J, *et al.* Enhanced tumor suppressor gene therapy via replication-deficient adenovirus vectors expressing an N-terminal truncated retinoblastoma protein. Cancer Res 1996, **56**, 2245–9.

229. Riley DJ, Nikitin AY, Lee WH. Adenovirus-mediated retinoblastoma gene therapy suppresses spontaneous pituitary melanotroph tumors in Rb+/–mice. Nat Med 1996, **2**, 1316–21.

230. Nikitin AY, Juarez-Perez MI, Li S, *et al.* RB-mediated suppression of Spontaneous multiple neuroendocrine neoplasia and lung metastases in Rb+/– mice. Proc Natl Acad Sci, USA 1999, **96**, 3916–21.

231. Eastham JA, Hall SJ, Sehgal I, *et al. In vivo* gene therapy with p53 or p21 adenovirus for prostate cancer. Cancer Res 1995, **55**, 5151–5.

232. Joshi US, Dergham ST, Chen YQ, *et al.* Inhibition of pancreatic tumor cell growth in culture by p21WAFl recombinant adenovirus. Pancreas 1998, **16**, 107–13.

233. Joshi US, Chen YQ, Kalemkerian GP, Adil MR, Kraut M, Sarkar FH, *et al.* Inhibition of tumor cell growth by p21WAFl adenoviral gene transfer in lung cancer. Cancer Gene Ther 1998, **5**, 183–91.

234. Cardinali M, Jakus J, Shah S, Ensley JF, Robbins KC, Yeudall WA. p21(WAPl/Cip1) retards the growth of human squamous cell carcinomas *in vivo.* Oral Oncol 1998, **34**, 211–18.

235. Ramondetta L, Mills GB, Burke TW, Wolf JK. Adenovirus-mediated expression of p53 or p21 in a papillary serous endometrial carcinoma cell line (SPEC-2) results in both growth inhibition and apoptotic cell death: potential application of gene therapy to endometrial cancer. Clin Cancer Res 2000, **6**, 278–84.

236. Parker LP, Wolf JK, Price JE. Adeno viral-mediated gene therapy with Ad5CMVp53 and Ad5CMVp21 in combination with standard therapies in human breast cancer cell lines. Ann Clin Lab Sci 2000, **30**, 395–405.

237. Hall MC, Li Y, Pong RC, Ely B, Sagalowsky AI, Hsieh JT. The growth inhibitory effect of p21 adenovirus on human bladder cancer cells. J Urol 2000, **63**, 1033–8.

238. Craig C, Wersto R, Kim M, *et al.* A recombinant adenovirus expressing p27Kip1 induces cell cycle arrest and loss of cyclin-Cdk activity in human breast cancer cells. Oncogene 1997, **14**, 2283–9.

239. Naruse I, Hoshino H, Dobashi K, Minato K, Saito R, Mori M. Over-expression of p27kipl induces growth arrest and apoptosis mediated by changes of pRb expression in lung cancer cell lines. Int J Cancer 2000, **88**, 377–83.

240. Patel SD, Tran AC, Ge Y, *et al.* The p53-independent tumoricidal activity of an adenoviral vector encoding a p27-pl6 fusion tumor suppressor gene. Mol Ther 2000, **2**, 161–9.

241. Park K, Young Seol J, Yoo C, *et al.* Adenovirus expressing p27(Kipl) induces growth arrest of lung cancer cell lines and suppresses the growth of established lung cancer xenografts. Lung Cancer 2001, **31**, 149–55.

242. Jin X, Nguyen D, Zhang WW, Kyritsis AP, Roth JA. Cell cycle arrest and inhibition of tumor cell proliferation by the pl6INK4 gene mediated by an adenovirus vector. Cancer Res 1995, **55**, 3250–3.

243. Fueyo J, Gomez-Manzano C, Yung WK, *et al.* Adenovirus-mediated p16/CDKN2 gene transfer induces growth arrest and modifies the transformed phenotype of glioma cells. Oncogene 1996, **12**, 103–10.

244. Schrump DS, Chen GA, Consuli U, Jin X, Roth JA. Inhibition of esophageal cancer proliferation by adenovirally mediated delivery of pl6INK4. Cancer Gene Ther 1996, **3**, 357–64.

245. Lee JH, Lee CT, Yoo CG, *et al.* The inhibitory effect of adenovirus-mediated p16INK4a gene transfer on the proliferation of lung cancer cell line. Anticancer Res 1998, **18**, 3257–61.

246. Frizelle SP, Grim J, Zhou J, *et al.* Re-expression of pl6INK4a in mesothehoma cell results in cell cycle arrest, cell death, tumor suppression and tumor regression. Oncogene 1998, **16**, 3087–95.

247. Rocco JW, Li D, Liggett WH, *et al.* pl6INK4A adenovirus-mediated gene therapy for human head and neck squamous cell cancer. Clin Cancer Res 1998, **4**, 1697–704.

248. Kobayashi S, Shirasawa H, Sashiyama H, *et al.* Pl6INK4a expression adenovirus vector to suppress pancreas cancer cell proliferation. Clin Cancer Res 1999, **5**, 4182–5.

249. Wolf JK, Kirn TE, Fightmaster D, Bodurka D. Gershenson DM, Mills G, Wharton JT. Growth suppression of human ovarian cancer cell lines by the intro-

duction of a p16 gene via a recombinant adenovirus. Gynecol Oncol 1999, **73**, 27–34.

250. Kawabe S, Roth JA, Wilson DR, Meyn RE. Adenovirus-mediated p16INK4a gene expression radiosensitizes non-small cell lung cancer cells in a p53-dependent manner. Oncogene 2000, **19**, 5359–66.

251. Steiner MS, Zhang Y, Farooq F, *et al.* Adenoviral vector containing wild-type p16 suppresses prostate cancer growth and prolongs survival by inducing cell senescence. Cancer Gene Ther 2000, **7**, 360–72.

252. Steiner MS, Wang Y, Zhang Y, *et al.* p16/MTS1/INK4A suppresses prostate cancer by both pRb dependent and independent pathways. Oncogene 2000, **19**, 1297–306.

253. Yang CT, You L, Yeh CC, *et al.* Adenovirus-mediated p14(ARF) gene transfer in human mesothelioma cells. J Natl Cancer Inst 2000, **92**, 636–41.

254. Castilla LH, Couch FJ, Erdos MR, *et al.* Mutations in the BRCA1 gene in family history with early-onset breast and ovarian cancer. Nat Genet 1994, **8**, 387–91.

255. Tait DL, Obermiller PS, Redlin-Frazier S, *et al.* A phase I trial of retroviral BRCA1sv gene therapy in ovarian cancer. Clin Cancer Res 1997, **3**, 1959–68.

256. Tait DL, Obermiller PS, Hatmaker AR, Redlin-Frazier S, Holt JT. Ovarian cancer BRCA1 gene therapy: phase I and II trial differences in immune response and vector stability. Clin Cancer Res 1999, **5**, 1708–14.

257. Le XF, Vallian S, Mu ZM, Hung MC, Chang KS. Recombinant PML adenovirus suppresses growth and tumorigenicity of human breast cancer cells by inducing G1 cell cycle arrest and apoptosis. Oncogene 1998, **16**, 1839–49.

258. He D, Mu ZM, Le X, *et al.* Adenovirus-mediated expression of PML suppresses growth and tumorigenicity of prostate cancer cells. Cancer Res 1997, **57**, 1868–72.

259. Cheney IW, Johnson DE, Vaillancourt MT, *et al.* Suppression of tumorigenicity of glioblastoma cells by adenovirus-mediated MMAC1/PTEN gene transfer. Cancer Res 1998, **58**, 2331–4.

260. Sakurada A, Hamada H, Fukushige S, *et al.* Adenovirus-mediated delivery of the PTEN gene inhibits cell growth by induction of apoptosis in endometrial cancer. Int J Oncol 1999, **15**, 1069–74.

261. Minaguchi T, Mori T, Kanamori Y, *et al.* Growth suppression of human ovarian cancer cells by adenovirus-mediated transfer of the PTEN gene. Cancer Res 1999, **59**, 6063–7.

262. Plendt F. Animal models of antisense oligonucleotides: lessons for use in humans. Mol Med Today 1996, **2**, 250–7.

263. Jen KY, Gewirtz AM. Suppression of gene expression by targeted disruption of messenger RNA: available options and current strategies. Stem Cells 2000, **18**, 307–19.

264. Kitajima I, Unoki K, Maruyama I. Phosphorothioate oligodeoxynucleotide inhibits basic fibroblast growth factor-induced angiogenesis *in vitro* and *in vivo*. Antisense Nucl Acid Drug Deliv 1999, **9**, 233–9.

265. Jansen B, Wadi H, Inoue SA, *et al.* Phosphorothioate oligonucleotides reduce melanoma growth in a SCID-hu mouse model by a nonantisense mechanism. Antisense Dev 1995, **5**, 271–7.

266. Tortora G, Bianco R, Damiano V, *et al.* Oral antisense that targets protein kinase A cooperates with taxol and inhibits tumor growth, angiogenesis, and growth factor production. Clin Cancer Res 2000, **6**, 2506–12.

267. Vooldridge JE, Ballas Z, Krieg AM, Weiner GJ. Immunostimulatory of oligodeoxynucleotides containing CpG motifs enhance the efficacy of monoclonal antibody therapy of lymphoma. Blood 1997, **89**, 2994–8.

268. Camerini-Otero RD, Hsieh P. Parallel DNA triplexes, homologous recombination, and other homology-dependent DNA interactions. Cell 1993, **73**, 217–23.

269. Morishita R, Gibbons GH, Horiuchi M, *et al.* A gene therapy strategy using a transcription factor decoy of the E2F binding site inhibits smooth muscle proliferation *in vivo*. Proc Natl Acad Sci, USA 1995, **92**, 5855–9.

270. Mann MJ, Whittemore AD, Donaldson MC, *et al.* Ex-vivo gene therapy of human vascular bypass grafts with E2F decoy: the PREVENT single-centre, randomised, controlled trial. Lancet 1999, **354**, 1493–8.

271. Aoki K, Yoshida T, Sugimura T, Terada M. Liposome-mediated in vivo gene transfer of antisense K-ras construct inhibits pancreatic tumor dissemination in the murine peritoneal cavity. Cancer Res 1995, **55**, 3810–16.

272. Dean N, McKay R, Miraglia L, *et al.* Inhibition of growth of human tumor cell lines in nude mice by an antisense of oligonucleotide inhibitor of protein kinase C-alpha expression. Cancer Res 1996, **56**, 3499–507.

273. Balaji KC, Koul H, Mitra S, *et al.* Antiproliferative effects of c-myc antisense oligonucleotide in prostate cancer cells: a novel therapy in prostate cancer. Urology 1997, **50**, 1008–15.

274. Geiger T, Muller M, Monia BP, Fabbro D. Antitumor activity of a C-raf antisense oligonucleotide in combination with standard chemotherapeutic agents against various human tumors transplanted subcutaneously into nude mice. Clin Cancer Res 1997, **3**, 1179–85.

275. Steiner MS, Anthony CT, Lu Y, *et al.* Antisense c-myc retroviral vector suppresses established human prostate cancer. Hum Gene Ther 1998, **9**, 747–55.

276. Jansen B, Schlagbauer-Wadl H, Brown BD, *et al.* bcl-2 antisense therapy chemosensitizes human melanoma in SCID mice. Nat Med 1998, **4**, 232–4.

277. Gleave M, Tolcher A. Miyake H, *et al.* Progression to androgen independence is delayed by adjuvant treatment with antisense Bcl-2 oligodeoxynucleotides after castration in the LNCaP prostate tumor model. Clin Cancer Res 1999, **5**, 2891–8.

278. Miyake H, Tolcher A, Gleave ME. Chemosensitization and delayed androgen; independent recurrence of prostate cancer with the use of antisense Bcl-2 oligodeoxynucleotides. J Natl Cancer Inst 2000, **92**, 34–41.

279. Schlagbauer-Wadl H, Klosner G, Heere-Ress E, *et al.* Bcl-2 antisense oligonucleotides (G3139) inhibit Merkel cell carcinoma growth in SCID mice. Invest Dermatol 2000, **114**, 725–30.

280. Bishop MR, Iversen PL, Bayever E, *et al.* Phase I trial of an antisense oligonucleotide OL(1)p53 in hematologic malignancies. J Clin Oncol 1996, **14**, 1320–6.

281. Webb A, Cunningham D, Cotter F, *et al.* BCL-2 antisense therapy in patients with non-Hodgkin lymphoma. Lancet 1997, **349**, 1137–41.

282. Nemunaitis J, Holmlund JT, Kraynak M, *et al.* Phase I evaluation of ISIS 3521, an antisense oligodeoxynucleotide to protein kinase C-alpha, in patients with advanced cancer. J Clin Oncol 1999, **17**, 3586–95.

283. Stevenson JP, Yao KS, Gallagher M, *et al.* Phase I clinicaVpharmacokinetic and pharmacodynamic trial of the c-raf-1 antisense oligonucleotide ISIS 5132 (CGP 69846A). J Clin Oncol 1999, **17**, 2227–36.

284. O'Dwyer PJ, Stevenson JP, Gallagher M, *et al.* C-raf-1 depletion and tumor responses in patients treated with the c-raf-1 antisense oligodeoxynucleotide ISIS 5132 (CGP 69846A). Clin Cancer Res 1999, **5**, 3977–82.

285. Yuen AR, Halsey J, Fisher GA, *et al.* Phase I study of an antisense oligonucleotide to protein kinase C-alpha (ISIS 3521/CGP 64128A) in patients with cancer. Clin Cancer Res 1999, **5**, 3357–63.

286. Cunningham CC, Holmlund JT, Schiller JH, *et al.* A phase I trial of c-Raf kinase antisense oligonucleotide ISIS 5132 administered as a continuous intravenous infusion in patients with advanced cancer. Clin Cancer Res 2000, **6**, 1259–66.

287. Waters JS, Webb A, Cunningham D. *et al.* Phase I clinical and harmacokinetic study of bcl-2 antisense oligonucleotide therapy in patients with non-Hodgkin's lymphoma. J Clin Oncol 2000, **18**, 1812–23.

288. Chen HX, Marshall JL, Ness E, *et al.* A safety and pharmacokinetic study of a mixed-backbone oligonucleotide (GEM231) targeting the type I protein kinase A by two-hour infusions in patients with refractory solid tumors. Clin Cancer Res 2000, **6**, 1259–66.

289. Dorai T, Perlman H, Walsh K, *et al.* A recombinant defective adenoviral agent expressing anti-bcl-2 ribozyme promotes apoptosis of bcl-2-expressing human prostate cancer cells. Int J Cancer 1999, **82**, 846–52.

290. Scherr M, Maurer AB, Klein S, *et al.* Effective reversal of a transformed phenotype by retrovirus-mediated transfer of a ribozyme directed against mutant N-ras. Gene Ther 1998, **5**, 1227–34.

291. Czubayko F, Downing SG, Hsieh SS, *et al.* Adenovirus-mediated transduction of ribozymes abrogates HER-2/neu and pleiotrophin expression and inhibits tumor cell proliferation. Gene Ther 1997, **4**, 943–9.

292. Tsuchida T, Kijima H, Hori S, *et al.* Adenovirus-mediated anti-K-ras ribozyme induces apoptosis and growth suppression of human pancreatic carcinoma. Cancer Gene Ther 2000, **7**, 373–83.

293. Irie A, Anderegg B, Kashani-Sabet M, *et al.* Therapeutic efficacy of an adenovirus-mediated anti-H-ras ribozyme in experimental bladder cancer. Antisense Nucleic Acid Drug Dev 1999, **9**, 341–9.

294. Suzuki T, Anderegg B, OhkawaT, et al. Adenovirus-mediated ribozyme targeting of HER-2/neu inhibits in, vivo growth of breast cancer cells. Gene Ther 2000, **7**, 241–8.

295. Zhang Y, Nemunaitis J, Scanlon KJ, Tong AW. Antitumorigenic effect of a K-ras ribozyme against human lung cancer cell line heterotransplants in nude mice. Gene Ther 2000, **7**, 2041–50.

296. Eamshaw DJ, Gait MJ. Hairpin ribozyme cleavage catalyzed by aminoglycoside antibiotics and the polyamine spermine in the absence of metal ions. Nucl Acids Res 1998, **26**, 5551–61.

297. Springer CJ, Niculescu-Duvaz I. Prodrug-activating systems in suicide gene therapy. J Clin Invest 2000, **105**, 1161–7.

298. Connors TA. The choice of prodrugs for gene directed enzyme prodrug therapy of cancer. Gene Ther 1995, **2**, 702.

299. Moolten FL. Tumor chemosensitivity conferred by inserted herpes thymidine kinase genes: paradigm for a prospective cancer control strategy. Cancer Res 1986, **46**, 5276–81.

300. Mullen CA, Kilstrup M, Blaese RM. Transfer of the bacterial gene for cytosine deaminase to mammalian cells confers lethal sensitivity to 5-fluorocytosine: a negative selection system. Proc Natl Acad Sci, USA 1992, **89**, 33–7.

301. Knox RJ, Friedlos F, Sherwood RF, Melton RG, Aniezark GM. The bioactivation of 5-(aziridin-l-yl)-2,4-dinitrobenzamide (CB1954)–II. A comparison of an *Escherichia coli* nitroreductase and Walker DT diaphorase. Biochem Pharmacol 1992, **44**, 2297–301

302. Anlezark GM, Melton RG, Sherwood RF, Coles B, Friedlos F. Knox RJ. The bioactivation of 5-(aziridin-l-yl)-2,4-dinitrobenzamide (CB1954)–I. Purification and properties of a nitroreductase enzyme from *Escherichia coli*–a potential enzyme for antibody-directed enzyme prodrug therapy (ADEPT). Biochem Pharmacol 1992, **44**, 2289–95.

303. Mroz PJ, Moolten FL. Retrovirally transduced *Escherichia coli* gpt genes combine selectability with chemosensitivity capable of mediating tumor eradication. Hum Gene Ther 1993, **4**, 589–95.

304. Sorscher EJ, Peng S, Bebok Z, Allan PW, Bennett LL Jr, Parker WB. Tumor cell bystander killing in colonic carcinoma utilizing the *Escherichia coli* DeoD gene to generate toxic purines. Gene Ther 1994, **1**, 233–8.

305. Patterson AV, Zhang H, Moghaddam A, *et al.* Increased sensitivity to the prodrug 5'-deoxy-5-fluorouridine and modulation of 5-fluoro-2'-deoxyuridine sensitivity in MCF-7 cells transfected with thymidine phosphorylase. Br J Cancer 1995, **72**, 669–75.

306. Danks MK, Morton CL, Pawlik CA, Potter PM. Overexpression of a rabbit liver cirbixylesterase sensitizes human tumor cells to CPT-11. Cancer Res 1998, **58**, 20–2.

307. Aghi M, Kramm CM, Breakefield XO. Folylpolyglutarnyl synthetase gene transfer and glioma antifolate sensitivity in culture and *in vivo*. J Natl Cancer Inst 1999, **91**, 1233–41.

308. Hamstra DA, Rehemtulla A. Toward an enzyme/prodrug strategy for cancer gene therapy: endogenous activation of carboxypeptidase A mutants by the PACE/Furin family of propeptidases. Hum Gene Ther 1999, **10**, 235–48.

309. Marais R, Spooner RA, Light Y, Martin J, Springer CJ. Gene-directed enzyme prodrug therapy with a mustard prodrug/carboxypeptidase G2 combination. Cancer Res 1996, **56**, 4735–42.

310. Chen L, Waxman DJ. Intratumoral activation and enhanced chemotherapeutic effect of oxazaphosphorines following cytochrome P-450 gene transfer: development of a combined chemotherapy/cancer gene therapy strategy. Cancer Res 1995, **55**, 581–9.

311. Greco 0, Dachs GU. Gene directed enzyme/prodrug therapy of cancer: historical appraisal and future prospectives. J Cell Physiol 2001, **187**, 22–36.

312. Ram Z, Culver KW, Oshiro EM, *et al.* Therapy of malignant brain tumors by intratumoral implantation of retroviral vector-producing cells. Nat Med 1997, **3**, 1354–61.

313. Sterman DH, Treat J, Litzky LA, *et al.* Adenovirus-mediated herpes simplex virus thymidine kinase/ganciclovir gene therapy in patients with localized malignancy: results of a phase I clinical trial in malignant mesothelioma. Hum Gene Ther 1998, **9**, 1083–92.

314. Klatzmann D, Valery CA, Bensimon G, *et al.* A phase I/II study of herpes simpfex virus type 1 thymidine kinase 'suicide' gene therapy for recurrent glioblastoma. Study Group on Gene Therapy for Glioblastoma. Hum Gene Ther 1998, **9**, 2595–604.

315. Klatzmann D, Cherin P, Bensimon G, *et al.* A phase I/II dose-escalation study of herpes simplex virus type 1 thymidine kinase 'suicide' gene therapy for metastatic melanoma. Study Group on Gene Therapy of Metastatic Melanoma. Hum Gene Ther 1998, **9**, 2595–604.

316. Herman JR. Adier HL, Aguilar-Cordova E, *et al. In situ* gene therapy for adenocarcinoma of the prostate: a phase I clinical trial. Hum Gene Ther 1999, **10**, 1239–49.

317. Shand N, Weber F, Mariani L, *et al.* A phase 1–2 clinical trial of gene therapy for recurrent glioblastoma multiforme by tumor transduction with the herpes simplex thymidine kinase gene followed by ganciclovir. GLI328 European–Canadian Study Group. Hum Gene Ther 1999, **10**, 2325–35.

318. Pandha HS, Martin LA, Rigg A, *et al.* Genetic prodrug activation therapy for breast cancer: a phase I clinical trial of erbB-2-directed suicide gene expression. J Clin Oncol 1999, **17**, 2180–9.

319. Packer RJ, Raffel C, Villablanca JG, *et al.* Treatment of progressive or recurrent pediiaric malignant supratentorial brain tumors with herpes simplex virus thymidine kinase gene vector-producer cells followed by intravenous ganciclovir administration. J Neurosurg 2000, **92**, 249–54.

320. Trask TW, Trask RP, Aguilar-Cordova E, *et al.* Phase I study of adenoviral delivery of the HSV-tk gene and ganciclovir administration in patients with current malignant brain tumors. Mol Ther 2000, **1**, 195–203.

321. Hasenburg A, Tong XW, Rojas-Martinez A *et al.* Thymidine kinase gene therapy with concomitant topotecan chemotherapy for recurrent ovarian cancer. Cancer Gene Ther 2000, **7**, 839–4.

322. Sandmair AM, Loimas S, Puranen P, *et al.* Thymidine kinase gene therapy for human malignant glioma, using replication-deficient retroviruses or adenoviruses. Hum Gene Ther 2000, **11**, 2197–205.

323. Evan G, Littlewood T. A matter of life and cell death. Science 1998, **281**, 1317–22.

324. Sato T, Yamauchi N, Sasaki H, *et al.* An apoptosis-inducing gene therapy for pancreatic cancer with a combination of 55-kDa tumor necrosis factor (TNF) receptor gene transfection and mutein TNF administration. Cancer Res 1998, **58**, 1677–83.

325. Griffith TS, Anderson RD, Davidson BL, Williams RD, Ratliff TL. Adenoviral-mediated transfer of the TNF-related apoptosis-inducing ligand/Apo-2 ligand gene induces tumor cell apoptosis. J Immunol 2000, **165**, 2886–94.

326. Arai H, Gordon D, Nabel EG, Nabel GJ. Gene transfer of Fas ligand induces tumor regression *in vivo.* Proc Natl Acad Sci, USA 1997, **94**, 13862–7.

327. Hofmann A, Blau HM. Death of solid tumor cells induced by Fas ligand expressing primary myoblasts. Somat Cell Mol Genet 1997, **23**, 249–57.

328. Hedlund TE, Meech SJ, Srikanth S, Kraft AS, Miller GJ, Schaack JB, Duke RC. Adenovirus-mediated expression of Fas ligand induces apoptosis of human prostate cancer cells. Cell Death Differ 1999, **6**, 175–82.

329. Ambar BB, Frei K, Malipiero U, Morelli AE, Castro MG, Lowenstein PR, Fontana A. Treatment of experimental glioma by administration of adenoviral vectors expressing Fas ligand. Hum Gene Ther 1999, **10**, 1641–8.

330. Aoki K, Akyurek LM, San H, *et al.* Restricted expression of an adenoviral vector encoding Fas ligand (CD95L) enhances safety for cancer gene therapy. Mol Ther 2000, **1**, 555–65.

331. Hyer ML, Voelkel-Johnson C, Rubinchik S, Dong J, Norris JS. Intracellular Fas ligand expression causes Fas-mediated apoptosis in human prostate cancer cells resistant to monoclonal antibody-induced apoptosis. Mol Ther 2000, **2**, 348–58.

332. Pataer A, Fang B, Yu R, *et al.* Adenoviral Bak overexpression mediates caspase-dependent tumor killing. Cancer Res 2000, **60**, 788–92.

333. Shinoura N, Saito K, Yoshida Y, *et al.* Adenovirus-mediated transfer of bax with caspase-8 controlled by myelin basic protein promoter exerts an enhanced cytotoxic effect in gliomas. Cancer Gene Ther 2000, **7**, 739–48.

334. Li X, Marani M, Yu J, Nan B, *et al.* Adenovirus-mediated Bax overexpression for the induction of therapeutic apoptosis in prostate cancer. Cancer Res 2001m **61**, 186–91.

335. Yu JS, Sena-Esteves M, Paulus W, Breakefield XO, Reeves SA. Retroviral delivery and tetracycline-dependent expression of GL-lbeta-con verting enzyme (ICE) in glioma model provides controlled induction of apoptotic death in tumor cells. Cancer Res 1996, **56**, 5423–7.

336. Marcelli M, Cunningham GR, Walkup M, *et al.* Signaling pathway activated during apoptosis of the prostate cancer cell line LNCaP: overexpression of caspase-7 as a new gene therapy strategy for prostate cancer. Cancer Res 1999, **59**, 382–90.

337. Yamabe K, Shimizu S, Ito T, *et al.* Cancer gene therapy using a pro-apoptotic gene, caspase-3. Gene Ther 1999, **6**, 1952–9.

338. Shariat SF, Desai S, Song W, *et al.* Adenovirus-mediated transfer of inducible caspases: a novel 'death switch' gene therapeutic approach to prostate cancer. Cancer Res 2001, **61**, 2562–71.

339. Desai SB, Libutti SK. Tumor angiogenesis and endothelial cell modulatory factors. J Immunother 1999, **22**, 186–211.

340. Harris SR, Thorgeirsson UP. Tumor angiogenesis: biology and therapeutic prospects. *In Vivo* 1998, **12**, 563–70.

341. Bergers G, Javaherian K, Lo KM, *et al.* Effects of angiogenesis inhibitors on multistage carcinogenesis in mice. Science 1999, **284**, 808–12.

342. Modhch U, Pugh CW, Bicknell R. Increasing endothelial cell specific expression by the use of heterologous hypoxic and cytokine-inducible enhancers. Gene Ther 2000, **7**, 896–902.

343. O'Reilly MS, Holmgren L, Shing Y, *et al.* Angiostatin: a novel angiogenesis inhibitor that mediates the suppression of metastases by a Lewis lung carcinoma. Cell 1994, **79**, 315–28.

344. O'Reilly MS, Holmgren L, Chen C, Folkman J. Angiostatin induces and sustains dormancy of human primary tumors in mice. Nat Med 1996, **2**, 689–92.

345. O'Reilly MS, Boehm T, Shing Y, *et al.* Endostatin: an endogenous inhibitor of angiogenesis and tumor growth. Cell 1997, **88**, 277–85.

346. O'Reilly MS, Pirie-Shepherd S, Lane WS, Folkman J. Antiangiogenic activity of the cleaved conformation of the serpin antithrombin. Science 1999, **285**, 1926–8.

347. Sauter BV, Martinet 0, Zhang WJ, Mandeli J, Woo SL. Adenovirus-mediated gene transfer of endostatin *in vivo* results in high level of transgene expression and inhibition of tumor growth and metastases. Proc Natl Acad Sci, USA 2000, **97**, 4802–7.

348. Chen CT, Lin J, Li Q, *et al.* Antiangiogenic gene therapy for cancer via systemic administration of adenoviral vectors expressing secretable endostatin. Hum Gene Ther 2000, **11**, 1983–96.

349. Felddman AL, Restifo NP, Alexander HR, *et al.* Antiangiogenic gene therapy of cancer utilizing a recombinant adenovirus to elevate systemic endostatin levels in mice. Cancer Res 2000, **60**, 1503–6.

350. Tanaka T, Manome Y, Wen P, *et al.* Viral vector-mediated transduction of a modified platelet factor 4 cDNA inhibits angiogenesis and tumor growth. Nat Med 1997, **3**, 437–42.

351. Li H, Griscelli F, Lindenmeyer F, *et al.* Systemic delivery of antiangiogenic adenovirus AdmATF induces liver resistance to metastasis and prolongs survival of mice. Hum Gene Ther 1999, **10**, 3045–53.

352. Goldman CK, Kendall TL, Cabrera G, *et al.* Paracrine expression of a native soluble vascular endothelial growth factor receptor inhibits tumor growth, metastasis, and mortality rate. Proc Natl Acad Sci, USA 1998, **95**, 8795–800.

353. Lin P, Buxton JA, Acheson A, *et al.* Antiangiogenic gene therapy targeting the endothelium-specific receptor tyrosine kinase Tie2. Proc Natl Acad Sci, USA 1998, **95**, 8829–34.

354. Boyd M, Cunningham SH, Brown MM, Mairs RJ, Wheldon TE. Noradrenaline transporter gene transfer for radiation cell kill by 1311 meta-iodobenzylguanidine. Gene Ther 1999, **6**, 1147–52.

355. Cunningham S, Boyd M, Brown MM. *et al.* A gene therapy approach to enhance the targeted radiotherapy of neuroblastoma. Med Pediatr Oncol 2000, **35**, 708–11.

356. Spitzweg C, Harrington KJ, Pinke LA, Vile RG, Morris JC. The sodium iodide symporter and its potential role in cancer therapy. J Clin Endocrinol Metab, 2001, **86**, 3327–35.

357. Boland A, Ricard M, Opolon P, *et al.* Adenovirus-mediated transfer of the thyroid sodium/iodide symporter gene into tumors for a targeted radiotherapy. Cancer Res 2000, **60**, 3484–92.

358. Melief CJ, Toes RE, Medema JP, van der Burg SH, Ossendorp F, Offringa R. Strategies for immunotherapy of cancer. Adv Immunol 2000, **75**, 235–82.

359. Tepper RI, Mule JJ. Experimental and clinical studies of cytokine gene-modified tumor cells. Hum Gene Ther 1994, **5**, 153–64.

360. Dohring C, Angman L, Spagnoli G, Lanzavecchia A. T-helper- and accessory-cell-independent cytotoxic responses to human tumor cells transfected with a B7 retroviral vector. Int J Cancer 1994, **57**, 754–9.

361. Dalgleish A. The case for therapeutic vaccines. Melanoma Res 1996, **6**, 5–10.

362. Hall SJ, Sanford MA, Atkinson G, Chen SH. Induction of potent antitumor natural killer cell activity by herpes simplex virus-thymidine kinase and ganciclovir therapy in an orthotopic mouse model of prostate cancer. Cancer Res 1998, **58**, 3221–5.

363. Wei C, Willis RA, Tilton BR, *et al.* Tissue-specific expression of the human prostate-specific antigen gene in transgenic mice: implications for tolerance and immunotherapy. Proc Natl Acad Sci, USA 1997, **94**, 6369–74.

364. Nabel GJ, Gordon D, Bishop DK, *et al.* Immune response in human melanoma after transfer of an allogeneic class I major histocompatibility complex gene with DNA–liposome complexes. Proc Natl Acad Sci, USA 1996, **93**, 15388–93.

365. Rubin J, Galanis E, Pitot HC, *et al.* Phase I study of immunotherapy of hepatic metastases of colorectal carcinoma by direct gene transfer of an allogeneic histocompatibility antigen, HLA-B7. Gene Ther 1997, **4**, 419–25.

366. Hui KM, Ang PT, Huang L, Tay SK. Phase I study of immunotherapy of cutaneous metastases of human carcinoma using allogeneic and xenogeneic MHC DNA–liposome complexes. Gene Ther 1997, **4**, 783–90.

367. Gleich LL, Gluckman JL, Armstrong S, *et al.* Alloantigen gene therapy for squamous cell carcinoma of the head and neck: results of a phase-1 trial. Arch Otolaryngol Head Neck Surg 1998, **124**, 1097–104.

368. Nemunaitis J, Fong T, Robbins JM, *et al.* Phase I trial of interferon-gamma (IFN-gamma) retroviral vector administered intratumorally to patients with metastatic melanoma. Cancer Gene Ther 1999, **6**, 322–30.

369. Nemunaitis J, Fong T, Burrows F, *et al.* Phase I trial of interferon gamma retroviral vector administered intratumorally with multiple courses in patients with metastatic melanoma. Hum Gene Ther 1999, **10**, 1289–98.

370. Stewart AK, Lassam NJ, Quirt 1C, *et al.* Adenovector-mediated gene delivery of interleukin-2 in metastatic breast cancer and melanoma: results of a phase 1 clinical trial. Gene Ther 1999, **6**, 350–63.

371. Gilly FN, Beaujard A, Bienvenu J, *et al.* Gene therapy with Adv-IL-2 in unresectable digestive cancer: phase I–II study, intermediate report. Hepatogastroenterology 1999, **46** (suppl. 1), 1268–73.

372. Nemunaitis J, Bohart C, Fong T, et al. Phase I trial of retroviral vector-mediated interferon (IFN)-gamma gene transfer into autologous tumor cells in patients with metastatic melanoma. Cancer Gene Ther 1998, **5**, 292–300.

373. Sun Y, Jurgovsky K, Moller P, *et al.* Vaccination with IL-12 gene-modified autologous melanoma cells: preclinical results and a first clinical phase I study. Gene Ther l998, **5**, 481–90.

374. Sobol RE, Shawler DL, Carson C, *et al.* Interleukin 2 gene therapy of colorectal carcinoma with autologous irradiated tumor cells and genetically engineered fibroblasts: a phase I study. Clin Cancer Res 1999, **5**, 2359–65.

375. Rochlitz C, Jantscheff P, Bongartz G, *et al.* Gene therapy study of cytokine-transected xenogeneic cells (Vero-interleukin-2) in patients with metastatic solid tumors. Cancer Gene Ther 1999, **6**, 271–81.

376. Palmer K, Moore J, Everard M, et al. Gene therapy with autologous, interleukin secreting tumor cells in patients .with malignant melanoma. Hum Gene Ther 1999, **10**, 1261–8.

377. Arienti F, Belli F, Napolitano F, *et al.* Vaccination of melanoma patients with interleukin 4 gene-transduced allogeneic melanoma cells. Hum Gene Ther 1999, **10**, 2907–16.

378. Schmidt-Wolf IG, Finke S, Trojaneck B, *et al.* Phase I clinical study applying autologous immunological effector cells transfected with the interleukin-2 gene in patients with metastatic renal cancer, colorectal cancer and lymphoma. Br J Cancer 1999, **81**, 1009–16.

379. Chang AE, Li Q, Bishop DK, Normolle DP, Redman BD, Nickoloff BJ. Immunogenetic therapy of human melanoma utilizing autologous tumor cells transduced to secrete granulocyte–macrophage colony-stimulating factor. Hum Gene Ther 2000, **11**, 839–50.

380. Plautz GE, Miller DW, Bamett GH, *et al.* T cell adoptive immunotherapy of newly diagnosed gliomas. Clin Cancer Res 2000, **6**, 2209–18.

381. Jaffee EM, Hruban RH, Biedrzycki B, *et al.* Novel allogeneic granulocyte–macrophage colony-stimulating factor-secreting tumor vaccine for pancreatic cancer: a phase I trial of safety and immune activation. J Clin Oncol 2001, **19**, 145–56.

9

Targeted genetic prodrug activation therapy

Anne Rigg and Hardev S. Pandha

Introduction

Genetically modifying a cell so that it gains sensitivity to a particular agent resulting in cell death is an attractive anticancer strategy, especially if the therapy is able to distinguish between tumor and normal tissues. More than a decade ago, Moolton described this concept of genetic prodrug activation therapy (GPAT; otherwise known as VDEPT, GDEPT, or suicide gene therapy) (1). GPAT involves the transfer of a gene encoding a drug-metabolizing enzyme (suicide gene) into the target cell to be killed. A nontoxic prodrug is then administered systemically and is converted into the toxic agent in any cells producing the enzyme. There is now considerable preclinical data to provide proof of principle and early clinical trials are in progress for a variety of tumor types.

Enzyme–prodrug systems

Ideally, a non-mammalian enzyme would be utilized for this strategy to avoid possible production of the toxic agent at sites of endogenous enzyme expression. Examples of non-mammalian enzymes are cytosine deaminase and viral thymidine kinase (Table 9.1). Although, human cells contain thymidine kinase, human thymidine kinase has far less specificity for the prodrug ganciclovir than herpes simplex virus thymidine kinase (HSVtk) (2). HSVtk catalyses the conversion of ganciclovir to ganciclovir monophosphate, which is then phosphorylated to the toxic metabolite ganciclovir triphosphate by cellular enzymes. Ganciclovir triphosphate inhibits DNA polymerase and is therefore toxic to cells in the S phase of the cell cycle (3). As a result the HSVtk/ganciclovir system is only suitable where the target cells are proliferating. Cytosine deaminase is an enzyme produced by bacteria and fungi and has the ability to convert the antifungal agent 5-fluorocytosine into the anticancer agent 5-fluorouracil (5FU). 5FU inhibits thymidylate synthetase resulting in prevention of DNA synthesis. Although 5FU is a well acknowledged cytotoxic agent, only certain tumor types are sensitive such as breast and gastrointestinal carcinomas. Therefore, the use of cytosine deaminase/5-fluorocytosine is limited to these tumors.

Table 9.1 Enzyme–prodrug systems under investigation for genetic prodrug activation therapy

Enzyme	Prodrug	Cytotoxic product
HSV thymidine kinase	Ganciclovir	Ganciclovir triphosphate
Cytosine deaminase	5-Fluorocytosine	5-Fluorouracil
Varicella zoster virus thymidine kinase	6-Methoxypurine arabinoside	Adenine arabinonucleoside triphosphate
Nitroreductase	CB1954	5-Aziridinyl-4-hydroxylamino-2-nitrobenzamide
Cytochrome p450 2B1	Cyclophosphamide	Acrolein and phosphoramide mustard
Thymidine phosphorylase	5'-Deoxy-5-fluorouridine	5-Fluorouracil
Purine nucleoside phosphorylase	6-Methylpurine-deoxyriboside	6-Methylpurine
Alkaline phosphatase	Etoposide phosphate	Etoposide
Carboxypeptidase A	Methotrexate-alanine	Methotrexate
Carboxypeptidase G2	Benzoic acid mustard-glucuronide	Benzoic acid mustard
Linamerase	Amygdalin	Cyanide
Xanthine oxidase	Xanthine	Oxygen radicals
D-lactamase	Cephalosporin-mustard-carbamate	Nitrogen mustard

There is research investigating the use of mammalian drug-metabolizing enzymes such as the cytochrome p450 family of enzymes. It is possible that genetic modification of target cells with a mammalian enzyme gene would produce far greater enzyme levels than those produced by endogenous tissues so that much lower prodrug doses could be given. The cytochrome p450 2B gene has been transfected into glioblastoma cells *in vitro* and *in vivo* conferring sensitivity to cyclophosphamide (4, 5).

The bystander effect

Initially, it was thought that all cells would need to be transduced with the suicide gene to achieve significant cell killing on administration of the prodrug. However, it was subsequently found that a phenomenon called the 'bystander effect' occurred. Initial experiments suggested that, if HSVtk-positive and HSVtk-negative cells were grown together, in the presence of ganciclovir both cell populations were killed (1). Interestingly, it was shown that the bystander effect with HSVtk/ganciclovir only occurred if the cells were grown at high density, suggesting that the bystander effect is related to the close proximity of cells. Mice inoculated with HSVtk-positive cells and then treated with ganciclovir showed death of adjacent non-transduced cells (6). The growth of varying proportions of transduced and non-transduced cells together *in vitro* showed that only 10 per cent of cells needed to be HSVtk-positive to achieve significant cell death on the administration of ganciclovir (7). BALB/c mice inoculated with tumor cells, varying proportions of which had been transduced with HSVtk, underwent complete remission if 50 per cent or more of the tumor cells were HSVtk-positive (7). The bystander effect has also been described for the cytosine deaminase/5-fluorocytosine system. Only 2 per cent of tumor cells needed to be cytosine deaminase-positive to induce significant tumor regressions *in vivo* on administration of the 5-fluorocytosine (8).

Several theories have evolved to explain the bystander effect. It is clear that for the HSVtk/ganciclovir system the close proximity of cells is critical to the bystander effect. Ganciclovir triphosphate is unable to diffuse across a cell membrane. *In vitro* and *in vivo* studies show that the degree of bystander killing attained is directly proportional to the expression of the gap junction connexin proteins by a cell (9, 10). Therefore, it has been proposed that ganciclovir triphosphate passes between adjacent cells via gap junctions. Alternatively, 5FU is soluble and probably passes between cells in close proximity by diffusion (8). Another explanation for the bystander effect relies on the apoptotic cell death of transduced cells in the presence of the prodrug. As the cells are destroyed, apoptotic vesicles are formed in which the toxic metabolite is concentrated. Adjacent non-transduced cells then take up the apoptotic vesicles by phagocytosis and are exposed to the toxin, thereby inducing their own death (7).

In vivo, the bystander effect has been observed to cause hemorrhagic tumor necrosis (HTN) within 24 hours of inoculation of HSVtk[+] tumor cells and prodrug administration (11). Packaging cells producing recombinant virus to transduce HSVtk have been injected directly into murine glioblastomas and administered into the peritoneal cavities of mice with peritoneal tumors (12, 13). In both cases, HTN occurred in the center of the tumors. In the experiment with intraperitoneal tumors, the packaging cells producing HSVtk virus were not injected into the tumor itself. Therefore, the peripheral tumor cell death and bystander effect must have caused central HTN indirectly, perhaps by release of a soluble cytokine. Mice harboring intraperitoneal tumors had enhanced survival if, at a later date, HSVtk[+] tumor cells were inoculated and ganciclovir given (7). There is now strong evidence of an immunological component to the *in vivo* bystander effect. Mice inoculated with cytosine deaminase-positive tumor cells achieved a complete response on administration of 5-fluorocytosine. When the mice were re-challenged with the wild-type tumor cells there was protective immunity (14). It was postulated that this protective immunity could be due to better antigen presentation by dying tumor cells, with cytosine deaminase acting as a super-antigen, or successful GPAT destruction of the tumor, producing immunity in the same way as in a surgical resection. Vile *et al* demonstrated that the HSVtk/ganciclovir GPAT system significantly reduced melanoma pulmonary metastases in immunocompetent mice but not in immunodeficient mice (15). This suggested a requirement for an effective immune system to aid the bystander effect.

Targeting strategies

Clearly, it is important to endeavor to restrict suicide gene expression to the target cells only. This has been attempted in a variety of different ways. Most simply, the suicide gene can be injected intratumorally so that it is localized at a specific site. Alternatively, the delivery vector can be modified to enhance genetic modification of a specific cell population. These two approaches are relevant to all gene therapy strategies that aim to target specific cell types and are described elsewhere in more detail. In the context of GPAT two other targeting strategies have evolved to allow selective gene transfer and expression in the target cells, and not in normal cells.

Transductional targeting

The first strategy is known as transductional targeting and utilizes differences in proliferation rates between cell populations. Transductional targeting relies on the use of a retroviral vector as retroviruses only infect dividing cells. This makes retroviruses ideal to deliver a suicide gene to a malignant brain tumor that is rapidly proliferating against a background of quiescent neural tissue. Potentially ideal targets would be glioblastomas, which proliferate rapidly but tend not to metastasize, making therapies that instill local control imperative.

Retroviral vectors encoding the HSVtk gene have been produced. It has often been difficult to achieve high enough levels of retrovirus within the tumor and therefore vector producer cells (VPCs) have also been used. It is possible that if VPCs survive as xenografts within the tumor they will continue to release retroviral particles. There has been considerable preclinical data to demonstrate that the injection of retroviral producer cells releasing HSVtk-encoding retroviruses within a brain tumor leads to significant tumor kill on administration of ganciclovir (13, 16–18).

The first clinical trial investigating transductional GPAT was published in 1997 (19). Fifteen patients (with a total of 19 tumors between them) were recruited with recurrent progressive malignant glioma, or cerebral metastatic melanoma or breast carcinoma. Murine VPCs for a Moloney murine leukemia virus vector (replication-incompetent) containing the HSVtk gene were injected stereotactically into the malignant brain tumors. The computerized tomography (CT)-guided stereotactic injections were performed in tracts 3 to 6 mm apart to ensure that the VPCs were well distributed throughout the tumor. Thirteen patients received ganciclovir from days 7 to 21. The other two patients underwent a tumor resection on day 7 after VPC injection. The resection bed was infiltrated with further VPCs. Ganciclovir was then given starting 1 week later. Four patients received a second treatment. There was an objective response in five of the smaller tumors (3 had a partial response; 2 had a complete response). Toxicity was limited to neurological symptoms in two patients related to the intratumoral injection procedure or tumor biopsies. The retroviral vector could not be detected in the blood mononuclear cells. Ten patients had antibodies to the murine VPCs in the blood. In the two resected tumors, HSVtk mRNA could be detected in tumor cells. HSVtk-positive cells were mostly in columns around the injection tracts with little sign of spread. There was a suggestion of transduction of endothelial cells in areas of angiogenesis, probably because endothelial cells proliferate, unlike most neural cells. The results of the *in situ* hybridization for HSVtk mRNA indicated that the transduction rate was very low. Therefore, another mechanism must have been involved for those tumors that responded. The bystander effect may account for the tumor responses. It is also possible that there was a local immunological reaction against non-human cells resulting in an antitumor effect.

Recently, two other groups have published phase I clinical trial data using a similar strategy of VPCs producing HSVtk-encoding retroviruses. Klatzmann and co-workers treated 12 patients with solitary recurrent primary glioblastoma (20). Only patients with potentially resectable tumors were eligible. At the time of tumor resection, murine VPCs (M11 cells) were injected into the cavity walls. Patients received ganciclovir treatment from day 7 to 21 after surgery. There was some toxicity related to the surgical procedures performed including one patient who developed a subarachnoid hemorrhage and one with aseptic meningitis. One patient demonstrated HSVtk by polymerase chain reaction (PCR) of blood mononuclear cells 1 hour after VPC injection and subsequently was no longer positive. It was interesting that, for the six patients who had intracranial drains postoperatively, fluid from three of the drains contained VPCs and these VPCs could be established *in vitro* and retained sensitivity to ganciclovir. This suggested that the VPCs might be surviving long enough within the tumors to produce retroviruses. Other than toxicity, the major endpoint was lack of disease progression. Four patients had lack of progression by day 120. One patient is disease-free at 2.8 years. Three patients progressed, all with recurrent tumor at the resection margins. Median survival was 206 days. Due to the experimental design there were no post-gene-therapy biopsies so there were no tissues to analyze for suicide gene expression or evidence of cell death.

Children with progressive or recurrent brain tumors have been treated with HSVtk gene therapy in the context of a phase I clinical trial (21). The HSVtk gene was incorporated into the murine Moloney leukemia virus. Twelve children who had progressive solitary malignant brain tumors were recruited for the study. The patients underwent surgical tumor debulking, which was as extensive as possible. VPCs were then injected into the resection margins. There were three dose levels for the VPCs: 10^7 cells/ml; 5×10^7 cells/ml; and 10^8 cells/ml. Ganciclovir was administrated from days 14 to 28.

Only four children experienced transient side-effects that the authors felt were attributable to the gene therapy. There were three episodes of seizures and one of raised intracranial pressure that may have been related to the recent surgery. Three of the four children developed these side-effects during the fortnight of ganciclovir, and only one prior to the commencement of the prodrug. Toxicity was not related to the dose of the VPCs given and no maximum tolerated dose was identified. Of five patients who had a tumor biopsy at a later date, one had a biopsy that was positive for vector DNA by PCR. This positive result occurred 6 months after the administration of the VPCs. As the tumors were resected prior to the administration of suicide gene therapy, radiological assessment was not particularly helpful. One child is still disease-free after 2 years. Of the other 11 children, one was not included in the evaluation as he received focal radiotherapy shortly after the VPC injections. All the remaining 10 children had progressive disease at a median time of 5 months.

These three phase I clinical trials of transductional targeting of GPAT have illustrated that toxicity is low and that the retroviral vectors are safe. There is no evidence of retroviruses regaining replication competency in any of these studies. However, these trials have provided little information on the efficiency of gene transfer. Although there is good proof of the principle of transductional GPAT in animal models, this has yet to be demonstrated in a clinical trial. This is a recurring problem for clinical trials of suicide gene therapy as it is difficult to justify repeated biopsies of the tumor in patients who are already unwell and have undergone multiple interventions.

Transcriptional targeting

The other GPAT targeting strategy is referred to as transcriptional targeting. This approach exploits differences in gene expression by target cells and other cells. An example of this is the expression of a tumor-specific oncogene that is not found in benign cells. As a result the appropriate transcriptional regulatory elements, such as the oncogene promoter and enhancers, can be used to construct a chimeric suicide gene under the control of the tumor-specific gene promoter. If the chimeric construct is inserted into a tumor cell expressing that oncogene and the prodrug given, cell death results. If the chimeric construct is inserted into benign cells, in the presence of the prodrug no toxin is produced (Fig. 9.1and Table 9.2). A variation on the theme is the use of tissue-specific transcriptional regulatory elements to distinguish between cell populations. Considerable *in vitro* and *in vivo* work has demonstrated that suicide genes can be engineered to be under the control of a tumor- or a tissue-specific promoter. When target cells are transfected with the chimeric suicide gene construct and the prodrug given, cell death results. The carcinoembryonic antigen (CEA) promoter element has been used to target suicide gene expression to CEA-positive gastric carcinoma cells (22). Likewise, the transcriptional regulatory elements of MUC1 and ERBB2 genes, which are overexpressed in some breast cancers, can reliably target prodrug activation to the MUC1- and ERBB2-positive cells only (23). Tissue-specific transcriptional regulatory elements are useful when a tumor arises from a particular type of cell. Hence, the tyrosinase promoter can target reporter gene and suicide gene expression to melanoma cells *in vitro* and in animal models (24).

To date, only one clinical trial of transcriptional targeting of GPAT has been conducted. In this phase I study the *Escherichia coli* cytosine deaminase (CDase) gene was placed under the control of the ERBB2 promoter in an expression plasmid vector (25). Twelve women with cutaneous metastatic ERBB2-positive breast cancer were recruited. Three cutaneous metastases were chosen as the treatment, placebo, and no-injection lesions, respectively. On day 1 the treatment lesion received an intratumoral injection of the plasmid encoding the CDase suicide gene. The placebo lesion was injected with an empty plasmid and the third lesion was left untreated. On day 2 the skin lesions were biopsied. The patients then received a 48-hour infusion of the prodrug 5-fluorocytosine. A second biopsy was performed on day 7. There was a dose escalation of the plasmid DNA with four patients treated at each dose level before proceeding to the next dose level. The doses of plasmid DNA ranged from 50 to 400 μg. No toxicity was identified clinically or serologically. No maximum tolerated dose of plasmid DNA was identified. Seventy-five per cent of the patients had evidence of CDase in day 2 biopsies and 25 per cent in day 7 biopsies as assessed by immunohistochemistry. In all cases the CDase immunoreactivity was limited to ERBB2-positive tumor cells. Intralesional CDase could also be detected by *in situ* hybridization in four patients. In three patients, conversion of 5-fluorocytosine to 5FU could be demonstrated by thin-layer chromatography. This study

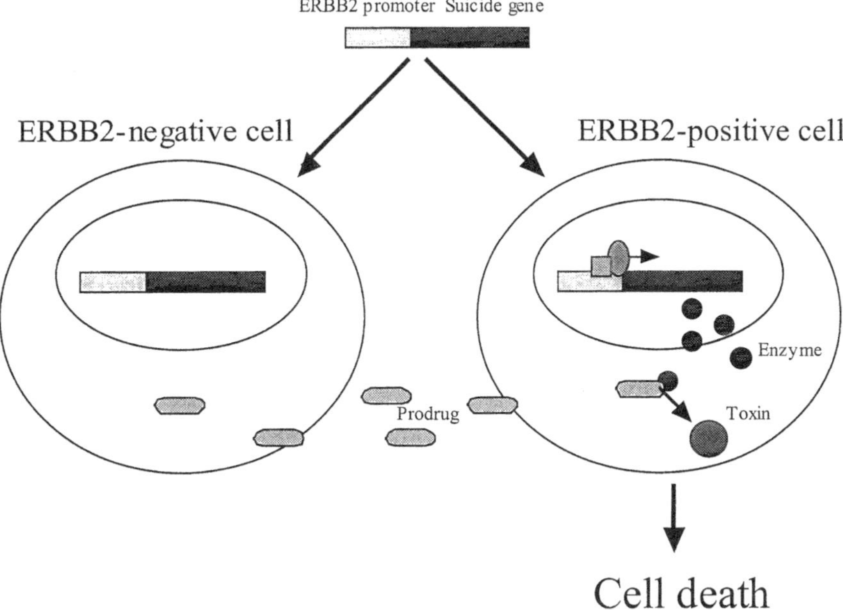

Fig. 9.1 Tumor-specific targeting of a suicide gene to a tumor cell that is ERBB2-positive by the creation of a chimeric construct whereby the suicide gene is under the control of the ERBB2 promoter element.

Table 9.2 Transcriptional regulatory elements under development for genetic prodrug activation therapy

Transcriptional regulatory elements	
Tumor-specific	Tissue-specific (tissue)
α-Fetoprotein	Albumin promoter element (liver)
Carcinoembryonic antigen	Tyrosinase (melanin-producing cells)
ERBB2	Tyrosinase-related protein 1 (melanin-producing cells)
ERBB3	MUC1 (simple ductal epithelium)
ERBB4	Prostate-specific antigen (prostate epithelium)

did investigate gene transfer and find evidence of CDase mRNA, and functional protein, although the number of patients studied was small. Given that plasmid DNA is not readily taken up into cells it was surprising to see targeted gene expression so clearly.

Clinical trials of non-targeted genetic prodrug activation therapy

Several other clinical trials have also been performed using GPAT, although specific targeting was not used. The efficacy of HSVtk gene transfer into donor lymphocytes has been evaluated (26, 27). Donor lymphocytes are often used after an allogeneic bone marrow transplant to promote a graft-versus-leukemia effect and boost immune recognition. However, a severe graft-versus-host reaction can occur. If the donor lymphocytes are transduced with HSVtk *ex vivo* then, if graft-versus-host disease (GVHD) occurs, ganciclovir can be given and the donor lymphocytes are selectively destroyed. A retroviral vector was developed that encoded the HSVtk gene. Eight patients with relapsed leukemia or an Epstein–Barr virus (EBV)-induced lymphoma after a T-cell depleted allograft were treated with these HSVtk-transduced donor lymphocytes. Modified donor lymphocytes could be demonstrated in the peripheral blood, the bone marrow, and tissues experiencing GVHD by PCR for up to 12 months. Five of the patients developed a graft-versus-leukemia effect with three complete responses. Two patients developed acute GVHD and were treated with ganciclovir. Both had a complete resolution of the GVHD with ganciclovir and remained in complete clinical remission. A third patient developed chronic skin GVHD and was treated with ganciclovir. A significant reduction of HSVtk-positive lymphocytes was achieved, although they could not be completely eliminated. It is possible that, as ganciclovir is active against proliferating cells, chronic GVHD may be less responsive to this approach. Another difficulty with the study was that two patients demonstrated a strong immune response against the genetically modified cells, which was thought to be due to the presence of the neomycin-resistance gene. Therefore, in a follow-up to the first study, the researchers have developed new retroviral vectors that do not contain the neomycin-resistance gene and are able to confer higher ganciclovir sensitivity to transduced cells. These new retroviral HSVtk vectors have not as yet been tested on human subjects.

Conclusions

Almost 15 years since the first description of genetic prodrug activation therapy, clinical trials are now underway to investigate the uses of this therapy for the treatment of human cancers. While preclinical studies have clearly demonstrated that targeting of GPAT is efficient and efficacious, the clinical data are not so convincing. As the trials described show, there are ethical constraints as to the type of patient that can be recruited. Patients have to have progressive tumors that have failed to respond to other treatments and often repeated biopsies that might have shown gene expression are not possible as the level of intervention is unacceptably high. There are advances in the field of real-time imaging of tumor metabolism that provide an alternative, non-invasive way of monitoring tumor responses to GPAT. Combinations of positron emission tomography (PET) tracers have been successfully used to monitor HSVtk/ganciclovir gene therapy *in vitro* and in rats bearing intracerebral tumors (28, 29).

Another limitation relates to the gene therapy delivery vectors currently available. More effective gene transfer would obviously aid GPAT suicide gene expression and many groups are now working on both viral and nonviral vectors to enhance delivery.

It would be unfair to dismiss GPAT for the treatment of human tumors as no large trials have been conducted and, traditionally, efficacy is not an end point of phase I studies. There are a number of interesting preclinical experiments that suggest that, when suicide gene therapy is given in conjunction with another modality of treatment, there is an additive therapeutic effect. Suicide genes have been combined with cytokine genes. Mullen and co-workers transduced a poorly immunogenic tumor cell line with the genes for CDase and interleukin-6 (IL-6). Mice already bearing the wild-type tumor had prolonged survival and in some cases cure when the transduced cells were given in the form of a vaccine compared to cells transduced with IL-6 alone (30). No prodrug had to be given for this effect and this emphasizes that the transfer of suicide genes is not an immunologically neutral event. Another group demonstrated that HSVtk gene therapy with IL-2 gene vaccine was more effective for hepatic metastases of a colorectal cancer than either treatment alone (31). Another approach relates to the use of 5FU as a radiosensitizing agent. Human squamous cancers were established as xenografts in immunodeficient mice. Adenoviruses were used to transduce the xenograft tumors with the CDase gene. The mice then received intraperitoneal 5-fluorocytosine and ionizing radiation to the tumors. Combination GPAT and radiation was more successful in terms of response and survival than either treatment alone (32). While current conventional anticancer treatment relies on chemotherapy, radiotherapy, and surgery, it is probable that suicide gene therapy will become an integral part of anticancer regimens for the future in combination with already existing options.

References

1. Moolton F. Tumor chemosensitivity conferred by inserted herpes thymidine kinase genes: paradigm for a prospective cancer control strategy. Cancer Res 1986, 46, 5276–81.
2. Roizman B, Sears AE. Herpes simplex viruses and their replication. In: Fields's virology (ed. BN Fields, DM Knipe, and PM Howley). Lippincott–Raven, New York, 1996, 2231–95.
3. Mar EC, Chiou JF, Cheng YC, Huang ES. Inhibition of cellular DNA polymerase α and human cytomegalovirus-induced DNA polymerase by the triphosphates of 9-(2-hydroxyethoxymethyl)guanine and 9-(1,3-dihydroxy-2-propoxymethyl)guanine. J Virol 1985, 53, 776–80.
4. Chang TKH, Weber GF, Crespi CL, Waxman DJ. Differential activation of cyclophosphamide and ifosphamide by cytochrome P-450 2B and 3A in human liver microsomes. Cancer Res 1993, 53, 5629–37.
5. Chen L, Waxman DJ. Intratumoral activation and enhanced chemotherapeutic effect of oxazaphosporine following chemotherapy/cancer gene therapy strategy. Cancer Res 1995, 55, 581–9.

6. Freeman SM, Whartenby KA, Koeplin DS, Moolten FA, Abboud CN, Abraham GN. Tumor regression when a fraction of tumor mass contains the HSV-TK gene. J Cell Biochem 1992, **16** (suppl.), 47.

7. Freeman SM, Abboud CN, Whartenby KA, Packman CH, Koeplin DS, Moolton FS, Abraham GN. The 'bystander effect': tumor regression when a fraction of the tumor mass is genetically modified. Cancer Res 1993, **53**, 5274–83.

8. Huber BE, Austin EA, Richards CA, Davis ST, Good SS. Metabolism of 5-fluorocytosine to 5-fluorouracil in human colorectal tumor cells transduced with the cytosine deaminase gene: significant antitumor effects when only a small percentage of tumor cells express cytosine deaminase. Proc Natl Acad Sci, USA 1994, **91**, 8302–6.

9. Dilber MS, Abedi MR, Christensson B, Bjorkstrand B, Kidder GM, Naus CCG, Gahrton G, Smith CIE. Gap junctions promote the bystander effect of herpes simplex thymidine kinase *in vivo*. Cancer Res 1997, **57**, 1523–8.

10. Yang L, Chiang Y, Lenz HJ, Danenberg KD, Spears CP, Gordon EM, Anderson WF, Parekh D. Intracellular communication mediates the bystander effect during herpes simplex thymidine kinase/ganciclovir-based gene therapy of human gastrointestinal tumor cells. Hum Gene Ther 1998, **9**, 719–28.

11. Freeman SM, McCune C, Robinson W, Abboud CN, Abraham GN, Angel C, Marrogi A. Treatment of ovarian cancer using a gene-modified vaccine. Hum Gene Ther 1995, **6**, 927–39.

12. Freeman SM, Ramesh R, Shastri M, Munshi A, Jensen AK, Marrogi AJ. The role of cytokines in mediating the bystander effect using HSV-TK xenogenic cells. Cancer Lett 1995, **92**, 167–74.

13. Ram Z, Walbridge S, Shawker T, Culver KW, Blaese RM, Oldfield EH. The effect of thymidine kinase transduction and ganciclovir therapy on tumor vasculature and growth of 9L gliomas in rats. J Neurosurg 1994, **81**, 256–60.

14. Mullen CA, Coale MM, Lowe R, Blaese RM. Tumors expressing the cytosine deaminase suicide gene can be eliminated *in vivo* with 5-fluorocytosine and induce protective immunity to wild type tumor. Cancer Res 1994, **54**, 1503–6.

15. Vile RG, Nelson JA, Castleden S, Chong H, Hart IR. Systemic gene therapy of murine melanoma using tissue specific expression of the HSVtk gene involves an immune component. Cancer Res 1994, **54**, 6228–34.

16. Barba D, Hardin J, Ray J, Gage FH. Thymidine kinase-mediated killing of rat brain tumours. J. Neurosurg 1993, **79**, 729–35.

17. Culver KM, Ram Z, Wallbridge S, Ishii H, Oldfield E, Blaese R. *In vivo* gene transfer with retroviral vector-producer cells for treatment of experimental brain tumours. Science 1992, **256**, 1550–2.

18. Ezzeddine Z, Martuza R, Platika D, Short M, Malick M, Choi A, Breakefield X. Selective killing of glioma cells in culture and *in vivo* by retrovirus transfer of the herpes simplex thymidine kinase gene. New Biol 1991, **3**, 608–14.

19. Ram Z, Culver KW, Oshiro EM, Viola JJ, DeVroom HL, Otto E, Long Z, Chiang Y, McGarrity GJ, Muul LM., Blaese RM., Oldfield EH. Therapy of malignant brain tumors by intratumoral implantation of vector-producing cells. Nat Med 1997, **3**, 1354–61.

20. Klatzmann D, Valery CA, Bensimon G, Marro B, Boyer O, Mokhtari K, Diquet B, Salzmann JL, Philippon J. A phase I/II study of herpes simplex virus type I thymidine kinase 'suicide' gene therapy for recurrent glioblastoma. Hum Gene Ther 1998, **9**, 2595–604.

21. Packer RJ, Raffel C, Villablanca JG, Tonn JC, Burdach SE, Burger K, LaFond D, McComb G, Cogen PH, Vezina G, Kapcala LP. Treatment of progressive or recurrent pediatric malignant supratentorial brain tumors with herpes simplex virus thymidine kinase gene vector-producer cells followed by intravenous ganciclovir administration. J Neurosurg 2000, **92**, 249–54.

22. Tanaka T, Kanai F, Okabe S, Yoshida Y, Wakimoto H, Hamada H, Shiratori Y, Lan KH, Ishitobi M, Omata M. Adenovirus-mediated prodrug gene therapy for carcinoembryonic antigen-producing human gastric carcinoma cells *in vitro*. Cancer Res 1996, **56**, 1341–5.

23. Ring CJA, Blouin P, Martin LA, Hurst HC, Lemoine NR. Use of transcriptional regulatory elements of the MUC1 and ERBB2 genes to drive tumour-selective expression of a prodrug activating enzyme. Gene Ther 1997, **4**, 1045–52.

24. Vile RG, Hart IR. *In vitro* and *in vivo* targeting of gene expression to melanoma cells. Cancer Res 1993, **53**, 962–7.

25. Pandha HS, Martin LA, Rigg A, Hurst HC, Stamp GWH, Sikora K, Lemoine NR. Genetic prodrug activation therapy for breast cancer: a phase I clinical trial of erbB-2-directed suicide gene expression. J Clin Oncol, 1999, **17**, 2180–9.

26. Bonini C, Ferrari G, Verzeletti S, Servida P, Zappone E, Ruggieri L, Ponzoni M, Rossini S, Mavilio F, Traversari C, Bordignon C. HSV-TK gene transfer into donor lymphocytes for control of allogeneic graft-versus-leukemia. Science 1997, **276**, 1719–24.

27. Verzeletti S, Bonini C, Marktel S, Nobili N, Ciceri F, Traversari C, Bordignon C. Herpes simplex virus thymidine kinase gene transfer for controlled graft-versus-host disease and graft-versus-leukemia: clinical follow-up and improved new vectors. Hum Gene Ther 1998, **9**, 2243–51.

28. Haberkorn U, Altmann A, Morr I, Germann C, Oberdorfer F, van Kaick G. Multitracer studies during gene therapy of hepatoma cells with herpes simplex virus thymidine kinase and ganciclovir. J Nucl Med 1997, **38**, 1048–54.

29. Tjuvajev JG, Stockhammer G, Desai R, Uehara H, Watanabe K, Gansbacher B, Blasberg RG. Imaging the expression of transfected genes *in vivo*. Cancer Res 1995, **55**, 6126–32.

30. Mullen CA, Petropoulos D, Lowe RM. Treatment of microscopic pulmonary metastases with recombinant autologous tumor vaccine expressing Interleukin 6 and *Escherichia coli* cytosine deaminase suicide genes. Cancer Res 1996, **56**, 1361–6.

31. Chen SH, Kosai K, Xu B, Pham-Nguyen K, Contant C, Finegold MJ, Woo SLC. Combination suicide and cytokine gene therapy for hepatic metastases of colon carcinoma: sustained antitumor immunity prolongs animal survival. Cancer Res 1996, **56**, 3758–62.

32. Hanna NN, Mauceri HJ, Wayne JD, Hallahan DE, Kufe DW, Weichselbaum RR. Virally directed cytosine deaminase/5-fluorocytosine gene therapy enhances radiation response in human cancer xenografts. Cancer Res 1997, **57**, 4205–9.

10 | *Antisense therapy as a targeted modality*

Justin Waters and David Cunningham

Introduction

Remarkable progress has been made over the course of the last 2 decades in elucidating the molecular basis of carcinogenesis. Many genes involved in this process have been characterized, and have naturally aroused interest as potential therapeutic targets. Oligonucleotide-based strategies exploit the sequence-specificity of the interaction between complementary deoxyribonucleic acid (DNA) and ribonucleic acid (RNA) molecules to inhibit the function of a particular gene. Although conceptually straightforward, this strategy has been hampered by a number of technical difficulties. Zamecnik and Stephenson first demonstrated a potential therapeutic effect of an antisense oligonucleotide in 1978 when they inhibited the replication of Rous sarcoma virus in culture with a 13-base DNA oligonucleotide complementary to a portion of the viral genome (1). A subsequent important discovery was that of naturally occurring antisense RNA molecules in prokaryotes that regulate the expression of their corresponding gene (2, 3). The inhibition of expression of a thymidine kinase reporter gene in eukaryotic cells by antisense RNA (4) further buttressed belief that human gene expression could potentially be regulated by an antisense approach. Further progress was initially slow, but the last few years have seen the fruition of many years' preclinical research, with the publication of encouraging results from several clinical trials of antisense oligonucleotide therapy.

Two basic strategies have been adopted to modify gene expression using antisense oligonucleotides. Firstly, molecules can be designed to target a DNA sequence, with the aim of inhibiting gene transcription, the so-called anti-gene strategy. This is a very attractive concept since only two target molecules are present within each cell. However, major difficulties have been encountered in translating this approach from cell-free systems to intact cells *in vitro*. As yet there have been no reports of successful *in vivo* application, and the use of this strategy in a therapeutic setting is not contemplated at present. In contrast, the second approach is to design antisense molecules to target an RNA sequence, with the aim of inhibiting translation. Many of the initial hurdles in this arena have now been overcome, and early clinical applications have shown a measure of success. The majority of this chapter will be devoted to this latter approach, but we will start with a brief discussion of anti-gene strategies.

Antisense oligonucleotides targeting DNA

DNA oligonucleotides are capable of binding to the major groove of double-stranded DNA by recognition of the oligopurine-rich strand, thus creating a triple helix. The triple helical structure depends on the base composition of the triplex-forming oligonucleotide (TFO) (5). Each base within the TFO forms two hydrogen bonds with the complementary purine base in the duplex, so-called Hoogsteen or reverse Hoogsteen bonds. A (T, C)-containing TFO binds in a parallel orientation with respect to the 5′–3′ orientation of the oligopurine strand in the duplex, T bonding to A, and C bonding to G in Hoogsteen configuration. The cytosine bases in the TFO must be protonated for this interaction, rendering these molecules less likely to be active at physiological pH. An (A, G)-containing TFO binds in an anti-parallel orientation with A bonding to A in the duplex, and G bonding to G in reverse Hoogsteen configuration. Finally, a (T, G)-containing TFO can bind in either parallel or anti-parallel orientation depending on the length of the poly-(A) tracts in the oligopurine target sequence. Bonding is between T and A, and between G and G, in either Hoogsteen or reverse Hoogsteen configuration (6).

The possible effects of triple helix formation include prevention of binding of transcription factors to the DNA molecule, thus inhibiting the initiation of transcription. Secondly, they may inhibit transcription elongation if the target sequence is within the transcribed part of the gene. The efficiency of either of these effects depends on the stability of the triplex, a significant problem in physiological conditions where high potassium concentrations inhibit triplex formation, particularly for G-rich TFOs (7). In addition, helicases, enzymes that unwind DNA duplexes for the processes of replication, transcription, and repair, have been reported to efficiently unwind triplexes as well (8). For these reasons, much of the initial work with TFOs has been conducted using cell-free systems, in non-physiological conditions. The other major limitation of this approach has been the requirement for a homopurine target sequence, of at least 13 nucleotides in length. The presence of a single pyrimidine base within the target sequence can decrease TFO affinity by 20- to 30-fold. Numerous chemical modifications to the base, the sugar, or the backbone of the TFO have been investigated to improve these inherently unfavorable properties, and thus introduce the possibility of intracellular applications. Backbone modification with N3′ Ø P5′ phosphoramidates has proven a useful strategy. This structure renders the oligonucleotide relatively resistant to nuclease degradation, and also increases the stability of triple helix formation (9). Oligonucleotides with this structure targeting the polypurine tract of human immunodeficiency virus (HIV) proviral DNA, have been demonstrated to arrest RNA polymerase II at the specific triplex site in a eukaryotic transcription assay (10). Increased affinity of the TFO for the DNA duplex has also been achieved by the conjugation of an intercalator molecule to the TFO. For instance, incorporation of acridine at the appropriate site allows the formation of a stable triplex despite the presence of a pyrimidine base within the target homopurine sequence (11). Tetracyclic aromatic compounds such as benzopyridoindole and benzopyridoquinoxaline derivatives have also been shown to increase triplex stability in both Hoogsteen and reverse Hoogsteen motifs (12). Such molecules have been used to stabilize TFO targeting sequences comprising oligopurine tracts on alternate strands of the duplex, the TFO zigzagging across the major groove, switching from one purine tract to the other (6). A similar outcome can be produced by the covalent linkage of two oligonucleotide sequences designed to bind to the target duplex in reverse orientations (13).

It has been established that these and other oligonucleotide modifications have allowed stable triplex formation with several gene targets in near-physiological conditions, and have inhibited transcription in cell-free systems (14). Triplexes formed between TFO and plasmid DNA can also remain stable, with continued inhibition of transcription of the plasmid gene after transfection into cells (15–18). However, there remains some doubt as to whether exogenously applied oligonucleotides can form triplexes with nuclear DNA in eukaryotic cells (15, 19). A number of groups have demonstrated inhibition of transcription of a target gene following the incubation of cells in culture with TFO (20–26). Although, in some cases, sequence specificity was established with the use of mismatched control oligonucleotides, these reports have been criticized for failing to verify that the mechanism is by triplex formation. Alternative, non-sequence-specific, though sequence-dependent effects of oligonucleotides, including binding to transcription factors, have been postulated to account for these results (14). Many TFO able to bind in physiological conditions contain G-rich sequences that have been shown to bind, and inhibit the function of several intra- and extracellular proteins, and it is therefore important to demonstrate triplex formation within the cell, in order to substantiate a true sequence-specific anti-gene effect. Despite these reservations, a number of investigators have provided compelling evidence for such an effect. The first report was of a 27-base oligonucleotide targeting the *c-myc* P1 promoter, investigated in HeLa cells (27). This was shown to be taken up into the nuclei of cells in culture. Nuclei harvested after incubation of the cells with oligonucleotide for 2.5 hours were subjected to a DNAase I assay. A hypersensitive site within the putative triplex region showed reduced cleavage compared with untreated cells, or those treated with a control oligonucleotide unable to form a triplex. There was a corresponding reduction in *c-myc* mRNA in the treated cells. Wang and colleagues have demonstrated an increased rate of mutagenesis around a target triplex site after exogenous application of the relevant TFO, but not controls. This was abrogated in cells deficient in certain DNA repair processes, and was consistent with the hypothesis that DNA repair coupled to transcription arrest was responsible for the increased mutation rate (28). These results provide the impetus for ongoing research in this field, although the therapeutic application of these molecules remains far off.

Antisense oligonucleotides targeting RNA

Oligonucleotides with a complementary sequence to an mRNA target are able to bind specifically to the target sequence by Watson–Crick base-pairing. This has the potential to specifically inhibit translation. At least two possible mechanisms may be involved. Firstly, the formation of the duplex may prevent the ribosomal complex from reading along the message by steric hindrance, thereby preventing assembly of the appropriate tRNA. Secondly, an RNA–DNA duplex can be a substrate for the ubiquitous nuclear enzyme RNAase H, which recognizes and cleaves the RNA strand in the duplex. Several considerations are fundamental to the success of antisense strategies. The oligonucleotide must be stable *in vitro* and, ultimately, *in vivo* if it is to be used for clinical purposes. It must be delivered to its site of action at a sufficient concentration and, once there, must hybridize successfully with its target sequence and inhibit translation by one of the mechanisms described above. Finally, an ideal antisense oligonucleotide should not cause any unpredictable effects as a consequence of interaction with molecules other than the intended target.

Oligonucleotide structure

Naturally occurring phosphodiester DNA oligonucleotides have a short half-life both *in vitro* and *in vivo* as a consequence of degradation by endonucleases and exonucleases (29, 30). The use of oligonucleotides with this chemical structure has, therefore, been limited to cell-free systems and some *in vitro* applications. Chemical modification of the sugar–phosphate backbone has been widely adopted to induce nuclease resistance. Two of the early modifications to be investigated involved replacing one of the non-bridging oxygen atoms in the phosphate group with a sulfur to produce a phosphorothioate molecule (31) or a methyl group to produce a methylphosphonate molecule (32) (Fig. 10.1). The relative simplicity of these chemical

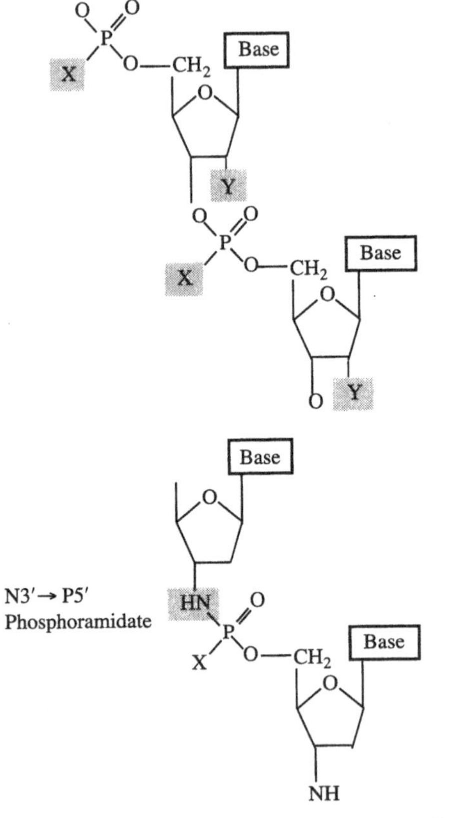

Fig. 10.1   Structural modifications to antisense oligonucleotides.

structures has meant that the manufacture of sufficient quantities of specific oligonucleotides for clinical applications has been economically viable. Methylphosphonates suffer from the disadvantage of failing to be recognized by RNAase H in the duplex with RNA, which may limit their effectiveness in producing an antisense effect. In addition, their lipophilic nature, while potentially enhancing cellular uptake, renders these molecules difficult to get into aqueous solution. For these reasons, they have not been widely used. In contrast, phosphorothioate oligonucleotides have several favorable properties, and have become the predominant tool for the *in vivo* investigation of antisense oligonucleotides, as well as for almost all clinical applications to date. The phosphorothioate bond is relatively nuclease-resistant, and the negative charge imparted to the phosphate backbone makes the molecule hydrophilic, and therefore water-soluble. In addition, phosphorothioate oligonucleotide–RNA duplexes are a substrate for RNAase H, although this is dependent on the relative concentration of antisense oligonucleotide and target RNA molecules. RNAase H activity is inhibited at high phosphorothioate concentrations (33). These molecules do have certain limitations. Firstly, the backbone is chiral, resulting in a racemic mixture of 2^n different oligonucleotide species (where *n* is the number of phosphorothioate internucleotide linkages). Consequently, the affinity of a phosphorothioate oligonucleotide for its target is lower than that for the corresponding phosphodiester (34). Secondly, at least *in vitro*, the cellular uptake of these molecules is limited by their polyanionic structure, with the resulting requirement for additional strategies to deliver the oligonucleotide to its target. Thirdly, it is recognized that phosphorothioate oligonucleotides interact in a non-sequence-specific manner with various proteins. This not only has the potential to produce undesirable side-effects when these molecules are used for therapeutic purposes, but also makes interpretation of their effects difficult (35). Two such non-sequence-specific effects, particularly relevant to the development of targeted anticancer antisense oligonucleotides, are the inhibition of angiogenesis and the activation of the immune system. Anti-angiogenic effects have been described as a result of binding of phosphorothioate oligonucleotides to basic fibroblast growth factor (bFGF) in both *in vitro* and *in vivo* models of angiogenesis (36). Such effects may have been responsible for the non-sequence-specific inhibition of melanoma growth in a severe combined immunodeficiency (SCID) mouse model (37). There have been a number of

reports of immunological effects of phosphorothioate oligonucleotides that have fuelled speculation that the antitumor activity of these molecules may result from immune stimulation rather than reduction of target protein expression (38). Though not sequence-specific, the presence of certain motifs within the oligonucleotide, such as CpG dinucleotides or G-quartets, appears to enhance these effects (39). Localized activation of natural killer (NK) cell lytic activity in the draining lymph nodes was reported in mice injected subcutaneously with CpG-containing oligonucleotides (40). Activation of NK cells was dependent on the production of interleukin (IL)-12, interferon (IFN)-$\alpha\beta$, and tumor necrosis factor (TNF)α by accessory cells. CpG-containing oligonucleotides have also been shown to activate dendritic cells in the skin of BALB/c mice following local injection, leading to a local T helper (Th1) response (41). These observations suggest that recognition of non-methylated CpG sequences, which evolved as antigen-independent immune mechanisms to protect against bacterial infection, may be responsible for these effects.

Numerous alternative chemical modifications of oligonucleotide structure have been investigated, with a view to improving the undesirable qualities of phosphorothioates. The properties of various compounds are summarized in Table 10.1, and the chemical structures of selected molecules are shown in Fig. 10.1. While some of these have achieved a measure of success, their use has been largely limited to preclinical applications. The main restriction has been the cost of manufacture of large quantities of these molecules. As with the phosphorothioates, the cost will undoubtedly come down in due course, at which point clinical use on a wide scale may become realistic. One strategy that has proven useful has been the design of chimeric oligonucleotides incorporating a mixture of backbone structures, such as phosphorothioate and phosphodiester linkages within the same molecule (42). Phosphorothioates positioned at the ends of the oligonucleotide provide resistance to exonucleases, while the reduced number of phosphorothioate bonds in these molecules lessens their propensity for non-specific binding, and therefore side-effects. Another chimeric design incorporates a modification of the sugar with a 2'-O-methyl group or a 2'-O-methoxyethyl group in the internucleoside linkages at the 3' and 5' ends of the molecule, with a phosphorothioate-modified deoxyribose core. Once again, the number of phosphorothioate bonds is reduced, but RNAase H activation is retained, and duplex stability

Table 10.1   Properties* of modified oligodeoxynucleotides

Structure	Site of modification	Nuclease stability[†]	Duplex stability	RNAase H activation	Entry into cell
Phosphodiester	Naturally occurring	−	++	++	+
Methylphosphonate	Phosphodiester bridge	++	+	−	+
Phosphorothioate	Phosphodiester bridge	+	+	++	+
N3′ → P5′ phosphoramidate	Phosphodiester bridge	++	+++	−	+
2′-O-methyl group	Sugar	++	++	−	+
2′-O-methoxyethyl group	Sugar	++	++	−	+
α-Anomeric glycosidic linkage	Sugar	++	+	−	+
Peptide nucleic acid	Sugar–phosphate backbone	+++	+/−	−	−
C5 propynyl substitution	Pyrimidine base	−	+++	++	−
Circular DNA	No 5′ or 3′ ends	++ (exo)	++	++	+

* Each property is graded from − (zero or poor quality) to +++ (excellent quality).
[†] exo, Stable to exonuclease-mediated degradation only.

is increased compared with that of a pure phosphorothioate (43, 44). Molecules of this type (referred to as mixed backbone oligonucleotides) have now entered clinical trials.

Other structures have relied on extremely stable hybridization with the target RNA. It is thought that inhibition of translation by a steric hindrance mechanism may be effective if the duplex is very stable. This must be sufficient to prevent its disruption by repair/editing enzymes such as helicase and RNA unwindase (45), or by the ribosomal complex itself (46). If this is the case, RNAase H may not be such an important mediator of antisense activity. An example of this kind of oligonucleotide is the N3′ → P5′ phosphoramidate, in which each 3′-oxygen is substituted with a 3′-amino group. The duplex thermal stability of these molecules is typically increased by 2.2–2.6°C per modified linkage, compared with phosphodiesters (9). Despite not supporting RNAase H-mediated RNA hydrolysis (47), these molecules do demonstrate antisense activity *in vitro*, where they have been reported to be more active than other chemistries (48). *In vivo*, the tissue distribution and cellular uptake is similar to that seen with phosphorothioates. Furthermore, the anti-leukemia effect of a *c-myc* antisense phosphoramidate oligonucleotide was greater than that produced by the corresponding phosphorothioate in a SCID mouse model (49).

Another approach to circumventing the requirement for RNAase H activity has been to synthesize a conjugate between an oligonucleotide and a molecule that can cause the destruction of the complementary RNA strand. For instance 5′-linked anthraquinone oligonucleotides deliver a reactive species to the target RNA (50). Other investigators have conjugated a 2′,5′-tetraadenylate to the 5′ end of an antisense oligonucleotide. 2′,5′-Oligoadenylates induce the activation of another ubiquitous endoribonuclease, RNAase L, which is present in many mammalian cell types. The resulting 2–5A antisense molecule acts as a sequence-specific endoribonuclease, and has been shown to produce cleavage of its target in cell-free systems (51), and in human cells *in vitro* (52). Inhibition of proliferation of chronic myelogenous leukemia (CML) cell lines and primary patient cultures was achieved with a 2–5A antisense molecule targeting *bcr/abl* mRNA, in a sequence-specific manner (52). Further modification of these molecules to enhance nuclease resistance is currently being undertaken (53).

Delivery of antisense oligonucleotides to the target site

In order to produce antisense effects, oligonucleotides must both enter cells, and become available to hybridize with their target RNA in the cytoplasm and possibly the nucleus. Two mechanisms of oligonucleotide uptake have been described, namely, passive, fluid-phase endocytosis (54) and receptor-mediated endocytosis. The latter mechanism is important for the uptake of negatively charged oligonucleotides such as phosphodiesters and phosphorothioates, and appears to have evolved as a mechanism to salvage nucleic acids from the extracellular milieu following their release from apoptotic cells (55). Phosphorothioates have been shown to bind to a number of cell-surface proteins, in a competitive and saturable manner (56, 57). Hence the uptake mechanism is concentration- and energy-dependent, with receptor-mediated endocytosis predominating at low concentrations of phosphorothioates (up to approximately 1 μM), and fluid-phase endocytosis becoming more important at higher concentrations (57). Uptake of oligonucleotide into cultured cells *in vitro* appears particularly inefficient, possibly due to binding of oligonucleotides to proteins within the culture medium such as bovine serum albumin (58). This phenomenon was the likely cause of many experimental failures during the early evaluation of antisense techniques to modify gene expression. It has been overcome by the use of methods to enhance uptake such as physical disruption of the cell membrane by electroporation (59, 60), or the use of streptolysin O, which permeabilizes the membrane (60). However, the technique that has proven most effective is the use of cationic lipids (61, 62). These coat the oligonucleotide in a charge-dependent interaction, imparting an overall positive charge to the oligonucleotide–lipid complex, and present a lipid tail to the exterior. This complex is able to associate with the negatively charged phospholipid bilayer forming the cell membrane. Uptake appears to be by endocytosis, followed by destabilization of the endosomal membrane by the cationic lipid, thus releasing the oligonucleotide into the cytoplasm (63). Uptake of phosphorothioate oligonucleotides complexed with cationic lipids is nevertheless affected by serum components, which can either prevent association of the complex with the cell membrane or displace oligonucleotide from the complex (64). More efficient delivery systems using cationic peptides (65) or combinations of lipid and peptide (66) are being developed to overcome some of these limitations.

Once internalized, the oligonucleotide is initially confined within the lysosomal and endosomal compartments. Electron microscope studies have shown that oligonucleotide can also be detected within the cytoplasm, but the majority of material released from endosomes or lysosomes is localized within the nucleus, primarily to the euchromatin/ heterochromatin interface (57, 67). Transport to the nucleus appears to be by passive diffusion (57, 68). Of note, Beltinger and colleagues failed to demonstrate any significant association between oligonucleotides and rough endoplasmic reticulum or ribosomes (57). These observations suggest that antisense oligonucleotides may exert their effects within the nucleus, rather than at the ribosome. However, the distribution of a particular oligonucleotide within the subcellular compartments is likely to be dependent on its chemical structure (69, 70), and also its nucleotide sequence (71). It has also been shown that uptake and subcellular distribution of a

c-myc antisense oligonucleotide was dependent on the phase of the cell cycle to which the cells were synchronized. Furthermore, downregulation of c-myc protein was correlated with the amount of oligonucleotide localized to the cytosolic compartment (72). Association of phosphorothioate oligonucleotides with subcellular structures such as intermediate filaments, cytoplasmic membranes, and the nuclear interior has also been described (69). Thus, it should not be assumed that all active molecules work in the same way. Some may exert an antisense effect predominantly in the nucleus, perhaps by interfering with mRNA transport or by inducing RNAase H-mediated cleavage of the target, while others may act within the cytoplasm, interfering with the interaction between mRNA and ribosome. The development of powerful techniques to follow hybridization of DNA oligonucleotides with RNA molecules in real time will doubtless shed further light on this question. One such is the use of so-called molecular beacons. These are oligonucleotides complementary to a target sequence of interest that adopt a stem-loop structure when unhybridized. Matched fluorescent donor and acceptor chromophores are attached to the 5′ and 3′ ends, respectively. When in the stem-loop conformation, fluorescence is quenched but, upon hybridization to the target RNA sequence, the distance between donor and acceptor chromophores is increased, and fluorescence is emitted. Using confocal microscopy, fluorescence was detected within 15 minutes of microinjection of such a molecular beacon targeting the *vav* protooncogene mRNA into K562 human leukemia cells. No fluorescence was detected when a mismatched molecular beacon control was injected (73).

Antisense oligonucleotide delivery *in vivo* presents somewhat different problems to *in vitro* delivery. An unexpected early finding was that chemically modified oligonucleotides such as phosphorothioates do appear to be taken up by cells after delivery to animals simply in saline solution. Reproducible, sequence-specific antisense effects have been shown in a number of animal models of human disease following intravenous (49, 74–78) and subcutaneous (79) injection of oligonucleotides. Nevertheless, there is little doubt that oligonucleotide delivery to the target cell population by this method is inefficient. Pharmacokinetic studies in rodents have demonstrated that the majority of retained oligonucleotide is located in certain organs, notably the liver, kidneys, spleen, and bone marrow (80, 81). Uptake into tumor was at a lower level in a murine pancreatic cancer model, amounting to only

2–3 per cent of the initial dose (82). Adaptation of lipid-based delivery systems appears to be a potential way forward. Cationic lipid/DNA complexes are cleared rapidly from the circulation and also accumulate in organs, and are therefore not suitable for delivery of oligonucleotides to tumor cells *in vivo*. An ideal carrier system would comprise small, neutral, serum-stable particles that are not recognized by cells of the reticuloendothelial system and yet are able to interact readily with cells and destabilize the cell membrane to allow intracellular delivery of the oligonucleotide molecule. Particles containing small amounts of positively charged lipid with a polyethylene glycol (PEG) coating have been described as fulfilling some of these requirements (83, 84). The introduction of fusogenic peptides from the hemagglutinating virus of Japan (HVJ) into a liposome complex has also been described to enhance uptake of nucleic acids to a variety of tissues following local or systemic delivery (85–89). Other investigators have attempted to target the oligonucleotide specifically to the cell of interest. For instance, by introducing a specific antibody into a liposome, uptake of oligonucleotide into myeloid or lymphoid leukemia cells was doubled when the appropriate antibody (CD2 or CD32) was incorporated, compared with using the liposome alone, or one incorporating an inappropriate antibody (90). Economic considerations will undoubtedly play a role in determining which, if any, of these strategies may be adopted in human antisense therapeutics. Collaboration and mergers between antisense oligonucleotide companies and companies developing delivery systems attest to the importance of this issue.

Choice of target sequence

The choice of a target sequence within the mRNA of interest is governed by several factors. Firstly, the length of the target (and consequently of the complementary oligonucleotide) is important. It is estimated on statistical grounds that an oligonucleotide of 12–15 bases is required to ensure that there will be a unique target sequence in the human genome (91). An oligonucleotide of this length is also required for the formation of a stable duplex between a phosphodiester and its target RNA in physiological conditions, and a larger molecule is probably required for phosphorothioates (92). However, if the oligonucleotide is too long, hybridization to partially complementary sequences may occur. Since human RNAase H is able to recognize as little as a single base-pair of RNA/DNA duplex, this could potentially lead to

cleavage of RNA molecules other than the desired target (93). In practice, antisense oligonucleotides between 14 and 27 bases in length have been used.

The region of mRNA to be targeted is a second important consideration. A considerable proportion of RNA sequence is likely to be inaccessible to a complementary oligonucleotide because of the presence of secondary and tertiary structure. Various approaches to identifying accessible sequence have been undertaken. Theoretical considerations have led researchers to target regions that are expected to be single-stranded because of their functional significance. Examples include the translation–initiation codon region (94, 95), the 5′ cap site (the site initially recognized by the ribosome) (96, 97), splice donor–acceptor sites (96), the polyadenylation signal 5′ to the poly-(A) tail (98), and the junctional sequences of tumor-associated chromosomal translocations (99). However, such considerations may not always be able to predict the optimal target site. A study comparing the ability of 13 20-mer oligonucleotides targeting different regions of the *bcl*-2 mRNA to reduce *bcl*-2 mRNA and protein expression in small-cell lung cancer cell lines demonstrated that the most effective oligonucleotide targeted an area of the coding region (100). This suggests that single-stranded regions of mRNA exist that are accessible for hybridization. Attempts to predict such regions by computer modeling of RNA structure have so far met with very limited success (101, 102). Advances in array technology allow the high volume screening of all possible complementary oligonucleotides up to a predetermined length, for any known mRNA sequence (103). The oligonucleotide array is synthesized on a solid support and a labeled mRNA transcript is allowed to hybridize to the array. After removing unbound transcript, the oligonucleotides able to hybridize successfully can be identified by the positions of greatest signal intensity. In the case of the rabbit β-globin mRNA, hybridization efficiency of an oligonucleotide in this assay was found to be correlated with antisense activity in an RNAase H assay and in an *in vitro* translation assay (104), suggesting this approach may be generally applicable. As with most screening methods carried out *in vitro*, there may not be a 100 per cent correlation with activity *in vivo*, due to differences in RNA folding, but this may at least narrow the field of potentially useful molecules for *in vivo* study. Another approach is to attempt to find sites within the mRNA molecule that are sensitive to RNAase H-mediated hydrolysis. The end-labeled mRNA molecule is incubated in a cell-free system with

RNAase H and random or semirandom libraries of oligonucleotides of a specified length. Sites of mRNA cleavage can be mapped by a number of techniques, and oligonucleotides targeting these sites are synthesized for further evaluation (102, 105–108).

Pharmacokinetics of antisense oligonucleotides in animal studies

The *in vivo* pharmacokinetics of antisense oligonucleotides have been extensively studied in rodents and, to a lesser extent, in primates. Phosphodiester oligonucleotides are cleared rapidly from the plasma with an elimination half-life of a few minutes (109). They are distributed widely to tissues but show little tissue accumulation. Metabolism to monomer is the primary mechanism responsible for clearance (30). Modification of the 3' and 5' end internucleoside linkages with a phosphorothioate or a methylphosphonate bond did not substantially improve these characteristics, with rapid clearance from the blood, little tissue accumulation, and rapid degradation to mononucleotides (110). Fully phosphorothioate-modified oligonucleotides display distinctly different pharmacokinetic behavior. Following intravenous (IV) bolus delivery to rodents, phosphorothioate oligonucleotides with a variety of sequences have shown broadly similar pharmacokinetics (Table 10.2) (80, 111–114). They are rapidly cleared from the plasma with bi- or tri-exponential kinetics representing distribution to tissues and elimination, respectively. In the plasma, oligonucleotide is highly protein-bound. Oligonucleotide is concentrated in specific tissues, predominantly the kidney, liver, spleen, lymph nodes, and bone marrow and, to a lesser extent, other highly vascular organs. Tissue uptake to high-affinity organs appears to be a saturable process.

At higher doses, a greater proportion of the dose is distributed to well-perfused, low-affinity sites (112). Very little or no uptake was demonstrated in brain and testis. Both full-length oligonucleotide and reduced chain-length metabolites can be recovered from plasma and tissues. Metabolism appears to result primarily from 3' exonuclease activity, with some 5' exonuclease-mediated degradation occurring in the liver and kidney (115). Excretion is largely via the urine, but different investigators have found variable proportions of intact oligonucleotide in the urine, ranging from very little (80, 113) to nearly 100 per cent (111). The pharmacokinetic behavior of phosphorothioate oligonucleotides administered by subcutaneous infusion or repeated IV bolus to rodents is similar to that of a single IV bolus (80, 111–113). Pharmacokinetic studies of phosphorothioate oligonucleotides administered to monkeys report a similar plasma elimination half-life to that seen in rodents, with accumulation to greatest levels in the kidney and liver, and excretion in the urine. Both intact and degraded species were detected in plasma, kidney, liver, spleen, and lymph nodes (116, 117).

A number of investigators have examined the nature of tissue uptake of phosphorothioate oligonucleotides to high-affinity sites in rodents. Kidney uptake occurs predominantly in the proximal tubule, and appears to occur by reabsorption following glomerular filtration (118–120). Liver uptake is mainly to Kupffer and endothelial cells with a small amount of oligonucleotide accumulating in parenchymal cells (81, 118). Subcellular fractionation demonstrated saturable uptake to nonparenchymal cells with oligonucleotide reaching the nuclear, cytosolic, and membrane fractions. Higher doses were required to produce nuclear uptake in parenchymal cells, with no evidence of saturable binding (121). Competition studies with dextran

Table 10.2 Pharmacokinetic properties of phosphorothioate oligonucleotides following intravenous injection in animal models

Ref.	Animal	Oligonucleotide	Dose range	$t_{1/2}\ \alpha$ (min)*	Elimination $t_{1/2}$ (hours)	Clearance (ml/min/kg)*
111	Sprague–Dawley rat	HIV-1 *rev*, 27-mer	35–3257 µg	20–25	27–41	5.31
112	Wistar rat	ISIS 5132 (*c-raf*), 20-mer	0.06–60 mg/kg	19–48	12.9	2.33
113	CD1 mouse	ISIS 5132 (*c-raf*), 20-mer	4–20 mg/kg	30–45	NR	9.3–14.3
80	Balb-C mouse	G3139 (*bcl-2*), 18-mer	5 mg/kg	37	11	6.4
114	Nude mouse	DNA methyl-transferase, 20-mer	10–300 mg/kg	NR	0.8–4.0	7.9–15.2
116	Cynomolgus monkey	GEM 91 (HIV-1 *gag*), 25-mer	4 mg/kg	NR	11–100	NR
126	Rhesus monkey	ISIS 2503 (*Ha-ras*) 17-mer	10 mg/kg	NR	1.1 ± 0.2 hrs	0.9 ± 0.2

* NR, Not reported; $t_{1/2}\ \alpha$, initial plasma half-life where biexponential kinetics were observed.

sulfate, polyinosinic acid, and fucoidan suggest that tissue uptake is mediated by class A type I/II scavenger receptors (81, 120). Uptake to mononuclear cells in the blood, bone marrow, and spleen has also been examined using fluorescence-labeled oligonucleotides in conjunction with fluorescence-activated cell sorting. This demonstrated greatest accumulation within the monocyte/macrophage population, with lower levels in B cells and the least uptake in T cells (122). Uptake into tumor tissue has also been demonstrated in a nude mouse xenograft model of human pancreatic cancer, with 2–3 per cent of the administered dose being associated with the tumor (82). Importantly, intact oligonucleotide was recoverable from tumor tissue.

Oligonucleotide sequence can influence its pharmacokinetic behavior. A 17-mer phosphorothioate-capped phosphodiester oligonucleotide comprising only deoxyguanosines and thymidines has shown markedly extended plasma and tissue half-lives in mice and cynomolgus monkeys. The sequence and composition of the 17-mer favors the formation of a compact, intramolecularly folded structure dominated by two stacked guanine quartet motifs that are connected by three loops of TGs. This provides nuclease resistance, and may result in tight binding to tissues (123–125). Clearly, the use of such sequences is limited by the availability of a suitable target sequence in the mRNA of interest. *In vivo* pharmacokinetics data has also been reported for a phosphorothioate oligonucleotide encapsulated in PEGylated liposomes delivered to rhesus monkeys by IV infusion. In comparison with the unencapsulated oligonucleotide, the plasma elimination half-life was increased approximately 50-fold to 57.8 hours. Tissue distribution was also affected by encapsulation, being mainly to tissues of the reticuloendothelial system rather than to the kidney and liver, and the extent of metabolism was reduced (126). The authors conclude that the reduced rate of plasma clearance and metabolism observed may favor the use of encapsulated oligonucleotides for their delivery to tissues with high blood flow, as expected for tumors and sites of inflammation. Altered *in vivo* pharmacokinetics have also been reported for oligonucleotides complexed with polyhexylcyanoacrylate nanoparticles, producing enhanced liver accumulation (127), and for oligonucleotides associated with sponge-like alginate nanoparticles, which accumulated in lungs, liver, and spleen (128).

The possibility of pharmacokinetic interactions between phosphorothioate oligonucleotides and other drugs has been investigated to a limited extent. Interactions with other highly protein-bound drugs may be predicted, and are supported by *in vitro* experiments showing up to 30 per cent displacement of a 27-mer oligonucleotide from human serum albumin by nifedipine, warfarin, midazolam, probenecid, indomethacin, and mitoxantrone (129). Furthermore, the pharmacokinetics of a phosphorothioate oligonucleotide were altered by prior administration of aspirin to rats (130). Metabolic interactions between phosphorothioate oligonucleotides and acetaminophen (131), or DNA-intercalating cytotoxic drugs (132, 133) have also been reported.

Preclinical toxicology of antisense oligonucleotides

Antisense oligonucleotides have the potential to produce toxicity as a result of their pharmacological effect on target gene expression. For molecules targeting oncogenes, such toxicity is clearly dependent on the importance of the target gene product for normal cellular physiology, as compared with its role in the oncogenic process. Many oncogenes for which antisense strategies have been adopted are members of gene families within which there is a degree of redundancy in the normal functioning of the cell. Hence, it may be expected that target-specific toxicity would be limited or absent in such cases. These considerations have been borne out in mouse studies in which the toxicity of an oligonucleotide antisense to a human gene sequence has been compared to that of an oligonucleotide targeting the murine homolog. Such experiments have been performed for phosphorothioate oligonucleotides targeting intercellular adhesion molecule-1 (ICAM-1) (134) and *c-raf-1* kinase (135) and have shown no differences in the toxicity profiles produced by the murine and human antisense sequences. While these results cannot be extrapolated to molecules with different gene targets, they serve to establish the likely sequence-independent toxic effects of this class of molecule.

The toxicity profile of phosphorothioate oligonucleotides as a class is well characterized in several species, including mice, rats, and monkeys. It has become apparent that transient changes in biochemical and hematological parameters occur that are related to peak plasma concentrations of oligonucleotide following IV injection or infusion. Of more concern, transient hemodynamic changes have been observed in monkeys, which in some cases have been sufficiently severe to cause sudden death (136, 137). These changes are predictable based on the dose delivered, and can be avoided by reducing the dose, or prolonging the duration of the infusion to reduce peak plasma levels. They are manifested as prolongation of clotting times, a phenomenon that has been observed in all species studied (125, 138), and activation of complement, an effect only observed in monkeys to date (135, 137, 139). In general, both complement activation and prolongation of clotting times appear independent of oligonucleotide sequence, but chemical structure is important. For instance, the use of mixed backbone oligonucleotides with fewer phosphorothioate bonds reduces the extent of these effects (140).

Inhibition of coagulation is thought to result from ionic interactions between the phosphorothioate molecule and proteins involved in the clotting cascade. This is suggested by reversal of the effect by protamine, and the demonstration that protamine binds to phosphorothioate oligonucleotides in a dose-dependent manner (141). The intrinsic pathway appears more sensitive to inhibition than the extrinsic pathway as reflected by greater prolongation of the activated partial thromboplastin time (APTT) than the prothrombin time (PT) (141, 142). The mechanism of inhibition was independent of that of heparin, and no direct inhibition of factors Xa, XIa, or thrombin was observed *in vitro* (142). However, the interaction between thrombin and fibrinogen was identified as a possible target.

Complement activation is measurable *in vivo* as an increase in plasma levels of complement split products C3a and C5a. *In vitro* studies have also shown that phosphorothioate treatment of normal human serum results in a concentration-dependent reduction in hemolytic complement activity with parallel increases in concentrations of complement fragment C4d, but with relatively minor increases in complement fragment Bb. These observations suggest that phosphorothioates activate complement via the classical pathway, thereby consuming complement components necessary for hemolytic activity (141). In contrast, other investigators report increases in complement split product Bb with no increase in C4a following a 10-minute infusion of 20 mg/kg of a phosphorothioate oligonucleotide to cynomolgus monkeys. Furthermore, plasma levels of the complement inhibitor, factor H, decreased in a dose-dependent manner following oligonucleotide administration. Factor H is a DNA-binding protein, and was found to bind to a phosphorothioate oligonucleotide *in vitro*. The authors conclude that complement activation occurs via the alternative pathway, possibly as a result of removal of the regulatory protein factor H. This may explain why complement activation only occurs once a threshold plasma level of oligonucleotide is exceeded (139). An alternative explanation of these data would be that factor H levels are reduced as a result of complement activation, since no mechanism is proposed for the reduction in factor H by oligonucleotide. Activation of complement has been postulated to be responsible for several of the clinical features that have been observed following bolus IV injections of phosphorothioates to monkeys. Production of C3a and C5a, which are chemotactic molecules, may account for observed fluctuations in circulating neutrophil counts characterized by a transient neutropenia followed by rebound neutrophilia. Activation of other cell types by these molecules, such as mast cells and basophils, with the subsequent release of vasoactive autocoids could lead to changes in vascular permeability and tone, resulting in the transient profound hypotension observed (136, 137, 139). However, an alternative explanation for these cardiovascular effects is that phosphorothioate oligonucleotides act as α_1-adrenergic receptor antagonists (143). Support for this hypothesis is provided by the observation that epinephrine (also called adrenaline) failed to reverse the hypotension, whereas administration of IV fluids was effective. A 15-mer phosphorothioate was found to compete with prazosin for binding to the α_1-adrenergic receptor with an IC_{50} (injected drug concentration corresponding to 50 per cent cell survival) of 14 μM. Mixing oligonucleotide with albumin prior to injection to macaque monkeys abrogated the cardiovascular effects. This suggests that interaction of unbound oligonucleotide with the receptor, before its association with plasma proteins, may lead to a reduction in sympathetic tone (143).

Subacute toxicity of phosphorothioate oligonucleotides, produced by repeated dosing for up to 2 weeks, is observed in all species studied, but only at doses in substantial excess of those required to produce pharmacological activity. Target organs for toxicity are those in which oligonucleotide is known to accumulate. Renal toxicity occurs in rodents at oligonucleotide doses of 100 mg/kg or greater, and in monkeys at doses of 80 mg/kg. It is characterized by proximal tubular and cortical necrosis, and may be associated with elevation of serum urea and creatinine levels, and with hematuria and proteinuria (138, 144). Lower doses of oligonucleotide produce milder renal histological changes in rodents, including renal tubule regeneration (145) and perivasculitis with diffuse interstitial mononuclear cell infiltrates, seen primarily in the cortex (134). In monkeys intracytoplasmic eosinophilic granules and vacuolation in proximal tubular epithelial cells, with free red blood cells in the proximal tubular lumen are observed (146). Other subacute toxic effects have been largely confined to rodents. Hepatic abnormalities are seen at moderate to high doses of oligonucleotide and consist of inflammatory changes, mixed mononuclear cell infiltrates, and focal hepatic necrosis (134, 135, 144, 145). This is associated with mild elevations in serum liver enzyme levels. Thrombocytopenia and anemia have also been documented and appear related in severity to dose and duration of treatment (134, 135, 144, 145). The exact mechanism for these changes is unclear, but depletion of megakaryocytes from the bone marrow has been reported, suggesting that platelet production may be impaired (144, 147). Increased sequestration of platelets and red blood cells in the spleen is another possible explanation.

Other abnormalities appear to represent an immunological response to phosphorothioate oligonucleotides to which mice and rats are particularly sensitive. The changes observed comprise splenomegaly, lymphoid hyperplasia, hypergammaglobulinemia, and a multiorgan mixed mononuclear cell infiltrate (135, 144, 145, 147–149). Oligonucleotide sequence is an important factor in determining the extent of immune stimulation. The presence of the so-called CpG motif, a palindromic sequence comprising a CpG dinucleotide flanked by two 5′ purines and two 3′ pyrimidines, confers a high degree of stimulatory activity, producing characteristic changes in mice at lower doses than needed for control oligonucleotides lacking such motifs (149). However, the presence of such motifs was not the sole factor determining the degree of immune stimulation. The mechanism of the changes observed has not been fully elucidated. B-lymphocyte proliferation accounts for the observation of splenomegaly (148, 150, 151), and has been shown to occur following incubation of spleen cells or peripheral blood leukocytes with oligonucleotides *in vitro* (138, 149, 152). NK-cell activation has also been reported (40, 153). The pattern of cytokine production observed following oligonucleotide administration to mice involves secretion of IL-6, IL-12, and IFN-γ (154, 155), consistent with activation of monocyte/macrophage and Th1 cells. Activation of dendritic cells in the skin of mice injected subcutaneously with CpG-containing oligonucleotides has also been demonstrated (41). Hence a complex, cell-mediated immune activation, possibly mediated by antigen-presenting cells and leading to B-cell proliferation, antibody and cytokine production, and NK-cell activation, appears to take place. The only observation in monkeys possibly relating to immune stimulatory effects of phosphorothioate oligonucleotides has been slight lymphoid hyperplasia in spleen and lymph nodes (146), but it is unknown why this phenomenon appears to be species-dependent.

Clinical development of antisense oligonucleotide therapy

Human pharmacokinetics of phosphorothioate oligonucleotides

Phase I clinical trials have evaluated the pharmacokinetics, toxicity, and pharmacology of several phosphorothioate oligonucleotides in healthy volunteers (156) and in patients with malignancy (157–161), HIV infection (162, 163), and Crohn's disease (164). These studies have differed in the mode and schedule of drug administration, the dose range employed, and in the method of pharmacokinetic analysis, factors that may account for the differences in the reported pharmacokinetic parameters (Table 10.3). The most reproducible factor is plasma clearance, which is generally somewhat lower than that observed in rodents but similar to that observed in monkeys. Some studies have reported evidence for a saturable component to clearance and distribution of oligonucleotide, as predicted by animal models (156, 161, 163, 164). Trials in which oligonucleotide is given as a 2-hour IV infusion every other day report a relatively short plasma elimination half-life, which probably represents rapid tissue uptake (156, 160, 161, 164). In contrast, trials in which oligonucleotide is administered as a continuous infusion over 10–14 days report a longer half-life, which is of a similar order of magnitude to the elimination half-life observed in animal studies using radiolabeled oligonucleotides (157, 159). The only clinical study able to characterize biexponential plasma disappearance behavior was that of Zhang and colleagues, which also used a radiolabeled oligonucleotide (162). This showed a short initial half-life of 11 minutes and a long terminal half-life of 26.7 hours. These studies are, therefore, generally consistent with the preclinical data showing fairly rapid clearance of the plasma by distribution of oligonucleotide to tissues, and relatively slow clearance from the body. After short IV infusion, maximum plasma levels are achieved at the end of the infusion, and are roughly proportional to dose. No plasma accumulation of oligonucleotide was observed

Table 10.3   Pharmacokinetic parameters of phosphorothioate oligonucleotides in human trials

Ref.	Oligonucleotide	Schedule*	Dose range	Half-life $t_{1/2}$	Clearance[†] (ml/min/kg)	C_{max}[‡] (µg/ml)
160	ISIS 5132 (*c-raf*), 20-mer	2-h IVI × 3/week for 3 weeks	0.5–6 mg/kg	60 (36–107) min	1.9 (1.2–2.4)	2.8–22.7
161	ISIS 3521 (PKC-α), 20-mer	2-h IVI × 3/week for 3 weeks	0.5–6 mg/kg	18–140 min	1.4–3.4	0.5–22.4
156	ISIS 2302 (ICAM-1), 20-mer	2-h IVI single dose or alt day dosing	0.06–2 mg/kg	53 ± 16 min	1.3–2.1	1.6–15.5
164	ISIS 2302 (ICAM-1), 20-mer	2-h IVI alt day × 26 days	0.5–2 mg/kg	34–56 min	Dose-dependent	1.4–18.1
162	GEM-91 (HIV-1 *gag*), labeled, 25-mer	^{35}S-2-h IVI	0.1 mg/kg	26.7 ± 1.7 h	0.4 ± 0.03	0.3 ± 0.04
157	OL(1)p53, 20-mer	10-day cont IVI	1.2–6 mg/kg/day	24.4–62.5 h	NR	2.1–4.2
159	G3139 (*bcl-2*), 18-mer	14-day cont SC	0.125–5.3 mg/kg/day	7.5 ± 4.3 h	1.5 ± 1.0	0.5–5.6

* IVI, Intravenous infusion; SC, subcutaneous; alt day, alternate day; cont, continuous.
[†] NR, Not reported.
[‡] C_{max}, Maximum concentration.

in these studies with alternate day dosing frequency (156, 160, 161, 164). Continuous infusion produced steady-state plasma levels within 24 hours for IV (157) and 48 hours for subcutaneous administration (159). Again, steady-state plasma level was dose-proportional, but we also identified renal function as a significant factor in predicting steady-state concentration. Detection of oligonucleotide in the urine was variable between studies, but a low or undetectable level of intact oligonucleotide was generally reported (156, 161). Higher levels of short-chain-length metabolites have been reported to appear in the urine, with a substantial proportion of the material appearing as monomer (157, 162). Degradation products also appeared in the plasma in most studies, but intact full-length oligonucleotide was the predominant species at this site (156, 159, 160, 162, 164). In summary, these studies have shown feasible pharmacokinetic parameters for the administration of phosphorothioate oligonucleotides to patients by both IV and subcutaneous routes, either by intermittent short infusion or continuous infusion.

Toxicity of phosphorothioate oligonucleotides in phase I trials

The toxicity that has been observed in the clinical trials of antisense oligonucleotides is consistent with the non-sequence-specific toxic effects of phosphorothioate molecules predicted from animal studies. Dose-limiting adverse events in patients with non-Hodgkin's lym-

phoma treated with an antisense molecule targeting *bcl-2* were fatigue, fever, hypotension, and thrombocytopenia (165). The maximum tolerated dose of a 14-day subcutaneous infusion of this 18-mer phosphorothioate oligonucleotide was 147.2 mg/m²/day (approximately 4 mg/kg/day). Thrombocytopenia was clearly related to dose and duration of treatment in this study (Fig. 10.2). Other studies have reported similar dose-limiting toxicity, including fatigue (160, 161, 166, 167), fever (160), fever and hypotension (167), and thrombocytopenia (161, 166, 167). None of these studies reached a maximum tolerated dose, but a dose of 2 mg/kg/day continuous IV infusion for 3 of every 4 weeks was selected for further phase II investigation on the basis of the more favorable pharmacokinetic profile of this administration method (166, 167). Schedule-dependent toxic effects have included prolongation of the activated partial thromboplastin time and elevation of complement split product C3a. These abnormalities were associated with peak plasma levels following short IV infusions of oligonucleotide, were transient in nature, and were not associated with any clinical sequelae (156, 160, 161, 163, 164). None of the trials in which oligonucleotides were delivered by protracted infusion reported clotting abnormalities or elevation of complement components. Continuous subcutaneous infusion resulted in inflammation of the skin at the infusion site, together with enlargement of the draining lymph nodes in some patients (165). Other non-dose-limiting toxic effects reported have been nausea and vomiting (161, 164), hyperglycemia (157, 158, 165), elevated liver enzymes

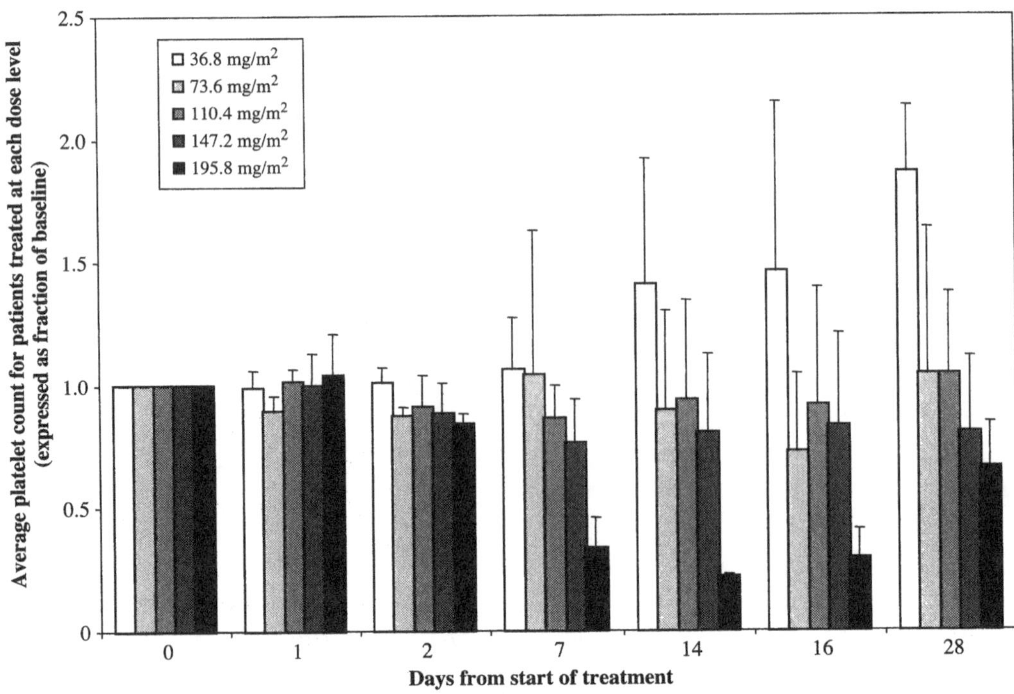

Fig. 10.2 Development of thrombocytopenia in patients treated at increasing dose levels of G3139, a phosphorothioate oligonucleotide targeting *bcl-2*. Treatment commenced on day 0 by continuous subcutaneous infusion for 14 days at the daily doses shown. Mean values for the patients treated at each dose level are given. N = 4, 4, 3, 5, and 2 for dose levels 36.8, 73.6, 110.4, 146.2, and 195.8 mg/m²/day, respectively. Error bars represent the standard deviation.

(157, 165), elevated blood urea nitrogen and creatinine (157, 165, 168), anemia (157, 160), and lymphopenia (165). In general, phosphorothioate oligonucleotides have been well-tolerated at doses predicted to be pharmacologically active. The spectrum of toxicity is favorable compared with that of conventional cytotoxic agents.

The development of antisense oligonucleotides for cancer therapy

In the preceding sections of this chapter we have discussed the development of antisense oligonucleotides as a general therapeutic class, with specific consideration of the problems unique to the use of these molecules as drugs. Clearly, the work described has not been carried out in an ivory tower, and much of it has been directed to the therapy of a particular disease by targeting a specific gene. In this final section, we will describe some of the approaches that may have promise for the treatment of cancer. Targets for anticancer therapy include

apoptosis (*bcl-2*, p53), protein kinases (for example, protein kinase C-α, protein kinase A, *c-raf*), transcription factors and nuclear proteins (for example, *c-myb*, *c-myc*), oncogenes (for example, *bcr-abl*, *ras*), growth factors, cytokines, and many others. Antisense oligonucleotides designed to inhibit the translation of several of these targets have been extensively investigated, and have shown sufficient activity in preclinical models to warrant clinical trials.

Apoptosis (Bcl-2)

The *bcl-2* gene provides a rational target for antisense strategies. Overexpression leads to cellular resistance to programed cell death (apoptosis) (169), resulting in chemoresistance *in vitro* (170). Bcl-2 was identified by virtue of its involvement in the t(14;18) translocation, in which the *bcl-2* gene is brought under the transcriptional control of the immunoglobulin heavy chain promoter. This accounts for the overexpression of Bcl-2 in 70–80 per cent of cases of follicular non-Hodgkin's lymphoma (NHL) (171). This and other mechanisms also lead to Bcl-2 upregulation in approximately 30–50 per cent of cases of diffuse large B-cell NHL (172–174), and in many other malignancies including small cell lung cancer (175), prostate cancer (176, 177), breast cancer (178–180), nasopharyngeal cancer (181), colorectal cancer (182, 183), gastric cancer (182), pancreatic cancer (184), multiple myeloma (185), acute myeloid leukemia (186), acute lymphoblastic leukemia (186), and melanoma (187). There is evidence for an etiological role of Bcl-2 overexpression in lymphoma. Transgenic mice with deregulated Bcl-2 expression initially develop lymphoid hyperplasia with extended B-cell survival (188). In some cases, this progresses to diffuse large B-cell lymphoma, often with the accumulation of additional genetic abnormalities such as rearrangement of the *c-myc* gene (189). Bcl-2 expression was also found to be an independent poor prognostic factor in patients with diffuse large B-cell NHL (172–174).

Antisense oligonucleotides targeting *bcl-2* have been shown to reduce *bcl-2* mRNA and protein levels *in vitro* (190), and to reverse chemoresistance of Bcl-2-expressing lymphoma cell lines (191). It has also been demonstrated that eradication of lymphoma can be achieved in a SCID-mouse model of human NHL by a 14-day subcutaneous infusion of an 18-mer phosphorothioate oligonucleotide targeting the first 6 codons of the *bcl-2* mRNA open reading frame (79). The antilymphoma effect was dependent on oligonucleotide dose and the duration of treatment, and was sequence-specific. Similar anti-lymphoma activity was observed in non-obese diabetic SCID mice that lack NK-cell activity as well as T and B lymphocytes, suggesting that antitumor activity was the result of specific Bcl-2 downregulation and not immune stimulation. The active dose achieved plasma levels of approximately 1 μg/ml. This oligonucleotide (G3139, Genta Inc, Lexington, MA) was administered to 21 patients with relapsed, pretreated NHL in dose-escalating cohorts from 4.6 to 195.8 mg/m^2/day as a 14-day continuous subcutaneous infusion. Antitumor activity was observed, with an objective complete response in one patient, and a minor response in two other patients. Reductions in the number of circulating lymphoma cells in the peripheral blood were seen in 10 of 14 patients with peripheral blood involvement, and lymphoma-related symptoms were improved in 6 of the 10 patients with such symptoms. Importantly, Bcl-2 protein levels in patients' tumor cells were assessed by fluorescence-activated cell sorting before and after treatment, and were found to be reduced by treatment in 7 of 16 evaluable cases (165). Correlation of steady-state plasma levels of G3139 with reduction in Bcl-2 protein expression reveals that plasma concentrations of 1 μg/ml are adequate to downregulate Bcl-2, and that further dose escalation does not appear to have an additional effect (Fig. 10.3). No evidence for a Th1-

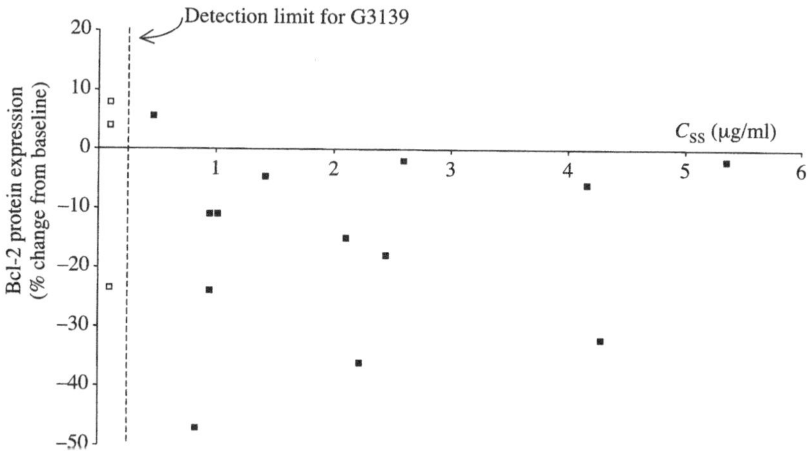

Fig. 10.3 Plasma level of G3139 associated with downregulation of Bcl-2 protein. Maximum observed reduction in Bcl-2 protein expression during the course of therapy with a 14-day subcutaneous infusion of G3139, a phosphorothioate oligonucleotide targeting *bcl-2*, is plotted against the steady-state plasma concentration, C_{SS}, of G3139. Bcl-2 protein expression was evaluated by fluorescence-activated cell sorting of peripheral blood or bone marrow mononuclear cells, and cells obtained from fine needle aspirates of involved lymph nodes. Plasma G3139 concentration was measured by high-performance liquid chromatography. Changes in Bcl-2 protein in patients with plasma G3139 levels below the detection limit of our assay (0.25 μg/ml) are represented by open symbols.

type immune response or NK-cell activation was found in 4 patients in whom this was investigated, suggesting that the antitumor effects observed were likely to be the result of Bcl-2 downregulation rather than a non-specific immune activation. A second phase I trial of G3139 therapy has been conducted in patients with advanced prostate or renal cell carcinoma. Treatment was given as a 14-day continuous IV infusion to 15 patients over a dose range of 0.6–2.3 mg/kg/day followed by 4 weeks' observation. Stable disease was seen in 3 patients (2 renal cell carcinoma, 1 prostate carcinoma) over 3, 3, and 2 cycles of treatment, respectively (192).

Bcl-2 antisense oligonucleotide therapy has also been investigated as a chemosensitizing strategy. Several *in vivo* xenograft models of human tumors have demonstrated accelerated apoptosis and reduced tumor viability following treatment with a combination of G3139 and conventional cytotoxic agents, compared with chemotherapy treatment alone (193–196). Preliminary reports of a clinical trial in which patients with treatment-refractory malignant melanoma were treated with a combination of G3139 and dacarbazine suggest that this may be a useful approach (197). Reductions in Bcl-2 protein levels and increased rates of apoptosis were observed in serial tumor biopsies following the initial *bcl-2* antisense therapy. Apoptosis was further enhanced following the addition of dacarbazine therapy at standard doses, and disappearance of select metastatic lesions was observed. Further clinical trials investigating combinations of *bcl-2* antisense therapy and chemotherapy are underway.

Signal transduction

Several proteins involved in the transduction of signals leading to cellular proliferation and differentiation have been extensively investigated as targets of antisense oligonucleotides for the treatment of cancer. Protein kinase C-α (PKC-α) is a phospholipid-dependent cytoplasmic serine-threonine kinase. It is activated by 1,2-diacylglycerol, which is generated by the cleavage of membrane phospholipids by phospholipases. Phospholipases are activated by a number of growth factors and hormones, and are responsible for the activation of several cytoplasmic PKC enzymes. These convey signals that lead to proliferation or differentiation, and their overactivity has been implicated in carcinogenesis (198). A 20-mer phosphorothioate oligonucleotide complementary to the 3'-untranslated region of PKC-α mRNA (ISIS 3521) specifically

reduced PKC-α mRNA expression *in vitro* (199). This molecule had antiproliferative activity in xenograft models of glioblastoma, breast cancer, bladder cancer, colon cancer, and lung cancer (76, 200). Three phase I trials of ISIS 3521 administered to patients with a variety of advanced solid tumors have been reported (161, 166, 201). No attempts were made to evaluate changes in target protein expression in these studies, which makes pharmacodynamic interpretation difficult. However, two patients with small lymphocytic lymphoma treated with alternate-day 2-hour IV infusions of ISIS 3521 for 3 of every 4 weeks achieved complete remissions after 17 and 9 cycles of therapy, respectively. An additional 8 patients of the 34 treated with this regimen had stable disease after 2 months (161). Of the 21 patients treated with a continuous IV infusion of ISIS 3521 for 3 of every 4 weeks, 3 patients with epithelial ovarian cancer had evidence for a tumor response. This comprised objective reduction in the size of an abdominal mass in one patient, as assessed by computerized tomography (CT) scan, and a sustained reduction in serum CA-125 levels in the other two (166). On the basis of these results, phase II trials of this agent have been initiated in ovarian cancer, low-grade NHL, and colorectal cancer.

Raf-1 is a serine/threonine protein kinase encoded by *c-raf*-1 that acts downstream of Ras in the mitogen-activated protein (MAP) kinase signal transduction pathway. This pathway is responsible for inducing cellular proliferation and differentiation in response to certain growth factors (202). Raf-1 is also activated independently of Ras by Bcl-2 (203) and by PKC-α (204) and promotes expression of the multidrug resistance gene *mdr1* (205). Constitutive expression of mutant Ras and Raf-1 occurs in many human tumors, and such mutations have oncogenic potential *in vitro* (206). ISIS 5132 is a 20-mer phosphorothioate oligonucleotide designed to hybridize to the 3'-untranslated region of the *c-raf*-1 mRNA, with sequence-specific activity in reducing *c-raf*-1 mRNA expression *in vitro* and *in vivo* (75). Antitumor activity *in vivo* was also observed against three human tumor xenograft models, A549 tumors (lung cancer), T24 tumors (bladder cancer), and MDA-MB-231 tumors (breast cancer), in nude mice (75). However, the oligonucleotide dose required for antitumor effects was probably higher than initially reported (207). Three phase I clinical trials employing ISIS 5132 have been reported to date (160, 167, 208). The first trial used a 3-week continuous IV infusion schedule, which was followed by a week off treatment before commencing the next cycle (167). Thirty-four patients with a variety of advanced cancers were treated with doses ranging from 0.5 to 5 mg/kg/day. Activity was reported in 2 patients, one with ovarian cancer who achieved a 97 per cent reduction in CA-125 levels and one with renal cancer who had stable disease for a period of 9 months on study. The effect of treatment on target mRNA or protein expression was not reported. The second study used a schedule of 2-hour IV infusion on 3 days each week for 3 of every 4 weeks (160). Thirty-one patients with refractory malignancies were treated at doses ranging from 0.5 to 6 mg/kg. C-*raf*-1 mRNA levels in peripheral blood mononuclear cells were evaluated by reverse transcriptase polymerase chain reaction (RT-PCR), and were found to be reduced by ISIS 5132 treatment in 13 out of the 14 patients treated at doses of 2.5 mg/kg or more, within 48 hours of the initial dose. Two patients were reported to have prolonged stable disease, one with metastatic colorectal cancer (8 months) and one with renal cell carcinoma (10 months). Interestingly, in these two patients the suppression of *c-raf*-1 mRNA levels mirrored the time-course of disease stabilization. The final trial, reported in preliminary form, used a 24-hour weekly IV infusion of ISIS 5132 at doses ranging from 6–24 mg/kg/week. Fourteen patients had been treated at the time of the report, but no objective responses had been observed (208).

ISIS 2503 is a 20-mer phosphorothioate oligonucleotide designed to bind to the translation–initiation region of H-*ras* mRNA. This has been shown *in vitro* to reduce H-*ras* mRNA expression and to inhibit proliferation of T24 cells that contain a codon 12 activating H-*ras* mutation (209). *In vivo* activity has also been demonstrated in a number of tumor types including pancreas, breast, lung, colon, and bladder cancers (209). Two phase I clinical trials of this oligonucleotide have been reported, in which ISIS 2503 was administered as a 14-day continuous IV infusion followed by a 7-day break (210) or as a 24-hour weekly infusion (211). A total of 36 patients with advanced cancer have been treated on the two protocols, with doses up to 10 mg/kg/day in the continuous infusion study and 18 mg/kg/week in the 24-hour infusion trial. Although no objective responses have been observed, disease stabilization was reported in 4 patients for 9, 18, 24, and 30 weeks, respectively. Northern blot assay was used to demonstrate a reduction in H-*ras* mRNA expression in peripheral blood mononuclear cells at the 1.0 and 2.0 mg/kg/day dose levels, with further analyses pending (210).

Suppression of the expression of a single signal transduction gene may not be sufficient to induce tumor regression in patients. Combination of *c-raf*-1 antisense therapy with radiotherapy has been investigated *in vivo* (212). Athymic mice bearing SQ-20B tumors (a cell line derived from a laryngeal squamous cell carcinoma in a patient who failed after radical radiotherapy) were treated with radiotherapy alone, ISIS 3521 liposomal formulation alone, or a combination of the two treatments. Either treatment alone caused a transient inhibition of tumor growth, but the combination of treatments led to significant and sustained tumor regression. A clinical trial combining PKC-α antisense therapy with carboplatin and paclitaxel chemotherapy produced 5 partial responses among 6 patients with non-small-cell lung cancer at the time of a preliminary report (213). The contribution of the antisense treatment to these results is being investigated in a randomized phase III trial that began in 2000. This antisense molecule has also been combined with 5-fluorouracil and leucovorin in a phase I trial, which was reported following the enrollment of 10 patients with advanced cancer (214). Two partial responses were observed in patients with colon cancer and adenocarcinoma of unknown primary site, respectively. Another approach being considered is the combination of two antisense oligonucleotides with different targets, for instance, *c-raf*-1 and PKC-α. This approach is rational in view of the multiple genetic abnormalities present in most malignant cells, which may allow them to overcome the effects of disruption of a single signaling pathway.

Bcr-abl

Chronic myelogenous leukemia (CML) is characterized by a chromosomal translocation involving the c-*abl* gene on chromosome 9,and the *bcr* gene on chromosome 22, resulting in the formation of the Philadelphia chromosome (Ph) and the neogene *bcr/abl*. The tyrosine kinase encoded by this gene has pleotropic activity on a number of downstream effector molecules including Ras, MAP kinase, and Bcl-2. This presents a unique, tumor-cell-specific target for antisense therapeutic approaches. Antisense oligonucleotides designed to bind to one of the three common *bcr-abl* junction sequences were able to reduce colony formation from primary leukemic blast cells, while having no effect on granulocyte–macrophage colony formation from normal marrow progenitors (99, 215). Such oligonucleotides also effectively eradicated Ph+ CML cells from SCID mice, and extended their survival (74). Ex-*vivo* bone marrow purging with *bcr-abl* antisense oligonucleotides has been investigated as a possible therapeutic strategy (216, 217). Eight patients with CML in second chronic phase or at the time of transformation in accelerated phase were treated with a standard conditioning chemotherapy regimen followed by autologous bone marrow transplantation. Prior to re-infusion, mononuclear bone marrow cells were treated *in vitro* for 24 or 72 hours with 150 μg/ml of a junction-specific antisense oligonucleotide. Hematological reconstitution occurred in all patients. Two patients had a complete karyotypic response, while the other 6 patients had a minimal or no response. Prolonged survival duration was reported for this small group of patients, suggesting a beneficial effect of bone marrow purging. A clinical study of IV administered antisense oligonucleotides targeting *bcr-abl* in patients with blast crisis CML has been initiated (218).

Transcription factors

The Myb protein is encoded by the *c-myb* proto-oncogene and acts as a regulator of the G_1/S transition in cycling hemopoietic cells. It probably also functions as a transactivator of a number of important cellular genes such as the Kit receptor, CD4, and CD34. As such it is critical for normal hemopoietic cell development, but it is also required for leukemic hemopoiesis, with evidence to suggest that leukemic cells are more dependent on Myb activity than are normal hemopoietic cells (reviewed in reference 219). Antisense oligonucleotides targeting *c-myb* mRNA have shown greater inhibitory activity against leukemia cell lines and primary patient leukemic cultures than against normal hemopoietic cells (220). Treatment of SCID mice previously engrafted with K562 leukemia cells with *c-myb* antisense oligonucleotides extended their survival and reduced the number of leukemic cells in the central nervous system and ovaries of these animals. Control oligonucleotides were ineffective (221). Clinical trials have evaluated the use of antisense oligonucleotides targeting *c-myb* for bone marrow purging prior to autologous bone marrow transplantation in patients with chronic phase or accelerated phase CML, and as IV treatment to patients with accelerated phase or blast crisis CML (168). Extending the exposure of bone marrow cells *ex vivo* to oligonucleotide from 24 to 72 hours resulted in poor engraftment, suggesting toxicity to normal bone marrow progenitors. Otherwise, the treatment was well tolerated, but clinical benefit to patients resulting from the antisense treatment was uncertain. C-Myc is a second nuclear transcription factor that has known oncogenic potential, which has been investigated as a potential target for antisense oligonucleotide therapeutics. As yet no clinical trials have been undertaken, but *in vitro* and *in vivo* activity of *c-myc* antisense oligonucleotides has been demonstrated in models of Burkitt's lymphoma (222), melanoma (223), and leukemia (223). Combination of antisense molecules targeting *bcr-abl* and *c-myc* was found to have synergistic antiproliferative effects in CML blast crisis primary cell cultures, and to enhance survival of SCID mice injected with CML blast crisis primary cells (224).

Conclusions

Antisense oligonucleotide therapy has come a long way from the initial experiments of Zamecnik and Stephenson. Fundamental issues of oligonucleotide stability and access to the target site have been addressed, and overcome to a certain extent. Non-sequence-specific effects of phosphorothioate oligonucleotides in particular, which threatened to cast doubt on the validity of many of the earlier positive results, have been recognized and measures taken to control for them. Fortunately, clinical trials have clearly demonstrated the tolerability of these molecules at doses exceeding those required for pharmacological activity, together with feasible pharmacokinetic behavior. Most importantly, specific downregulation of target mRNA and protein has been demonstrated in clinical trials, providing evidence that this treatment approach is tenable. Future developments likely to enhance the utility of antisense molecules include the further chemical modification of the oligonucleotide backbone, and the development of effective delivery systems, areas of research that are already making good progress. These refinements have the potential to substantially increase the activity of antisense oligonucleotides. The best way to use particular oligonucleotides in the treatment of various malignancies has also yet to be established. While the specific downregulation of a single target gene is an attractive concept, it is likely to be inadequate to control tumor growth in view of the multiple genetic abnormalities present in most human cancers. In this regard, combinations of antisense oligonucleotides with other treatment modalities such as chemotherapy, radiotherapy, or even other 'biological' therapies may prove useful. Downregulation of multiple genes by antisense techniques is another interesting possibility. The evidence for a relatively wide therapeutic window for phosphorothioate oligonucleotides means that several genes could potentially be targeted without exceeding tolerable total phosphorothioate doses.

References

1. Zamecnik PC, Stephenson ML. Inhibition of Rous sarcoma virus replication and cell transformation by a specific oligodeoxynucleotide. Proc Natl Acad Sci, USA 1978, **75**, 280–4.
2. Simons RW, Kleckner N. Translational control of IS10 transposition. Cell 1983, **34**, 683–91.
3. Mizuno T, Chou MY, Inouye M. A unique mechanism regulating gene expression: translational inhibition by a complementary RNA transcript (micRNA). Proc Natl Acad Sci, USA 1984, **81**, 1966–70.
4. Izant JG, Weintraub H. Inhibition of thymidine kinase gene expression by anti-sense RNA: a molecular approach to genetic analysis. Cell 1984, **36**, 1007–15.
5. Plum GE, Pilch DS, Singleton SF, et al. Nucleic acid hybridization: triplex stability and energetics. Annu Rev Biophys Biomol Struct 1995, **24**, 319–50.
6. de Bizemont T, Duval Valentin G, Sun JS, et al. Alternate strand recognition of double-helical DNA by (T,G)-containing oligonucleotides in the presence of a triple helix-specific ligand. Nucl Acids Res 1996, **24**, 1136–43.
7. Olivas WM, Maher LJ, 3rd. Overcoming potassium-mediated triplex inhibition. Nucl Acids Res 1995, **23**, 1936–41.
8. Maine IP, Kodadek T. Efficient unwinding of triplex DNA by a DNA helicase. Biochem Biophys Res Commun 1994, **204**, 1119–24.
9. Gryaznov SM, Lloyd DH, Chen JK, et al. Oligonucleotide N3′ → P5′ phosphoramidates. Proc Natl Acad Sci, USA 1995, **92**, 5798–802.
10. Escude C, Giovannangeli C, Sun JS, et al. Stable triple helices formed by oligonucleotide N3′ → P5′ phosphoramidates inhibit transcription elongation. Proc Natl Acad Sci, USA 1996, **93**, 4365–9.
11. Kukreti S, Sun JS, Garestier T, et al. Extension of the range of DNA sequences available for triple helix formation: stabilization of mismatched triplexes by acridine-containing oligonucleotides. Nucl Acids Res 1997, **25**, 4264–70.
12. Silver GC, Nguyen CH, Boutorine AS, et al. Conjugates of oligonucleotides with triplex-specific intercalating agents. Stabilization of triple-helical DNA in the promoter region of the gene for the alpha-subunit of interleukin 2 (IL-2R alpha). Bioconjug Chem 1997, **8**, 15–22.
13. de Bizemont T, Sun JS, Garestier T, et al. New junction models for alternate-strand triple-helix formation. Chem Biol 1998, **5**, 755–62.
14. Giovannangeli C, Helene C. Progress in developments of triplex-based strategies. Antisense Nucl Acid Drug Dev 1997, **7**, 413–21.
15. Bailey CP, Dagle JM, Weeks DL. Cationic oligonucleotides can mediate specific inhibition of gene expression in Xenopus oocytes. Nucl Acids Res 1998, **26**, 4860–7.
16. Joseph J, Kandala JC, Veerapanane D, et al. Antiparallel polypurine phosphorothioate oligonucleotides form stable triplexes with the rat alpha1(I) collagen gene promoter and inhibit transcription in cultured rat fibroblasts. Nucl Acids Res 1997, **25**, 2182–8.
17. Kim HG, Reddoch JF, Mayfield C, et al. Inhibition of transcription of the human c-myc protooncogene by intermolecular triplex. Biochemistry 1998, **37**, 2299–304.
18. Musso M, Wang JC, Van Dyke MW. *In vivo* persistence of DNA triple helices containing psoralen-conjugated oligodeoxyribonucleotides. Nucl Acids Res 1996, **24**, 4924–32.
19. Debin A, Malvy C, Svinarchuk F. Investigation of the formation and intracellular stability of purine (purine/pyrimidine) triplexes. Nucl Acids Res 1997, **25**, 1965–74.
20. Orson FM, Thomas DW, McShan WM, et al. Oligonucleotide inhibition of IL2R alpha mRNA transcription by promoter region collinear triplex formation in lymphocytes. Nucl Acids Res 1991, **19**, 3435–41.
21. Ing NH, Beekman JM, Kessler DJ, et al. *In vivo* transcription of a progesterone-responsive gene is specifically inhibited by a triplex-forming oligonucleotide. Nucl Acids Res 1993, **21**, 2789–96.
22. Thomas TJ, Faaland CA, Gallo MA, et al. Suppression of c-myc oncogene expression by a polyamine-complexed triplex forming oligonucleotide in MCF-7 breast cancer cells. Nucl Acids Res 1995, **23**, 3594–9.
23. Tu GC, Cao QN, Israel Y. Inhibition of gene expression by triple helix formation in hepatoma cells. J Biol Chem 1995, **270**, 28402–7.
24. Porumb H, Gousset H, Letellier R, et al. Temporary *ex vivo* inhibition of the expression of the human oncogene HER2 (NEU) by a triple helix-forming oligonucleotide. Cancer Res 1996, **56**, 515–22.
25. Kochetkova M, Shannon MF. DNA triplex formation selectively inhibits granulocyte–macrophage colony-stimulating factor gene expression in human T cells. J Biol Chem 1996, **271**, 14438–44.
26. Kochetkova M, Iversen PO, Lopez AF, et al. Deoxyribonucleic acid triplex formation inhibits granulocyte macrophage colony-stimulating factor gene expression and suppresses growth in juvenile myelomonocytic leukemic cells. J Clin Invest 1997, **99**, 3000–8.
27. Postel EH, Flint SJ, Kessler DJ, et al. Evidence that a triplex-forming oligodeoxyribonucleotide binds to the c-myc promoter in HeLa cells, thereby reducing c-myc mRNA levels. Proc Natl Acad Sci, USA 1991, **88**, 8227–31.
28. Wang G, Seidman MM, Glazer PM. Mutagenesis in mammalian cells induced by triple helix formation and transcription-coupled repair. Science 1996, **271**, 802–5.
29. Plenat F. Animal models of antisense oligonucleotides: lessons for use in humans. Mol Med Today 1996, **2**, 250–7.

30. Sands H, Gorey-Feret LJ, Cocuzza AJ, *et al.* Biodistribution and metabolism of internally 3H-labeled oligonucleotides. I. Comparison of a phosphodiester and a phosphorothioate. Mol Pharmacol 1994, **45**, 932–43.

31. Stein C, Cohen J: Phosphorothioate oligodeoxynucleotide analogues. In: Oligodeoxynucleotides: antisense inhibitors of gene expression (ed. J Cohen). Macmillan, London, 1989, 97–117.

32. Crooke ST. Antisense technology. Curr Opin Biotechnol 1991, **2**, 282–7.

33. Gao WY, Han FS, Storm C, *et al.* Phosphorothioate oligonucleotides are inhibitors of human DNA polymerases and RNAase H: implications for antisense technology. Mol Pharmacol 1992, **41**, 223–9.

34. LaPlanche LA, James TL, Powell C, *et al.* Phosphorothioate-modified oligodeoxyribonucleotides. III. NMR and UV spectroscopic studies of the Rp–Rp, Sp–Sp, and Rp–Sp duplexes, [d(GGSAATTCC)]2, derived from diastereomeric O-ethyl phosphorothioates. Nucl Acids Res 1986, **14**, 9081–93.

35. Stein CA. Does antisense exist? Nat Med 1995, **1**, 1119–21.

36. Kitajima I, Unoki K, Maruyama I. Phosphorothioate oligodeoxynucleotides inhibit basic fibroblast growth factor-induced angiogenesis *in vitro* and *in vivo*. Antisense Nucl Acid Drug Dev 1999, **9**, 233–9.

37. Jansen B, Wadl H, Inoue SA, *et al.* Phosphorothioate oligonucleotides reduce melanoma growth in a SCID-hu mouse model by a nonantisense mechanism. Antisense Res Dev 1995, **5**, 271–7.

38. Wooldridge JE, Ballas Z, Krieg AM, *et al.* Immunostimulatory oligodeoxynucleotides containing CpG motifs enhance the efficacy of monoclonal antibody therapy of lymphoma. Blood 1997, **89**, 2994–8.

39. Pisetsky DS, Reich CF, 3rd. The influence of base sequence on the immunological properties of defined oligonucleotides. Immunopharmacology 1998, **40**, 199–208.

40. Ballas ZK, Rasmussen WL, Krieg AM. Induction of NK activity in murine and human cells by CpG motifs in oligodeoxynucleotides and bacterial DNA. J Immunol 1996, **157**, 1840–5.

41. Jakob T, Walker PS, Krieg AM, *et al.* Activation of cutaneous dendritic cells by CpG-containing oligodeoxynucleotides: a role for dendritic cells in the augmentation of Th1 responses by immunostimulatory DNA. J Immunol 1998, **161**, 3042–9.

42. Thierry AR, Dritschilo A. Intracellular availability of unmodified, phosphorothioated and liposomally encapsulated oligodeoxynucleotides for antisense activity. Nucl Acids Res 1992, **20**, 5691–8.

43. Zhou W, Agrawal S. Mixed-backbone oligonucleotides as second-generation antisense agents with reduced phosphorothioate-related side effects. Bioorg Med Chem Lett 1998, **8**, 3269–74.

44. Agrawal S, Jiang Z, Zhao Q, *et al.* Mixed-backbone oligonucleotides as second generation antisense oligonucleotides: *in vitro* and *in vivo* studies. Proc Natl Acad Sci, USA 1997, **94**, 2620–5.

45. Nellen W, Lichtenstein C. What makes an mRNA antisense-itive? Trends Biochem Sci 1993, **18**, 419–23.

46. Shakin SH, Liebhaber SA. Destabilization of messenger RNA/complementary DNA duplexes by the elongating 80 S ribosome. J Biol Chem 1986, **261**, 16018–25.

47. DeDionisio L, Gryaznov SM. Analysis of a ribonuclease H digestion of N3′ → P5′ phosphoramidate–RNA duplexes by capillary gel electrophoresis. J Chromatogr B Biomed Appl 1995, **669**, 125–31.

48. Boulme F, Freund F, Moreau S, *et al.* Modified (PNA, 2′-O-methyl and phosphoramidate) anti-TAR antisense oligonucleotides as strong and specific inhibitors of *in vitro* HIV-1 reverse transcription. Nucl Acids Res 1998, **26**, 5492–500.

49. Skorski T, Perrotti D, Nieborowska-Skorska M, *et al.* Antileukemia effect of c-myc N3′ → P5′ phosphoramidate antisense oligonucleotides *in vivo*. Proc Natl Acad Sci, USA 1997, **94**, 3966–71.

50. Mori K, Subasinghe C, Cohen JS. Oligodeoxynucleotide analogs with 5′-linked anthraquinone. FEBS Lett 1989, **249**, 213–18.

51. Maitra RK, Li G, Xiao W, *et al.* Catalytic cleavage of an RNA target by 2–5A antisense and RNAse L. J Biol Chem 1995, **270**, 15071–5.

52. Maran A, Waller CF, Paranjape JM, *et al.* 2′,5′-Oligoadenylate-antisense chimeras cause RNAse L to selectively degrade bcr/abl mRNA in chronic myelogenous leukemia cells. Blood 1998, **92**, 4336–43.

53. Xiao W, Li G, Player MR, *et al.* Nuclease-resistant composite 2′,5′-oligoadenylate-3′,5′-oligonucleotides for the targeted destruction of RNA: 2–5A-iso-antisense. J Med Chem 1998, **41**, 1531–9.

54. Shoji Y, Akhtar S, Periasamy A, *et al.* Mechanism of cellular uptake of modified oligodeoxynucleotides containing methylphosphonate linkages. Nucl Acids Res 1991, **19**, 5543–50.

55. Bennett RM. As nature intended? The uptake of DNA and oligonucleotides by eukaryotic cells. Antisense Res Dev 1993, **3**, 235–41.

56. Yakubov LA, Deeva EA, Zarytova VF, *et al.* Mechanism of oligonucleotide uptake by cells: involvement of specific receptors? Proc Natl Acad Sci, USA 1989, **86**, 6454–8.

57. Beltinger C, Saragovi HU, Smith RM, *et al.* Binding, uptake, and intracellular trafficking of phosphorothioate-modified oligodeoxynucleotides. J Clin Invest 1995, **95**, 1814–23.

58. Geselowitz DA, Neckers LM. Bovine serum albumin is a major oligonucleotide-binding protein found on the surface of cultured cells. Antisense Res Dev 1995, **5**, 213–17.

59. Bergan R, Hakim F, Schwartz GN, *et al.* Electroporation of synthetic oligodeoxynucleotides: a novel technique for *ex vivo* bone marrow purging. Blood 1996, **88**, 731–41.

60. Flanagan WM, Wagner RW. Potent and selective gene inhibition using antisense oligodeoxynucleotides. Mol Cell Biochem 1997, **172**, 213–25.

61. Juliano RL, Akhtar S. Liposomes as a drug delivery system for antisense oligonucleotides. Antisense Res Dev 1992, **2**, 165–76.

62. Lewis JG, Lin KY, Kothavale A, *et al.* A serum-resistant cytofectin for cellular delivery of antisense oligo-

deoxynucleotides and plasmid DNA. Proc Natl Acad Sci, USA 1996, **93**, 3176–81.

63. Zelphati O, Szoka FC, Jr. Mechanism of oligonucleotide release from cationic liposomes. Proc Natl Acad Sci, USA 1996, **93**, 11493–8.

64. Zelphati O, Uyechi LS, Barron LG, *et al*. Effect of serum components on the physico-chemical properties of cationic lipid/oligonucleotide complexes and on their interactions with cells. Biochim Biophys Acta 1998, **1390**, 119–33.

65. Wyman TB, Nicol F, Zelphati O, *et al*. Design, synthesis, and characterization of a cationic peptide that binds to nucleic acids and permeabilizes bilayers. Biochemistry 1997, **36**, 3008–17.

66. Kim JS, Kim BI, Maruyama A, *et al*. A new non-viral DNA delivery vector: the terplex system. J Controlled Release 1998, **53**, 175–82.

67. Li B, Hughes JA, Phillips MI. Uptake and efflux of intact antisense phosphorothioate deoxyoligonucleotide directed against angiotensin receptors in bovine adrenal cells. Neurochem Int 1997, **31**, 393–403.

68. Clarenc JP, Lebleu B, Leonetti JP. Characterization of the nuclear binding sites of oligodeoxyribonucleotides and their analogs. J Biol Chem 1993, **268**, 5600–4.

69. Shoeman RL, Hartig R, Huang Y, *et al*. Fluorescence microscopic comparison of the binding of phosphodiester and phosphorothioate (antisense) oligodeoxyribonucleotides to subcellular structures, including intermediate filaments, the endoplasmic reticulum, and the nuclear interior. Antisense Nucl Acid Drug Dev 1997, **7**, 291–308.

70. Corrias MV, Guarnaccia F, Ponzoni M. Bioavailability of antisense oligonucleotides in neuroblastoma cells: comparison of efficacy among different types of molecules. J Neurooncol 1997, **31**, 171–80.

71. Etore F, Tenu JP, Teiger E, *et al*. Sequence dependency of the internalization and distribution of phosphorothioate oligonucleotides in vascular smooth muscle cells. Biochem Pharmacol 1998, **55**, 1465–73.

72. Wu-Pong S, Bard J, Huffman J, *et al*. Oligonucleotide biological activity: relationship to the cell cycle and nuclear transport. Biol Cell 1997, **89**, 257–61.

73. Sokol DL, Zhang X, Lu P, *et al*. Real time detection of DNA·RNA hybridization in living cells. Proc Natl Acad Sci, USA 1998, **95**, 11538–43.

74. Skorski T, Nieborowska-Skorska M, Nicolaides NC, *et al*. Suppression of Philadelphia 1 leukemia cell growth in mice by BCR-ABL antisense oligodeoxynucleotide. Proc Natl Acad Sci, USA 1994, **91**, 4504–8.

75. Monia BP, Johnston JF, Geiger T, *et al*. Antitumor activity of a phosphorothioate antisense oligodeoxynucleotide targeted against C-raf kinase. Nat Med 1996, **2**, 668–75.

76. Dean N, McKay R, Miraglia L, *et al*. Inhibition of growth of human tumor cell lines in nude mice by an antisense oligonucleotide inhibitor of protein kinase C-alpha expression. Cancer Res 1996, **56**, 3499–507.

77. McGraw K, McKay R, Miraglia L, *et al*. Antisense oligonucleotide inhibitors of isozymes of protein kinase C: *in vitro* and *in vivo* activity, and clinical development as anti-cancer therapeutics. Anticancer Drug Des 1997, **12**, 315–26.

78. Bennett CF, Kornbrust D, Henry S, *et al*. An ICAM-1 antisense oligonucleotide prevents and reverses dextran sulfate sodium-induced colitis in mice. J Pharmacol Exp Ther 1997, **280**, 988–1000.

79. Cotter FE, Johnson P, Hall P, *et al*. Antisense oligonucleotides suppress B-cell lymphoma growth in a SCID-hu mouse model. Oncogene 1994, **9**, 3049–55.

80. Raynaud FI, Orr RM, Goddard PM, *et al*. Pharmacokinetics of G3139 a phosphorothioate oligodeoxynucleotide antisense to bcl-2 following intravenous administration or continuous subcutaneous infusion to mice. J Pharmacol Exp Ther 1997, **281**, 420–7.

81. Bijsterbosch MK, Manoharan M, Rump ET, *et al*. *In vivo* fate of phosphorothioate antisense oligodeoxynucleotides: predominant uptake by scavenger receptors on endothelial liver cells. Nucl Acids Res 1997, **25**, 3290–3296.

82. DeLong RK, Nolting A, Fisher M, *et al*. Comparative pharmacokinetics, tissue distribution, and tumor accumulation of phosphorothioate, phosphorodithioate, and methylphosphonate oligonucleotides in nude mice. Antisense Nucl Acid Drug Dev 1997, 7, 71–7.

83. Maurer N, Mori A, Palmer L, *et al*. Lipid-based systems for the intracellular delivery of genetic drugs. Mol Membr Biol 1999, **16**, 129–40.

84. Wheeler JJ, Palmer L, Ossanlou M, *et al*. Stabilized plasmid-lipid particles: construction and characterization. Gene Ther 1999, **6**, 271–81.

85. Aoki M, Morishita R, Muraishi A, *et al*. Efficient *in vivo* gene transfer into the heart in the rat myocardial infarction model using the HVJ (hemagglutinating virus of Japan)—liposome method. J Mol Cell Cardiol 1997, **29**, 949–59.

86. Kaneda Y. Development of a novel fusogenic viral liposome system (HVJ–liposomes) and its applications to the treatment of acquired diseases. Mol Membr Biol 1999, **16**, 119–22.

87. Uehara T, Honda K, Hatano E, *et al*. Gene transfer to the rat biliary tract with the HVJ–cationic liposome method. J Hepatol 1999, **30**, 836–42.

88. Yamada K, Moriguchi A, Morishita R, *et al*. Efficient oligonucleotide delivery using the HVJ–liposome method in the central nervous system. Am J Physiol 1996, **271**, R1212–20.

89. Yonemitsu Y, Kaneda Y, Muraishi A, *et al*. HVJ (Sendai virus)–cationic liposomes: a novel and potentially effective liposome-mediated technique for gene transfer to the airway epithelium. Gene Ther 1997, **4**, 631–8.

90. Ma DD, Wei AQ. Enhanced delivery of synthetic oligonucleotides to human leukaemic cells by liposomes and immunoliposomes. Leuk Res 1996, **20**, 925–30.

91. Helene C, Toulme JJ. Specific regulation of gene expression by antisense, sense and antigene nucleic acids. Biochem Biophys Acta 1990, **1046**, 99–125.

92. Khan IM, Coulson JM. A novel method to stabilise antisense oligonucleotides against exonuclease degradation. Nucl Acids Res 1993, **21**, 2957–8.

93. Eder PS, Walder JA. Ribonuclease H from K562 human erythroleukemia cells. Purification, characterization, and substrate specificity. J Biol Chem 1991, **266**, 6472–9.

94. Reed JC, Cuddy M, Haldar S, *et al*. Bcl-2-mediated tumorigenicity of a human T-lymphoid cell line: synergy

with *myc* and inhibition by bcl-2 antisense. Proc Natl Acad Sci, USA 1990, **87**, 3660–4.

95. Reed JC, Stein C, Subasighe C, *et al*. Antisense mediated inhibition of bcl-2 protooncogene expression and leukemic cell growth and survival: Comparisons of phosphodiester and phosphorothioate oligodeoxynucleotides. Cancer Res 1990, **50**, 6565–70.

96. Daaka Y, Wickstrom E. Target dependence of antisense oligonucleotide inhibition of c-Ha-ras p21 expression and focus formation in T24-transformed NIH3T3 cells. Oncogene Res 1990, **5**, 267–75.

97. Bacon T, Wickstrom E. Walking along the human c-myc mRNA with antisense oligodeoxynucleotides: maximum efficacy at the 5′ cap region. Oncogene Res 1991, **6**, 13–19.

98. Goodchild J. Inhibition of human immunodeficiency virus replication by antisense oligodeoxynucleotides. Proc Natl Acad Sci, USA 1988, **85**, 5507–11.

99. Szczylik C, Skorski T, Nicolaides N, *et al*. Selective inhibition of leukemia cell proliferation by BCR-ABL antisense oligodeoxynucleotides. Science 1991, **253**, 562–5.

100. Ziegler A, Luedke GH, Fabbro D, *et al*. Induction of apoptosis in small-cell lung cancer cells by an antisense oligonucleotide targeting the bcl-2 coding sequence. J Natl Cancer Inst 1997, **89**, 1027–36.

101. Sczakiel G, Homann M, Rittner K. Computer-aided search for effective antisense RNA target sequences of the human immunodeficiency virus type 1. Antisense Res Dev 1993, **3**, 45–52.

102. Ho SP, Bao Y, Lesher T, *et al*. Mapping of RNA accessible sites for antisense experiments with oligonucleotide libraries. Nat Biotechnol 1998, **16**, 59–63.

103. Southern EM, Case-Green SC, Elder JK, *et al*. Arrays of complementary oligonucleotides for analysing the hybridisation behaviour of nucleic acids. Nucl Acids Res 1994, **22**, 1368–73.

104. Milner N, Mir KU, Southern EM. Selecting effective antisense reagents on combinatorial oligonucleotide arrays. Nat Biotechnol 1997, **15**, 537–41.

105. Lima WF, Brown-Driver V, Fox M, *et al*. Combinatorial screening and rational optimization for hybridization to folded hepatitis C virus RNA of oligonucleotides with biological antisense activity. J Biol Chem 1997, **272**, 626–38.

106. Ho SP, Britton DH, Stone BA, *et al*. Potent antisense oligonucleotides to the human multidrug resistance-1 mRNA are rationally selected by mapping RNA-accessible sites with oligonucleotide libraries. Nucl Acids Res 1996, **24**, 1901–7.

107. Matveeva O, Felden B, Audlin S, *et al*. A rapid *in vitro* method for obtaining RNA accessibility patterns for complementary DNA probes: correlation with an intracellular pattern and known RNA structures. Nucl Acids Res 1997, **25**, 5010–16.

108. Matveeva O, Felden B, Tsodikov A, *et al*. Prediction of antisense oligonucleotide efficacy by *in vitro* methods. Nat Biotechnol 1998, **16**, 1374–5.

109. Reyderman L, Stavchansky S. Pharmacokinetics and biodistribution of a nucleotide-based thrombin inhibitor in rats. Pharm Res 1998, **15**, 904–10.

110. Sands H, Gorey-Feret LJ, Ho SP, *et al*. Biodistribution and metabolism of internally 3H-labeled oligonu-cleotides. II. 3′,5′-blocked oligonucleotides. Mol Pharmacol 1995, **47**, 636–46.

111. Iversen PL, Mata J, Tracewell WG, *et al*. Pharmacokinetics of an antisense phosphorothioate oligodeoxynucleotide against rev from human immunodeficiency virus type 1 in the adult male rat following single injections and continuous infusion. Antisense Res Dev 1994, **4**, 43–52.

112. Phillips JA, Craig SJ, Bayley D, *et al*. Pharmacokinetics, metabolism, and elimination of a 20-mer phosphorothioate oligodeoxynucleotide (CGP 69846A) after intravenous and subcutaneous administration. Biochem Pharmacol 1997, **54**, 657–68.

113. Geary RS, Leeds JM, Fitchett J, *et al*. Pharmacokinetics and metabolism in mice of a phosphorothioate oligonucleotide antisense inhibitor of C-raf-1 kinase expression. Drug Metab Dispos 1997, **25**, 1272–81.

114. Qian M, Chen SH, Von Hofe E, *et al*. Pharmacokinetics and tissue distribution of a DNA-methyltransferase antisense (MT-AS) oligonucleotide and its catabolites in tumor-bearing nude mice. J Pharmacol Exp Ther 1997, **282**, 663–70.

115. Temsamani J, Roskey A, Chaix C, *et al*. *In vivo* metabolic profile of a phosphorothioate oligodeoxyribonucleotide. Antisense Nucl Acid Drug Dev 1997, **7**, 159–65.

116. Grindel JM, Musick TJ, Jiang Z, *et al*. Pharmacokinetics and metabolism of an oligodeoxynucleotide phosphorothioate (GEM91) in cynomolgus monkeys following intravenous infusion. Antisense Nucl Acid Drug Dev 1998, **8**, 43–52.

117. Iversen PL, Copple BL, Tewary HK. Pharmacology and toxicology of phosphorothioate oligonucleotides in the mouse, rat, monkey and man. Toxicol Lett 1995, **82–83**, 425–30.

118. Butler M, Stecker K, Bennett CF. Cellular distribution of phosphorothioate oligodeoxynucleotides in normal rodent tissues. Lab Invest 1997, **77**, 379–88.

119. Carome MA, Kang YH, Bohen EM, *et al*. Distribution of the cellular uptake of phosphorothioate oligodeoxynucleotides in the rat kidney *in vivo*. Nephron 1997, **75**, 82–7.

120. Steward A, Christian RA, Hamilton KO, *et al*. Co-administration of polyanions with a phosphorothioate oligodeoxynucleotide (CGP 69846A): a role for the scavenger receptor in its *in vivo* disposition. Biochem Pharmacol 1998, **56**, 509–16.

121. Graham MJ, Crooke ST, Monteith DK, *et al*. *In vivo* distribution and metabolism of a phosphorothioate oligonucleotide within rat liver after intravenous administration. J Pharmacol Exp Ther 1998, **286**, 447–58.

122. Zhao Q, Zhou R, Temsamani J, *et al*. Cellular distribution of phosphorothioate oligonucleotide following intravenous administration in mice. Antisense Nucl Acid Drug Dev 1998, **8**, 451–8.

123. Wallace TL, Bazemore SA, Holm K, *et al*. Pharmacokinetics and distribution of a 33P-labeled anti-human immunodeficiency virus oligonucleotide (AR177) after single- and multiple-dose intravenous administration to rats. J Pharmacol Exp Ther 1997, **280**, 1480–8.

124. Wallace TL, Bazemore SA, Kornbrust DJ, *et al*. Repeat-dose toxicity and pharmacokinetics of a partial phos-

phorothioate anti-HIV oligonucleotide (AR177) after bolus intravenous administration to cynomolgus monkeys. J Pharmacol Exp Ther 1996, **278**, 1313–17.

125. Wallace TL, Bazemore SA, Kornbrust DJ, *et al*. Single-dose hemodynamic toxicity and pharmacokinetics of a partial phosphorothioate anti-HIV oligonucleotide (AR177) after intravenous infusion to cynomolgus monkeys. J Pharmacol Exp Ther 1996, **278**, 1306–12.

126. Yu RZ, Geary RS, Leeds JM, *et al*. Pharmacokinetics and tissue disposition in monkeys of an antisense oligonucleotide inhibitor of Ha-ras encapsulated in stealth liposomes. Pharm Res 1999, **16**, 1309–15.

127. Zimmer A. Antisense oligonucleotide delivery with polyhexylcyanoacrylate nanoparticles as carriers. Methods 1999, **18**, 286–295, 322.

128. Aynie I, Vauthier C, Chacun H, *et al*. Spongelike alginate nanoparticles as a new potential system for the delivery of antisense oligonucleotides. Antisense Nucl Acid Drug Dev 1999, **9**, 301–12.

129. Srinivasan SK, Tewary HK, Iversen PL. Characterization of binding sites, extent of binding, and drug interactions of oligonucleotides with albumin. Antisense Res Dev 1995, **5**, 131–9.

130. Agrawal S, Zhang X, Cai Q, *et al*. Effect of aspirin on protein binding and tissue disposition of oligonucleotide phosphorothioate in rats. J Drug Target 1998, **5**, 303–12.

131. Copple BL, Gmeiner WM, Iversen PL. Reaction between metabolically activated acetaminophen and phosphorothioate oligonucleotides. Toxicol Appl Pharmacol 1995, **133**, 53–63.

132. Blagosklonny MV, Neckers LM. Oligonucleotides protect cells from the cytotoxicity of several anti-cancer chemotherapeutic drugs. Anticancer Drugs 1994, **5**, 437–42.

133. Stull RA, Zon G, Szoka FC, Jr. Single-stranded phosphodiester and phosphorothioate oligonucleotides bind actinomycin D and interfere with tumor necrosis factor-induced lysis in the L929 cytotoxicity assay. Antisense Res Dev 1993, 3, 295–300.

134. Henry SP, Taylor J, Midgley L, *et al*. Evaluation of the toxicity of ISIS 2302, a phosphorothioate oligonucleotide, in a 4-week study in CD-1 mice. Antisense Nucl Acid Drug Dev 1997, 7, 473–81.

135. Monteith DK, Geary RS, Leeds JM, *et al*. Preclinical evaluation of the effects of a novel antisense compound targeting C-raf kinase in mice and monkeys. Toxicol Sci 1998, **46**, 365–75.

136. Cornish KG, Iversen P, Smith L, *et al*. Cardiovascular effects of a phosphorothioate oligonucleotide with sequence antisense to p53 in the conscious rhesus monkey. Pharmacol Commun 1993, 3, 239–47.

137. Galbraith WM, Hobson WC, Giclas PC, *et al*. Complement activation and hemodynamic changes following intravenous administration of phosphorothioate oligonucleotides in the monkey. Antisense Res Dev 1994, 4, 201–6.

138. Henry SP, Monteith D, Levin AA. Antisense oligonucleotide inhibitors for the treatment of cancer: 2. Toxicological properties of phosphorothioate oligodeoxynucleotides. Anticancer Drug Des 1997, **12**, 395–408.

139. Henry SP, Giclas PC, Leeds J, *et al*. Activation of the alternative pathway of complement by a phosphorothioate oligonucleotide: potential mechanism of action. J Pharmacol Exp Ther 1997, **281**, 810–16.

140. Henry SP, Monteith D, Bennett F, *et al*. Toxicological and pharmacokinetic properties of chemically modified antisense oligonucleotide inhibitors of PKC-alpha and C-raf kinase. Anticancer Drug Des 1997, **12**, 409–20.

141. Shaw DR, Rustagi PK, Kandimalla ER, *et al*. Effects of synthetic oligonucleotides on human complement and coagulation. Biochem Pharmacol 1997, **53**, 1123–32.

142. Henry SP, Novotny W, Leeds J, *et al*. Inhibition of coagulation by a phosphorothioate oligonucleotide. Antisense Nucl Acid Drug Dev 1997, 7, 503–10.

143. Iversen PL, Cornish KG, Iversen LJ, *et al*. Bolus intravenous injection of phosphorothioate oligonucleotides causes hypotension by acting as alpha(1)-adrenergic receptor antagonists. Toxicol Appl Pharmacol 1999, **160**, 289–96.

144. Sarmiento UM, Perez JR, Becker JM, *et al*. *In vivo* toxicological effects of rel A antisense phosphorothioates in CD-1 mice. Antisense Res Dev 1994, 4, 99–107.

145. Agrawal S, Zhao Q, Jiang Z, *et al*. Toxicologic effects of an oligodeoxynucleotide phosphorothioate and its analogs following intravenous administration in rats. Antisense Nucl Acid Drug Dev 1997, 7, 575–84.

146. Henry SP, Bolte H, Auletta C, *et al*. Evaluation of the toxicity of ISIS 2302, a phosphorothioate oligonucleotide, in a four-week study in cynomolgus monkeys. Toxicology 1997, **120**, 145–55.

147. Henry SP, Grillone LR, Orr JL, *et al*. Comparison of the toxicity profiles of ISIS 1082 and ISIS 2105, phosphorothioate oligonucleotides, following subacute intradermal administration in Sprague–Dawley rats. Toxicology 1997, **116**, 77–88.

148. Branda RF, Moore AL, Mathews L, *et al*. Immune stimulation by an antisense oligomer complementary to the *rev* gene of HIV-1. Biochem Pharmacol 1993, **45**, 2037–43.

149. Monteith DK, Henry SP, Howard RB, *et al*. Immune stimulation—a class effect of phosphorothioate oligodeoxynucleotides in rodents. Anticancer Drug Des 1997, **12**, 421–32.

150. McIntyre KW, Lombard-Gillooly K, Perez JR, *et al*. A sense phosphorothioate oligonucleotide directed to the initiation codon of transcription factor NF-kappa B p65 causes sequence-specific immune stimulation. Antisense Res Dev 1993, 3, 309–22.

151. Zhao Q, Temsamani J, Iadarola PL, *et al*. Effect of different chemically modified oligodeoxynucleotides on immune stimulation. Biochem Pharmacol 1996, **51**, 173–82.

152. Krieg AM, Yi AK, Matson S, *et al*. CpG motifs in bacterial DNA trigger direct B-cell activation. Nature 1995, **374**, 546–9.

153. Boggs RT, McGraw K, Condon T, *et al*. Characterization and modulation of immune stimulation by modified oligonucleotides. Antisense Nucl Acid Drug Dev 1997, 7, 461–71.

154. Klinman DM, Yi AK, Beaucage SL, *et al*. CpG motifs present in bacteria DNA rapidly induce lymphocytes to

secrete interleukin 6, interleukin 12, and interferon gamma. Proc Natl Acad Sci, USA 1996, **93**, 2879–83.

155. Zhao Q, Temsamani J, Zhou RZ, *et al.* Pattern and kinetics of cytokine production following administration of phosphorothioate oligonucleotides in mice. Antisense Nucl Acid Drug Dev 1997, **7**, 495–502.

156. Glover JM, Leeds JM, Mant TG, *et al.* Phase I safety and pharmacokinetic profile of an intercellular adhesion molecule-1 antisense oligodeoxynucleotide (ISIS 2302). J Pharmacol Exp Ther 1997, **282**, 1173–80.

157. Bishop MR, Iversen PL, Bayever E, *et al.* Phase I trial of an antisense oligonucleotide OL(1)p53 in hematologic malignancies. J Clin Oncol 1996, **14**, 1320–6.

158. Webb A, Cunningham D, Cotter F, *et al.* Bcl-2 antisense therapy in patients with non Hodgkin's lymphoma. Lancet 1997, **349**, 1137–41.

159. Raynaud FI, Foster L, Judson I, *et al.* Clinical pharmacokinetics of G3139, oligonucleotide antisense to bcl-2 [abstract]. Proc Am Assoc Cancer Res 1998, **39**, 3543.

160. Stevenson JP, Yao KS, Gallagher M, *et al.* Phase I clinical/pharmacokinetic and pharmacodynamic trial of the c-raf-1 antisense oligonucleotide ISIS 5132 (CGP 69846A). J Clin Oncol 1999, **17**, 2227.

161. Nemunaitis J, Holmlund JT, Kraynak M, *et al.* Phase I evaluation of ISIS 3521, an antisense oligodeoxynucleotide to protein kinase C-alpha, in patients with advanced cancer. J Clin Oncol 1999, **17**, 3586–95.

162. Zhang R, Yan J, Shahinian H, *et al.* Pharmacokinetics of an anti-human immunodeficiency virus antisense oligodeoxynucleotide phosphorothioate (GEM 91) in HIV-infected subjects. Clin Pharmacol Ther 1995, **58**, 44–53.

163. Sereni D, Tubiana R, Lascoux C, *et al.* Pharmacokinetics and tolerability of intravenous trecovirsen (GEM 91), an antisense phosphorothioate oligonucleotide, in HIV-positive subjects. J Clin Pharmacol 1999, **39**, 47–54.

164. Yacyshyn BR, Bowen Yacyshyn MB, Jewell L, *et al.* A placebo-controlled trial of ICAM-1 antisense oligonucleotide in the treatment of Crohn's disease. Gastroenterology 1998, **114**, 1133–42.

165. Waters JS, Webb A, Cunningham D, *et al.* Results of a phase I clinical trial of Bcl-2 antisense molecule G3139 (Genta) in patients with non-Hodgkin's lymphoma [abstract]. Proc Am Soc Clin Oncol 1999, **18**, 4a.

166. Sikic BI, Yuen AR, Advani R, *et al.* Antisense oligonucleotide therapy targeted to protein kinase C-alpha (ISIS 3521/CGP 64128A) by 21-day infusion: results of the phase I trial and activity in ovarian carcinomas [abstract]. Proc Am Soc Clin Oncol 1998, **17**, 429a.

167. Holmlund J, Nemunaitis J, Schiller J, *et al.* Phase I trial of c-raf antisense oligonucleotide ISIS 5132 (CGP 69846A) by 21-day continuous intravenous infusion in patients with advanced cancer [abstract]. Proc Am Soc Clin Oncol 1998, **17**, 210a.

168. Gewirtz AM, Luger S, Sokol D, *et al.* Oligodeoxynucleotide therapeutics for human myelogenous leukemia: interim results [abstract]. Blood 1996, **88** (suppl. 1), 270a.

169. Hockenbery D, Nunez G, Milliman C, *et al.* Bcl-2 is an inner mitochondrial membrane protein that blocks programmed cell death. Nature 1990, **348**, 334–6.

170. Miyashita T, Reed JC. Bcl-2 gene transfer increases relative resistance of S49.1 and WEHI7.2 lymphoid cells to cell death and DNA fragmentation induced by glucocorticoids and multiple chemotherapeutic drugs. Cancer Res 1992, **52**, 5407–11.

171. Pezzella F, Jones M, Ralfkiaer E, *et al.* Evaluation of bcl-2 protein expression and 14;18 translocation as prognostic markers in follicular lymphoma. Br J Cancer 1992, **65**, 87–9.

172. Hermine O, Haioun C, Lepage E, *et al.* Prognostic significance of bcl-2 protein expression in aggressive non-Hodgkin's lymphoma. Groupe d'Etude des Lymphomes de l'Adulte (GELA). Blood 1996, **87**, 265–72.

173. Hill ME, MacLennan KA, Cunningham DC, *et al.* Prognostic significance of BCL-2 expression and bcl-2 major breakpoint region rearrangement in diffuse large cell non-Hodgkin's lymphoma: a British National Lymphoma Investigation Study. Blood 1996, **88**, 1046–51.

174. Gascoyne RD, Adomat SA, Krajewski S, *et al.* Prognostic significance of Bcl-2 protein expression and Bcl-2 gene rearrangement in diffuse aggressive non-Hodgkin's lymphoma. Blood 1997, **90**, 244–51.

175. Ikegaki N, Katsumata M, Minna J, *et al.* Expression of bcl-2 in small cell lung carcinoma cells. Cancer Res 1994, **54**, 6–8.

176. McDonnell TJ, Troncoso P, Brisbay SM, *et al.* Expression of the protooncogene bcl-2 in the prostate and its association with emergence of androgen-independent prostate cancer. Cancer Res 1992, **52**, 6940–4.

177. Colombel M, Symmans F, Gil S, *et al.* Detection of the apoptosis-suppressing oncoprotein bc1–2 in hormone-refractory human prostate cancers. Am J Pathol 1993, **143**, 390–400.

178. Bhargava V, Kell DL, van de Rijn M, *et al.* Bcl-2 immunoreactivity in breast carcinoma correlates with hormone receptor positivity. Am J Pathol 1994, **145**, 535–40.

179. Silvestrini R, Veneroni S, Daidone MG, *et al.* The Bcl-2 protein: a prognostic indicator strongly related to p53 protein in lymph node-negative breast cancer patients. J Natl Cancer Inst 1994, **86**, 499–504.

180. Leek RD, Kaklamanis L, Pezzella F, *et al.* bcl-2 in normal human breast and carcinoma, association with oestrogen receptor-positive, epidermal growth factor receptor-negative tumours and *in situ* cancer. Br J Cancer 1994, **69**, 135–9.

181. Lu QL, Elia G, Lucas S, *et al.* Bcl-2 proto-oncogene expression in Epstein–Barr-virus-associated nasopharyngeal carcinoma. Int J Cancer 1993, **53**, 29–35.

182. Ayhan A, Yasui W, Yokozaki H, *et al.* Loss of heterozygosity at the bcl-2 gene locus and expression of bcl-2 in human gastric and colorectal carcinomas. Jpn J Cancer Res 1994, **85**, 584–91.

183. Sinicrope FA, Ruan SB, Cleary KR, *et al.* bcl-2 and p53 oncoprotein expression during colorectal tumorigenesis. Cancer Res 1995, **55**, 237–41.

184. Sinicrope FA, Evans DB, Leach SD, *et al.* bcl-2 and p53 expression in resectable pancreatic adenocarcinomas: association with clinical outcome. Clin Cancer Res 1996, **2**, 2015–22.

185. Sangfelt O, Osterborg A, Grander D, *et al*. Response to interferon therapy in patients with multiple myeloma correlates with expression of the Bcl-2 oncoprotein. Int J Cancer 1995, **63**, 190–2.

186. Maung ZT, MacLean FR, Reid MM, *et al*. The relationship between bcl-2 expression and response to chemotherapy in acute leukaemia. Br J Haematol 1994, **88**, 105–9.

187. Cerroni L, Soyer HP, Kerl H. bcl-2 protein expression in cutaneous malignant melanoma and benign melanocytic nevi. Am J Dermatopathol 1995, **17**, 7–11.

188. McDonnell TJ, Nunez G, Platt FM, *et al*. Deregulated Bcl-2-immunoglobulin transgene expands a resting but responsive immunoglobulin M- and D-expressing B-cell population. Mol Cell Biol 1990, **10**, 1901–7.

189. McDonnell TJ, Korsmeyer SJ. Progression from lymphoid hyperplasia to high-grade malignant lymphoma in mice transgenic for the t(14; 18). Nature 1991, **349**, 254–6.

190. Kitada S, Miyashita T, Tanaka S, *et al*. Investigations of antisense oligonucleotides targeted against bcl-2 RNAs. Antisense Res Dev 1993, **3**, 157–69.

191. Kitada S, Takayama S, de Riel K, *et al*. Reversal of chemoresistance of lymphoma cells by antisense-mediated reduction of bcl-2 gene expression. Antisense Res Dev 1994, **4**, 71–9.

192. Morris MJ, Tong W, Osman I, *et al*. A phase I/IIA dose-escalating trial of bcl-2 antisense (G3139) treatment by 14-day continuous intravenous infusion for patients with androgen-independent prostate cancer or other advanced solid tumor [abstract]. Proc Am Soc Clin Oncol 1999, **18**, 323a.

193. Jansen B, Schlagbauer Wadl H, Brown BD, *et al*. Bcl-2 antisense therapy chemosensitizes human melanoma in SCID mice. Nat Med 1998, **4**, 232–4.

194. Tolcher A, Miyake H, Gleave M. Downregulation of bcl-2 expression by antisense-oligonucleotide treatment enhances mitoxantrone cytotoxicity in the androgen-dependent Shionogi tumor model [abstract]. Proc Am Assoc Cancer Res 1999, **40**, 3198a.

195. Wong F, Bally M, Klasa R. Antisense oligonucleotides to bcl-2 with low-dose cyclophosphamide cures SCID/Rag-2 mice with a human B-cell lymphoma [abstract]. Proc Am Assoc Cancer Res 1999, **40**, 131a.

196. Yang D, Ling Y, Almazan M, *et al*. Tumor regression of human breast carcinomas by combination therapy of anti-bcl-2 antisense oligonucleotides and chemotherapeutic drugs [abstract]. Proc Am Assoc Cancer Res 1999, **40**, 4814a.

197. Jansen B, Wacheck V, Heere-Ress E, *et al*. A phase I–II study with dacarbazine and bcl-2 antisense oligonucleotide G3139 (Genta) as a chemosensitizer in patients with advanced malignant melanoma [abstract]. Proc Am Soc Clin Oncol 1999, **18**, 531a.

198. Blobe GC, Obeid LM, Hannun YA. Regulation of protein kinase C and role in cancer biology. Cancer Metastasis Rev 1994, **13**, 411–31.

199. Dean NM, McKay R, Condon TP, *et al*. Inhibition of protein kinase C-alpha expression in human A549 cells by antisense oligonucleotides inhibits induction of intercellular adhesion molecule 1 (ICAM-1) mRNA by phorbol esters. J Biol Chem 1994, **269**, 16416–24.

200. Yazaki T, Ahmad S, Chahlavi A, *et al*. Treatment of glioblastoma U-87 by systemic administration of an antisense protein kinase C-alpha phosphorothioate oligodeoxynucleotide. Mol Pharmacol 1996, **50**, 236–42.

201. Advani R, Fisher GA, Grant P, *et al*. A phase I trial of an antisense oligonucleotide targeted to protein kinase C-alpha (ISIS 3521/ISI641A) delivered as a 24-hour continuous infusion [abstract]. Proc Am Soc Clin Oncol 1999, **18**, 158a.

202. Nishida E, Gotoh Y. The MAP kinase cascade is essential for diverse signal transduction pathways. Trends Biochem Sci 1993, **18**, 128–31.

203. Wang HG, Rapp UR, Reed JC. Bcl-2 targets the protein kinase Raf-1 to mitochondria. Cell 1996, **87**, 629–38.

204. Kolch W, Heidecker G, Kochs G, *et al*. Protein kinase C alpha activates RAF-1 by direct phosphorylation. Nature 1993, **364**, 249–52.

205. Cornwell MM, Smith DE. A signal transduction pathway for activation of the mdr1 promoter involves the proto-oncogene c-raf kinase. J Biol Chem 1993, **268**, 15347–50.

206. Stanton VP, Jr., Cooper GM. Activation of human raf transforming genes by deletion of normal amino-terminal coding sequences. Mol Cell Biol 1987, **7**, 1171–9.

207. Monia BP. Anti-tumor activity of C-raf antisense—correction [letter]. Nat Med 1999, **5**, 127.

208. Holmlund JT, Rudin CM, Mani S, *et al*. Phase I trial of ISIS 5132/ODN 698A, a 20-mer phosphorothioate antisense oligonucleotide inhibitor of C-raf kinase, administered by a 24-hour weekly intravenous infusion to patients with advanced cancer [abstract]. Proc Am Soc Clin Oncol 1999, **18**, 157a.

209. Cowsert LM. *In vitro* and *in vivo* activity of antisense inhibitors of ras: potential for clinical development. Anticancer Drug Des 1997, **12**, 359–71.

210. Dorr A, Bruce J, Monia B, *et al*. Phase I and pharmacokinetic trial of ISIS 2503, a 20-mer antisense oligonucleotide against H-ras, by 14-day continuous infusion in patients with advanced cancer [abstract]. Proc Am Soc Clin Oncol 1999, **18**, 157a.

211. Gordon MS, Sandler AB, Holmlund JT, *et al*. A phase I trial of ISIS 2503, an antisense inhibitor of H-ras, administered by a 24-hour weekly infusion to patients with advanced cancer [abstract]. Proc Am Soc Clin Oncol 1999, **18**, 157a.

212. Gokhale PC, McRae D, Monia BP, *et al*. Antisense raf oligodeoxyribonucleotide is a radiosensitizer *in vivo*. Antisense Nucl Acid Drug Dev 1999, **9**, 191–201.

213. Sikic IB, Yuen AR, Advani R, *et al*. A phase I trial of ISIS 3521 (ISI 641A), an antisense inhibitor of protein kinase C alpha, combined with carboplatin and paclitaxel in patients with cancer [abstract]. Proc Am Soc Clin Oncol 1999, **18**, 445a.

214. Mani S, Shulman K, Kunkel K, *et al*. Phase I trial of protein kinase C-alpha antisense oligonucleotide (ISIS 3521; ISI 641A) with fluorouracil and leucovorin in patients with advanced cancer [abstract]. Proc Am Soc Clin Oncol 1999, **18**, 158a.

215. de Fabritiis P, Amadori S, Calabretta B, *et al*. Elimination of clonogenic Philadelphia-positive cells

using BCR-ABL antisense oligodeoxynucleotides. Bone Marrow Transplant 1993, **12**, 261–5.

216. de Fabritiis P, Amadori S, Petti MC, *et al. In vitro* purging with BCR-ABL antisense oligodeoxynucleotides does not prevent haematologic reconstitution after autologous bone marrow transplantation. Leukemia 1995, **9**, 662–4.

217. de Fabritiis P, Petti MC, Montefusco E, *et al.* BCR-ABL antisense oligodeoxynucleotide *in vitro* purging and autologous bone marrow transplantation for patients with chronic myelogenous leukemia in advanced phase. Blood 1998, **91**, 3156–62.

218. Kronenwett R, Haas R. Antisense strategies for the treatment of hematological malignancies and solid tumors. Ann Hematol 1998, **77**, 1–12.

219. Gewirtz AM, Sokol DL, Ratajczak MZ. Nucleic acid therapeutics: state of the art and future prospects. Blood 1998, **92**, 712–36.

220. Calabretta B, Sims RB, Valtieri M, *et al.* Normal and leukemic hematopoietic cells manifest differential sensi-tivity to inhibitory effects of c-myb antisense oligodeoxynucleotides: an *in vitro* study relevant to bone marrow purging. Proc Natl Acad Sci, USA 1991, **88**, 2351–5.

221. Ratajczak MZ, Kant JA, Luger SM, *et al. In vivo* treatment of human leukemia in a scid mouse model with c-myb antisense oligodeoxynucleotides. Proc Natl Acad Sci, USA 1992, **89**, 11823–7.

222. McManaway ME, Neckers LM, Loke SL, *et al.* Tumour-specific inhibition of lymphoma growth by an antisense oligodeoxynucleotide. Lancet 1990, **335**, 808–11.

223. Putney SD, Brown J, Cucco C, *et al.* Enhanced anti-tumor effects with microencapsulated c-myc antisense oligonucleotide. Antisense Nucl Acid Drug Dev 1999, **9**, 451–8.

224. Skorski T, Nieborowska-Skorska M, Wlodarski P, *et al.* Antisense oligodeoxynucleotide combination therapy of primary chronic myelogenous leukemia blast crisis in SCID mice. Blood 1996, **88**, 1005–12.

11 | *Dendritic cells—targeting the antitumor immune response*

Alan Melcher, Richard G. Vile, Andrew Bateman, and Kevin J. Harrington

Introduction

Stimulating the patient's immune system to attack malignant cells has long been the goal of tumor immunologists, and is currently an established, though small, component of oncological practice. Most current approaches rely on nonspecific activation of the immune system against the cancer—for example, the chronic bladder inflammation triggered by intravesical BCG (bacille Calmette–Guérin) given for superficial bladder cancer, or the general immune activation by systemic interleukin 2 (IL-2) in the treatment of melanoma or renal cell carcinoma (1). The problem with such treatments, and in particular with systemic cytokine delivery, is the toxicity that follows when the immune system is thrown into such nonspecific overdrive. More desirable by far would be to target particular components of immunity that are specific for the tumor, but that would spare normal tissue. Until recently, such a targeted approach to cancer immunotherapy was impossible, but the identification and characterization of relatively specific tumor-associated antigens has opened up a new field for tumor immunotherapy. This overview will discuss such targeted treatment, specifically using dendritic cells (DCs) to prime specific antitumor T-cell immunity against defined tumor antigens. The first part describes the nature of the novel antigenic targets for tumor immunologists, and the second discusses the basic biology of DCs and their application for the delivery of such antigens to the immune system, to generate a specific, nontoxic therapeutic response against the tumor.

Tumor antigens recognized by T cells—a target for immunotherapy

The identification of tumor antigens that can prime cytotoxic T lymphocytes (CTLs) and provide targets for the elimination of malignant cells provides the basis for activation of cell-mediated immunity by DCs as a rational strategy for cancer therapy. Antigens comprise short peptides, or epitopes, that bind to major histocompatibility complex (MHC) molecules on the cell surface, where they can be recognized by specifically reactive T cells. The presentation of such antigens to T cells can occur via several pathways. Firstly, there are antigens presented by MHC class I molecules (potentially on any nucleated cell), which prime and stimulate a cytotoxic T-cell (CD8+) response against that antigen. Specific CTLs then expand and potentially kill any antigen-expressing target cell. In contrast, MHC class II molecules are expressed only on so-called 'professional' antigen-presenting cells (APCs) such as DCs. MHC class II antigen presentation is to CD4+ 'helper' T cells, and results in secretion by the T cell of cytokines (such as IL-2), which help propagate and activate a CD8 response. Professional APCs are also uniquely capable of sampling their environment for antigens, which are taken up and presented via both MHC class I pathways to CD8 T cells (so-called cross-priming) and MHC class II pathways to CD4 helper T cells. Hence APCs, and DCs in particular, are central to the initiation of an effective immune response against an antigen. APCs have other features that equip them for this role. In particular, they express a high level of 'co-stimulatory' molecules, such as the B7 family of proteins, that are essential for T-cell activation. Without co-stimulation, antigen presentation to T cells may result in anergy rather than activation, allowing antigen-expressing targets to escape immune attack. For these reasons, APCs such as DCs are the ideal cell type for loading with antigen prior to presentation and activation of T cells.

To turn first to the antigens themselves, these can be divided into a number of categories, namely, tumor-specific antigens, differentiation antigens, antigens unique to individual tumors, viral antigens, and antigens arising from oncogenic products:

Tumor-specific shared antigens are antigens that are expressed specifically on tumors, but not by the majority of normal tissue. They include the melanoma antigens, MAGE-1 and MAGE-3, that encode peptides expressed on a large proportion of melanomas as well as on other tumor types (2, 3). They are not, however, found on normal tissue other than the testis. Two other gene families, GAGE (4) and BAGE (5), that are similarly expressed by malignant, but not normal cells have been described.

Aberrant glycosylation of the mucin encoded by MUC-1 exposes novel CTL epitopes in some adenocarcinomas that can act as tumor-specific antigens (6). Presentation of MUC-1 epitopes may allow novel therapeutic strategies in a wide variety of tumors such as carcinomas of the breast, gastrointestinal tract, and ovary.

The advantage of these tumor-specific antigens is that their targeted destruction by the immune system should not result in any damage to normal tissue.

Differentiation antigens are antigens, again described in melanoma, that are expressed only in cells of the melanocytic lineage. They include tyrosinase, which encodes epitopes presented by both MHC class I (7) and MHC class II (8) molecules; Melan-A/MART-1 (9); Pmel17/gp100 (10); and gp75/TRP-1 (11). In melanoma such differentiation antigens hold particular promise for immunotherapy as destruction of melanocytes leading to clinical vitiligo has been reported as associated with regression of melanomas (12). Hence, an immune response restricted to antigens expressed only by normal or malignant melanocytes may achieve therapeutic results without initiating toxic autoimmunity. Interestingly, immune-mediated damage to melanocytes in the retina has not been reported in melanoma regression associated with skin vitiligo.

Antigens unique to individual tumors are antigens that arise from point mutations in malignant cells resulting in novel epitopes for CTL recognition. As these epitopes are unique to the tumor from which they are identified their widespread clinical use may be problematical. However, definition of such mutations may suggest novel potential mechanisms for oncogenesis. Examples include point mutations in the cyclin-dependent kinase 4 (CDK4) gene (13), MUM-1 (14), β-catenin (15), and CASP-8 (16). Of more clinical interest are the unique tumor antigens arising from the idiotypic determinants of individual B-cell malignancies, which have already been tested as targets in the clinical setting (17, 18).

Viral antigens are oncogenic viruses implicated in a wide variety of cancers, which may encode potential tumor antigens. For example, human papilloma viruses (HPV)-16 and HPV-18 are strongly implicated in the etiology of carcinoma of the cervix. The E6 and E7 oncogenic protein products of these viruses inhibit function of the tumor suppressor genes p53 and RB, respectively, and may encode peptides recognized by CTLs (19). Other viruses encoding potential tumor antigens include Epstein–Barr virus (EBV), implicated in Burkitt's lymphoma, nasopharyngeal carcinoma, immunoblastic B-cell lymphoma, and Hodgkin's disease, and HTLV-1 responsible for adult T-cell leukemia (20).

Antigens arising from oncogenic products comprise a final class of potential tumor antigens derived from the protein products of oncogenes or tumor suppressor genes (21). Such products may be recognized by the immune system due to overexpression or mutation, and represent potentially useful therapeutic targets, particularly if they are directly implicated in transformation of the cell to a malignant phenotype. CTLs have been generated that recognize mutated human p53 (22), and both CD4 and CD8 T cells directed against mutated ras have been isolated from pancreatic and colon carcinoma patients (23, 24). Other sites for T-cell recognition are the breakpoint of the BCR-ABL gene translocation of chronic myelogenous leukemia (CML) (25) and the overexpressed HER-2/neu oncogene of breast and ovarian carcinomas (26).

The identification and characterization of tumor antigens described above have led to enthusiasm for immune-mediated therapies designed to instigate and augment effective T-cell responses against such antigens. The prediction has been that such targeted stimulation of T cells will create effective treatment strategies with minimal toxicity. The question of how best to generate a potent immune response against tumor antigens has been most effectively addressed using the most powerful APC cell of the immune system, the dendritic cell.

Dendritic cells—the most potent cellular approach to stimulating antitumor immunity

DCs are the most powerful APCs at initiating T-cell responses (27). Originally described by Steinman and

Cohn (28), they are a leukocyte population uniquely capable of presenting novel antigens to naive T cells *in vivo* as well as *in vitro* to generate effective immune responses (29, 30). DCs are able to take up antigens from a variety of sources, and process them for presentation to both CD4 (helper) and CD8 (cytotoxic) T cells. The uptake of antigens into the MHC class I-processing pathways of the DCs (cross-priming), for stimulation of CTLs, seems to be absolutely key to generating antitumor immunity (31). Hence, experimental strategies that place the DC at the center of antigen presentation to T cells may hold the greatest promise for therapy. Because of this, there has been an explosion in research into the basic science and clinical application of DCs in the last 2 decades, which is only now beginning to be applied in the clinical setting. An understanding of DC biology, including the uncertainties surrounding DC lineage, antigen processing, and culture for clinical use, highlights the current limitations, as well as potential, of antigen-loaded DC for cancer therapy.

Isolation of dendritic cells

Although DCs were first identified as Langerhans cells (LCs) more than 100 years ago, their characterization has only been possible over the last 25 years as techniques have developed for the isolation and culture of DCs in sufficient numbers for experimentation. DCs of various subtypes are found in multiple organs, and can be isolated directly from the skin (as LCs), spleen, blood, or lymphoid tissue. One challenge in the study of these cells is that their phenotype is never static. Hence DCs from different sites will inherently differ according to their functional role and, as soon as DCs are isolated, manipulated, or cultured *in vitro*, their surface molecular markers and behavior inevitably alter. This makes extrapolation of *in vitro* data to *in vivo* relevance particularly difficult in DC biology. It is imperative to acknowledge all experimental data specifically in the light of the conditions used to generate the DCs under study.

The isolation of fresh DCs from a variety of tissues has been achieved by a combination of density centrifugation techniques and depletion of other cell types (32). DCs are of low density and various gradient media have been used for their collection. The lack of specific cell markers for DCs (see below) makes their positive selection from a mixed cell population problematical. However, both for fresh

isolation and culture techniques, other cell types such as T cells, B cells, natural killer (NK) cells, monocytes, macrophages, and granulocytes can be routinely depleted using specific antibodies. Using such methods fresh DCs have been isolated from many tissues, particularly blood, skin, spleen, thymus, and lymphoid tissue (33–36). Indeed, DCs have been identified in almost all organs with the exception of the brain, parts of the eye, and the testis. Within DC populations specific terms may be applied to DCs from a particular source, for example, Langerhans cells of the skin, veiled cells within afferent lymph, and interdigitating, follicular, and germinal center DC isolated from lymphoid tissue (33, 35, 37). Within secondary lymphoid tissue, interdigitating DCs are found in T-cell-rich zones, follicular DCs interact with B cells in B-cell-rich areas, and the more recently described germinal center DCs present antigen to T cells, despite being located in germinal centers (37).

Culture of dendritic cells

As well as isolation of fresh DCs, many techniques have been developed for the culture of large numbers of DCs *in vitro*. Linked to these studies is an emerging lineage for DCs, although the precise origin and fate of specific DC subtypes remain, for the most part, unclear. Two central paradigms are, however, emerging that provide a useful framework into which new data can be incorporated. The first is that DCs arise from either a myeloid precursor (which can also differentiate into granuloctyes or monocytes/macrophages) or a lymphoid precursor, from which T cells, B cells, or NK cells can also be cultured (38). The second paradigm is the importance in any culture system of defining the maturation status of the DCs that emerge. DCs functionally mature from a high-antigen-acquiring, low-antigen-presentation phenotype to become low-acquisition/high-presentation APCs. This change reflects the *in vivo* necessity for DCs first to take up antigens, particularly at peripheral sites of potential invasion (such as the skin or mucosal surfaces), and then to migrate and mature to APCs equipped to present these antigens to reactive T cells in draining lymphoid tissue (39–41). This migrational, fuctional maturation is reflected in various DC culture conditions *in vitro*, and is critical to the potential uses of cultured DCs for various immunotherapeutic strategies *in vivo*.

Human DCs have been cultured from two main sources, CD34+ stem cells (from peripheral blood or bone marrow) and monocytes. Culture of monocytes in granulocyte–macrophage colony-stimulating factor (GM-CSF) and IL-4 produces a myeloid-derived population of immature DCs (42, 43). These cells are functionally equipped for antigen acquisition rather than presentation, and so exhibit significant levels of macropinocytosis, and express low levels of antigen presentation molecules such as MHC class II and B7. These immature DCs retain the ability to differentiate into macrophages under the influence of macrophage colony-stimulating factor (MCSF). If additional maturation signals, such as tumor necrosis factor α (TNFα), lipopolysaccharide (LPS), or monocyte-conditioned medium, are added to immature DC cultures, emerging cells become irreversibly committed to mature DC differentiation and their phenotype changes (44, 45). Macropinocytosis falls and expression of MHC class II/B7 increases.

The differentiation of DCs from human CD34+ stem cells is more complex than culture from monocytes as it can proceed down two distinct pathways (46). Culture of CD34+ cells with GM-CSF and TNFα first gives rise to two DC precursor cell types, characterized as CD1a+CD14− and CD1a−CD14+. On further culture with the same cytokines, the CD1a+ population differentiates into DCs with typical features of Langerhans cells, such as Birbeck granules and expression of Lag antigen. In contrast the CD14+ precursor differentiates into DCs more typical of those found in the dermis, which express CD68 and factor XIIIa and are functionally distinct (47). The CD14+s, but not the CD1a+ precursors retain the ability to differentiate into macrophages on addition of MCSF. Hence, even within the myeloid pathway of DC differentiation, there are alternative routes for the culture of populations of cells all classified as DCs.

These myeloid pathways of DC culture and differentiation all depend on the presence of GM-CSF as a critical cytokine. However, there are also precursor cells of lymphoid origin that can differentiate into DCs without GM-CSF. These have been identified within mouse and human thymus (48, 49) and human bone marrow (50). Such precursors can give rise to T, B, and NK cells as well as DCs, and their DC progeny in the mouse characteristically express CD8 as an $\alpha\alpha$ homodimer. Intriguingly, lymphoid DCs may have functions quite distinct from those of myeloid-derived DCs, directed more at downregulation of immune responses rather than activation. Hence CD8+ DCs can inhibit

proliferation of allogeneic T cells in a mixed lymphocyte reaction by blocking secretion of IL-2, and can trigger apoptosis of CD4+ T cells by a Fas-mediated mechanism (51, 52). These DCs have also been referred to as type 2 DCs (monocyte-derived DCs are type 1) and have an additional role in secreting type 1 interferons in response to viral infections (53).

In the mouse, DCs have similarly been cultured from myeloid and lymphoid origin, although there is no equivalent of the CD1a+ and CD14+ intermediates of human CD34+ cell culture. GM-CSF is again critical to murine myeloid DC differentiation and, used as a single cytokine, generates an immature DC population (54, 55). The same pattern of additional cytokines driving DCs towards a more mature phenotype is apparent. In particular, the addition of IL-4 or TNFα to GM-CSF-driven bone marrow cultures generates a more mature population of DCs (56, 57). For experiments testing the potential of DCs in the immunotherapy of tumors, cells are cultured most commonly from bone marrow or spleen (58, 59), although peripheral blood and liver have also been demonstrated as potential sources (60, 61).

There remain many unresolved questions surrounding the source, culture, lineage, and function of different DC subtypes. For example the role of endogenous GM-CSF in DC development is uncertain, since DCs from transgenic mice in which levels of the cytokine or its receptor have been altered show few differences from normal mouse DCs (62). Further complexity in pathways of DC development is illustrated by the potential of the tonsillar plamacytoid T cell as a further precursor for lymphoid type 2 DCs (63), and neutrophils can surprisingly be driven to differentiate towards DCs (64). The diversity of cytokine combinations used for DC culture is wide, and novel cytokines such as the hemopoietic growth factor FLT3 ligand (FLT3L) can increase both basal and cultured yields of DCs (65) and suggest further subtypes into which DC can be classified (66). Additional factors within DC cultures may promote or inhibit DC differentiation. Hence, addition of transforming growth factor (TGF)β-1 or triggering of CD40 can promote DC culture from CD34+ stem cells (67, 68), whereas IL-10 or vascular endothelial growth factor (VEGF) can be inhibitory (69, 70).

If DCs are to be used clinically for the treatment of cancer and other diseases, it is imperative to define optimal culture conditions. Encouragingly, although DCs isolated directly from human tumors are functionally impaired (71), efficient APCs can nevertheless be cultured from the blood of cancer patients (72). However, in one study, DCs cultured from CD34+ cells were more potent than monocyte-derived DCs at eliciting CTL responses against tumor antigens in melanoma patients (73), suggesting that precise culture conditions may critically affect clinical efficacy. A further study directly comparing DCs cultured in various ways from different precursors gave a different result, suggesting few significant differences (74).

The efficacy of DCs in a particular therapeutic protocol and the optimal conditions for their culture are likely to depend on the strategy to be employed. There is evidence that, if DC are required to process antigenic proteins before priming T cells, an immature phenotype is best, whereas, if DCs are pulsed with peptide epitopes that have already been defined and synthesized, mature DCs high in antigen-presenting capacity are more potent (75). A two-stage approach is to deliver antigens to an immature DC population and then provide additional signals for maturation before using them to elicit immune responses (76, 77).

Migration of dendritic cells

The maturation of DCs during *in vitro* culture from an antigen acquisition to an antigen presentation phenotype is mirrored by the migratory capacity of DCs *in vivo*. Immature DCs such as LCs are able to take up antigens in peripheral sites such as the skin and then migrate to draining lymph nodes where they can present these antigens to reactive T cells (78). Signals, including TNFα and IL-1β, can cause such migration as well as maturation of DCs (79, 80). In addition, a growing number of chemokines and their receptors that are likely to control DC trafficking into and out of lymphoid tissue have been identified (81–83). For potential therapeutic application, macrophage inflammatory protein 3α has been expressed in tumor cells and shown to attract DCs into established tumors and suppress their growth (84). During such trafficking specific changes are required to facilitate the retention of antigens by DCs until such time as they come into contact with potentially reactive T cells. Hence, immature DCs can retain antigen for significant periods of time before maturation, at which point MHC class II is redistributed to the cell surface for interaction with T cells (85, 86).

The fate of exogenous DCs injected subcutaneously and intravenously, such as might be used for clinical immunotherapy, has been tracked in mice and primates.

These studies have shown that DCs do migrate from the injection site to the T-cell areas of lymph nodes and spleen, supporting the therapeutic potential of DC treatment for modulating immune responses (87, 88). In addition, radiolabeled DCs injected subcutaneously into cancer patients have been shown to track to draining lymph nodes, but this depended on an intradermal route of administration (89).

Surface molecular markers for dendritic cells

Amongst the many subtypes of DCs from various tissues and culture systems at differing stages of maturation, there is a significant lack of specific cell surface markers. This makes comparisons between DCs often problematical. Cellular morphology and functional assays can help characterize DC subtypes, but only into broad categories. As described above, the presence or absence of lineage-specific markers can help description of DCs during development, as with the CD1a+ and CD14+ intermediates of CD34+-derived human DCs (46), or the CD4lo progenitors that have been described for lymphoid DCs (49). In addition, markers of antigen-presenting capacity (such as MHC class II and B7 expression) are often used to define DC, although these may be expressed only at low levels by immature DCs, and are expressed by other types of APCs such as macrophages and activated B cells.

Nevertheless, a number of cell surface molecules have been defined that have some specificity for staining of DCs. In the human these include CMRF-44 and CD83, both markers of activated DCs (90, 91). The integrin CD11c is commonly used as a DC marker in the mouse, as is the mannose receptor DEC205 (recognized by the antibody NLDC145), which is involved in endocytosis (33, 92). Both CD11c and DEC205 are not entirely specific to DCs and are accepted as markers of mature, rather than immature DCs, reflecting a fundamental lack of molecules useful in the definition of immature murine DCs or their precursors (93).

Mechanisms of antigen uptake and presentation by dendritic cells

If DCs are to be used to present tumor-associated antigens to T cells for therapy, they need to be optimally loaded with antigen from the most practical source. DCs are able to take up exogenous antigens by a variety of mechanisms for presentation to CD4 cells and, via the phenomenon of cross-priming, to MHC class I-restricted CD8 cells (94). Although initially DCs were thought to be non-phagocytic, it is now clear that immature DCs can take up antigen in this way for channeling into both MHC class I and class II pathways (76, 95, 96). Macropinocytosis can also serve as a source of antigens for both DC MHC class I and class II presentation pathways (97, 98). Receptor-mediated antigen capture through the mannose receptor, for example, is another source of potential antigens for DCs (97, 99). It has also been shown that immature DCs can process and present antigens entirely extracellularly (100).

The precise mechanism by which exogenous antigens access the MHC class I processing pathway of DCs is uncertain, as shown by the varying dependence of cross-priming on different components of the class I pathway in different model systems (98, 101). However, the importance of cross-priming for instigating antitumor immune responses has been clearly shown in animal models (31). These experiments involved the reconstitution of bone marrow in mice such that bone-marrow-derived host APCs and vaccinating tumor cells carried different MHC class I phenotypes able to prime CTL responses against different epitopes of a model influenza nucleoprotein tumor antigen. A CD8 response was detected only against the epitope presented by host APCs and not against that presented directly by the tumor vaccine, demonstrating that the antigen must have been cross-primed into host APCs before presentation to the immune system. Further studies showed that, if the tumor vaccine was engineered to express B7, direct priming of CD8 responses did now occur, although cross-priming into host APCs remained more efficient (102). These key experiments suggest that the best approach for clinical tumor vaccines is to design and develop those cellular or genetic therapies that are most potent at delivering antigens into patients' APC for cross-priming and subsequent presentation to reactive T cells.

Another area of critical importance to the acquisition and presentation of antigens by DCs is the range of live or dying cells that may be a target for uptake. There has been controversy over whether apoptotic or necrotic tumor cells are most potent at priming DCs for T-cell activation, and results vary with different experimental conditions. While apoptotic tumor cells can deliver antigens to DCs for cross-priming (103), particularly when normal immunosuppressive mechanisms for the clearance of apoptotic bodies are overwhelmed (104), there is accumulating evidence that necrotic death may be more immunostimulatory to DCs when tumors die (105, 106). Inevitably, the distinction between apoptotic and necrotic cell death is not absolute, but this area of research is critical for defining signals that may activate DCs *in vivo* when tumor cells die, and has profound implications for the design of novel strategies that aim optimally to load DCs for immune priming in patients (107).

One signal linking the mode of tumor cell death to antigen acquisition by DCs is heat shock proteins (HSPs). In murine models of suicide gene therapy, induction of HSPs was immunogenic and associated with necrotic, but not apoptotic, tumor cell death (108). HSP expression recruited DCs into growing tumors *in vivo* (109), and *in vitro* HSPs have been shown to deliver model antigens into APCs for presentation to T cells, probably through a receptor-mediated mechanism (110, 111). Defined receptors for HSPs so far are CD14 and CD91 (112). Hence, therapeutic strategies that stress tumor cells to express HSPs may be potent at delivering antigens to DCs for priming of antitumor immunity in patients.

Antigens delivered by genetic means *in vivo* serve as another potential source of epitopes for presentation by DCs. DNA vaccinations have been shown to rely on host DCs for presentation of their encoded antigen, although it is not entirely resolved whether DCs are directly transfected themselves by the vaccine, or are cross-primed with antigen initially expressed in other host cell types such as myocytes (113–115). The deliberate transfection of DCs for immunotherapy as a defined strategy is considered separately below.

Hence, antigens from a variety of sources can be delivered to DCs extracellularly, through phagocytosis, macropinocytosis, or receptor-mediated mechanisms, in some cases chaperoned by specific carriers such as HSPs. By routes that remain to be elucidated in detail, these antigens access both MHC class I and class II presentation pathways within DCs for eventual presentation to CD4 and CD8 T cells, respectively.

Priming dendritic cells with tumor antigens for immunotherapy

The use of DCs for the immunotherapy of cancer has been widely explored in murine tumor models. The central theme is to load DCs with tumor antigens and then rely on the antigen-processing and/or presentation capacity of DCs to initiate T cell-mediated antitumor immune responses. DCs are able to acquire, process, and present antigens at diverse stages of their differentiation and maturation, so that such antigens can be fed to DCs in a variety of ways. Techniques used have ranged from genetic delivery of antigenic genes by DNA, RNA, or viral vectors, through pulsing DCs with proteins or tumor cell lysates, to coating DCs with peptide epitopes either of known antigenicity or eluted from the MHC class I molecules of tumor cells. In addition, DCs have been adoptively transferred or fused with tumor cells to create therapeutic vaccines, and exosomes derived from DCs have shown benefit in murine models.

Genetic modification of dendritic cells for immunotherapy

DCs have been successfully transfected with DNA using liposomes or viral vectors. One comparative study with human DCs suggested that adenoviral-mediated delivery of a reporter gene was the most effective means of transduction, although a relatively high multiplicity of infection (MOI) was required (116). Other groups have had success with liposomal or gene gun-mediated delivery of DNA to DCs for subsequent presentation of antigens to CTL clones or generation of primary CTL responses *in vitro* (117, 118). There is also evidence that DNA vaccines given intramuscularly may transfect DCs *in vivo* (115).

Adenovirally transfected DCs are effective *in vivo* at generating CTL responses and protecting against tumors expressing either model tumor antigens, such as OVA (119) and β-gal (120), or human tumor antigens, such as MART-1/Melan-A (121) and MUC-1 (122). Although the MOI required to transduce DCs with adenovirus is high in some murine studies (since mouse cells are relatively resistant to infection with adenovirus), for clinical application lipofectamine can facilitate efficient transduction of human DCs (123). Adenoviruses have been used to transfect cytokines as well as model antigens into DCs. For example, DCs expressing GM-CSF were found to be more potent for immunotherapy *in vivo* than unmodified DCs (124).

Retroviruses have similarly been shown to be capable of transfecting DCs, although a somewhat technically complex co-culture of DCs with retroviral producer cells may be required (125). Again, *in vivo* benefit against tumor cells expressing the antigen expressed by the vaccinating DCs has been demonstrated, with asso-

ciated induction of CTL activity (126). Vaccinia viruses have also been successfully used to deliver antigen genes to DCs (119).

A novel way genetically to modify DCs has been to transfect them with RNA rather than DNA. This approach allows all transcribed RNA from a tumor cell to be delivered to DC, so that potentially multiple, undefined epitopes can be translated, processed, and presented to the immune system. DCs pulsed with RNA in this way have shown antitumor effects even against the poorly immunogenic murine melanoma B16 (127, 128). Moreover, such RNA-transfected DCs have been shown to elicit CTL *in vitro* against a human prostate-specific cancer antigen (129).

Dendritic cells pulsed with tumor cell lysates, proteins, or peptides for immunotherapy

Loading DCs with tumor cell lysates relies on uptake of cell fragments by DCs and subsequent processing and presentation of potentially antigenic epitopes both to CD4 cells via MHC class II pathways and, through cross-priming, to CD8 cells via MHC class I. The use of entire tumor cells in this way is appealing, since all potential epitopes are made available to the DCs for immune priming, and exact definition and characterization of the antigens responsible for initiating an immune response is unnecessary. Conversely, there is the concern that any relevant antigen that is expressed by tumor cells will be present at too low a level in crude lysates to allow effective immune activation. Nevertheless, DCs pulsed with tumor cell lysates have been shown to generate antitumor immunity (130, 131).

DCs have also been pulsed with antigenic proteins to elicit antitumor immune responses (98, 132). Of particular clinical relevance was the finding that DC pulsed with the unique idiotypic antigen of a murine B-cell lymphoma could generate protection against challenge *in vivo* (133). This approach has already been translated into a clinical protocol (18).

Many different characterized antigenic tumor peptide epitopes have been pulsed on to DCs to generate antitumor immunity. These include peptides from model tumor antigens such as OVA (30, 134), epitopes previously defined in mouse tumors (135), and antigenic peptides of clinical relevance from p53 (136), E7 (137), and melanoma antigens (138). In a different approach, all MHC class I-bound peptides have been eluted from the surface of tumor cells, pulsed on to DCs, and utilized for therapy (139).

As regards the mechanisms responsible for the efficacy of DCs pulsed with cell lysates, proteins, or peptides and delivered *in vivo*, the data is unclear. Empirically, the uptake of crude cell lysates or proteins may be more efficient using immature rather than mature DCs. Although it is known that DCs lose phagocytic capacity with maturation (95), there is a lack of evidence on the precise mechanisms of antigen uptake responsible for the immune activity of DCs administered *in vivo*, or comparing DCs of differing maturational status in the same therapeutic protocol. One study has, however, compared the importance of DC maturation when loading DCs with different forms of antigen for presentation to a carcinoembryonic antigen (CEA)-specific CTL clone *in vitro*. If DCs were pulsed with CEA as peptide, optimal presentation was achieved when DCs were matured through CD40 ligation prior to addition of antigen. In contrast, when CEA was delivered as RNA, the clone was maximally activated if immature DCs were first transfected and only then matured with CD40L (75). For phagocytic loading of DCs it was shown that pulsing DCs in an immature state and then allowing them to mature was optimal for priming anti-mycobacterial immunity (76). Hence, for clinical therapy, the ideal maturational state of the DCs to be used is likely to depend on the individual therapeutic immune strategy. If DCs are required to take up and process particulate cellular debris (for example, from autologous tumor lysates), immature DCs may be most potent, whereas, if DCs are to be pulsed with defined antigenic peptides (such as melanoma antigens), it may be best to mature DCs *in vitro* before loading them.

Other therapeutic strategies using dendritic cells for immunotherapy

Alternative methods of utilizing the antigen-presenting capacity of DCs for immunotherapy have been developed. One approach is to fuse DCs with tumor cells using polyethylene glycol (PEG) or electrofusion techniques. Such hybrids then express all potential tumor antigens within the hybrid cell, whilst at the same time maintaining the ability to process and present such antigens to generate immunity (140, 141). However, a further study has suggested, at least in mouse models, that DCs mixed with tumor cells can be as effective a vaccine as these fused hybrids in eliciting CTLs and protecting against tumor challenge (142). Recently, a

clinical trial in renal cell carcinoma using autologous tumor cells fused to allogeneic DCs produced encouraging results (143).

In a different strategy, exosomes secreted by DCs have been shown to elicit potent antitumor immunity (144). These are vesicles, initially identified in transformed B lymphocytes, that derive from direct fusion between the plasma membrane and endosomal/lysosomal compartments. Exosomes secreted by DCs were rich in MHC class I, class II, and B7 and, when isolated from DCs pulsed with eluted tumor peptides, they caused T-cell-mediated regression of established mouse tumors. These exosomes were more potent than whole DCs pulsed with eluted peptides, and were secreted more by immature than mature DCs. The role of endogenous exosomes from DCs is unclear, but they may provide a useful new tool for immunotherapy.

One approach that has received little attention is the adoptive transfer of DCs with tumor cells or directly into tumors as a potential therapeutic vaccine. The advantage of such an approach is that DCs have access to multiple potential antigens that do not need to be identified. Mixing DCs with irradiated tumor cells as an *in vivo* vaccine has generated some immune responses (142, 145), as has combining allogeneic tumor cells with syngeneic DCs for vaccination (146). When DCs have been directly injected into established tumors, it has usually been necessary to boost their function (for example, by transfection with IL-7 or IL-12) for tumor regression to follow (147–149).

There is evidence that immunotherapeutic approaches that do not directly use cultured DCs may nevertheless employ endogenous DCs to elicit an immune response. Hence successful gene therapy strategies using genetic modification of tumor cells with the immunostimulatory genes IL-4, GM-CSF, or MCSF have all been shown to increase numbers of DCs at the vaccine site (150–152), and systemic administration of the hemopoietic growth factor FLT3L slowed the growth of tumors within which DCs accumulated (153). Interestingly, FLT3L treatment has been shown to synergize with radiotherapy in a metastatic lung cancer model, suggesting combined modality approaches incorporating DCs may be effective for immune priming and activation (154). Tumors expressing both GM-CSF and CD40 ligand (a key stimulatory signaling model between T cells and DCs) attracted a significant influx of DCs, which were shown to have acquired and been cross-primed by an antigen specifically expressed by the tumor (155).

This shows directly that attracting endogenous DCs into tumors can be effective for delivering antigen to APCs *in vivo*. In clinical trials vaccines expressing GM-CSF have shown DC accumulation at the vaccine site in both prostate cancer and melanoma (156, 157).

Another promising approach is systemic therapy with immunostimulatory DNA sequences containing unmethylated CpG dinucleotides. These motifs are thought to mimic bacterial DNA sequences that the immune system recognizes, resulting in expansion of a variety of immune cells, including DCs. Hence CpG can act as an effective adjuvant for antitumor therapy, in part by activating the APC compartment (158).

In contrast to these various cytokines that may enhance DC activation *in vivo*, there are factors that inhibit DC function, such as IL-10 (159) and VEGF (69). Both of these may be produced by malignant cells *in vivo* to prevent DCs effectively initating a response against the tumor (160).

Dendritic cells in clinical oncology

If DCs are to be used effectively for cancer therapy it is important to characterize their function in patients with the disease. This is particularly so as DCs have the potential to downregulate the immune response (52) and in some cases lead to anergy (161). Since cancer patients have a variety of immunological dysfunctions (162), the functions of DCs in the context of malignancy and the optimal activating capacity of DCs to be used for therapy need careful consideration.

DCs isolated directly from tumors are poor at antigen presentation. This has been shown in both rodent and human malignancies (71, 163). DCs from progressive melanoma lesions were less potent at stimulating allogeneic T cells than DCs from tumors in the same patient that were responding to therapy (164). Nevertherless, in colorectal tumors that did have a significant DC infiltrate, this finding correlated with an improved clinical prognosis (165). DCs isolated fresh from the spleens of tumor-bearing mice (166) or the blood of breast cancer patients (167) were also dysfunctional. Further evidence of a specific effect of the tumor microenvironment on DCs comes from the observation that DCs in different maturational states are distributed differently within tumors. Immature DCs have been documented specifically in the centers of breast cancers, with more mature DCs distributed preferentially around the tumor periphery (168). However, regardless of the state of endogenous DCs within tumor-bearing individuals, it has been shown that functional DCs for therapy can be successfully cultured from the blood of patients with cancer (72, 167). Importantly, it has also been shown in such patients that cultured DCs can track from potentially therapeutic injection sites (intradermal, subcutaneous, and intravenous) to sites where immune priming of T cells is likely to occur, in particular, lymph nodes (89).

Although clinical application of DCs for cancer therapy is still at an early stage, some data are available on the ability of DCs to instigate immune responses *in vitro* or *in vivo* in cancer patients. For example, therapy with DC pulsed with peptides of prostate-specific membrane antigen (PSMA) has led to six partial and two complete responses in 33 patients with advanced, metastatic, hormone-refractory prostate cancer, with some responses being relatively durable (169). In this palliative setting, it has also been shown that the dose of DCs can be increased, and the frequency of treatment decreased, without impairing response rate or causing unacceptable toxicity (170). In a similar trial in locally recurrent prostate cancer, one complete and ten partial responses were seen amongst 37 patients (171). In these prostate trials and, indeed, in all DC clinical applications tried to date, no major toxicity has been reported.

A range of other malignancies has also been targeted with DC-based therapies. Pulsing DCs with idiotypic protein for administration to patients with low-grade B-cell lymphoma produced evidence of a cell-mediated immune response in all of four patients (18). There was one complete and two partial responses. In melanoma, injection into lymph nodes of DCs pulsed with peptide epitopes or autologous lysed tumor cells produced two complete and three partial responses amongst 15 patients, with infiltration of CD8 cells into delayed-type hypersensitivity (DTH) challenge sites that, on culture, generated CTLs capable of lysing peptide-pulsed target cells (172). In other melanoma trials using DCs pulsed with known antigenic epitopes, specific CTL responses have been generated, in some cases associated with clinical remission (173, 174). For therapy of tumors expressing CEA, vaccination with CEA peptide-pulsed DCs has also been shown to stimulate immune responses against the peptide (175, 176). However, the demonstration of such immune reactivity *in vitro* is of uncertain clinical significance, and does not inevitably correlate with any clinical tumor regression. Perhaps the most impressive clinical activity seen so far using DCs has been the four complete and two partial responses seen amongst 17 patients with metastatic renal cell carcinoma treated with a hybrid vaccine of autologous tumor cells fused with allogeneic DCs (143).

Although no significant adverse effects have been seen in DC clinical trials to date, there remain at least theoretical concerns about their safety. Specifically, generating a potent immune response against a tumor-associated antigen that may also be expressed by normal tissue could result in autoimmunity, a possibility that has been demonstrated in a mouse model system (177). Most tumor antigens defined so far are neither mutated nor tumor-specific, increasing the likelihood of immune cross-reactivity between tumor and normal tissue leading to significant toxicity on immune priming. For DC approaches using multiple potential antigens (such as tumor cell/DC hybrids or tumor-lysate-pulsed DCs), there is undoubtedly the risk of priming immunity against some eptiopes in the tumor that are also expressed by nonmalignant cells. This concern is not restricted to the use of DCs, and also applies to other strategies (such as genetically modified autologous or allogeneic tumor cell vaccines) designed to stimulate potent immunity against antigens that are unlikely to be entirely tumor-specific. If the normal tissue from which a tumor arises is expendable, for example, prostate, ovary, or breast, autoimmunity may be an acceptable price to pay for potent immune priming against the tumor. For other diseases, such as colon cancer or brain tumors, autoimmune consequences could be devastating. However, to date no such side-effects have been seen in treated patients, and the risk remains theoretical only.

Hence, early DC-based trials provide encouragement for the use of DCs as APCs to load with antigen for effective immune priming in cancer patients. However, many questions remain unanswered, both in preclinical and clinical models, which may have profound effects on the efficacy of treatment strategies. These include the following.

- The optimal culture conditions for growing DCs. These may vary depending on the role that the DC is being asked to play *in vivo* (that is, antigen acquisition, presentation, or both).
- Definition of the most useful antigens to deliver to DCs. Whether it is more effective to use a single/few epitopes that are known to act as targets for CTLs, or to load DCs with multiple potential

rejection antigens using cell fusion, cell lysates, or RNA transfection, is unclear.

- Understanding the most potent way to load DCs with antigens, by genetic modification, pulsing with whole apoptotic/necrotic cells, cell lysates, proteins, or peptides, or adoptively transferring or recruiting DC *in vivo*.
- Which route to use when administering DCs *in vivo*. There is currently no consensus between the options of intradermal, subcutaneous, intraperitoneal, intravenous, intratumoral, or intralymphoid delivery. Direct comparisons between vaccination routes have been made in animal models, but with conflicting results (178, 179).
- Which immunological read-outs to measure in clinical trials. Significant gross tumor shrinkage remains the gold standard, but the demonstration and significance of CTL responses, DTH reactions, and other in vitro assays remains problematic.

Conclusion

Our understanding of the antigens expressed by tumors and the mechanisms by which they may or may not be presented to the immune system in cancer patients has increased dramatically in recent years. This has led to the development, in animal models and early clinical studies, of ways to stimulate an effective immune response against a tumor, which, by definition, has managed to remain immunologically hidden during its development. The development of treatment strategies targeted to defined tumor antigens, rather than relying on nonspecific immune activation by, for example, systemic administration of cytokines, is likely to lead to novel therapies with an improved therapeutic index between efficacy and toxicity. APCs such as DCs are the key players in presenting such target antigens to the immune system in a stimulatory fashion. An improved understanding of the basic science of DCs and how best to harness them for clinical benefit remains a significant challenge for the next decade. To date, limited clinical information suggests that DCs can achieve tumor-targeted immune therapy without any major toxicity. However, an expanding world of basic tumor immunology is emerging—its application for patient benefit remains the clinical challenge.

References

1. Rosenberg SA. The immunotherapy and gene therapy of cancer. J Clin Oncol 1992, **10**, 180–99.

2. van der Bruggen P, Traversari C, Chomez P, *et al*. A gene encoding an antigen recognized by cytolytic T lymphocytes on a human melanoma. Science 1991, **254**, 1643–7.

3. Van der Bruggen P, Szikora JP, Boel P, *et al*. Autologous cytolytic T lymphocytes recognize a MAGE-1 nonapeptide on melanoma expressing HLA-Cw*1601. Eur J Immunol 1994, **24**, 2134–40.

4. Van den Eynde B, Peeters O, De Backer O, *et al*. A new family of genes coding for an antigen recognized by autologous cytolytic T lymphocytes on a human melanoma. J Exp Med 1995, **182**, 689–98.

5. Boel P, Wildmann C, Sensi ML, *et al*. BAGE: a new gene encoding an antigen recognized on human melanomas by cytolytic T lymphocytes. Immunity 1995, **2**, 167–75.

6. Taylor-Papadimitriou J, Stewart L, Burchell J, *et al*. The polymorphic epithelial mucin as a target for immunotherapy. Ann NY Acad Sci 1993, **690**, 69–79.

7. Brichard V, Van Pel A, Wolfel T, *et al*. The tyrosinase gene codes for an antigen recognised by autologous cytotoxic T lymphocytes on HLA-A2 melanomas. J Exp Med 1993, **178**, 489–95.

8. Topalian SL, Rivoltini L, Mancini M, *et al*. Human CD4+ T cells specifically recognize a shared melanoma-associated antigen encoded by the tyrosinase gene. Proc Natl Acad Sci, USA 1994, **91**, 9461–5.

9. Coulie PG, Brichard V, Van Pel A, *et al*. A new gene coding for a differentiation antigen recognized by autologous cytolytic T lymphocytes on HLA-A2 melanomas. J Exp Med 1994, **180**, 35–42.

10. Cox AL, Skipper J, Chen Y, *et al*. Identification of a peptide recognized by five melanoma-specific human cytotoxic T cell lines. Science 1994, **264**, 716–18.

11. Wang RF, Robbins PF, Kawakami Y, *et al*. Identification of a gene encoding a melanoma tumor antigen recognized by HLA-A31-restricted tumor-infiltrating lymphocytes. J Exp Med 1995, **181**, 799–804.

12. Rosenberg SA and White DE. Brief report: vitiligo in patients with melanoma: normal tissue antigens can be targets for cancer immunotherapy. J Immunother 1996, **183**, 1131–40.

13. Wolfel T, Hauer M, Schneider J, *et al*. A p16^{INK4a}-insensitive CDK4 mutant targeted by cytolytic T lymphocytes in a human melanoma. Science 1995, **269**, 1281–4.

14. Coulie PG, Lehmann F, Lethe B, *et al*. A mutated intron sequence codes for an antigenic peptide recognized by cytolytic T lymphocytes on a human melanoma. Proc Natl Acad Sci, USA 1995, **92**, 7976–80.

15. Robbins PF, El-Gamil M, Li YF, *et al*. A mutated beta-catenin gene encodes a melanoma-specific antigen recognised by tumor infiltrating lymphocytes. J Exp Med 1996, **183**, 1185–92.

16. Mandruzzato S, Brasseur F, Andry G, *et al*. A CASP-8 mutation recognised by cytolytic T lymphocytes on a human head and neck carcinoma. J Exp Med 1997, **186**, 785–93.

17. Kwak LW, Taub DD, Duffey PL, *et al*. Transfer of myeloma idiotype-specific immunity from an actively immunised marrow donor. Lancet 1995, **345**, 1016–20.

18. Hsu FJ, Benike C, Fagnoni F, *et al*. Vaccination of patients with B-cell lymphoma using autologous antigen-pulsed dendritic cells. Nat Med 1996, **2**, 52–8.

19. Ressing ME, Sette A, Brandt RM, *et al*. Human CTL epitopes encoded by human papillomavirus type 16 E6 and E7 identified through *in vivo* and *in vitro* immunogenicity studies of HLA-A*0201-binding peptides. J Immunol 1995, **154** (11), 5934–43.

20. Rickinson AB. Immune intervention against virus-associated human cancers. Ann Oncol 1995, **6** (suppl. 1), S69–S71.

21. Melief JM, Kast WM. Potential immunogenicity of oncogene and tumor suppressor gene products. Curr Opin Immunol 1993, **5**, 709–13.

22. Yanuck M, Carbone DP, Pendleton CD, *et al*. A mutant p53 tumor suppressor protein is a target for peptide-induced CD8+ cytotoxic T-cells. Cancer Res 1993, **53**, 3257–61.

23. Fossum B, Olsen AC, Thorsby E, *et al*. CD8$^+$ T cells from a patient with colon carcinoma, specific for a mutant p21-Ras-derived peptide (GLY^{13} to ASP), are cytotoxic towards a carcinoma cell line harbouring the same mutation. Cancer Immunol Immunother 1995, **40**, 165–72.

24. Qin H, Chen W, Takahashi M, *et al*. CD4+ T-cell immunity to mutated ras protein in pancreatic and colon cancer patients. Cancer Res 1995, **55**, 2984–7.

25. Chen W, Peace DJ, Rovira DK, *et al*. T-cell immunity to the joining region of p210BCR-ABL protein. Proc Natl Acad Sci, USA 1992, **89**, 1468–72.

26. Peoples GE, Goedegebuure PS, Smith R, *et al*. Breast and ovarian cancer-specific cytotoxic T lymphocytes recognize the same HER2/neu-derived peptide. Proc Natl Acad Sci, USA 1995, **92**, 432–6.

27. Banchereau J, Steinman RM. Dendritic cells and the control of immunity. Nature 1998, **392**, 245–52.

28. Steinman RM, Cohn ZA. Identification of a novel cell type in peripheral lymphoid organs of mice. I. Morphology, quantitation, tissue distribution. J Exp Med 1973, **137**, 1142–62.

29. Inaba K, Metlay JP, Crowley MT, *et al*. Dendritic cells pulsed with protein antigens *in vitro* can prime antigen-specific, MHC-restricted T cells *in situ*. J Exp Med 1990, **172**, 631–40.

30. Celluzzi CM, J.I. M, Storkus WJ, *et al*. Peptide-pulsed dendritic cells induce antigen specific, CTL-mediated protective tumor immunity. J Exp Med 1996, **183**, 283–7.

31. Huang AYC, Golumbek P, Ahmadzadeh M, *et al*. Role of bone marrow-derived cells in presenting MHC class 1-restricted tumor antigens. Science 1994, **264**, 961–4.

32. Hart DNJ. Dendritic cells: unique leukocyte population which control the primary immune response. Blood 1997, **90**, 3245–87.

33. Krall G, Breel M, Janse M, *et al.* Langerhans cells, veiled cells, interdigitating cells in the mouse recognised by a monoclonal antibody. J Exp Med 1986, **163**, 981–97.

34. O'Doherty U, Peng M, Gezelter S, *et al.* Human blood contains two subsets of dendritic cells, one immunologically mature and the other immature. Immunology 1994, **82**, 487–93.

35. Vremec D, Shortman K. Dendritic cells subtypes in mouse lymphoid organs. Cross-correlation of surface markers, changes with incubation, and differences among thymus, spleen, and lymph nodes. J Immunol 1997, **159**, 565–73.

36. Salomon B, Cohen JL, Masurier C, *et al.* Three populations of mouse lymph node dendritic cells with different origins and dynamics. J Immunol 1998, **160**, 708–17.

37. Grouard G, Durand I, Filgueira L, *et al.* Dendritic cells capable of stimulating T cells in germinal centres. Nature 1996, **384**, 364–7.

38. Cella M, Sallusto F, Lanzavecchia A. Origin, maturation and antigen presenting function of dendritic cells. Curr Opin Immunol 1997, **9**, 10–16.

39. Kampgen E, Koch N, Koch F, *et al.* Class II major histocompatibility complex molecules of murine dendritic cells: synthesis, sialylation of invariant chain, and antigen processing capacity are down-regulated upon culture. Proc Natl Acad Sci, USA 1991, **88**, 3014–18.

40. Pure E, Inaba K, Crowley MT, *et al.* Antigen processing by epidermal Langerhans cells correlates with the level of biosynthesis of major histocompatibility complex class II molecules and expression of invariant chain. J Exp Med 1990, **172**, 1459–69.

41. Stossel H, Koch F, Kampgen E, *et al.* Disappearance of certain acidic organelles (endosomes and Langerhans cell granules) accompanies loss of antigen processing capacity upon culture of epidermal Langerhans cells. J Exp Med 1990, **172**, 1471–82.

42. Chapuis F, Rosenzwajg M, Yagello M, *et al.* Differentiation of human dendritic cells from monocytes *in vitro*. Eur J Immunol 1997, **27**, 431–41.

43. Zhou L-J, Tedder TF. CD14+ blood monocytes can differentiate into functionally mature CD83+ dendritic cells. Proc Natl Acad Sci, USA 1996, **93**, 2588–92.

44. Romani N, Reider D, Heuer M, *et al.* Generation of mature dendritic cells from human blood. An improved method with special regard to clinical applicability. J Immunol Methods 1996, **196**, 137–51.

45. Sallusto F, Lanzavecchia A. Efficient presentation of soluble antigen by cultured human dendritic cells is maintained by granulocyte/macrophage colony-stimulating factor plus interleukin 4 and downregulated by tumor necrosis factor alpha. J Exp Med 1994, **179**, 1109–18.

46. Caux C, Vanbervliet B, Massacrier C, *et al.* CD34⁺ haematopoietic progenitors from human cord blood differentiate along two independent dendritic cell pathways in response to GM-CSF + TNFα. J Exp Med 1996, **184**, 695.

47. Caux C, Massacrier C, Vanbervliet B, *et al.* CD34⁺ haematopoietic progenitors from human cord blood differentiate along two independent dendritic cell pathways in response to granulocyte–macrophage colony-stimulating factor plus tumor necrosis factor α: II. Functional analysis. Blood 1997, **90**, 1458–70.

48. Marquez C, Trigueros C, Fernandez E, *et al.* The development of T and non-T cell lineages from CD34⁺ human thymic precursors can be traced by the differential expression of CD44. J Exp Med 1995, **181**, 475–83.

49. Saunders D, Lucas K, Ismaili J, *et al.* Dendritic cell development in culture from thymic precursors in the absence of granulocyte/macrophage colony-stimulating factor. J Exp Med 1996, **184**, 2185–96.

50. Galy A, Travis M, Cen D, *et al.* Human T, B, natural killer, and dendritic cells arise from a common bone marrow progenitor cell subset. Immunity 1995, **3**, 459–73.

51. Kronin V, Winkel K, Suss G, *et al.* A subclass of dendritic cells regulates the response of naive CD8 T cells by limiting their IL-2 production. J Immunol 1996, **157**, 3819–27.

52. Suss G, Shortman K. A subclass of dendritic cells kills CD4 T cells via Fas/Fas-ligand-induced apoptosis. J Exp Med 1996, **183**, 1789–96.

53. Siegal FP, Kadowaki N, Shodell M, *et al.* The nature of the principal type 1 interferon-producing cells in human blood. Science 1999, **284**, 1835–7.

54. Scheicher C, Mehlig M, Dienes H-P, *et al.* Uptake of microparticle-adsorbed protein antigen by bone marrow-derived dendritic cells results in up-regulation of interleukin-1α and interleukin-12 p40/p35 and triggers prolonged, efficient antigen presentation. Eur J Immunol 1995, **25**, 1566–72.

55. Sparwasser T, Koch E-S, Vabulas RM, *et al.* Bacterial DNA and immunostimulatory CpG oligonucleotides trigger maturation and activation of murine dendritic cells. Eur J Immunol 1998, **28**, 2045–54.

56. Lu L, McCaslin D, Starzl TE, *et al.* Bone marrow-derived dendritic cell progenitors (NLDC 145+, MHC class II+, B7-1dim, B7-2–) induce alloantigen-specific hyporesponsiveness in murine T lymphocytes. Transplantation 1995, **60**, 1539–45.

57. Yamaguchi Y, Tsumura H, Miwa M, *et al.* Contrasting effects of TGF-β1 and TNF-α on the development of dendritic cells from progenitors in mouse bone marrow. Stem Cells 1997, **15**, 144–53.

58. Inaba K, Inaba M, Romani N, *et al.* Generation of large numbers of dendritic cells from mouse bone marrow cultures supplemented with granulocyte/macrophage colony-stimulating factor. J Exp Med 1992, **176**, 1693–702.

59. Lu L, Hsieh M, Oriss TB, *et al.* Generation of DC from mouse spleen cell cultures in response to GM-CSF: immunophenotypic and functional analyses. Immunology 1995, **84**, 127–34.

60. Inaba K, Steinman RM, Pack MW, *et al.* Identification of proliferating dendritic cell precursors in mouse blood. J Exp Med 1992, **175**, 1157–67.

61. Lu L, Woo J, Rao AS, *et al.* Propagation of dendritic cell progenitors from normal mouse liver using granulocyte/macrophage colony-stimulating factor and their maturational development in the presence of type-1 collagen. J Exp Med 1994, **179**, 1823–34.

62. Vremec D, Lieschke GJ, Dunn AR, *et al.* The influence of granulocyte/macrophage colony-stimulating factor on dendritic cell levels in mouse lymphoid organs. Eur J Immunol 1997, **27**, 40–4.

63. Grouard G, Rissoan M-C, Filgueira L, *et al.* The enigmatic plasmacytoid T cells develop into dendritic cells with interleukin (IL)-3 and CD40-ligand. J Exp Med 1997, **185**, 1101–11.

64. Oehler L, Majdic O, Pickl WF, *et al.* Neutrophil granulocyte-committed cells can be driven to acquire dendritic cell characteristics. J Exp Med 1998, **187**, 1019–28.

65. Shurin MR, Pandharipande PP, Zorina TD, *et al.* FLT3 ligand induces the generation of functionally active dendritic cells in mice. Cell Immunol 1997, **179**, 174–84.

66. Pulendran B, Lingpappa J, Kennedy MK, *et al.* Developmental pathways of dendritic cells *in vivo*. Distinct function, phenotype, and localization of dendritic cell subsets in FLT3 ligand-treated mice. J Immunol 1997, **159**, 2222–31.

67. Flores-Romo L, Bjorck P, Duvert V, *et al.* CD40 ligation on human cord blood CD34+ haematopoietic progenitors induces their proliferation and differentiation into functional dendritic cells. J Exp Med 1997, **185**, 341–9.

68. Riedl E, Strobl H, Majdic O, *et al.* TGF-β1 promotes *in vitro* generation of dendritic cells by protecting progenitor cells from apoptosis. J Immunol 1997, **158**, 1591–7.

69. Gabrilovich DI, Chen HL, Girgis KR, *et al.* Production of vascular endothelial growth factor by human tumors inhibits the functional maturation of dendritic cells. Nat Med 1996, **2**, 1096–103.

70. Buelens C, Verhasselt V, De Groote D, *et al.* Interleukin-10 prevents the generation of dendritic cells from human peripheral blood mononuclear cells cultured with interleukin-4 and granulocyte/macrophage-colony-stimulating factor. Eur J Immunol 1997, **27**, 756–62.

71. Nestle FO, Burg G, Fah J, *et al.* Human sunlight-induced basal-cell-carcinoma-associated dendritic cells are deficient in T cell co-stimulatory molecules and are impaired as antigen-presenting cells. Am J Pathol 1997, **150**, 641–51.

72. Tjoa B, Erickson S, Barren R, *et al. In vitro* propagated dendritic cells from prostate cancer patients as a component of prostate cancer immunotherapy. Prostate 1995, **27**, 63–9.

73. Mortarini R, Anichini A, Di Nicola M, *et al.* Autologous dendritic cells derived from CD34$^+$ progenitors and from monocytes are not functionally equivalent antigen-presenting cells in the induction of melan-A/Mart-1$_{27-35}$-specific CTLs from peripheral blood lymphocytes of melanoma patients with low frequency of CTL precursors. Cancer Res 1997, **57**, 5534–41.

74. Herbst B, Kohler G, Mackensen A, *et al.* CD34$^+$ peripheral blood progenitor cell and monocyte derived dendritic cells: a comparative analysis. Br J Haematol 1997, **99**, 490–9.

75. Morse MA, Lyerly HK, Gilboa E, *et al.* Optimization of the sequence of antigen loading and CD40-ligand-induced maturation of dendritic cells. Cancer Res 1998, **58**, 2965–8.

76. Inaba K, Inaba M, Naito M, *et al.* Dendritic cell progenitors phagocytose particulates, including Bacillus Calmette–Guerin organisms, and sensitize mice to mycobacterial antigens *in vivo*. J Exp Med 1993, **178**, 479–88.

77. Herbst B, Kohler G, Mackensen A, *et al. In vitro* differentiation of CD34$^+$ haematopoietic progenitor cells toward distinct dendritic cell subsets of the Birbeck granule and MIIC-positive Langerhans cell and the interdigitating dendritic cell type. Blood 1996, **88**, 2541–8.

78. De Smedt T, Pajak B, Muraille E, *et al.* Regulation of dendritic cells numbers and maturation by lipopolysaccharide *in vivo*. J Exp Med 1996, **184**, 1413–24.

79. Larsen CP, Steinman RM, Witmer-Pack M, *et al.* Migration and maturation of Langerhans cells in skin transplants and explants. J Exp Med 1990, **172**, 1483.

80. Roake JA, Rao AS, Morris PJ, *et al.* Dendritic cell loss from nonlymphoid tissues after systemic administration of lipopolysaccharide, tumor necrosis factor, and interleukin 1. J Exp Med 1995, **181**, 2237–47.

81. Godiska R, Chantry D, Raport CJ, *et al.* Human macrophage-derived chemokine (MDC), a novel chemoattractant for monocytes, monocyte-derived dendritic cells, and natural killer cells. J Exp Med 1997, **185**, 1595–604.

82. Sozzani S, Luini W, Borsatti A, *et al.* Receptor expression and responsiveness of human dendritic cells to a defined set of CC and CXC chemokines. J Immunol 1997, **159**, 1993–2000.

83. Kellermann S-A, Hudak S, Oldham ER, *et al.* The CC chemokine receptor-7 ligands 6Ckine and macrophage inflammatory protein 3b are potent chemoattractants for *in vitro*- and *in vivo*-derived dendritic cells. J Immunol 1999, **162**, 3859–64.

84. Fushimi T, Kojima A, Moore MA, *et al.* Macrophage inflammatory protein 3 alpha transgene attracts dendritic cells to established murine tumors and suppresses tumor growth. J Clin Invest 2000, **105** (10), 1383–93.

85. Cella M, Engering A, Pinet V, *et al.* Inflammatory stimuli induce accumulation of MHC class II complexes on dendritic cells. Nature 1997, **388**, 782–7.

86. Pierre P, Turley SJ, Gatti E, *et al.* Developmental regulation of MHC class II transport in mouse dendritic cells. Nature 1997, **388**, 787–92.

87. Austyn JM, Kupiec-Weglinski JW, Hankins DF, *et al.* Migration patterns of dendritic cells in the mouse. Homing to T cell-dependent areas of spleen, and binding within marginal zone. J Exp Med 1988, **167**, 646–51.

88. Barratt-Boyes SM, Zimmer MI, Harshyne LA, *et al.* Maturation and trafficking of monocyte-derived dendritic cells in monkeys: implications for dendritic cell-based vaccines. J Immunol 2000, **164** (5), 2487–95.

89. Morse MA, Coleman RE, Akabani G, *et al.* Migration of human dendritic cells after injection in patients with metastatic malignancies. Cancer Res 1999, **59**, 56–8.

90. Hock BD, Starling GC, Daniel PB, *et al.* Characterization of CMRF-44, a novel monoclonal antibody to an activation antigen expressed by the allostimulatory cells within peripheral blood, including dendritic cells. Immunology 1994, **83**, 573–81.

91. Zhou L-J and Tedder TF. Human blood dendritic cells selectively express CD83, a member of the immunoglobulin superfamily. J Immunol 1995, **154**, 3821–35.

92. Jiang W, Swiggard WJ, Heufler C, *et al.* The receptor DEC-205 expressed by dendritic cells and thymic epithelial cells is involved in antigen processing. Nature 1995, **375**, 151–5.

93. Kato M, Neil TK, Clark G, *et al.* cDNA cloning of human DEC-205, a putative antigen-uptake receptor on dendritic cells. Immunogenetics 1998, **47**, 442–50.

94. Lanzavecchia A. Mechanisms of antigen uptake for presentation. Curr Opin Immunol 1996, **8**, 348–54.

95. Reis e Sousa C, Stahl PD, Austyn JM. Phagocytosis of antigens by Langerhans cells *in vitro*. J Exp Med 1993, **178**, 509–19.

96. Svensson M, Stockinger B, Wick MJ. Bone marrow-derived dendritic cells can process bacteria for MHC-I and MHC-II presentation to T cells. J Immunol 1997, **158**, 4229–36.

97. Sallusto F, Cella M, Danieli C, *et al.* Dendritic cells use macropinocytosis and the mannose receptor to concentrate macromolecules in the major histocompatibility complex class II compartment: downregulation by cytokines and bacterial products. J Exp Med 1995, **182**, 389–400.

98. Norbury CC, Chambers BJ, Prescott AR, *et al.* Constitutive macropinocytosis allows TAP-dependent major histocompatibility complex class I presentation of exogenous soluble antigen by bone marrow-derived dendritic cells. Eur J Immunol 1997, **27**, 280–8.

99. Engering AJ, Cella M, Fluitsma D, *et al.* The mannose receptor functions as a high capacity and broad specificity antigen receptor in human dendritic cells. Eur J Immunol 1997, **27**, 2417–25.

100. Santambrogio L, Sato AK, Carven GJ, *et al.* Extracellular antigen processing and presentation by immature dendritic cells. Proc Natl Acad Sci, USA 1999, **96** (26), 15056–61.

101. Bachmann ME, Lutz MB, Layton GT, *et al.* Dendritic cells process exogenous viral proteins and virus-like particles for class I presentation to CD8+ cytotoxic T lymphocytes. Eur J Immunol 1996, **26**, 2595–600.

102. Huang AYC, Bruce AT, Pardoll DM, *et al.* Does B7-1 expression confer antigen-presenting capacity to tumors *in vivo*? J Exp Med 1996, **183**, 769–76.

103. Albert ML, Sauter B, Bhardwaj N. Dendritic cells acquire antigen from apoptotic cells and induced class I-restricted CTLs. Nature 1998, **392**, 86–9.

104. Ronchetti A, Rovere P, Iezzi G, *et al.* Immunogenicity of apoptotic cells *in vivo*: role of antigen load, antigen-presenting cells, and cytokines. J Immunol 1999, **163**, 130–6.

105. Gallucci S, Lolkema M, Matzinger P. Natural adjuvants: endogenous activators of dendritic cells. Nat Med 1999, **5**, 1249–55.

106. Sauter B, Albert ML, Francisco L, *et al.* Consequences of cell death. Exposure to necrotic tumor cells, but not primary tissue cells or apoptotic cells, induces the maturation of immunostimulatory dendritic cells. J Exp Med 2000, **191** (3), 423–34.

107. Melcher A, Gough M, Todryk S, *et al.* Apoptosis or necrosis for tumor immunotherapy: what's in a name? J Mol Med 1999, **77**, 824–33.

108. Melcher AA, Todryk S, Hardwick N, *et al.* Tumor immunogenicity is determined by the mechanism of cell death via induction of heat shock protein expression. Nat Med 1998, **4**, 581–7.

109. Todryk S, Melcher AA, Hardwick N, *et al.* Heat shock protein 70 induced during tumor cell killing induces Th1 cytokines and targets immature dendritic cell precursors to enhance antigen uptake. J Immunol 1999, **163**, 1398–408.

110. Castellino F, Boucher PE, Eichelberg K, *et al.* Receptor-mediated uptake of antigen/heat shock protein complexes results in major histocompatibility complex class I antigen presentation via two distinct processing pathways. J Exp Med 2000, **191** (11), 1957–64.

111. Singh-Jasuja H, Toes RE, Spee P, *et al.* Cross-presentation of glycoprotein 96-associated antigens on major histocompatibility complex class I molecules requires receptor-mediated endocytosis. J Exp Med 2000, **191** (11), 1965–74.

112. Binder RJ, Han DK, Srivastava PK. CD91: a receptor for heat shock protein gp96. Nat Immunol 2000, **1**, 151–5.

113. Condon C, Watkins SC, Celluzzi CM, *et al.* DNA-based immunization by *in vivo* transfection of dendritic cells. Nat Med 1996, **2**, 1122–8.

114. Corr M, Lee DJ, Carson DA, *et al.* Gene vaccination with naked plasmid DNA: mechanism of CTL priming. J Exp Med 1996, **184**, 1555–60.

115. Casares S, Inaba K, Brumeanu T-D, *et al.* Antigen presentation by dendritic cells after immunization with DNA encoding a major histocompatibility complex class II-restricted viral epitope. J Exp Med 1997, **186**, 1481–6.

116. Arthur JF, Butterfield LH, Roth MD, *et al.* A comparison of gene transfer methods in human dendritic cells. Cancer Gene Ther 1997, **4**, 17–25.

117. Alijagic S, Moller P, Artuc M, *et al.* Dendritic cells generated from peripheral blood transfected with human tyrosinase induce specific T cell activation. Eur J Immunol 1995, **25**, 3100–7.

118. Tuting T, Wilson CC, Martin DM, *et al.* Autologous human monocyte-derived dendritic cells genetically modified to express melanoma antigens elicit primary cytotoxic T cell responses *in vitro*: enhancement by cotransfection of genes encoding the Th1-biasing cytokines IL-12 and IFN-α. J Immunol 1998, **160**, 1139–47.

119. Brossart P, Goldrath AW, Butz EA, *et al.* Virus-mediated delivery of antigenic epitopes into dendritic cells as a means to induce CTL. J Immunol 1997, **158**, 3270–6.

120. Song W, Kong H-L, Carpenter H, *et al.* Dendritic cells genetically modified with an adenovirus vector encoding the cDNA for a model antigen induce protective and therapeutic antitumor immunity. J Exp Med 1997, **186**, 1247–56.

121. Ribas A, Butterfield LH, McBride WH, *et al.* Genetic immunization for the melanoma antigen MART-1/Melan-A using recombinant adenovirus-transduced murine dendritic cells. Cancer Res 1997, **57**, 2865–9.

122. Gong J, Chen L, Chen D, *et al.* Induction of antigen-specific antitumor immunity with adenovirus-transduced dendritic cells. Gene Ther 1997, **4**, 1023–8.

123. Dietz AB, Vuk-Pavlovic S. High efficiency adenovirus-mediated gene transfer to human dendritic cells. Blood 1998, **91**, 392–8.

124. Curiel-Lewandrowski C, Mahnke K, Labeur M, *et al.* Transfection of immature murine bone marrow-derived dendritic cells with the granulocyte–macrophage colony-stimulating factor gene potently enhances their *in vivo* antigen-presenting capacity. J Immunol 1999, **163**, 174–83.

125. Reeves ME, Royal RE, Lam JS, *et al.* Retroviral transduction of human dendritic cells with a tumor-associated antigen gene. Cancer Res 1996, **56**, 5672–7.

126. Specht JM, Wang G, Do MT, *et al.* Dendritic cells retrovirally transduced with a model antigen gene are therapeutically effective against established pulmonary metastases. J Exp Med 1997, **186**, 1213–21.

127. Boczkowski D, Nair SK, Snyder D, *et al.* Dendritic cells pulsed with RNA are potent antigen-presenting cells *in vitro* and *in vivo*. J Exp Med 1996, **184**, 465–72.

128. Ashley DM, Faiola B, Nair S, *et al.* Bone marrow-generated dendritic cells pulsed with tumor extracts or tumor RNA induce antitumor immunity against central nervous system tumors. J Exp Med 1997, **186**, 1177–82.

129. Heiser A, Dahm P, D RY, *et al.* Human dendritic cells transfected with RNA encoding prostate-specific antigen stimulate prostate-specific CTL responses *in vitro*. J Immunol 2000, **164** (10), 5508–14.

130. Nair SK, Boczkowski D, Snyder D, *et al.* Antigen-presenting cells pulsed with unfractionated tumor-derived peptides are potent tumor vaccines. Eur J Immunol 1997, **27**, 589–97.

131. Fields RC, Shimizu K, Mule JJ. Murine dendritic cells pulsed with whole tumor lysates mediate potent antitumor immune responses *in vitro* and *in vivo*. Proc Natl Acad Sci, USA. 1998, **95**, 9482–7.

132. De Bruijn MLH, Schuurhuis DH, Vierboon MPM, *et al.* Immunization with human papillomavirus type 16 (HPV16) oncoprotein-loaded dendritic cells as well as protein in adjuvant induces MHC class I-restricted protection to HPV16-induced tumor cells. Cancer Res 1998, **58**, 724–31.

133. Flamand V, Sornasse T, Thielemans K, *et al.* Murine dendritic cells pulsed *in vitro* with tumor antigen induce tumor resistance *in vivo*. Eur J Immunol 1994, **24**, 605–10.

134. Porgador A, Gilboa E. Bone marrow-generated dendritic cells pulsed with a class I-restricted peptide are potent inducers of cytotoxic T lymphocytes. J Exp Med 1995, **182**, 255–60.

135. Mayordormo JI, Zorina T, Storkus WJ, *et al.* Bone marrow-derived dendritic cells pulsed with synthetic tumor peptides elicit protective and therapeutic antitumor immunity. Nat Med 1995, **1**, 1297–302.

136. Mayordomo JI, Loftus DJ, Sakamoto H, *et al.* Therapy of murine tumors with p53 wild-type and mutant sequence peptide-based vaccines. J Exp Med 1996, **183**, 1357–65.

137. Ossevoort MA, Feltkamp MCW, van Veen KJH, *et al.* Dendritic cells as carriers for a cytotoxic T-lymphocyte epitope-based peptide vaccine in protection against a human papillomavirus type 16-induced tumor. J Immunother 1995, **18**, 86–94.

138. Bakker ABH, Marland G, de Boer AJ, *et al.* Generation of antimelanoma cytotoxic T lymphocytes from healthy donors after presentation of melanoma-associated antigen-derived epitopes by dendritic cells *in vitro*. Cancer Res 1995, **55**, 5330–4.

139. Zitvogel L, Mayordormo JI, Tjandrawan T, *et al.* Therapy of murine tumors with tumor peptide-pulsed dendritic cells: dependence on T cells, B7 costimulation, and T helper cell 1-associated cytokines. J Exp Med 1996, **183**, 87–97.

140. Gong J, Chen D, Kashiwaba M, *et al.* Induction of antitumor activity by immunization with fusions of dendritic and carcinoma cells. Nat Med 1997, **3**, 558–61.

141. Lespagnard L, Mettens P, Verheyden A-M, *et al.* Dendritic cells fused with mastocytoma cells elicit therapeutic antitumor immunity. Int J Cancer 1998, **76**, 250–8.

142. Celluzzi CM, Falo LD. Physical interaction between dendritic cells and tumor cells results in an immunogen that induces protective and therapeutic tumor rejection. J Immunol 1998, **160**, 3081–5.

143. Kugler A, Stuhler G, Walden P, *et al.* Regression of human metastatic renal cell carcinoma after vaccination with tumor cell-dendritic cell hybrids. Nat Med 2000, **6** (3), 332–6.

144. Zitvogel L, Regnault A, Lozier A, *et al.* Eradication of established murine tumors using a novel cell-free vaccine: dendritic cell-derived exosomes. Nat Med 1998, **4**, 594–600.

145. Coveney E, Wheatley GH, Lyerly HK. Active immunisation using dendritic cells mixed with tumor cells inhibits the growth of primary breast cancer. Surgery 1997, **122**, 228–34.

146. Melcher A, Todryk S, Bateman A, *et al.* Adoptive transfer of immature dendritic cells with autologous or allogeneic tumor cells generates systemic antitumor immunity. Cancer Res 1999, **59** (12), 2802–5.

147. Nishioka Y, Hirao M, Robbins PD, *et al.* Induction of systemic and therapeutic antitumor immunity using intratumoral injection of dendritic cells genetically modified to express interleukin 12. Cancer Res 1999, **59**, 4035–41.

148. Melero I, Duarte M, Ruiz J, *et al.* Intratumoral injection of bone-marrow derived dendritic cells engineered to produce interleukin-12 induces complete regression of established murine transplantable colon adenocarcinomas. Gene Ther 1999, **6**, 1779–84.

149. Miller PW, Sharma S, Stolina M, *et al.* Intratumoral administration of adenoviral interleukin 7 gene-

modified dendritic cells augments specific antitumor immunity and achieves tumor eradication. Hum Gene Ther 2000, **11** (1), 53–65.

150. Lee C-T, Wu S, Ciernik F, *et al.* Genetic immunotherapy of established tumors with adenovirus-murine granulocyte–macrophage colony-stimulating factor. Human Gene Ther 1997, **8**, 187–93.

151. Stoppacciaro A, Paglia P, Lombardi L, *et al.* Genetic modification of a carcinoma with the IL-4 gene increases the influx of dendritic cells relative to other cytokines. Eur J Immunol 1997, **27**, 2375–82.

152. Kim JJ, Yang JS, Lee DJ, *et al.* Macrophage colony-stimulating factor can modulate immune responses and attract dendritic cells *in vivo*. Hum Gene Ther 2000, **11** (2), 305–21.

153. Esche C, Subbotin VM, Maliszewski C, *et al.* FLT3 ligand administration inhibits tumor growth in murine melanoma and lymphoma. Cancer Res 1998, **58**, 380–3.

154. Chakravarty PK, Alfieri A, Thomas EK, *et al.* Flt3-ligand administration after radiation therapy prolongs survival in a murine model of metastatic lung cancer. Cancer Res 1999, **59** (24), 6028–32.

155. Chiodoni C, Paglia P, Stoppacciaro A, *et al.* Dendritic cells infiltrating tumors cotransduced with granulocyte/macrophage colony-stimulating factor (GM-CSF) and CD40 ligand genes take up and present endogenous tumor-associated antigens, and prime naive mice for a cytotoxic T lymphocyte response. J Exp Med 1999, **190** (1), 125–34.

156. Simons JW, Mikhak B, Chang JF, *et al.* Induction of immunity to prostate cancer antigens: results of a clinical trial of vaccination with irradiated autologous prostate tumor cells engineered to secrete granulocyte-macrophage colony-stimulating factor using *ex vivo* gene transfer. Cancer Res 1999, **59** (20), 5160–8.

157. Chang AE, Li Q, Bishop DK, *et al.* Immunogenetic therapy of human melanoma utilizing autologous tumor cells transduced to secrete granulocyte–macrophage colony-stimulating factor. Hum Gene Ther 2000, **11** (6), 839–50.

158. Krieg AM. The role of CpG motifs in innate immunity. Curr Opin Immunol 2000, **12** (1), 35–43.

159. Steinbrink K, Wolfl M, Jonuleit H, *et al.* Induction of tolerance by IL-10-treated dendritic cells. J Immunol 1997, **159**, 4772–80.

160. Qin Z, Noffz G, Mohaupt M, *et al.* Interleukin-10 prevents dendritic cell accumulation and vaccination with granulocyte–macrophage colony-stimulating factor gene-modified tumor cells. J Immunol 1997, **159**, 770–6.

161. Grohmann U, Bianchi R, Ayroldi E, *et al.* A tumor-associated and self antigen peptide presented by dendritic cells may induce T cell anergy *in vivo*, but IL-12 can prevent or revert the anergic state. J Immunol 1997, **158**, 3593–602.

162. Kananaugh DY, Carbone DP. Immunologic dysfunction in cancer. Hematol Oncol Clin North Am 1996, **10**, 927–51.

163. Chaux P, Favre N, Martin M, *et al.* Tumor-infiltrating dendritic cells are defective in their antigen-presenting function and inducible B7 expression in rats. Int J Cancer 1997, **72**, 619–24.

164. Enk AH, Jonuleit H, Saloga J, *et al.* Dendritic cells as mediators of tumor-induced tolerance in metastatic melanoma. Int J Cancer 1997, **73**, 309–16.

165. Ambe K, Mori M, Enjoji M. S-100 protein-positive dendritic cells in colorectal adenocarcinomas. Cancer 1989, **63**, 496–503.

166. Gabrilovich DI, Ciernik F, Carbone DP. Dendritic cells in antitumor immune responses. 1. Defective antigen presentation in tumor-bearing hosts. Cell Immunol 1996, **170**, 101–10.

167. Gabrilovich DI, Corak J, Ciernik IF, *et al.* Decreased antigen presentation by dendritic cells in patients with breast cancer. Clinical Cancer Res 1997, **3**, 483–90.

168. Bell D, Chomarat P, Broyles D, *et al.* In breast carcinoma tissue, immature dendritic cells reside within the tumor, whereas mature dendritic cells are located in peritumoral areas. J Exp Med 1999, **190**, 1417–26.

169. Murphy GP, Tjoa BA, Simmons SJ, *et al.* Infusion of dendritic cells pulsed with HLA-A2-specific prostate-specific membrane antigen peptides: a phase II prostate cancer vaccine trial involving patients with hormone-refractory metastatic disease. Prostate 1999, **38**, 73–8.

170. Murphy GP, Tjoa BA, Simmons SJ, *et al.* Higher-dose and less frequent dendritic cell infusions with PSMA peptides in hormone-refractory metastatic prostate cancer patients. Prostate 2000, **43**, 59–62.

171. Murphy GP, Tjoa BA, Simmons SJ, *et al.* Phase II prostate cancer vaccine trial: report of a study involving 37 patients with disease recurrence following primary treatment. Prostate 1999, **39** (1), 54–9.

172. Nestle FO, Alijagic S, Gilliet M, *et al.* Vaccination of melanoma patients with peptide- or tumor lysate-pulsed dendritic cells. Nat Med 1998, **4**, 328–32.

173. Mackensen A, Herbst B, Chen JL, *et al.* Phase I study in melanoma patients of a vaccine with peptide-pulsed dendritic cells generated *in vitro* from CD34 (+) hematopoietic progenitor cells. Int J Cancer 2000, **86** (3), 385–92.

174. Thurner B, Haendle I, Roder C, *et al.* Vaccination with mage-3A1 peptide-pulsed mature, monocyte-derived dendritic cells expands specific cytotoxic T cells and induces regression of some metastases in advanced stage IV melanoma. J Exp Med 1999, **190** (11), 1669–78.

175. Morse MA, Deng Y, Coleman D, *et al.* A phase I study of active immunotherapy with carcinoembryonic antigen peptide (CAP-1)-pulsed, autologous human cultured dendritic cells in patients with metastatic malignancies expressing carcinoembryonic antigen. Clin Cancer Res 1999, **5**, 1331–8.

176. Nair SK, Hull S, Coleman D, *et al.* Induction of carcinoembryonic antigen (CEA)-specific cytotoxic T-lymphocyte responses *in vitro* using autologous dendritic cells loaded with CEA peptide or CEA RNA in patients with metastatic malignancies expressing CEA. Int J Cancer 1999, **82**, 121–4.

177. Ludewig B, Ochsenbein AF, Odermatt B, *et al.* Immunotherapy with dendritic cells directed against

tumor antigens shared with normal host cells results in severe autoimmune disease. J Exp Med 2000, **191** (5), 795–804.

178. Eggert AA, Schreurs MW, Boerman OC, *et al.* Biodistribution and vaccine efficiency of murine dendritic cells are dependent on the route of administration. Cancer Res 1999, **59**, 3340–5.

179. Wang TL, Ling M, Shih IM, *et al.* Intramuscular administration of E7-transfected dendritic cells generates the most potent E7-specific anti-tumor immunity. Gene Ther 2000, **7** (9), 726–33.

12 | *Cell carriers for cancer gene therapy: bridging the gap between targeted vectors and systemic delivery?*

Rosa Maria Diaz, Heung Chong, and Richard G. Vile

Introduction

The success of gene therapy as a treatment for cancer will eventually be underpinned by an ability to deliver genes specifically and accurately directly to tumour cells *in vivo* (1–3). To date, the majority of the experiments in which gene delivery by both viral and non-viral vectors has been described in animal models have used direct intratumoral injection of vector. Only a few experiments have shown truly systemic delivery of genes in which a vector is injected at a site distant from its target tissue/cells (4–6). Even in these cases, 'successful therapy' of tumors has often been associated with either highly locoregional (rather than truly systemic) vector administration (5) or with the recruitment of immune stimulatory effectors to compensate for the poor efficiency of gene delivery directly into tumor cells (4, 7, 8).

There have recently been highly significant advances in the understanding and engineering of tropism-determining proteins to target vectors for *in vivo* delivery (9–15). However, it still remains to be shown that targeted, recombinant vectors such as those currently in use can truly attain titers that will have therapeutic value in patients with disseminated disease through systemic administration. Realization of this fact has recently led to increasing advocacy of the use of replicating viruses for delivery to both local and disseminated tumors (16–22). However, problems associated with achieving genuine and realistic tumor targeting, along with immune inactivation of freely circulating virus, remain even with replicating constructs (2).

Therefore, there is real need now to develop methods by which surface targeting of vector5 particles may be complemented in order to localize viral vectors/therapeutic genes to the sites of tumor growth. Thus, instead of diluting and exposing valuable stocks of vector to neutralizing circulating immune effectors, it would be preferable to package the vectors within carriers that serve themselves as the primary delivery vehicle. These carriers would serve two principal purposes: the first would be *protective*—preserving the integrity of the vectors until they can be released at high concentration locally at the tumor site(s); the second would be *targeting*—by exploiting the intrinsic abilities of the cell carriers to get to sites of tumor growth in ways that surface-targeted vectors may be unable to do at high efficiency. This concept is analogous to the function of an aircraft carrier that transports its expensive payload of fighters and bombers (the vector particles) to the proximity of a war zone (the tumor site) prior to their release at high local concentrations to seek and destroy their own targets.

Here, we propose the use of cells of a variety of different types to deliver genes and vectors directly to sites of tumor growth. In particular, we will discuss the prospects of using autologous or allogeneic cells as homing vehicles that stand a better chance of reaching tumor sites intact than do recombinant viral vectors.

The need for vector carriers

In a perfect world, oncologists would launch a 'tactical strike' against metastatic cancer deposits from a single intravenous injection of vector. The vector, once released into the blood stream, would remain untouched by any of the body's own anti-invader armoury—antibodies and immune effector cells that patrol the circulation constantly for viral or pathogenic raiders (23–28). Not only would the vector particles remain unmolested by these defence mechanisms, but they would also remain oblivious to the many opportunities for nonspecific adhesion (29) and sequestration (30) that would be put in their way—such as adhesion to vessel walls and uptake by non target cells such as the Kuppfer cells of the liver. Thereafter, the vector particles would require specific radar systems that locate their primary strike sites—usually, but not necessarily, the tumor cells sitting behind endothelial and matrix barriers outside of the circulation. These radar systems would have to include guidance systems that allow the vectors to extravasate out of the circulation and home into the direct target area, leading to infection of the cancer cells. The vectors must include sufficiently sophisticated software to allow high-level expression of the therapeutic genes following infection. However, further fail-safe mechanisms must be incorporated in the vector design to minimize the collateral damage to innocent cells that would result from poor targeting of the vector. This should include the incorporation of transcriptional targeting to ensure a lack of expression in non tumor cells that inadvertently become infected (31) and the inclusion, if possible, of self-destruct switches that could be used to abort the treatment if it should become necessary (32).

Unfortunately, this dream of vectors as precisely targeted missile systems is sadly lacking (Fig. 12.1). In reality, we are still very much at the stage where viral and non viral vectors can be engineered to hit specific targets with very high efficiency on the testing ground (*in vitro*) but at only very poor efficiencies on the battlefield (*in vivo*). The reasons for this are plentiful. Most significantly, the vector systems currently being developed for most gene therapy applications simply cannot be produced to levels that are high enough to tolerate the losses that will be incurred during their circulation, attempts at localization and extravasation, and, finally, infection of the tumor cells. Experiments in immunodeficient mice, where most of the major immune effects that act to reduce viral titers *in vivo* are absent, have shown that, even without anti vector immune responses being taken into consideration, the levels of virus that can be administered are still too low

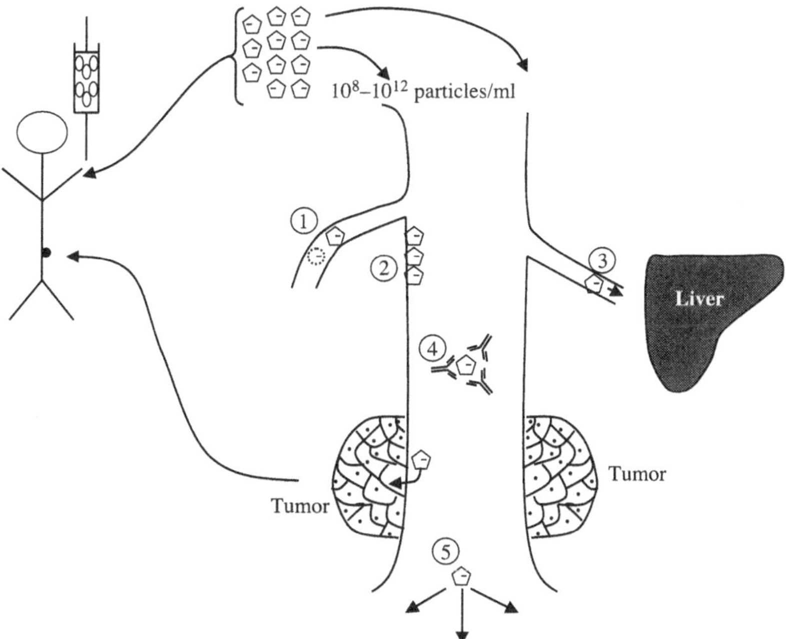

Fig. 12.1 Mechanisms by which viral titers administered systemically into patients will be reduced *in vivo*. The highly purified and concentrated viral stocks that are injected systemically into patients can typically reach titers of between 10^8 (retroviral vectors) to 10^{13} (adenoviral vectors) infectious units per ml as judged by *in vitro* titrations. However, once in the circulation, virus will be lost through: (1) normal degradation of particles (viral half-lives) before they reach the target area; (2) nonspecific adsorption to the surface of cells and tissues that are not the target cells; (3) clearance by cells of, for example, the reticuloendothelial system, such as Kuppfer cells in the liver or other organs; (4) neutralization by antibodies and/or other systems such as complement activation; (5) lack of ability to sense the sites of tumor growth and appropriate arrest of the particles, effective extravasation, and penetration into the tumor site. Thus, only a very small proportion of the vector stocks initially administered as free virus are likely to reach the tumor site itself if the site of administration is significantly far from the desired site of action.

to achieve really meaningful infection of tumors (4). To address the issue of dilution of viral particles by non specific adhesion and binding, extensive efforts have been made to alter the envelope proteins of vectors so that (1) the natural tropism of the envelope protein is removed and (2) a new binding specificity—which will be furnished predominantly by the surface of the tumor cells—is introduced (9–15). These twin aims prevent loss of vector titer through unwanted adhesion to cells that are not the target for transduction and clearly aim to provide a safety component that prevents toxicity of gene delivery to uninvolved normal cells. However, disquieting findings have recently suggested that surface targeting of retroviral vectors may be even more complex that originally thought. Very high levels of non specific adhesion of viral particles to the cell surface appear to occur *before* the envelope–receptor interaction becomes involved (29). If such non specific adsorption to cell surfaces also occurs *in vivo* and/or is extended also to other viruses such as adenoviruses, the reduction in viral titers that occurs on *in vivo* administration would be extensive (Fig. 12.1) and will require some radical rethinking in the field of surface targeting. Moreover, present studies on envelope re-direction have not seriously addressed the issue of how the circulating vector particles can effectively extravasate selectively at the site of tumor growth in order to gain access to the tumor cells. Indeed, appreciation of this fact has focused work on the targeting of tumor endothelial cells rather than the tumor cells themselves. Tumor endothelial cells are 'activated' in many cases relative to normal endothelium (33, 34) and express surface ligands that may form targets for re-directed envelope attachments (9, 35). Nonetheless, the surface targeting of viral sectors and their subsequently modified tropism remains very much at the experimental level. Alterations of binding specificity are clearly achievable in retroviral, adenoviral, and other viral systems; however, these alterations rarely significantly *increase* the already low viral titers. Moreover, sometimes, altering the binding specificity of a viral protein leads to unexpected changes in the pathways of cellular infection. For example, redirecting retroviral envelopes to new ligands by display of novel ligand-binding domains can uncouple the binding and fusion functions of the viral envelope— with the result that only cells no longer expressing the target ligand are infectable by the modified virus (9). Although this is the reverse effect to that initially planned, it can still be used to advantage in so-called inverse targeting strategies (36).

However, these envelope modification experiments, impressive as they are, still address only the issues of re-directing binding specificties. They do not look to the other issues of how to evade incoming patient immune responses exquisitely evolved to eradicate invading viral particles or to how to target selective arrest of vector circulation and efficient extravasation at tumor sites. With respect to the first issue, patients are actually very well equipped to repel systemic vector delivery, since the body's immune systems cannot distinguish a well-intentioned viral onslaught from a pathogenic attack. Circulating antibodies and the human complement system have evolved to neutralize invaders very rapidly. Other immune effectors can also see the vectors and the cells that they have infected and will often clear them (Fig. 12.1). So far, efforts to overcome some of these problems have been made using immunosuppression at the time of vector administration, new components in vectors to block immune responses, removal of viral genes that enhance vector immunogenicity, repeat dosings through the use of different vector serotypes and/or vector types , and plasmapheresis to deplete blocking antibodies (23–28). Very little work has been done on specifically engineering vectors to be able to arrest and extravasate at tumor sites. In general, *in vivo* targeting has relied mainly upon the enhanced leakiness of tumor vasculature to allow extravasation and access to the tumor cells, although this is still far from a foolproof way to ensure that the vectors go only to sites of tumor metastases.

Therefore, the inability to incorporate the combined elements of *tropism redirection, immune evasion, tumor site arrest* and *extravasation* into engineered viral vectors means that genuine *in vivo*, systemic delivery of high titer vector stocks that can reach dispersed tumor deposits has not yet proven possible with any of the principal vector types (Fig. 12.1). Nonetheless, the advances in understanding of how viral vectors can be redirected to certain cell types remains a potentially very powerful technology. It would be lamentable if it were to become of only academic interest rather than of practical clinical value. Hence, it would be highly valuable if strategies could be devised by which these relatively fragile and vulnerable vectors could be carried directly to the vicinity of their sites of action, to be released there in an environment where the molecular alterations conferring tropism redirection have a realistic chance of working. In this context, the time would seem ripe to use carriers that would steathily carry the vectors into the tumor deposits where they

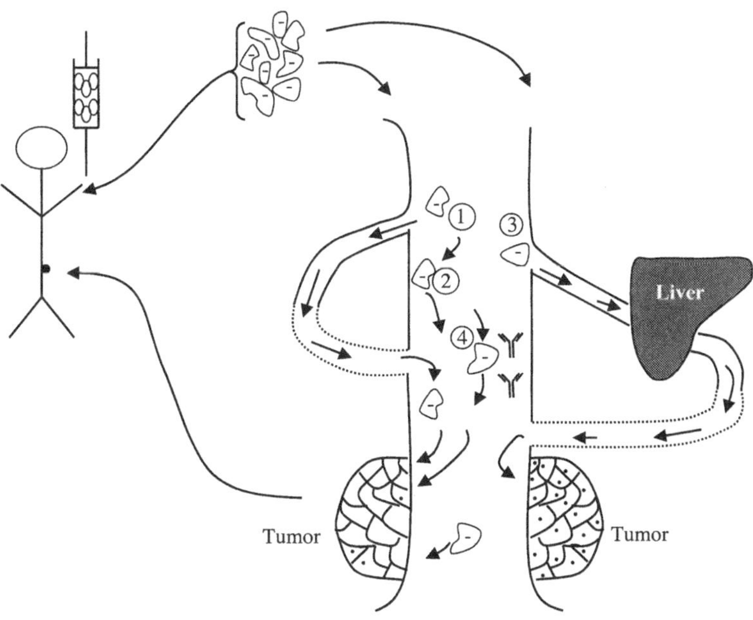

Fig. 12.2 Cell carriers have stability and tumor-homing properties that can be used to protect and target vectors to tumor sites. Autologous cell carries, preloaded with vector genomes, can be injected systemically into the patient. (1) In general, the half-life of such cells will be longer than that of viral particles, allowing misdirected cells to remain viable long enough to circulate and find the appropriate target sites. (2) Such cells will adhere to vessel walls but have generally developed mechanisms to avoid non-specific arrest in the absence of specific signals from surrounding tissues. (3) Similarly, cells that are autologous and normally circulate will not be cleared by the reticuloendothelial system. (4) Autologous cells will not be the target of immune attack, provided that the encoded genes are silent until they reach the tumor site. Cell carriers will be selected to be able to respond to environmental cues and signals produced by the tumor that stimulate site-specific arrest, extravasation, and permeation into the tumor.

could be released in response to externally applied signals (such as drugs) or environmental cues supplied by the biological properties of the tumor itself. The best candidates for such stealthy delivery of the tumor-targeted missiles, which themselves cannot make the hazardous journey through the circulation, would be immune-invisible, tumor-homing cells (Fig. 12.2).

Cell-based vector carriers for cancer gene therapy

Several different cell types exist with natural biological properties that allow them to home to sites of tumor growth. If these cell types are autologous to the patient, they will not be subject to immune clearance whilst circulating. In principle, it would be possible to recover such cells from the patient, load them *ex vivo* with their vector payloads, and then return them *in vivo* to localize specifically to tumor deposits. Alternatively, in some cases, it may be possible to use non-patient-derived cell carriers that can last long enough in the patient's circulation to locate to tumors and allow release of vector at the site. The most obvious choice of the cell carriers would be certain immune cells whose natural function is to travel to tumors. These include macrophages, T cells, natural killer (NK) cells, and eosinophils (37, 38). However, other non-immune populations are also candidates for use in this way. These include allogeneic tumor cells, which can 'chase' autologous tumor cells *in vivo*, and most exciting, stem cells, which can, in theory at least, be incorporated into tumor vasculature as a source of therapeutic genes or vectors.

Macrophages

Macrophages normally circulate through tissues sampling the local environment for evidence of cell death, either physiological or pathological (39), or other signs of infection and stress (40) (Fig. 12.3). In healthy tissues, there are no signals to cause their retention within the tissue and they pass on by, possibly back

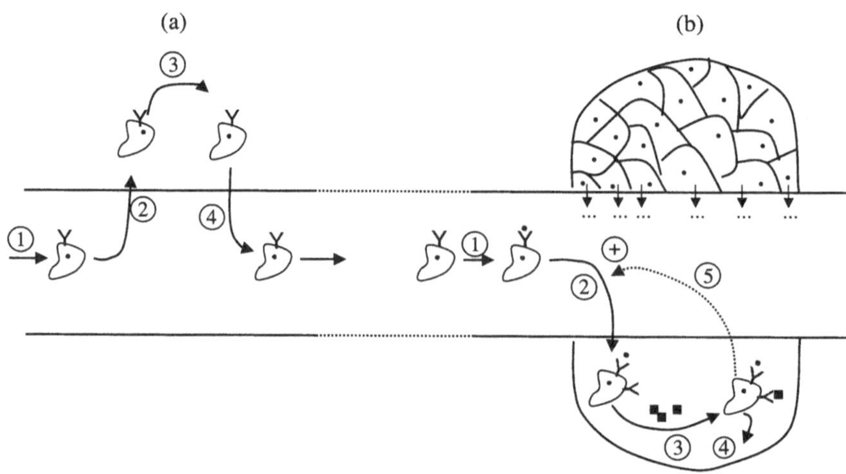

Fig. 12.3 Macrophages concentrate within tumors by sensing tumorderived factors and centers of hypoxia. (a) Macrophages circulate normally (1), extravasate (2), and pass through healthy tissues sampling the environment (3). In the absence of signals of infection, cell killing, or stress they return to the circulation (4) and pass to other areas of the body. (b) When they reach areas of pathology, such as a tumor (1), they detect growth factors, cytokines, or other signals that promote extravasation (2). Within the tissue they sample the environment (3), and further signals promote their retention in the tissue/tumor. In this case, areas of hypoxia are sensed through low oxygen tension (4), which activates the macrophages and promotes them to secrete further cytokines to attract more immune cells to the site of pathology (5).

into the circulation. However, if they detect appropriate signals, such as the results of infection, cell death, or hypoxia, they will be detained within the tissue to fulfill a variety of functions including antigen ingestion, cytokine production, and, under certain circumstances, (tumor) cell killing (Fig. 12.3). Macrophages are, therefore, potentially attractive for use as cell-based carriers of vectors and therapeutic genes because they have a well established natural targeting capacity for areas of necrosis associated with hypoxia (41–45). Many tumors contain areas of acute and chronic hypoxia, caused by the inability of the tumor to supply its rapidly expanding cell population with sufficient blood supply. Moreover, tumor cells within such regions of the tumor mass are usually resistant to radiation and chemotherapy (46), and it is these cells that are believed to pose the gravest threat of relapse following treatment. Macrophages comprise a large proportion of the tumor mass in many tumor types (41), again demonstrating their intrinsic ability to traffic to sites of neoplastic disease, although this observation is also associated with an adverse outcome for patients (45, 47–51). Therefore, purely as carriers of therapeutic genes (44) or of viral vectors (52), macrophages seem to offer the potential of natural targeting to tumors and to areas of tumors where vector delivery would be most welcome.

In addition to their abilities to concentrate within tumors, macrophages have a history, albeit chequered

and controversial, of being able to kill tumor cells directly and/or inhibit tumor growth (45, 53–58). For example, clinical trails of interferon (IFN)-γ-activated macrophages have reported minimal toxicities and tumor localization—although clinical benefit was not observed (59). Our own recent data has also shown that adoptive transfer of murine macrophages can provide clinical benefit against both pre-established disease and in a vaccination setting (60), although probably not in this context as a result of trafficking to the tumor sites. These experiments show that macrophages can be induced to respond to tumor cell killing in either an immunosuppressive or an immunostimulatory manner, through secretion of cytokines such as interleukin (IL)-10 or tumor necrosis factor (TNF)-γ, respectively. By manipulating the tumor environment to activate the immunostimulatory response of the macrophages, we have shown that they can stimulate other immune effector cells to lead to tumor eradication.

Therefore, there is very powerful evidence to support the localization of macrophages to sites of tumor growth and a body of less definitive observations indicating that they can act as tumoricidal agents, both directly and indirectly, under certain circumstances. Taken together, these results suggest that macrophages are excellent candidates for use as vector carriers *in vivo* (Fig. 12.3). In this respect, it has already been

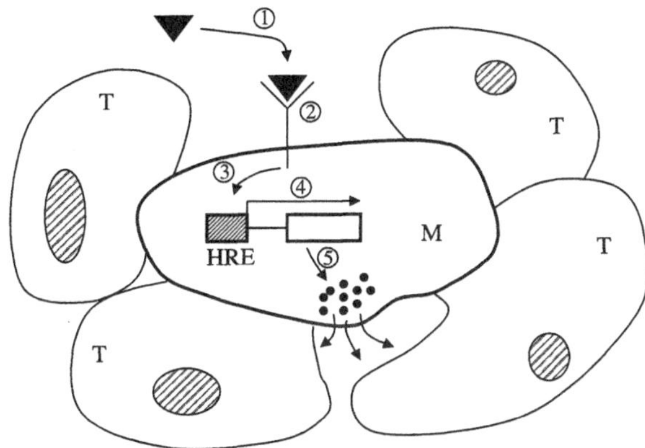

Fig. 12.4 Tumor-specific activation of therapeutic gne expression from macrophage cell carriers. Tumor-derived environment cues (1), such as low oxygen tension, are sensed by macrophages (M) infiltrating the tumor (2). Signal transduction pathways within the macrophage (3) are transmitted to the nucleus and activate transcription factors, which bind to hypoxia-responsive (promoter) elements (HRE) controlling expression of the therapeutic construct pre-loaded into the macrophage. Transcription of the therapeutic cassette occurs in response to the tumor-associated hypoxia (4) leading to production of therapeutic proteins (5), which may be directly cytotoxic, secreted cytokines, or viral proteins (see text) leading to tumor cell (T) killing.

shown that macrophages can be 'armed' (44) with transcriptionally targeted vectors expressing a suicide gene to enhance any tumoricidal activity that they may possess (Fig. 12.4). Human macrophages, infected with an adenoviral vector in which the human cytochrome P4502B6 gene was transcriptionally controlled by a hypoxia response element (HRE) (44, 61), were able to infiltrate into tumor spheroids. Moreover, gene expression within the macrophages was shown to be activated by hypoxia either artifically applied to the entire spheroid or within areas of the spheroid itself. Finally, killing of both macrophages and tumor cells was seen when the prodrug was applied. Thus, tumor targeting was provided on the one hand by the ability of macrophages to traffic to hypoxic sites and on the other hand by transcriptional activation of the toxic gene only once the macrophages had reached the target (Fig. 12.4). Since these studies were not carried out in tumor-bearing animals, the body-wide distribution of the macrophages was not assessed. Nor were the levels of gene expression resulting from macrophage trafficking and deposition into other organs and tissues where hypoxia may be present monitored. These considerations are important for understanding the possible toxicities of such approaches and also underscore

the need for thoughtful design of the vectors that would be carried by the macrophage carriers (see below).

Further refinements of macrophages targeting could be possible by adding additional levels of targeting. For example, Paul *et al.* used a modified vaccinia Ankaravirus-based vector to deliver a membrane-anchored single-chain variable fragment of an antibody (scF$_V$) that recognizes the tumor antigen MUC-1 to activated human macrophages (62). They demonstrated that the lytic function of these activated macrophages could be targeted to MUC-expressing tumor cells *in vitro*. Therefore, the possibilities open up of combining surface targeting of macrophage cell carriers with their inherent abilities to traffic to hypoxic tumor sites. However, although this study *added* a level of targeting to the macrophages, it did not address the issue of *blocking* their ability to travel to other locations in the body. Hence, this dual-level targeting may help to lessen, but will not remove, some of the concerns described above relating to increasing the localization of the macrophages to specific sites of tumor growth.

T cells

Just as macrophages patrol peripheral tissues, sample their environment, and either are retained or move on, so T cells circulate through the body and will be arrested prior to extravasating at sites in which there are cytokine signals from sites of infection or cell killing. If there are sufficient cytokine and activatory signals at tumor sites (and this is not necessarily so), T cells, including natural killer T cells, will extravasate from the circulation and pass into the site to sample it for antigens. Many groups have, therefore, sought to use the presumed ability of tumor-cell-specific T cells to home to tumors for therapeutic purposes (63–71).

In its simplest form, tumour-infiltrating lymphocytes (TILs) have been recovered from patient tumors, expanded *in vitro*, and then re-infused to the patient. The rationale is that the specificity of the T-cell receptors (TCRs) expressed on such TILs for tumor-associated antigens (TAAs) must be responsible for their initial location to the tumor. Thereafter, following expansion in numbers and activation with cytokine (often IL-2), they could be re-infused and will target sites of metastatic tumor through the continued expression of the TAA. In the early trails, it was the intrinsic target cell killing capability of the T cells that was used to lead to therapeutic benefits (63, 64, 66–68, 72). However, such trials have not been trouble-free but did show localization of adoptively transferred T cells to sites of tumor growth. Unfortunately, there was also extensive localization to other organs—such as the liver and spleen. More recent advances have built on earlier experiences and have fortified the intrinsic tumoricidal capabilities of the T cells through gene transfer of cytokines such as IL-2 or granulocyte—macrophage colony-stimulating factor (GM-CSF) (73). In addition, the identification of different subsets of T cells that infiltrate into tumors has become more sophisticated. As well as major histocompatibility complex (MHC)-restricted T cells (presumably tumor-antigen-specific), clinical trials have been carried out using NK cell subsets with additional activation by cytokines such as IL-2 (69, 74, 75).

These experiments and clinical trials have demonstrated that it is possible to recover tumor-infiltrating immune T cells of various types and that such cells can be transduced with viral vectors to encode potentially therapeutic genes. In addition, related studies on the identification of TAAs have shown that certain cancer patients carry peripheral T cells that have specificity for specific TAAs (76, 77), which can also be recovered and manipulated *ex vivo*. However, it has also become clear that it would be advantageous if it were to be possible to manipulate the specificity of peripheral T cells *in vitro* in order to recognize specific TAAs of choice. Expansion of these MHC-restricted, antigen-specific T-cell populations, would allow re-infusion of a highly targeted population of T cells that could kill target tumor cells *in vivo*. To this end, it has been shown that T cells can be engineered to express chimeric TCRs in which ligand binding/targeting is accomplished by, for example, a single-chain Fv (scFv) molecule against a known target antigen. Complexing of the scFV molecule to the intracytoplasmic domain of the zeta or gamma chain of the TCRs or FcgRIII receptors allows legitimate T-cell activation signals to be passed to the nucleus on ligand binding, with subsequent initiation of T-cell effector functions (78–86).

Hence, it should be possible to use T cells, either freshly recovered from patients' tumors or periphery and/or engineered previously to incorporate specific target-binding and T-cell activation properties, to serve as cell platforms for the delivery of vectors/vector packaging functions. Indeed, provided that one believes in the existence of TAAs that can be recognized by natural TCRs or even artificially manipulated TCRs, T cells provide one of the most attractive forms of carrying vector functions directly to sites of tumor growth.

Once there, they provide two attractive possible functions: (1) the release of vectors in an antigen-binding-specific manner (see below) and (2) the direct cytotoxic killing of the target tumor cells.

Obvious problems remain. The biggest is obtaining truly tumor-specific T cells. The TIL populations extracted from patient tumors do clearly contain T cells with TCRs with specificity for TAAs within the tumor; however, they also contain a variety of other cells that may not be so specific for tumor cells. Expanding sufficient numbers of the truly tumor-specific cells remains a challenging task and then transducing them with the packaging plasmids is far from trivial. In addition, re-infused T cells with circulate but may not necessarily extravasate and migrate into tumor sites in the patients unless there are chemoattractive signals to direct them there. Many tumors are actually immunosuppressive, thereby decreasing the chances that appropriately targeted T cells will actually reach the tumors at all or, if they do, that once there they will be functional (87).

Despite these misgivings, the T cell remains a very attractive vehicle for vector delivery to tumors given its natural abilities to (1) circulate freely, (2) bind specifically to target molecules, such as TAA, and (3) to initiate effector functions following that binding.

Tumor cells

Some of the earliest gene therapy trials for cancer involved the injection of murine retroviral producer cells into brain tumor deposits with the aim of releasing retrovirus encoding the herpes simplex virus thymidine kinase (HSVtk) suicide gene (88, 89). Infection of surrounding tumor cells (the only cells that should be replicating in that site and, therefore, susceptible to C-type retroviral infection) should lead to a conferred susceptibility to the prodrug ganciclovir. This would, in turn, lead to killing of both the cell carriers, the infected tumor cells, and any neighboring tumor cells that are close enough to be killed by the local bystander killing effect. The results of these trials showed very little toxicity (90) and some infection of both tumor cells and tumor-associated endothelial cells (91), but the gene transfer efficiency was very poor indeed and unlikely to lead to therapeutic gains (92, 93). It was, in part, from these results that the enthusiasm for the use of replicating viruses arose since it was clear that dramatic improvements in viral gene transfer and spread of the transgene would be required to confer clinical benefits (3).

One of the problems associated with the transfer of murine packaging cells is that they are rapidly rejected *in vivo*. In addition, direct stereotactic injection of the producer cells may not allow optimal dispersal of the tumor cells into the tumor to allow efficient cell–cell contacts and viral release. Therefore, there is still a rational reason to believe that it may be possible to use tumor cells as cell carriers to deliver vectors and viruses to tumors in patients. In general, this is based upon the observation that (tumor) cells of a particulr histological cell type will bind preferentially to (tumor) cells of the same histological type (94, 95). Hence, infusion of a cell carrier line into a localized organ area where tumor is known to exist can lead to tracking of those carrier cells to sites of dispersed tumor, cell–cell adhesion, and localized delivery of vector. Glioma and epithelial ovarian cancer represent excellent examples where the tumor to be treated remains in a relatively localized area (the brain or the peritoneal cavity, respectively) but consists of tumor cells actively migrating and dispersed through the area.

Thus, the administration of a selectively replicating HSV intraperitoneally (IP) in animals bearing a xenograft model of epithelial ovarian cancer was able to reduce tumor volume significantly (94). However, using the observation that an epithelial ovarian tumor cell line, PA-1, bound selectively to other human ovarian carcinoma cells compared to mesothelial surfaces, Coukos *et al.* (94) showed that these therapeutic effects were dramatically enhanced by delivering the replicating virus via locally administrated PA-1 cells loaded with the virus *in vitro*. The PA-1 cells localized very well to sites of established tumor rather than to areas of normal peritoneum through mechanisms that were not determined but that probably depend upon the surface expression of adhesion molecules that are specific for the epithelial ovarian cells.

A similar strategy and principle has been used in the treatment of experimental gliomas by Namba *et al.* (95). Here, autologous glioma cells transduced with the HSVtk gene were administered *in vivo* to 'chase' pre-existing tumor cells. The authors showed that good therapeutic effects were achieved on administration of ganciclovir through the prior adhesion of the glioma tumor and chaser cells. Thereafter, this adhesion facilitated the bystander effect of ganciclovir-mediated killing. Chasing established tumor cells with HSVtk+ fibroblasts was far less effective, presumably because of the reduced cell–cell adhesion between fibroblasts and glioma cells and the reduced migratory capacity of the fibroblasts, leading to less targeting and reduced bystander effects *in vivo*.

These examples show that autologous or even allogeneic tumor cell lines (95) could be used to track patient tumor cells *in vivo*, adhere to them, and then be used to deliver vector and/or therapeutic genes. As with all of the cell carrier systems, cell–cell virus spread may be more effective than free viral release both through proximity of virus and receptors and through the partial protection of the virus from host antiviral antibodies. This approach would be most valuable for tumor types where the neoplastic cells adopt a migratory behavior that is, nonetheless, still restricted to a localized compartment.

Clearly, the problems with such a strategy focus upon the ability to kill the adoptively transferred cells. If the HSVtk system, or something similar, is being used as in the glioma studies above, killing of the carrier cells is central to the therapeutic strategy. However, if the carrier cells are being used to deliver vector *per se*, then there may have to be other ways to ensure their killing, such as irradiation prior to *in vivo* administration (94). Conversely, if the cell chaser line cannot be autologous to the patient (which is most probable), actually *prolonging* the survival of the allogeneic line becomes an issue. If the carrier line does not last long enough to seek out tumor deposits, because of its allogeneicity, its value as a vector delivery vehicle will be greatly reduced. Nonetheless, there will also be added value from an immunological vaccination point of view in the use of allogeneic 'chaser' cells—based on evidence that allergenic vaccines can have immunological benefit to antitumor immune responses (96–98).

Hence, the use of histologically matched, or possibly allergenic tumor cell lines as cell carriers for tumor therapy may be an effective way to target vectors to tumor cells prior to their release. Since irradiated allogeneic tumor cells are already clinically used as cancer vaccines, such a concept—that is, using tumor cells to treat tumors—is not as radical as it might at first sound.

Other non-immune differentiated cell types

Several types of tumor are often associated with infiltration of normal cell types, as evidenced by T cell, macrophage, and other immune infiltrates (see above). However, in certain cases, tumors can also be the target for homing by non-immune cells that may, or may not contribute to the pathogenesis of the disease. One particular example is the cancer-induced bone destruction that is promoted by osteoclast homing, accumulation, and activation at the site of bone metastases (99). Therefore, the accumulation of osteoclasts at sites of metastatic disease could, in theory, be used as an ideal way to concentrate vector production at the very sites that threaten the life of patients.

Although the technology for the harvest, transduction, and re-infusion of non-immune cells is generally less advanced than it is for immune cell types, the opportunities presented by the infiltration of tumors by normal cell types, such as osteoclasts, are great if those cells can be subverted to act as gene and vector delivery carriers.

Stem cells

The demonstration that stem cells, from any of a variety of sources, can be induced to differentiate into any of several lineages of choice opens an enormous vista of opportunity for all types of cell-based therapy (100–110). The possibility is raised by these remarkable findings that the plasticity of the stem cell could be used to create to order any cell type that is required for any particular application. If this turns out to be true in the long term, then the issues of *ex vivo* harvest of sufficient numbers of, for example, macrophages or T cells or osteoclasts or whatever may become moot. It may be possible to isolate stem cell populations, engineer them with the vectors required to deliver therapeutic genes/viruses to tumors and their metastases, differentiate the manipulated stem cells down the appropriate pathway, and re-infuse them into the patient.

At present, such complete plasticity has not been shown, although new examples of stem cell differentiation to different histological types are continually being described. One example that is already clearly described in the literature is the ability to differentiate bone-marrow-derived stem cells into endothelial cells (104, 105, 111).This provides one clear opportunity for cancer gene therapy and vector delivery since the vasculature of developing tumors is continually expanding (112) and because, as described earlier, vectors released from the endothelial cells at sites of tumor growth are significantly closer to the tumor cells than vectors circulating in the bloodstream. Moreover, sites of tumor growth are one of the relatively few sites of active angiogenesis in a healthy adult (113, 114). Hence, modified stem/endothelial cells administered to a patient with metastatic deposits should be incorporated into relatively few sites of vessel growth apart from the tumor vasculature.

The differentiation of stem cells into endothelial cells, and the incorporation of those stem cells into sites of active angiogenesis has been demonstrated in animal models (115), including incorporation into sites of tumor growth (111). The obvious problem is currently the numbers of stem cells that can successfully populate the vascular bed of a tumor deposit. The animal models where successful incorporation has been reported with any appreciable frequency have mostly used models of angiogenesis that are probably more potent that any that may exist in a tumor itself, especially in human tumors. For example, most encouragingly, Gomez-Navvarro *et al.* showed that stem cells could populate skin autografts or matrigel pellets that were spiked with vascular growth factors (115). Such sites are physiologically much more potently pro-angiogenic than human tumors are likely to be. Our own experience with tumor models to date has been that such incorporation is possible, but at a very low frequencies (Chong *et al.*, unpublished data). Nonetheless, the prospect that stem cells can be used to infiltrate the vessels that form the very life blood of the tumor is tremendously encouraging and, as stem cell technology grows, the likelihood is that such efficiencies will improve to levels where stem cells armed with vectors and vector packaging functions can populate significant proportions of the tumor blood supply.

If, indeed, stem cells can be used to deliver genes and vectors to sites of tumor blood vessels, then a range of therapeutic genes could be delivered including suicide genes (to kill both the vasculature and adjoining tumor), anti-angiogenic genes, and, of course, tumor-targeted viruses (see below).

Biological activities of cell carriers

It is important to remember, however, that none of the cell types that are proposed here to serve as carriers of genes and packaging functions are themselves biologically inert. Therefore, their subversion for use as delivery vehicles may itself not be without risk. A prime example of this concern is in the proposed use of macrophages for delivery to hypoxic regions of tumors. The data showing macrophage accumulation within tumors is compelling and therefore promising for the strategies described above. However, many investigators have documented a pro-tumorigenic role for macrophages at the tumor site (43, 45, 47–50, 53–58, 116, 117). These tumor-promoting activities stem from a variety of reported properties of macrophages within the tumor microenvironment, including the promotion of angiogenesis (118), suppression of T and NK cells, and a response to tumor-derived molecules that leads to a generalized macrophage 'suppressor phenotype'. Alternatively, other groups have already sought to use adoptive transfer of macrophages as a tumor therapy, exploiting the clearly documented activity of these cells as tumoricidal agents (59).

Similarly, previous experience with the adoptive transfer of T cells has shown that, whilst a certain proportion of T cells do indeed traffic to tumor sites, a large number still end up at sites completely uninvolved with metastatic disease. The uncontrolled release of vector at these sites—such as the liver or the spleen—could lead to highly toxic effects on patient health. Finally, the use of adoptively transferred, vector-engineered stem cells intentionally to promote angiogenesis within tumors is itself counterintuitive to some extent. If the angiogenic properties of tumors already present a significant threat to patient survival, why intentionally feed the fire with extra endothelial cells? Counter to this argument is the fact that the tumor will feed itself anyway and by supplying the gene-modified stem/endothelial cells that angiogenic. Achilles heel of the tumor will be able to subverted to therapeutic, rather than deleterious, ends. There is also the risk that the modified stem cells will be incorporated elsewhere in the patient—at sites of angiogenesis involved in wound healing or placental development, for example.

These considerations raise important concerns about the subversion of cell functions to attack tumors. However, they can be relatively easily countered, at least in principle, by careful design of the vectors that will be carried by the cells (see below). Thus, the cell carriers themselves can be sent on Bellerophonic missions into the tumor such that they will themselves be destroyed by the therapies they deliver. That is, the vectors carried and released by the carriers, be they T cells, stem cells, or macrophages, should ideally kill the messenger as well as the largest tumor cells. In this context, the adoptive transfer of such cells to inappropriate sites may lead to only transient toxic activities in the patient. However, this strategy will itself set up conflicting requirements of the system. In the first place, persistence of the carriers *in situ* must be sufficient to release appreciable amounts of vector particles to the tumor cells; conversely, the killing of the carriers is required to prevent adverse toxicities. Some of the strategies by which controlled vector release with tumor-specific killing of target cells can be achieved are discussed below. Nonetheless, a full

appreciation of the biology of the cell types and their *in vivo* routing is important to predict and understand the possibilities of adverse events *in vivo*, which understanding in turn as important as the design of the vector-carrying strategy.

Therapeutic strategies

Direct cytotoxicity

In the simplest form of therapy, cell carriers could carry a gene that would kill both carrier and surrounding tumor cells (Fig. 12.5(a). This is the principle behind the treatment of gliomas with HSVtk-transduced tumor cells as described above (89, 95). In such instances, to have an appreciable antitumor effect the killing of the carrier cells would have to be closely linked to a potent bystander killing of nearby (tumor) cells (32, 119). Alternatively, if the carrier cells were endothelial cells carrying a toxic gene, the killing would have to be sufficient to lead to appreciable destruction of the vascular cells around the transduced cells. Such genes could include suicide genes (HSVtk, cytosine deaminase (32)), or other types of potent cytotoxic genes (such as the fusogenic membrane glycoproteins, FMG) (120, 121) or surface proteins that mark the cells as targets for immune destruction through, for example, complement-mediated lysis (23).

Secreted gene products

Alternatively, the vectors expressed by the carrier cells could encode a secreted protein that might have local cytotoxic effects but that might also have more fat-reaching, systemic effects to amplify the therapeutic benefits (Fig. 12.5(b). Obvious examples include cytokines that, if secreted a the tumor site could have potent immune stimulating and therefore antitumor activity (7, 122). Alternatively, the secreted protein may have anti-angiogenic effects (123), such as endostatin (124) or angiostatin (125).

Viral vectors

Since it is likely that, at least in the short term, the efficiency of incorporation of any particular type of cell carrier into the tumor environment will be at relatively low efficiency, converting these cells into virus-vector-producing cells is the most attractive strategy (Fig. 12.5(c)). This means that, for each cell that accumu-

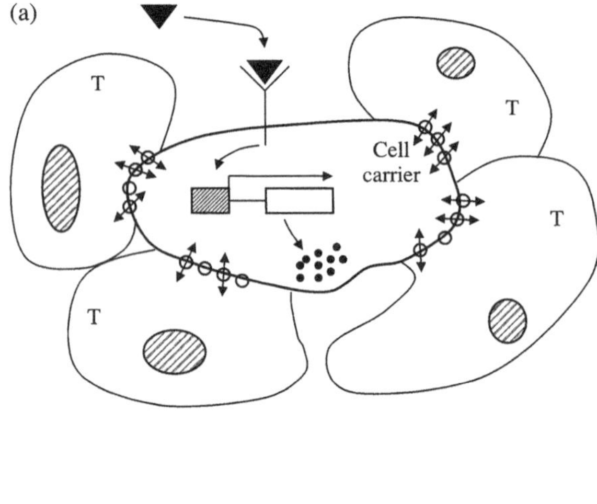

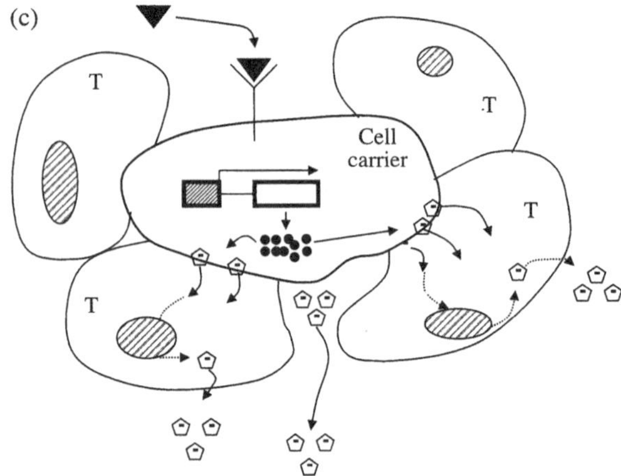

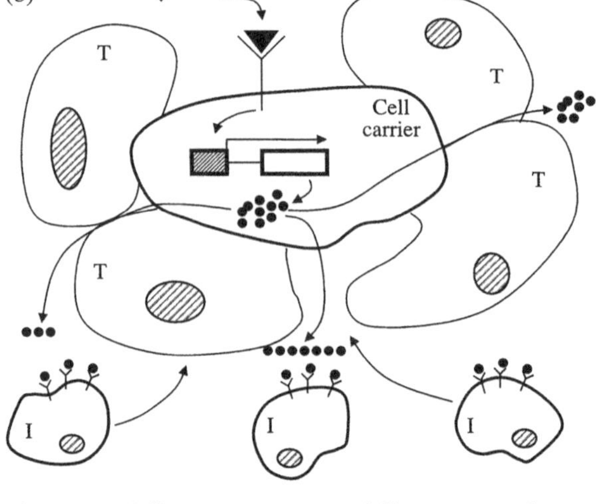

Fig. 12.5 Cell carriers can carry different types of genetic payloads into tumors. Tumor-specific gene activation signals (for example, hypoxia via the HRE, T-cell activation signals, or angiogenic signals) will initiate transcription of the genes previously loaded into the cell carrier. (a) Cytotoxicity. This could be a single cytotoxic gene whose expression leads to direct killing of both cell carrier and directly adjacent tumor cells through a local bystander killing effect. (b) Secreted immune activating proteins. Alternatively, the cell carrier could release secreted proteins—such as cytokines and chemokines—that attract immune cells (I) into the tumor deposit and lead to activation of tumor-specific immune responses and tumor cell killing. (c) Cell carriers as *in situ* viral-producing cells. For maximal efficiency of gene transfer into the tumor, the cell carriers would encode the genes for production of viral particles. These viruses, when released, would infect the surrounding tumor cells either through direct cell–cell transmission or through short-range diffusion mechanisms. The cell carriers could produce either recombinant virus (one hit) or replicating viruses both with tumor-specific targeting and expression mechanisms. In the latter case, the carrier cells would serve as foci of virus spread through the tumor (dashed lines).

lates at the tumor site, multiple viruses can be released. This amplification of the initial delivery frequency will itself be amplified if the therapeutic gene within the vector itself has a local (for example, HSVtk) or immune-mediated (for example, a cytokine) bystander effect. Moreover, if these cells can be effectively converted into vector producers, then the array of strategies that has been developed for surface targeting can be incorporated into these locally produced vectors, which no longer have to run the gauntlet of circulation in the bloodstream.

The viruses produced by the cell carriers could either be replication-defective or replication-competent, the latter providing a further amplification of the efficiency of gene delivery to tumor cells.

Vector design for cell-based carriers

The efficacy and safety of the strategies described above, especially of the release of viral vectors from the cell carriers, depend heavily upon the design of the vectors with which the cells are loaded. In principle, these vectors must permit:

- *tumor-site-inducible expression* of the therapeutic gene, vector genome, and/or packaging functions;
- *tumor-cell-specific expression* of the therapeutic gene and/or replicating viral genome from released viral vectors.

To illustrate the principles involved, we will describe a strategy based upon the release of a retroviral vector from a cell-based carrier that has reached the tumor environment through any of the biological properties described above. The generic vector would be constructed on the lines shown in Fig. 12.6.

Thus, the vector genome, *within the cell carrier*, would be expressed from transcription unit 1. This would control expression of the therapeutic gene and/or the viral genome depending on the strategy being used (see above). Transcription unit 1 would be the key switch by which the therapeutic gene/vector genome would be kept silent in the cell carrier until it had arrived and lodged at the site of tumor growth. It would then be activated by some signal specific to the tumor environment in order to turn on therapeutic gene expression or viral production. In the context of the cell carriers discussed above, this tumor-specific signal could be, for example:

(a) Carrier cell

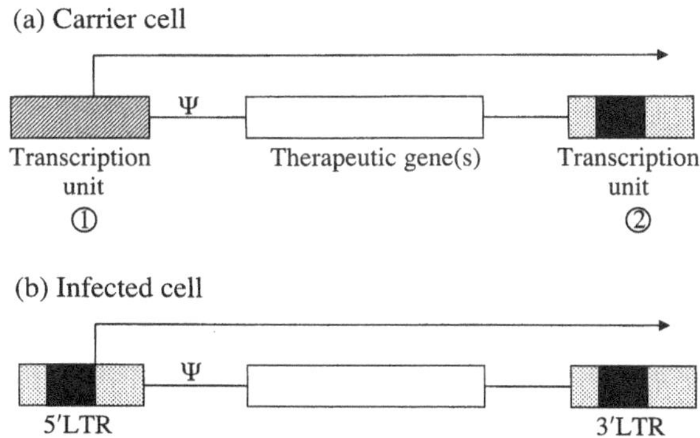

Fig. 12.6 Double targeted retroviral vector design for cell carrier delivery of viral vectors to tumors. (a) A generalized retroviral vector that would be used to transduce a cell carrier is shown. Transcription unit 1 would control expression of the therapeutic gene(s) within the cell carrier (macrophage, T cell, stem cell, etc.) This would be a promoter/enhancer element activated by tumor-specific signals such as an HRE (hypoxia-responsive element, the IL-2 promoter (T-cell receptor ligation), or by exogenously applied signals such as rapamycin. The therapeutic gene(s) expressed would vary from single cytotoxic genes or secreted cytokines to those encoding all the viral packaging functions to make the cell carrier a viral producer cell *in situ*. Transcription unit 2 would be a hybrid viral LTR in which a tissue or tumor-specific promoter/enhancer combination replaced the viral enhancer—for example, the tyrosinase, CEA, or PSA promoters to treat melanoma, colorectal, or prostate cancers, respectively. (b) Hence, in the case of production of recombinant virus from the cell carrier, the virus released would infect target cells and the therapeutic gene(s) would only be expressed in target tumor cells under control of transcription unit 2, which reverse transcription would have placed in the 5′ LTR.

- hypoxia-inducible promoter element (HRE), activatable in macrophages arriving at the site of tumor growth and hypoxia;
- promoter that is activated on ligation of the T cell receptor with its target (tumor-associated) antigen—such as the Il-2 promoter (126, 127);
- a promoter that is activated by angiogenic factors that are released at the site of tumor growth.

Alternatively, in the absence of a biological inducible signal to the cell carrier on arrival at the tumor, or even additionally, transcription unit 1 could be under inducible control through the administration of small molecules, such as tetracycline (128, 129) or rapamycin (130–132). This would allow *temporal* control of vector expression. In such circumstances, release of vector would be achieved after a predetermined time period when it was known that the cell carriers had reached their tumor targets. The use of such a system would have the added safety benefit of being able to extinguish vector production by removal of the inducing drug molecule (132). Moreover, we and others have shown recently that it is possible to combine tissue-specific promoters with a drug-inducible element to provide double levels of control gene induction (Chong *et al.*, unpublished observations).

The virus that is released at the tumor site will exit the carrier cell and will, therefore, be available to infect surrounding tumor and/or stromal cells. It is very improbable, with any of the putative systems described earlier, that 100 per cent of the cell carriers will localize only to tumor. Therefore, to prevent toxicity from localization of cell carriers at non tumor sites, it is necessary to build in designs that lead to tumor-specific infection or tumor-specific expression or both (Fig. 12.6). In the context of the retroviral structure depicted in Fig. 12.6, this can be achieved using transcription unit 2. A result of the retroviral life cycle through reverse transcriptase is that any control elements placed in the 3′LTR (long terminal repeat) of a retroviral vector will be transferred into the 5′LTR in the provirus that integrates into the infected cell (133–135). Therefore, transcription unit 2 offers the opportunity to control expression of the therapeutic gene/vector genome in a tumor-specific manner. Thus, transcription unit 2 would contain the viral transcriptional control elements replaced by transcriptional elements from genes that confer tissue- or tumor-specific gene expression (136). Examples would include the tyrosinase promoter (for targeting melanomas), the erb-B2 promoter for breast tumors, the carcinoembryonic antigen (CEA) promoter for colorectal tumors, the prostate-specific antigen (PSA) promoter for prostate cancers, and so on (31, 137). In addition, it may yet prove possible to use pan-tumor-specific promoters (as opposed to just tissue-specific promoters) such as the telomerase promoter, which is active in the majority of transformed cells but only in a very few normal cell types (138). This hybrid LTR design is a tried and tested method by which tissue-specific expression can be achieved from retroviral vectors (135, 136, 139) and will allow the virus released from the carriers to be expressed only in tumor-associated tissue. Thus, if, as is inevitable, some of the carrier cells traffic to normal tissues and virus is released from them there, although it may infect normal surrounding tissue it should not express its toxic/viral genes (Fig. 12.7).

A further means to ensure correct targeting of carrier-released virus to target tumor cells is to incorporate any surface-targeting elements that are possible in the viral packaging functions that are included in the gene unit of Fig. 12.6. As discussed earlier, modifications of retro-, adeno-, and other viral tropisms have been described through genetic engineering of envelope or knob and fiber proteins (9–15). Therefore, if the cell carrier is to serve as an *in situ* viral producer cell, the packaging functions carried within could include such modified envelope genes (Fig. 12.6).

In summary, the use of the double targeted retroviral vector design depicted in Fig. 12.6 would allow tumor targeting to be achieved with multiple levels of safety built into the system. These would, depending upon each individual example, include the following.

- The natural tumor-targeting properties of the cell carrier—such as hypoxia (macrophages), antigen specificity (engineered T cells), or angiogenesis (endothelial progenitor cells).

- Tumor-site-specific induction of gene expression (cytotoxicity or cytokine release) or viral production, through biological activation signals specific to the cell carrier cell type acting on transcription unit 1.

- The release of retroviral particles in the direct vicinity of cells surrounding the cell carriers which, if they are not tumor cells, may not be actively dividing. Therefore, these innocent cells would not be infected by release of C-type particles (140). Tumor cells, would, however, be cycling and would therefore be productively infected by the released viruses. The use of cell carriers to generate other types of virus particles—such as adenoviruses—would not have the benefit of this level of targeting.

- Envelope-specific target-cell binding/infection if possible using the envelope redirection strategies

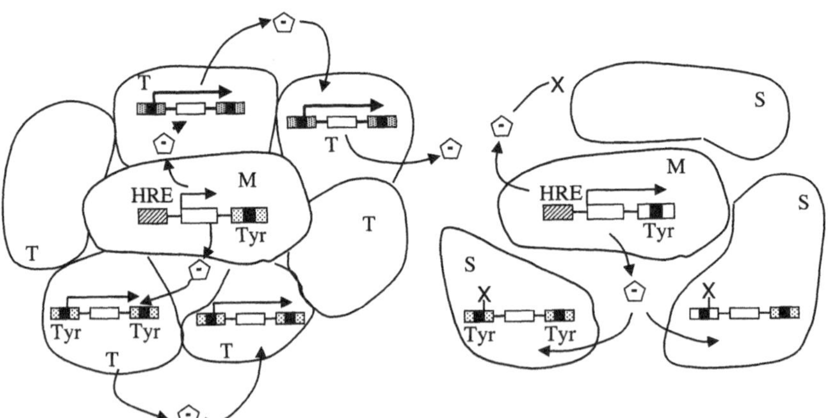

Fig. 12.7 Transcriptional controls incorporated in the vector design can ensure that toxicity associated with inappropriate localization of a cell carrier can be minimized. In the case of a macrophage (M) delivering a replicating virus construct to a melanoma deposit, the macrophage will lodge in the tumor (T). The hypoxia of the tumor will activate expression of the viral genes through the HRE. Virus will be produced and released from the macrophage and will infect dividing tumor cells around the cell carrier. The tyrosinase (Tyr) promoter in the 3' LTR will be transferred to the 5' LTR (see text) and will drive expression of the viral genes in the tumor cells leading to therapy. If the macrophages located to other sites in the body, for example, in the spleen (S), the HRE element may not be activated if there is no pathological hypoxia. Even if it is, the released virus may not infect the surrounding cells if they are quiescent. Even if they do, the tyrosinase promoter would be silent in these cells so the spread of virus and therapy would be halted.

already developed but which are difficult to achieve through genuinely systemic delivery of virus alone.

- Tumor-cell-specific expression of the therapeutic gene and/or replicating viral genome from released viral vectors using defined tissue/tumor-specific promoters to drive further gene/viral expression from transcription unit 2.

- Rheostat control of expression of cell-carrier-specific induction of viral production (transcription unit 1) and/or of tumor-specific gene expression (transcription unit 2) using small drug control elements such as the tetracycline or rapamycin systems.

The examples above have been based on the use and release of retroviral vectors/particles from the cell carriers used to infiltrate tumor sites. However, similar molecular control strategies can readily be translated in the generation of adenoviral vectors or, indeed, other types of viruses (115). Thus, tissue-specific promoters have been included in E1-deleted and later-generation adenoviral vectors with good retention of tissue specificity of expression (6, 141) as have inducible elements such as the tetracycline and rapamycin control elements (132). For example, hypoxia-induced expression of a suicide gene has been described from an adenoviral vector (44, 61). Replication of virus loaded into the cell carriers could readily be induced by placing essential viral genes (such as E1) under control of such elements as described for transcription unit 1 in Fig. 12.6. Similarly, replicating virus that is released could be tumor-specific through inclusion of genetic controls that allow replication only in cells carrying oncogenic mutations, or further inclusion of promoters that are characteristic of transcription unit 2 above could be used to drive the essential viral genes (18–22, 142, 143). In such a case, it would be necessary to transduce the cell carriers with two transcription units:

(1) one vector in which viral replication could be induced from the cell carrier by a first signal (hypoxia, rapamycin, etc.), such as HRE-E1 or Rapa-E1 encoding cassettes for replicating adenoviral vectors;

(2) a second vector—the adenoviral genome—in which the E1 region is controlled by a tissue/tumor-specific promoter.

We have described systems by which cell carriers of various types can be converted into effective suicide bombers and/or virus-producing factories with multiple levels of targeting and safety features built into the molecular constructs that they would carry to the tumor site. Such strategies would be applicable to retroviral or adenoviral release at the tumor site and would use vector designs already well established within different contexts.

Practicalities of cell isolation, loading and delivery

The use of cells as carriers for gene therapy vectors obviously requires expertise in cell harvest, *in vitro* transduction, and re-infusion into patients (Fig. 12.8). For the most part, the candidate cell types would be autologous, patient-derived cells that would need to be modified relatively rapidly before being returned to the patient (144). There are examples where allogeneic cell types might be used as discussed in detail earlier. In particular, a major attraction of the use of stem cells is that they do not express MHC molecules, making the immunologically silent. This may be very valuable—stem cells for *in vivo* transfer may not necessarily have to be patient-specific, making their prior preparation and storage for use much easier.

Cell-based therapies are now commonplace in the clinic (144) and harvest of T cells, stem cells, and macrophages now presents few technical problems. Of more importance from the pragmatic aspect is the ability to transduce these cells *in vitro* to high efficiency and rapidly enough to allow sufficient numbers of

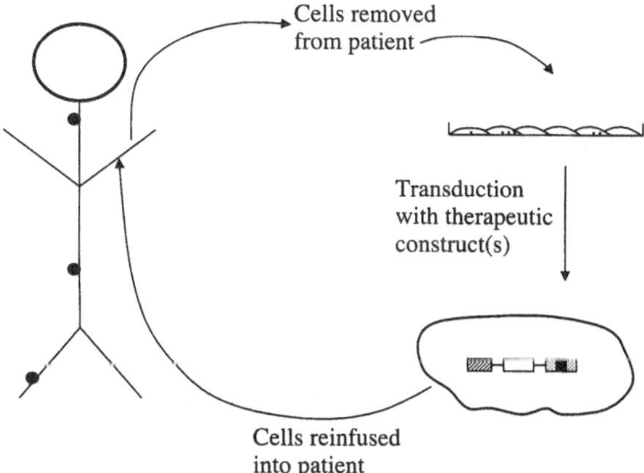

Fig. 12.8 Generation of cell carriers for gene and vector delivery. The production of genetically modified cell carriers involves well-established technologies of cell harvest, transduction *in vitro*, and return to the patient.

vector-carrying cells to be re-infused. This point is made more complex by the numbers of vectors that would have to be loaded into the cell targets. Where the aim is simply to load the carrier cell with a single vector that will, on tumor-site-specific activation, express a cytotoxic gene to kill both carrier and surrounding cells, the transduction event should be relatively simple. However, in the more complex case where the cell carrier is to become an *in situ* viral producer, multiple genes must be transferred on either single or multiple separate vectors. Wherever there is a need to achieve transduction of the same cell with more than a single vector, the efficiency of productive transduction will fall off. Nonetheless, there are already well described systems in which a single cell can be converted into a viral producer cell (145–147). For example, delivery of three separate adenoviral vectors can be used to transfer the retroviral *gag* and *pol* genes (virus 1), the retroviral envelope gene (virus 2), and the retroviral vector itself encoding the possible therapeutic gene (virus 3) (147). By placing all the retroviral packaging genes (*gag, pol,* and *env*) on a single vector (146), the number of input vectors required to transduce the cell carrier can be reduced to two. Furthermore, it is possible to construct adenoviral vectors multiply deleted in adenoviral genes to carry both the retroviral packaging functions (*gag, pol,* and *env*) and the retroviral vector itself. To release replicating retroviruses from the cell carriers, these two units would be included within the same retroviral LTR cassette.

In the case of converting the cell carriers into producers of adenoviral vectors a two-vector system is readily attainable. Thus, in the first, the essential replicative viral genes (usually E1) would be transferred under the transcriptional control of a promoter that would be activated at the tumor site (for example, a hypoxia-inducible element or a rapamycin switch). In the second vector, the adenoviral genome, containing the therapeutic gene under the tumor-cell-specific promoter control (transcription unit 2 in the examples above), would be transferred and would be released on expression of the E1 proteins. Once again, the use of multiply deleted adenoviruses would allow both of these cassettes to be transferred into the cell carrier by a single adenoviral vector if necessary. Since it is unlikely that the cell types used for *in vivo* transfer would divide to a great extent before reaching the tumor sites, transfer of the vectors into the carriers would probably be best achieved with adenoviral transfer as described. However, if longer-term incorporation of the vector genome(s) were required, then

similar strategies would have to be developed to obtain integrated copies of therapeutic and/or viral-producing vector cassettes.

Therefore, the technology to construct the appropriate vectors to load cells to fulfill the roles described for them already exists. Rapid *in vitro* transduction of the appropriately harvested cell types should be possible at high levels using adenoviral or other viral-based vectors (144). Optimization of such protocols would yield high levels of transduction of the cell carriers ready for return to the patient (Fig. 12.8).

Results from our own laboratory, as well as others, demonstrate that rapid transduction of most cell types is possible to generate *de novo* viral-producing cells from a variety of histological sources. Along with rapid advances in the technology associated with cell harvest, expansion, and re-infusion, the technical barriers to the use of cell-based carriers of gene and virus delivery to tumors will be significant but readily soluble.

Summary

It seems probable that the simple, systemic administration of currently manufactured viral stocks to patients is not likely to achieve high enough circulating titers of surviving vector particles to allow therapeutic targeting of metastatic disease. Targeting strategies that have been incorporated into viral vectors, including transcriptional and surface, allow highly targeted *delivery in vitro* but not so far in patients. Problems, such as low titers, immune inactivation, nonspecific adhesion, and loss of particles, mean that, realistically, it is difficult to see how such vector stocks will be able to reach tumor deposits in sufficient numbers to produce therapeutic gains.

One way to exploit the elegant molecular manipulations that have been made to increase vector targeting is to protect these vectors until they reach the local sites of tumor growth. Various cell types that home preferentially to tumors based on the biological properties and functions of the cells have been described. Such cells can readily be loaded with the constructs required to produce targeted vectors. Such vectors can easily incorporate mechanisms to achieve tumor-site-inducible expression of the therapeutic gene and/or packaging functions along with tumor-cell-specific expression of the therapeutic gene and/or replicating viral genome from released viral vectors. Along with advances in cell harvest and manipulation, stem cell differentiation, and cell transduction technology, it is already possible to generate cell carriers with tumor-homing properties that can protect vector stocks until they can be released locally at tumor sites in a controlled and targeted manner. We propose that, by mobilizing a fleet of potential cell carriers that can be used to chaperone precious vectors directly to the battleground, that is, into the tumors, the great advances that have so far been made with the engineering of vector tropisms may be exploited and converted into clinical benefit.

References

1. Verma I, Somia N. Gene therapy—promises, problems and prospects. Nature 1997, **389**, 239–42.
2. Peng K-W, Vile R. Vector development for cancer gene therapy. Tumor Targeting 1994, **4**, 3–11.
3. Vile RG, Russell S, Lemoine N. Cancer gene therapy: hard lessons and new courses. Gene Ther. 2000, **7**, 2–8.
4. Vile RG, Nelson JA, Castleden S, *et al.* Systemic gene therapy of murine melanoma using tissue specific expression of the HSVtk gene involves an immune component. Cancer Res. 1994, **54**, 6228–34.
5. Hurford JRK, Dranoff G, Mulligan RC, *et al.* Gene therapy of metastatic cancer by *in vivo* retroviral gene targeting. Nat Gen 1995, **10**, 430–5.
6. Reynolds PN, Zinn KR, Gavrilyuk VD, *et al.* A targetable, injectable adenoviral vector for selective gene delivery to pulmonary endothelium *in vivo*. Mol Ther 2000, **2**, 562–78.
7. Pardoll DM. Paracrine cytokine adjuvants in cancer immunotherapy. Annu Rev Immunol 1995, **13**, 399–415.
8. Melcher AA, Todryk S, Hardwick N, *et al.* Tumor immunogenicity is determined by the mechanism of cell death via induction of heat shock protein expression. Nat Med 1998, **4**, 581–7.
9. Russell SJ, Cosset F-J. Modifying the host range properties of retroviral vectors. J Gene Med 1999, **1**, 300–11.
10. Grill J, Van Beussechem VW, Van Der Valk P, *et al.* Combined targeting of adenoviruses to integrins and epidermal growth factor receptors increases gene transfer into primary glioma cells and spheroids. Clin Cancer Res 2001, **7**, 641–50.
11. Krasnykh V, Belousova N, Korokhov N, *et al.* Genetic targeting of an adenovirus vector via replacement of the fiber protein with the phage T4 fibritin. J Virol 2001, **75**, 4176–83.
12. Curiel DT. Strategies to adapt adenoviral vectors for targeted delivery. Ann NY Acad Sci 1999, **886**, 158–71.
13. Girod A, Ried M, Wobus C, *et al.* Genetic capsid modifications allow efficient retargeting of adeno-associated virus type 2. Nat Med 1999, **5**, 1438.
14. Wu P, Xiao W, Conlon T, *et al.* Mutational analysis of the adeno-associated virus type 2 (AAV2) capsid gene and construction of AAV2 vectors with altered tropism. J Virol 2000, **74**, 8635–47.
15. Bartlett JS, Kleinschmidt J, Boucher RC, *et al.* Targeted adeno-associated virus vector transduction of nonpermissive cells mediated by a bispecific F (ab′γ)₂ antibody. Nat Biotechnal 1999, **17**, 181–6.
16. Russell SJ. Replicating vectors for cancer therapy: a question of strategy. Sem Cancer Biol 1994, **5**, 437–43.
17. Russell SJ. Replicating vectors for gene therapy of cancer: risks, limitations and prospects. Eur J Cancer 1994, **30A**, 1165–71.
18. Alemany R, Balague C, Curiel DT. Replicative adenoviruses for cancer therapy. Nat Biotechnol 2000, **18**, 723–7.
19. Curiel DT. The development of conditionally replicative adenoviruses for cancer therapy. Clin Cancer Res 2000, **6**, 3395–9.
20. Nemunaitis J, Khuri F, Ganly I, *et al.* Phase II trial of intratumoral administration of ONYX-015, a replication-selective adenovirus, in patients with refractory head and neck cancer. J Clin Oncol 2001, **19**, 289–98.
21. Heise C, Hermiston T, Johnson L, *et al.* An adenovirus EIA mutant that demonstrates potent and selective systemic anti-tumoral efficacy. Nat Med 2000, **6**, 1134–9.
22. Kirn DH. A tale of two trials: selectively replicating herpesviruses for brain tumors. Gene Ther 2000, **7**, 815–16.
23. Takeuchi Y, Porter CD, Strahan KM, *et al.* Sensitization of cells and retroviruses to human serum by (α1-3) galactosyltransferase. Nature 1996, **379**, 85–8.
24. Yang Y, Ertl HCJ, Wilson JM. MHC-class I-restricted cytotoxic T lymphocytes to viral antigens destroy hepatocytes in mice infected with E1-deleted recombinant adenoviruses. Immunity 1994, **I**, 433–42.
25. Chirmule N, Raper SE, Burkly L, *et al.* Readministration of adenovirus vector in nonhuman primate lungs by blockade of CD40–CD40 ligand interactions. J Virol 2000, **74**, 3345–52.
26. Ilan Y, Prakash D, Davidson A, *et al.* Oral tolerization to adenoviral antigens permits long term gene expression using recombinant adenoviral vectors. J Clin Invest 1997, **99**, 1098–106.
27. Paillard F.Circumventing adenovirus immune response to achieve long-term correction of genetic diseases. Hum Gene Ther 1998, **9**, 454–6.
28. Yang Y, Nunes FA, Berencsi, K, *et al.* Cellular immunity to viral antigens limits E1-deleted adenoviruses for gene therapy. Proc Natl Acad Sci, USA 1994, **91**, 4407–11.
29. Pizzato M, Marlow SA, Blair ED, *et al.* Initial binding of murine leukemia virus particles to cells does not require specific Env–receptor interaction. J Virol 1999, **73**, 8599–611.
30. Alemany R, Suzuki K, Curiel DT. Blood clearance rates of adenovirus type 5 in mice. J Gen Virol 2000, **81** (pt. 11), 2605–9.
31. Harrington KJ, Linardakis E, Vile RG.Transcriptional control: an essential component of cancer gene therapy strategies? Adv Drug Delivery Rev 2000, **44**, 167–84.
32. Moolten FL.Drug sensitivity ('suicide') genes for selective cancer chemotherapy. Cancer Gene Ther 1994, **1**, 279–87.
33. Folkman J. Angiogenesis research: from laboratory to clinic. Forum (Genova) 1999, **9**, 59–62.

34. Sunassee K, Vile RG. Tumour angiogenesis: hitting cancer where it hurts. Curr Biol 1997, **7**, R282–R5.

35. Gottstein C, Wels W, Ober B, *et al.* Generation and characterization of recombinant vascular targeting agents from hybridoma cell lines. Biotechniques 2001, **30**, 190–4,6, 8, *passim.*

36. Fielding AK, Maurice M, Morling FJ, *et al.* Inverse targeting of retroviral vectors: selective gene transfer in a mixed population of hematopoietic and nonhematopoietic cells. Blood 1998, **91**, 1802–9.

37. Di Carlo E, Forni G, Lollini P, *et al.* The intriguing role of polymorphonuclear neutrophils in antitumor reactions. Blood 2001, **97**, 339–45.

38. Rosenberg SA. The immunotherapy and gene therapy of cancer. J Clin Oncol 1992, **10**, 180–99.

39. Fadok VA, McDonald PP, Bratton DL, *et al.* Regulation of macrophage cytokine production by phagocytosis of apoptotic and post-apoptotic cells. Biochem Soc Trans 1998, **26**, 653–6.

40. Savill J, Fadok V. Corpse clearance defines the meaning of cell death. Nature 2000, **407**, 784–8.

41. Normann SJ. Macrophage infiltration and tumor progression. Cancer Metastasis Rev 1985, **4**, 277–91.

42. Negus RP, Turner L, Burke F, *et al.* Hypoxia downregulates MCP-1 expression: implications for macrophage distribution in tumors. J Leukoc Biol 1998, **63**, 758–65.

43. Mantovani A, Bottazzi B, Colotta F, *et al.* The origin and function of tumor-associated macrophages. Immunol Today 1992, **13**, 265–70.

44. Griffiths L, Binley K, Iqball S, *et al.* The macrophages—a novel system to deliver gene therapy to pathological hypoxia. Gene Ther 2000, **7**, 255–62.

45. Elgert KD, Alleva DG, Mullins DW. Tumor-induced immune dysfunction: the macrophage connection. J Leukoc Biol 1998, **64**, 275–90.

46. Rockwell S, Knisely JP. Hypoxia and angiogenesis in experimental tumor models: therapeutic implications. EXS 1997, **79**, 335–60.

47. Evans R. Macrophage requirement for growth of a murine fibrosarcoma. Br J Cancer 1978, **37**, 1086–9.

48. Sunderkotter C, Steinbrink K, Goebeler M, *et al.* Macrophages and angiogenesis. J Leukocyte Biol 1994, **55**, 410–22.

49. Aoe T, Okamoto Y, Saito T. Activated macrophages induce structural abnormalities of the T cell receptor–CD3 complex. J Exp Med 1995, **181**, 1881–6.

50. Parajuli P, Singh SM. Alteration in IL-1 and arginase activity of tumor-associated macrophages: a role in the promotion of tumor growth. Cancer Lett 1996, **107**, 249–56.

51. Leek RD, Lewis CE, Whitehouse R, *et al.* Association of macrophage infiltration with angiogenesis and prognosis in invasive breast carcinoma. Cancer Res 1996, **56**, 4625–9.

52. Pastorino S, Massazza S, Cilli M, *et al.* Generation of high-titer retroviral vector-producing macrophages as vehicles for *in vivo* gene transfer. Gene Ther 2001, **8**, 431–41.

53. Mills CD, Shearer J, Evans R, *et al.* Macrophage arginine metabolism and the inhibition or stimulation of cancer. J Immunol 1992, **149**, 2709–14.

54. Herberman RB, Holden HT, Djeu JY, *et al.* Macrophages as regulators of immune responses against tumors. Adv Exp Med Biol 1980, **121B**, 361–79.

55. Fidler IJ, Schroit AJ. Recognition and destruction of neoplastic cells by activated macrophages: discrimination of altered self. Biochem Biophys Acta 1988, **948**, 151–73.

56. Bonta IL, Ben-Efraim S. Involvement of inflammatory mediators in macrophage antitumor activity. J Leukocyte Biol 1993, **54**, 613–26.

57. Grabbe S, Bruvers S, Beissert S, *et al.* Interferon-gamma inhibits tumor antigen presentation by epidermal antigen-presenting cells. J Leukocyte Biol 1994, **55**, 695–701.

58. Blachere NE, Li Z, Chandawarkar RY, *et al.* Heat shock protein-peptide complexes, reconstituted *in vitro*, elicit peptide-specific cytotoxic T lymphocyte response and tumor immunity. J Exp Med 1997, **186**, 1315–22.

59. Andreesen R, Scheibenbogen C, Brugger W, *et al.* Adoptive transfer of tumor cytotoxic macrophages generated *in vitro* from circulating blood monocytes: a new approach to cancer immunotherapy. Cancer Res 1990, **50**, 7450–6.

60. Gough MJ, Melcher AA, Ahmed A, *et al.* Macrophages orchestrate the immune response to tumor cell death. Cancer Res 2001, **61**, 7240–7.

61. Binley K, Iqball S, Kingsman A, *et al.* An adenoviral vector regulated by hypoxia for the treatment of ischaemic disease and cancer. Gene Ther 1999, **6**, 1721–7.

62. Paul S, Snary D, Hoebeke J, *et al.* Targeted macrophage cytotoxicity using a nonreplicative live vector expressing a tumor-specific single-chain variable region fragment. Hum Gene Ther 2000, **11**, 1417–28.

63. Rosenberg SA. Immunotherapy of cancer by systemic administration of lymphoid cells plus interleukin-2. J Biol Response Modifiers 1984, **3**, 501–11.

64. Rosenberg SA. Adoptive immunotherapy of cancer: accomplishments and prospects. Cancer Treat Rep 1984, **68**, 233–55.

65. Ioannides CG, Whiteside TL. T cell recognition of human tumors: implications for molecular immunotherapy of cancer. Clin Immunol Immunopathol 1993, **66**, 91–106.

66. Rosenberg SA, Packard BS, Aebersold PM, *et al.* Use of tumor-infiltrating lymphocytes and interleukin-2 in the immunotherapy of patients with metastatic melanoma, special report. New Engl J Med 1988, **319**, 1676–80.

67. Kjaergaard J, Shu S. Tumor infiltration by adoptively transferred T cells is independent of immunologic specificity but requires down-regulation of L-selectin expression. J Immunol 1999, **163**, 751–9.

68. Melief CJ. Tumour eradication by adoptive transfer of cytotoxic T lymphocytes. Adv Cancer Res 1992, **58**, 143–75.

69. Basse PH, Whiteside TL, Herberman RB. Use of activated natural killer cells for tumor immunotherapy in mouse and human. Methods Mol Biol 2000, **121**, 81–94.

70. Whiteside TL. Monitoring of antigen-specific cytolytic T lymphocytes in cancer patients receiving immunotherapy. Clin Diagn Lab Immunol 2000, **7**, 327–32.

71. Ribeiro U, Whiteside TL, Basse PH, *et el*. Activated natural killer cell tumor retention and cytokine production in colon tumor using a tissue-isolated model. J Surg Res 1999, **82**, 78–87.

72. Rosenberg SA, Lotze MT, Muul LM, *et al*. A progress report on the treatment of 157 patients with advanced cancer using lymphokine-activated killer cells and interleukin-2 or high-dose interleukin-2 alone. New Engl J Med 1987, **316**, 889–97.

73. Chang AE, Li Q, Bishop DK, *et al*. Immunogenetic therapy of human melanoma utilizing autologous tumor cells transduced to secrete granulocyte–macrophage colony-stimulating factor. Hum Gene Ther 2000, **11**, 839–50.

74. Rosenberg SA, Lotze MT, Yang JC, *et al*. Prospective randomised trial of high-dose interleukin-2 alone or in conjunction with lymphokine activated killer cells for the treatment of patients with advanced cancer. J Natl Cancer Inst 1993, **85**, 622–32.

75. de Magalhaes-Silverman M, Donnenberg A, Lembersky B, *et al*. Posttransplant adoptive immunotherapy with activated natural killer cells in patients with metastatic breast cancer. J Immunother 2000, **23**, 154–60.

76. Boon T, De Plaen E, Lurguin C, *et al*. Identification of tumour rejection antigens recognised by T lymphocytes. Cancer Surveys 1992, **13**, 23–37.

77. Boon T, van der Bruggen P. Human tumor antigens recognized by T lymphocytes. J Exp Med 1996, **183**, 725–9.

78. Altenschmidt U, Klundt E, Groner B. Adoptive transfer of *in vitro*-targeted, activated T lymphocytes results in total tumor regression. J Immunol 1997, **159**, 5509–15.

79. Bolhuis RL, Gratama JW. Genetic re-targeting of T lymphocyte specificity. Gene Ther 1998, **5**, 1153–5.

80. Brocker T, Riedinger M, Karjalainen K. Redirecting the complete T cell receptor/CD3 signaling machinery towards native antigen via modified T cell receptor. Eur J Immunol 1996, **26**, 1770–4.

81. Eshhar Z, Waks T, Gross G, *et al*. Specific activation and targeting of cytotoxic lymphocytes through chimeric single chains consisting of antibody-binding domains and the gamma or zeta subunits of the immunoglobulin and T-cell receptors. Proc Natl Acad Sci, USA 1993, **90**, 720–4.

82. Hombach A, Koch D, Sircar R, *et al*. A chimeric receptor that selectively targets membrane-bound carcinoembryonic antigen (mCEA) in the presence of soluble CEA. Gene Ther 1999, **6**, 300–4.

83. Weijtens ME, Willemsen RA, Valerio D, *et al*. Single chain Ig/gamma gene-redirected human T lymphocytes produce cytokines, specifically lyse tumor cells, and recycle lytic capacity. J Immunol 1996, **157**, 836–43.

84. Wang G, Chopra RK, Royal RE, *et al*. A T cell-independent antitumor response in mice with bone marrow cells retrovirally transduced with an antibody/Fc-gamma chain chimeric receptor gene recognizing a human ovarian cancer antigen. Nat Med 1998, **4**, 168–72.

85. Alvarez-Vallina L, Agha-Mohammadi S, Hawkins RE, *et al*. Pharmacological control of antigen responsiveness in genetically modified T lymphocytes. J Immunol 1997, **159**, 5889–95.

86. Alvarez-Vallina L, Yanez R, Blanco B, *et al*. Pharmacologic suppression of target cell recognition by engineered T cells expressing chimeric T-cell receptors. Cancer Gene Ther 2000, **7**, 526–9.

87. Whiteside TL. Signaling defects in T lymphocytes of patients with malignancy. Cancer Immunol Immunother 1999, **48**, 346–52.

88. Culver KW, Ram Z, Wallbridge S, *et al In vivo* gene transfer with retroviral vector-producer cells for treatment of experimental brain tumors. Science 1992, **256**, 1550–2.

89. Oldfield EH, Ram Z, Culver KW, *et al*. Clinical protocol: gene therapy for the treatment of brain tumors using intra-tumoral transduction with the thymidine kinase gene and intravenous ganciclovir. Hum Gene Ther 1993, **4**, 39–69.

90. Ram Z, Culver KW, Walbridge S, *et al*. Toxicity studies of retroviral-mediated gene transfer for the treatment of brain tumors. J Neurosurg 1993, **79**, 400–7.

91. Ram Z, Culver KW, Walbridge S, *et al*. *In situ* retroviral mediated gene transfer for the treatment of brain tumors in rats. Cancer Res 1993, **53**, 83–8.

92. Ram Zea. Summary of results and conclusions of the gene therapy of malignant brain tumors: clinical study. J Neurosurg 1995, **82**, 343A.

93. Ram Z, Culver KW, Oshiro EM, *et al*. Therapy of malignant brain tumors by intratumoral implantation of retroviral vector-producing cells. Nat Med 1997, **3**, 1354–61.

94. Coukos G, Makrigiannakis A, Kang EH, *et al*. Use of carrier cells to deliver a replication-selective herpes simplex virus-1 mutant for the intraperitoneal therapy of epithelial ovarian cancer. Clin Cancer Res 1999, **5**, 1523–37.

95. Namba H, Tagawa M, Iwadate Y, *et al*. Bystander-effect-mediated therapy of experimental brain tumor by genetically engineered tumor cells. Hum Gene Ther 1998, **9**, 5–11.

96. Dalgleish A. The case for therapeutic vaccines. Melanoma Res 1996, **6**, 5–10.

97. Morton DL, Foshag LJ, Hoon DSB, *et al*. Prolongation of survival in metastatic melanoma after active specific immunotherapy with a new polyvalent melanoma vaccine. Ann Surg 1993, **216**, 463–82.

98. Hsueh EC, Gupta RK, Qi K, *et al*. Correlation of specific immune responses with survival in melanoma patients with distant metastases receiving polyvalent melanoma cell vaccine. J Clin Oncol 1998, **16**, 2913–20.

99. Clohisy DR, Ramnaraine ML. Osteoclasts are required for bone tumors to grow and destroy bone. J Orthoped Res 1998, **16**, 660–6.

100. Brustle O, Jones KN, Learish RD, *et al*. Embryonic stem cell-derived glial precursors: a source of myelinating translants. Science 1999, **285**, 754–6.

101. Pereira RF, Halford KW, O'Hara MD, *et al*. Cultured adherent cells from marrow can serve as long-lasting precursor cells for bone, cartilage, and lung in irradiated mice. Proc Natl Acad Sci, USA 1995, **92**, 4857–61.

102. Saito T. Myogenic expression of mesenchymal stem cells within myotubes of mdx mice *in vitro* and *in vivo*. Tissue Eng 1995, **1**, 327–43.

103. Prockop DJ. Marrow stromal cells as stem cells for non-hematopoietic tissues. Science 1997,. **276**, 71–4.

104. Asahara T, Murohara T, Sullivan A, *et al.* Isolation of putative progenitor endothelial cells for angiogenesis. Science 1997, **275**, 964–7.

105. Shi Q, Rafii S, Hong-De Wu M, *et al.* Evidence for circulating bone marrow-derived endothelial cells. Blood 1998, **92**, 362–7.

106. Bjornson CR, Rietze RL, Reynolds BA, *et al.* Turning brain into blood: a hematopoietic fate adopted by adult neural stem cells *in vivo*. Science 1999, **283**, 534–7.

107. Ferrari G, Cussella-De Angelis G, Coletta M, *et al.* Muscle regeneration by bone marrow-drived myogenic progenitors. Science 1998, **279**, 1528–30.

108. Bittner RE, Schofer C, Weipoltshammer K, *et el.* Recruitment of bone-marrow-derived cells by skeletal and cardiac muscle in adult dystrophic mdx mice. Anat Embryol (Berl) 1999, **199**, 391–6.

109. Goodell MA, Brose K, Paradis G, *et al.* Isolation and functional properties of murine hematopoietic stem cells that are replicating *in vivo*. J Exp Med 1996, **183**, 1797–806.

110. Shamblott MJ, Axelman J, Wang S, *et al.* Derivation of pluripotent stem cells from cultured human primordial germ cells. Proc Natl Acad Sci, USA 1998, **95**, 13726–31.

111. Asahara T, Masuda H, Takahashi T, *et al.* Bone marrow origin of endothelial progenitor cells responsible for postnatal vasculogenesis in physiological and pathological neovascularization. Circ Res 1999, **85**, 221–8.

112. Isner JM, Asahara T. Angiogenesis and vasculogenesis as therapeutic strategies for postnatal neovascularization. J Clin Invest 1999, **103**, 1231–6.

113. Fidler IJ, Ellis LM. The implications of angiogenesis for the biology and therapy of cancer metastasis. Cell 1994, **79**, 185–8.

114. Risau W. Mechanisms of angiogenesis. Nature 1997, **386**, 671–4.

115. Gomez-Navarro J, Contreras JL, Arafat W, *et al.* Genetically modified CD34+ cells as cellular vehicles for gene delivery into areas of angiogenesis in a rhesus model. Gene Ther 2000, **7**, 43–52.

116. Elgert KD, Farrar WL. *In vitro* immune blastogenesis during contact sensitivity in tumor-bearing mice. I. Description of progressive impairment and demonstration of splenic suppressor cells. Cell Immunol 1978, **40**, 356–64.

117. Aso H, Tamura K, Yoshie O, *et al.* Impaired NK response of cancer patients to IFN-alpha but not to IL-2: correlation with serum immunosuppressive acidic protein (IAP) and role of suppressor macrophage. Microbiol Immunol 1992, **36**, 1087–97

118. Knighton DR, Hunt TK, Scheuenstuhl H, *et al.* Oxygen tension regulates the expression of angiogenesis factor by macrophages. Science 1983, **221**, 1283–5.

119. Freeman SM, Abboud CN, Whartenby KA, *et al.* The 'bystander effect': tumor regression when a fraction of the tumor mass is genetically modified. Cancer Res 1993, **53**, 5274–83.

120. Diaz RM, Bateman A, Emiliusen L, *et al.* A lentiviral vector expressing a fusogenic glycoprotein for cancer gene therapy. Gene Ther 2000, **7**, 1656–63.

121. Bateman A, Bullough F, Murphy S, *et al.* Fusogenic membrane glycoproteins as a novel class of genes for the local and immune-mediated control of tumor growth. Cancer Res 2000, **60**, 1492–7.

122. Forni G, Lollini PL, Musiani P, *et al.* Immunoprevention of cancer: is the time ripe? Cancer Res 2000, **60**, 2571–5.

123. Folkman J. Antiangiogenic gene therapy. Proc Natl Acad Sci, USA 1998, **95**, 9064–6.

124. O'Reilly MS, Boehm T, Shing Y, *et al.* Endostatin: an endogenous inhibitor of angiogenesis and tumor growth. Cell 1997, **88**, 277–85.

125. O'Reilly MS, Holmgren L, Shing Y, *et al.* Angiostatin: a novel angiogenesis inhibitor that mediates the suppression of metastases by a Lewis lung carcinoma. Cell 1994, **79**, 315–28.

126. Chen L, Rao A, Harrison SC. Signal integration by transcription-factor assemblies: interactions of NF-AT1 and AP-1 on the IL-2 promoter. Cold Spring Harb Symp Quant Biol 1999, **64**, 527–31.

127. Yui MA, Hernandez-Hoyos G, Rothenberg EV. A new regulatory region of the IL-2 locus that confers position-independent transgene expression. J Immunol 2001, **166**, 1730–9.

128. Gossen M, Bonin AL, Freundlieb S, *et al.* Inducible gene expression systems for higher eukaryotic cells. Curr Opin Biotechnol 1994, **5**, 516–20.

129. Gossen M, Freundlieb S, Bender G, *et al.* Transcriptional activation by tetracyclines in mammalian cells. Science 1995, **268**, 1766–9.

130. Rivera VM, Clackson T, Natesan S, *et al.* A humanized system for pharmacologic control of gene expression. Nat Med 1996, **2**, 1028–32.

131. Rivera VM, Wang X, Wardwell S, *et al.* Regulation of protein secretion through controlled aggregation in the endoplasmic reticulum [see comments]. Science 2000, **287**, 826–30.

132. Ye X, Rivera VM, Zoltick P, *et al.* Regulated delivery of therapeutic proteins after *in vivo* somatic cell gene transfer.Science 1999, **283**, 88–91.

133. Varmus HE. Retroviruses. Science 1988, **240**, 1427–35.

134. Vile RG, Russell SJ. Retroviruses as vectors. B Med Bull 1995, **51**, 12–30.

135. Vile RG, Diaz RM, Miller N, *et al.* Tissue specific gene expression from Mo-MLV retroviral vectors with hybrid LTRs containing the murine tyrosinase enhancer/promoter. Virology 1995, **214**, 307–13.

136. Diaz RM, Eisen T, Hart IR, *et al.* Exchange of viral promoter/enhancer elements with heterologous regulatory sequences generates targeted hybrid long terminal repeat vectors for gene therapy of melanoma. J Virol 1998, **72**, 789–95.

137. Nettelbeck DM, Jerome V, Muller R. Gene therapy: designer promoters for tumour targeting. Trends Genet 2000, **16**, 174–81.

138. Koga S, Hirohata S, Kondo Y, *et al.* A novel telomerase-specific gene therapy: gene transfer of caspase-8 utilizing the human telomerase catalytic subunit gene promoter

[in process citation]. Hum Gene Ther 2000, **11**, 1397–406.

139. Gough MJ, Emiliusen L, Bateman A, *et al.* A transcriptional feedback loop for tissue specific expression of highly cytotoxic genes which incorporates an immunostimulatory component. Gene Ther 2001, **8**, 987–98.

140. Miller DG, Adam MA, Miller AD. Gene transfer by retrovirus vectors occurs only in cells that are actively replicating at the time of infection. Mol Cell Biol 1990, **10**, 4239–42.

141. Ring CJA, Harris JD, Hurst HC, *et al.* Suicide gene expression induced in tumour cells transduced with recombinant adenoviral, retroviral and plasmid vectors containing the ERBB2 promoter. Gene Ther 1996, **3**, 1094–103.

142. Rodriguez R, Schuur ER, Lim HY, *et al.* Prostate attenuated replication competent adenovirus (ARCA) CN706: a selective cytotoxic for prostate-specific antigen-positive prostate cancer cells. Cancer Res 1997, **57**, 2559–63.

143. Alemany R, Lai S, Lou YC, *et al.* Complementary adenoviral vectors for oncolysis. Cancer Gene Ther 1999, **6**, 21–5.

144. Bordignon C, Carlo-Stella C, Colombo MP, *et al.* Cell therapy: achievements and perspectives. Haematologica 1999, **84**, 1110–49.

145. Noguiez-Hellin P, Meur MR-L, Salzmann J-L, *et al.* Plasmoviruses: nonviral/viral vectors for gene therapy. Proc Natl Acad Sci, USA 1996, **93**, 4175–80.

146. Feng M, Jackson WH, Goldman CK, *et al.* Stable *in vivo* transduction via a novel adenoviral/retroviral chimeric vector. Nat Biotechnol 1997, **15**, 866–70.

147. Duisit G, Salvetti A, Moullier P, *et al.* Functional characterization of adenoviral/retroviral chimeric vectors and their use for efficient screening of retroviral producer cell lines. Hum Gene Ther 1999, **10**, 189–200.

Liposomal targeting of cytotoxic drugs

Kevin J. Harrington and Konstantinos N. Syrigos

Introduction

Despite the fact that the armamentarium of available agents for the treatment of cancer continues to expand, none of the new agents has resulted in dramatic changes in the prognosis of patients with the common types of solid cancers. To some extent, this failure may be seen to be the result of the inability of cytotoxic agents to kill cancer cells selectively. Therefore, current clinical practice involves the administration of compounds at 'tolerable' doses that cause significant normal tissue toxicity, although this is below a certain threshold of acceptability. One potential means of circumventing this limitation on cytotoxic chemotherapy is to deliver it in the form of vehicles, such as liposomes, with the capacity to target tumors. Liposomes are phospholipid vesicles composed of lipid bilayer membranes entrapping a central aqueous core. They were first described more than 30 years ago, at which time they were called phospholipid spherules (1). The term liposome was coined in 1968 (2), and the first suggestions that liposomes might have potential as vehicles for targeted drug delivery for a range of diseases, including cancer, appeared shortly thereafter (3–5). The subsequent pathway to clinical application has taken more than a quarter of a century and has involved the generation and testing of a diverse array of liposomes in order to select formulations with optimal *in vivo* pharmacokinetics and biodistribution patterns (6).

The history of liposome development

The early development of liposomal therapeutics was dogged by a number of formidable problems (7). Difficulties were presented by the need to produce stable drug-containing liposomes in a reliable, reproducible way. The entrapment conditions for any particular agent needed to be optimized individually. Because liposomes can carry drugs in one of three potential compartments (water-soluble agents in the central aqueous core, lipid-soluble agents in the membrane, peptides and small proteins at the lipid–aqueous interface), a diverse range of optimal encapsulation conditions may exist for different agents. Furthermore, the release kinetics of the entrapped agents depend on the liposomal formulation and this factor can affect the therapeutic efficacy. Therefore, development of agents for preclinical and clinical use can be both laborious and expensive. In early *in vivo* studies, the liposomes that were tested had very short circulation half-lives, due to rapid liposomal opsonization by plasma proteins and phagocytosis by fixed tissue macrophages of the reticuloendothelial system (RES). In addition, lipid exchange with plasma lipoproteins destablized the liposomes leading to intravascular rupture with rapid release of the entrapped drug. Taken together, these various problems meant that the available liposomal formulations offered few advantages over the administration of the unencapsulated drug. As a result, the early clinical applications of liposomes were largely restricted to situations in which targeting of the RES was seen as an advantage (for example, treating systemic protozoal and fungal infections) (8–11).

In the search for liposomes with improved pharmacokinetic profiles, the effect of adding various components to the lipid membrane has been evaluated. In part, this work has been driven by the discovery that the stability of red cells in the blood is mediated by their hydrophilic, sialic-acid-rich glycocalyx (12). By incorporating different purified glycolipids, a new class of so-called sterically stabilized liposomes has been generated, and the pharmacokinetics and biodistribution of these agents have been evaluated *in vivo* in murine models (13). Significant enhancement of circulation half-life was achieved with a ganglioside (mono-sialoganglioside GM1) that is extracted from bovine brain tissue. This agent was considered unsuitable for clinical use, a fortunate decision when viewed in the light of the recent outbreak of new variant Creutzfeldt–Jakob disease in Europe. At about the same time, hydrogenated phosphatidylinositol (HPI), a molecule extracted from soybean oil, was shown to achieve similar results to GM1 (14). Unfortunately, the extraction process for HPI proved to be prohibitively expensive and its development was halted. A significant advance came with the discovery that liposomes with methoxypolyethylene glycol (MPEG)-derivatised lipids in their membranes had prolonged circulation half-lives and could be readily produced in large quantities (15, 16). MPEG is thought to act by providing a steric barrier against interactions with plasma proteins, such as opsonins and lipoproteins, and cell surface receptors such that PEGylated liposomes evade clearance by the RES (17). Subsequent research effort has helped to define the optimal formulation (including choice of MPEG-derivative) of such liposomes (18), and this area represents an extremely active field of research.

Although the PEG barrier may have beneficial effects in terms of extending the circulation half-life and increasing the area under the curve (AUC) of drug exposure, there is evidence that its presence may impede drug release/delivery to the target cell population. Attempts have been made to circumvent this problem by generating liposomes that can be dePEGylated *in vivo* (19, 20). One such system uses PEG–phosphatidylethanolamine with acyl chains of varying lengths, which determine the rate of exchange of the PEG component out of the liposome membrane. In effect, such liposomes are fitted with a 'timer' that determines how long they will remain functionally PEGylated (19). An alternative approach uses MPEG attached to the liposome membrane by linkers that are cleavable under mildly reducing conditions, such as those found within the tumor environment (20). Such studies are likely to represent just the beginning of a trend towards rational design of the components of the lipid membrane in order to influence favorably the behavior of liposomes *in vivo*.

Classification of liposomes

There are a number of classification schemes for liposomes. One system uses the simple physical characteristics of lamellarity (the number of phospholipid membrane layers) and diameter to divide liposomes into unilamellar vesicles (UV) and multilamellar vesicles (MLV) (21). UV have a single phospholipid bilayer membrane and a diameter of 50–250 nm. These liposomes can be further split into small UV (SUV) with a diameter of 50–100 nm and large UV (LUV) with a diameter of 100–250 nm. Because UV contain a large central aqueous compartment, they are particularly suitable for the encapsulation of water-soluble agents. Passive drug encapsulation is a relatively inefficient means of loading these liposomes and, more frequently, a gradient-driven system is used to achieve efficient entrapment. MLV are composed of concentric phospholipid bilayer membranes in an onion-skin arrangement and have a diameter of 100–500 nm. In contrast to UV, they contain a small aqueous compartment (*bl 10 per cent), which means that they preferentially entrap lipid-soluble drugs. This fact is likely to assume great importance in the future because a number of active cytotoxic drugs are highly lipid-soluble, a fact that has sometimes hampered their clinical development (22). An alternative classification scheme (as it relates specifically to liposomal anthracycline formulations) has been proposed (7). This categorization draws on both physical and physiological features of the liposomal formulations. The physical characteristic relates to whether, or not, the lipid membrane has been modified (so-called pure lipid (conventional) and surface-altered (sterically stabilized liposomes). The physiological division describes the relative extent of uptake of the liposomes by the RES (so-called RES-targeted and RES-avoiding liposomes).

There is an enormous published literature dealing with the preclinical and, to a lesser extent, the clinical evaluation of a diverse range of liposomal agents. In this review we will concentrate on those agents that appear to have found a niche in current clinical practice. In the interests of clarity, the data from biodistribution and pharmacokinetic studies will be considered separately from those derived from therapeutic studies.

Preclinical biodistribution and pharmacokinetic studies

Conventional liposomes

A summary of the published preclinical studies on the biodistribution and pharmacokinetics of those conventional liposomes that have reached clinical trials is pre-

Table 13.1 Preclinical *in vivo* biodistribution and pharmacokinetic studies of conventional liposomes that are currently undergoing clinical trials*

Liposome	Tracer model	Tumor	Comments	Reference
SUV	Doxorubicin	J-6456 (lymphoma)	There are decreased cardiac uptake with PS:PC:Chol (but not DPG:PC:Chol) liposomes with no loss of antitumor efficacy	23
SUV	^{111}In-NTA	EMT6	This study compared the tumor targeting achieved by various liposome formulations with neutral, positive, and negative surface charge. The highest tumor and lowest RES uptakes were documented for neutral SUV composed of 2:1 ratio of DSPC/Chol. There was significant RES uptake of all formulations, although this was lowest for neutral liposomes	24
SUV	Doxorubicin	J-6456 (lymphoma)	There was increased liver/spleen uptake with PS:PC:Chol liposomes compared with the unencapsulated drug. Increased drug levels were documented in J-6456 cells isolated from the liver after liposomal drug delivery.	25
SUV	Vincristine	P388 (leukemia) L1210 (leukemia)	A comparison between egg PC/Chol and DSPC/Chol liposomes containing vincristine was performed. The LD50 of the DSPC/Chol preparation was significantly lower than that of unencapsulated vicristine	30
SUV	^{111}In-NTA daunorubicin	P-1798 (lymphosarcoma) MA16C (breast)	Tumor deposition of ^{111}In-NTA and daunorubicin were 2.5 to 20-fold greater for liposomal compared with unencapsulated agents in both the P-1798 and MA16C models. The tumor AUC was 10-fold greater for liposomal as compared with unencapsulated daunorubicin in the P-1798 model	26
MLV	NDDP	None	The serum AUC after IV or IP injection was significantly higher for liposomal NDDP compared with unencapsulated CDDP. The AUC in the peritoneum was greater after IP liposomal NDDP compared with IP unencapsulated CDDP	34
SUV	Daunorubicin	P-1798 (lymphosarcoma)	There was a 2.5-fold increase in the tumor AUC of liposomal as compared with unencapsulated daunorubicin	27
SUV	^{67}Ga-or ^{111}In-NTA, ^{67}Ga-or ^{111}In-DF, ^{99m}Tc-HMPAO	Mouse sarcoma 180 Ehrlich tumor	This study was designed to define the optimal size and phospholipid/cholesterol content for tumor targeting by SUV. For DSPC/Chol (ratio 2:1) SUV, the optimal size was found to be 80–250 nm. The optimal phospholipid was DSPC and the optimal ratio of DSPC/Chol was 1:1 or 2:1	28
SUV	Doxorubicin	B16/BL6 (melanoma) L1210 (leukemia)	Maximum drug deposition was seen at 1 hour and 48 hours for unencapsulated and liposomal drugs, respectively. The tumor drug exposure was increased 2–3-fold (melanoma) and 10-fold (leukemia). respectively, for liposomal as compared with unencapsulated doxorubicin	29
MLV	NDDP	B16 (melanoma) VX2 (hepatic cancer)	There was no difference in tumor uptake after IV injection of unencapsulated or liposomal NDDP (MLV composed of 7:3 ratio of DMPC:DMPG) in a B16 melanoma model. There was significantly greater tumor uptake after IV and IA injection of the liposomal as compared with the unencapsulated drug in the VX2 model	

* AUC, Area under the curve; CDDP, cis-dichlorodiammine platinum (II); Chol, cholesterol; DMPC, dim myristoyl phosphatidylcholine; DMPG, dimyristoyl phosphatidylglycerol, DF, defer-oxamine; DPG, diphosphatidylglycerol; DSPC, distearoyl phosphatidylcholine; HMPAO, hexamethylpropyleneamine oxime; IA, intraarterial; IP, intraperitoneal; IV, intravenous; MLV, mul-tilamellar vesicle; NDDP, cis-bis-neodecanoato trans-R, R-1, 2 diaminocyclohexane platinum (II): NTA, nitrilotriacetic acid; PC, phosphatidylcholine; PS, phosphatidylserine; RES, reticuloendothelial system; SUV, small unilamellar vesicle.

sented in Table 13.1. The earliest studies defined SUV formulations that reduced normal tissue deposition but retained equivalent antitumor activity to the unencapsulated drug (23). Subsequently, liposomes with both favorable patterns of normal tissue distribution and improved tumor targeting were described (24, 25). One such neutral SUV, composed of a 2:1 ratio of distearoyl phosphatidylcholine (DSPC) and cholesterol, has been extensively evaluated because of its ability to target tumor tissue with only modest levels of RES uptake (26, 27). A systematic evaluation of SUV formulations composed of phospholipid and cholesterol has shown that DSPC in a ratio of 1:1 or 2:1 relative to cholesterol is optimal (28). As a consequence of these studies, a DSPC/cholesterol liposomal preparation of daunorubicin has entered clinical studies as DaunoXome (see below). An alternative formulation composed of egg phosphatidylcholine (PC) and cholesterol (ratio 1.2:1) has also been shown to deliver anthracyclines effectively to solid and intraperitoneal tumor xenografts (29). This formulation has been taken into clinical studies as TLC D-99 (see below). In addition to studies with anthracyclines, DSPC/cholesterol liposomes containing vincristine have been developed through preclinical studies. Liposome-encapsulated vincristine has been shown to be more active and less toxic than the unencapsulated agent in a number of murine models (30–32). The end result of these studies has been the development of a DSPC/cholesterol liposome formulation of vincristine (ONCO-TCS) which has entered phase I trials (see below).

In contrast to liposomal anthracycline and vinca alkaloid preparations, the development of conventional liposomal platins has involved the use of MLV rather than SUV. This choice has been guided by the desire to generate clinically applicable preparations encapsulating lipophilic platinum compounds, which are poorly encapsulated in the aqueous phase of SUV. MLV composed of dimyristoyl phosphatidylcholine (DMPC) and dimyristoyl phosphatidylglycerol (DMPG) (7:3 ratio) containing the lipophilic platin *cis*-bis-neodecanoata *trans*-R, R-1, 2 diaminocyclohexane platinum (II) (NDDP) have been shown to yield equivalent or increased tumor levels compared to the unencapsulated drug after intravenous administration (33). In addition, this agent appeared to have particularly attractive pharmacokinetics after intraperitoneal injection (34), which has promoted its use as an intracavitary agent in patients with malignant pleural and peritoneal effusions in early clinical trials (see below).

Sterically stabilized liposomes

A summary of the published preclinical data on the biodistribution and pharmacokinetics of sterically stabilized liposomes is presented in Table 13.2. As has been detailed above, sterically stabilized liposomes evolved from studies in which various components were added to the membrane and their effect on *in vivo* longevity was measured (13–15). Of the three agents, GM1, HPI, and MPEG, only the latter has given rise to a family of liposomal agents that have entered clinical usage. Klibanov *et al.* (15) were the first to show that incorporation of polyethylene glycol-conjugated phosphatidylethanolamine (PEG–PE) into LUV composed of egg PC and cholesterol (ratio 1:1) increased the blood circulation half-life by more than 10-fold compared to unPEGylated liposomes ($t_{1/2}$ = 5 h versus < 30 min). A number of subsequent studies have confirmed these data and have demonstrated the ability of liposomes to accumulate in tumor tissues in rodent models (35–43). Studies using intravenous injections of gold particles entrapped in egg PC/cholesterol liposomes containing GM1 or a PEG–PE derivative have shed light on the microbiodistribution of these agents. At electron microscopy, intracytoplasmic colloidal gold was observed in hepatic Kuppfer cells and bone marrow macrophages, confirming their role in clearing circulating liposomes. In xenograft solid tumors and Kaposi's sarcoma-like dermal lesions in transgenic mice, gold particles were seen in blood vessels and in a perivascular cuff beyond the endothelium (36, 37). There was no sign of colloidal gold in the cytoplasm of tumor cells suggesting that, at least in the case of PEGylated liposomes, endocytosis by tumor cells does not occur to a significant extent (36). Uptake was more pronounced in the Kaposi's sarcoma-like lesions than in the adjacent normal skin (37). More recently, the liposomal formulation has been adjusted to contain hydrogenated soy PC and microfluorometric studies have provided elegant data that show PEGylated liposomes accumulating in the extracellular space of tumors, where they release their contents, which are subsequently distributed throughout the tumor (38, 39). Furthermore, a recent study has determined the detailed biodistribution and pharmacokinetics of radiolabeled liposomes in tumor and a range of normal tissues in mice (42). As a direct consequence of these studies, PEGylated liposomes incorporating methoxypolyethylene glycol-derivatized phosphatidylethanolamine (MPEG-DSPE) have been developed for clinical use with doxorubicin (Caelyx/Doxil) and cis-

Table 13.2 Preclinical *in vivo* biodistribution and pharmacokinetic studies using sterically stabilized liposomal agents that are currently undergoing clinical evaluation

Liposomes	Tracer	Tumor model	Comments	Reference
PC:Chol:HPI PC:Chol:GM1	^{67}Ga-DF	J-6456 (lymphoma)	Optimal tumor targeting was seen with 100 nm liposomes containing a neutral phospholipid and a negatively charged glycolipid (HP1 or GM1). Blood (60-fold) and tumor (25-fold) levels were increased and RES levels were decreased (4-fold)	14
DSPC:Chol DSPC:Chol:GM1 DSPC:Chol: PEG-PE	^{67}Ga-DF	C-26 (colon)	The AUC in tumor tissue was increased 2–3-fold and the AUC in the RES was decreased 2-fold for PEGylated compared with conventional liposomes	35
EPC:Chol:GM1 EPC:Chol: MPEG-DSPE	Colloidal gold Rhodamine B	C-26 (colon)	Electron microscopy demonstrated deposition of gold-containing liposomes in perivascular space in tumors. Colloidal gold particles were seen in Kuppfer cells but not within liver parenchyma or tumor cells	36
EPC:Chol:MPEG-DSPE	Colloidal gold	KS-like lesions	Extravasation and transcytosis of liposomes were significantly increased in KS-like dermal lesions compared to adjacent normal skin of transgenic mice bearing the human immunodeficiency virus *tat* gene	37
HSPC:Chol: MPEG-DSPE	Doxorubicin	PC-3 (prostate)	Microfluorometry demonstrated 25-fold increase in the tumor AUC with liposomal compared with unencapsulated drug	38
HSPC:Chol: MPEG-DSPE	Doxorubicin	MFH (sarcoma)	Increased drug deposition was seen in tumor compared with adjacent normal brain tissue with liposomal but not unencapsulated drug. Peak tumor deposition of doxorubicin was 14-fold greater with the liposomal drug	40
HSPC:Chol: MPEG-DSPE	Doxorubicin Texas Red	AsPC-1 (pancreas)	Microfluorometry demonstrated a 6–16-fold increase in tumor AUC for liposomal compared with unencapsulated drug. Diffusion of drug from perivascular liposomes to nuclei of stromal and tumor cells was demonstrated	39
HSPC:Chol: MPEG-DSPE	Cisplatin	C-26 (colon) Lewis lung tumor	The tumor AUC was 28-fold higher for liposomal compared with unencapsulated cisplatin. There was a 4-fold reduction in renal drug deposition with the liposomal agent	41
HSPC:Chol: MPEG-DSPE	^{111}In-DTPA	KB (head and neck)	There was prolonged circulation of the radiotracer in liposomes compared with the unencapsulated agent with an approximately 10-fold increase in circulation half-life. Maximum tumor uptake was seen at 24 hours (5.5 ± 3.0% i.d./g) and 5 minutes (1.0 ± 0.2% i.d./g) for encapsulated and unencapsulated radiolabel, respectively.	42
HSPC:Chol: MPEG-DSPE	^{111}In-DTPA	KB (head and neck)	There was an inverse correlation between uptake of radiolabelled liposomes and tumor size with significant reduction of liposome uptake in areas of tumor necrosis.	43

* % i.d/g, per cent injected dose per gram; AUC, area under the curve; Chol, cholesterol; DF, deferoxamine; DSPC, distearoyl phosphatidylcholine; EPC, egg phosphatidylcholine; GM1, monoganglioside; HP1, hydrogenated phosphatidylinositine; HSPC, hydrogenated soy phosphatidylcholine; KS, Kaposi's sarcoma; MPEG-DSPE, pegylated distearoyl phosphatidylethanolamine; PC, phosphatidylcholine; PEG-PE, pegylated phosphatidylethanolamine; RES, reticuloendothelial system.

platin (SPI-077) and another formulation containing vincristine is under development (44).

Preclinical therapeutic studies

Conventional liposomes

The main emphasis of development of conventional liposomal agents was initially directed towards the anthracyclines (Table 13.3). The reasons for this selection are easy to understand: (1) they exhibit a broad range of antitumor activity; (2) they cause a relatively predictable dose-limiting cardiotoxicity, which provides a powerful model for studying the effect of liposomal encapsulation on the toxicity profile of drugs; (3) they are relatively easy to incorporate in liposomes. The earliest studies demonstrated the ability of liposomes containing doxorubicin to reduce cardiac drug localization without reducing the antitumor efficacy of the entrapped agent (23, 45, 46). Further studies identified liposomal preparations that enhanced the therapeutic effect relative to the unencapsulated agent by increasing drug delivery within tumor cells. This effect was achieved at the same time as reducing treatment-related toxicity (47–50). For example, in these studies, toxic death, cardiomyopathy, and renal, hepatic, and biochemical (hyperlipidemias and hypoglycemia) toxicities were appreciable for the unencapsulated drug but negligible for liposomal doxorubicin (49). Data such as these provided the background for the development of PC: cholesterol liposomes containing doxorubicin (TLC-D99) for clinical study. The activity of daunorubicin in a liposome composed of DSPC: cholesterol was also reported (26, 27). This agent has been shown to yield superior response rates to those seen with the unencapsulated agent and is undergoing clinical evaluation as DaunoXome.

Two issues have dominated the preclinical therapeutic assessment of conventional liposomal platinum compounds: (1) the need to reduce the systemic toxicity of the available platins (cisplatin, carboplatin); (2) the desire to encapsulate novel lipophilic platinum analogs that cannot be formulated in the aqueous phase (Table 13.4). Regarding the first of these issues, liposomal preparations of cisplatin have been shown to have reduced nephrotoxicity and to have higher maximum tolerated doses than the unencapsulated agent, although this effect has been achieved at the expense of some clinical activity (51, 52). As for the second issue, in recent years the development of novel lipophilic plat-

inum analogs has concentrated on examination of various *cis*-bis-carboxylato(*trans*-R, R-1, 2-diaminocyclohexane) platinum (II) complexes (53–55). A number of such compounds encapsulated in liposomes composed of DMPC and DMPG (in a 7:3 molar ratio) have been shown to exhibit activity in *in vivo* studies using rodent models. NDDP appears to be most promising with either equivalent or superior antitumor activity to cisplatin but significantly reduced nephrotoxicity. This agent has entered clinical studies as both an intravenous and intraperitoneal/intrapleural therapeutic agent.

Sterically stabilized liposomes

As with the conventional liposomes, most of the published studies on the therapeutic efficacy of sterically stabilized liposomal agents concern the anthracyclines (Table 13.5). The formulation that has become Caelyx/Doxil has been shown to exert significant activity against a broad range of syngeneic and xenograft tumors in rodent models. In general, these effects have been shown to exceed those of comparable conventional liposomal formulations with appreciable amelioration of treatment-related toxicity (35, 38–40, 56–63).

In addition, the therapeutic efficacy of a number of non-anthracycline compounds encapsulated in sterically stabilized liposomes has been assessed (Table 13.6). Studies have been performed with vincristine (44, 58), mitoxantrone (64), and platinum analogs (41, 63, 65–67). In the cases of vincristine and mitoxantrone, liposomal encapsulation was shown to significantly increase their antitumor activity while, for vincristine, reducing the toxicity of treatment. As yet, neither of these agents has been further developed towards clinical trials. The activity of PEGylated liposome-encapsulated cisplatin (SPI-077) has also been reported in a number of studies. This agent has been shown to be more active than unencapsulated cisplatin with a greatly reduced toxicity profile. However, the degree of enhancement of the activity of the parent compound appeared to be less than that reported for PEGylated liposomal doxorubicin (63).

Clinical pharmacokinetic and biodistribution studies

As described above, an enormous number of liposomal preparations have been subjected to preclinical

Table 13.3 Preclinical *in vivo* therapeutic studies of conventional liposomal anthracyclines*

Liposome	Agents	Tumor model	Outcome	Reference
PS:PC:Chol SA:PC:Chol	DOX	Lewis lung cancer P388 ascitic leukemia	A comparison was performed between positively and negatively charged liposomes. Positively charged (SA:PC:Chol) liposomes had equivalent therapeutic activity but reduced cardiotoxicity compared with unencapsulated drug	45
PS:PC:Chol PC:Chol DPG:PC:Chol	DOX	J-6456 (lymphoma)	There was significantly increased survival for animals treated with PS:PC:Chol liposomal doxorubicin compared with the unencapsulated drug. Survival after PC:Chol and DPG:PC:Chol liposomal doxorubicin was equivalent to that seen with the unencapsulated drug	24
PS:PC:Chol	DOX	Lewis lung cancer Mouse sarcoma 180	In comparison with unencapsulated doxorubicin, liposomal doxorubicin was significantly more effective against Lewis lung cancer and had equivalent activity against mouse sarcoma 180	48
PS:PC:Chol SA:PC:Chol	DOX	IgM immunocytoma	Negatively charged (PS:PC:Chol) liposomes had equivalent activity and decreased cardiotoxicity compared with unencapsulated doxorubicin. Positively charged (SALPC:Chol) liposomes had reduced therapeutic effect	46
PS:PC:Chol PG:PC:Chol	DOX	J-6456 (lymphoma)	There was significantly increased survival with liposomal compared with unencapsulated drug	47
PG:PC:Chol	DOX	None	The rate of drug-related deaths in mice treated with liposomal compared to unencapsulated doxorubicin was significantly reduced. There was reduced cardiac, renal hepatic, and biochemical (hyperlipidemia, hypoglycemia) toxicity with liposomal doxorubin	49
PG:PC:Chol: α-Toc	DOX	CT38LD (colon) CT26 (colon)	The CT38LD cell line was more sensitive than CT26 to doxorubicin *in vitro*. Liposomal doxorubicin was significantly more active than the unencapsulated agent when administered according to a protracted dose schedule against CT38LD and CT26 tumors *in vivo*	50
DSPC:Chol	DNR	P-1798 (lymphosarcoma) MA16C (breast)	Liposomal DNR was more active than the unencapsulated agent against both P-1798 and MA16C models. At the MTD, there were 100% cures for liposomal DNR compared with 40% for unencapsulated DNR against MA16C. In the P-1798 model, the liposomal agent was only more effective than the unencapsulated drug at lower doses	26

* α-Toc, α-Tocopherol; Chol, cholesterol; DNR, daunorubicin; DOX, doxorubicin; DPG, diphosphatidylglycerol; DSPC, distearoyl phosphatidylcholine; MTD, maximum tolerated dose; PC, phosphatidylcholine; PG, phosphatidylglycerol; PS, phosphatidylserine; SA, stearylamine.

Table 13.4 Preclinical *in vivo* therapeutic studies of conventional liposomal platinum analogs*

Liposomes	Agents	Tumor model	Outcome	Reference
DMPC:DMPG (L-NDDP)	NDDP CDDP	L1210 (leukemia) M5076 (reticulosarcoma)	L-NDDP was more active than unencapsulated NDDP or CDDP administered by the IP route against IP L1210 tumors, L-NDDP administered by the IP route retained its activity against platin-resistant IP L1210 tumors. L-NDDP was more active than unencapsulated CDDP when administered IV against the M5076 liver metastasis model	53
PS/PC/Chol (L-CDDP1) DPPC:DPPG:Chol (L-CDDP2)	CDDP	IgM immunocytoma	Both L-CDDP1 and L-CDDP2 were less effective than unencapsulated CDDP. Increased platinum levels were documented in renal tissue with L-CDDP1 but this was associated with less nephrotoxicity than unencapsulated CDDP	51
DMPC:DMPG (L-NDDP)	NDDP	L-1210 (leukemia) L-1210/PDD (leukemia) M5076 (reticulosarcoma)	L-NDDP was more active than unencapsulated NDDP or CDDP *in vitro*. L-NDDP was more active than unencapsulated NDDP administered by the IP route against IP L1210 and L1210/PDD tumors *in vivo*. L-NDDP was more active than unencapsulated NDDP administered by the IV route against M5076 liver metastases *in vivo*.	54
DMPC-DMPG (L-NPDP, L-NDDP, L-DEDP)	NPDP NDDP DEDP	L-1210 (leukemia) M5076 (reticulosarcoma) B16 (melanoma)	L-NDDP, L-NDDP and L-DEDP had equivalent activity to unencapsulated CDDP as single injections by the IP route against IP L1210 tumors. L-NPDP, L-NDDP and L-DEDP were more active than unencapsulated CDDP as multiple IP injections against IP L1210 tumors. Only IV L-NDDP demonstrated any activity against intravenously administered L1210 tumors. L-NDDP, and L-DEDP were more effective than unencapsulated CDDP against liver metastases of M5076. L-NPDP, L-NDDP, and L-DEDP demonstrated activity against IP implanted B16 tumors.	55
PC/PS/Chol (L-CDDP)	CDDP	L1210 (leukemia) NIH OVCAR (ovary)	There was no difference between unencapsulated CDDP and L-CDDP in terms of *in vivo* cytotoxicity or *invivo* activity after IV injection. Significantly increased antitumor activity was demonstrated for L-CDDP compared with unencapsulated CDDP after IP injection *in vivo*. L-CDDP caused a significantly lower rate of fatal toxicity than unencapsulated CDDP *in vivo*.	52

* CDDP, cis-dichlorodiammine platinum (II); Chol, cholesterol; DEDP, cis-bis-*n*-decanoato trans-R, R-1,2 diaminocyclohexane platinum (II); DMPC, dimyristoyl phosphatidylocholine; DMPG, dimyristoyl phosphatidylglycerol; DPPC, dipalmitoyl phosphatidylcholine; DPPG, dipalmitoyl phosphatidylglycerol; IP, intraperitoneal; IV, intravenous; L, liposomal; NDDP, cis-bis-neodecanoato trans-R, R-1,2 diaminocyclohexane platinum (II); NPDP, cis-bis-neopentanoato trans-R, R-1,2 diaminocyclohexane platinum (II); PC, phosphatidylcholine; PS, phosphatidylserine.

Table 13.5 Preclinical *in vivo* therapeutic studies of sterically stabilized liposomal anthracyclines*

Liposomes	Agent	Tumor model	Comments	Reference
HPC:Chol:HP1 (PL-DOX, PL-EPI) PC:PG:Chol (L-DOX, L-EPI)	DOX EPI	J-6456 (lymphoma)	PL-DOX was significantly more effective than L-DOX or unencapsulated DOX, L-DOX, in turn, was significantly more effective than encapsulated DOX	56
PC/PG:Chol:BHT (L-DOX), HSPC:Chol:PEG-DSPE:Toc (PL-DOX)	DOX	MC19/MC65/MC2A/ MC2B (breast)	Therapy was associated with reduced metastasis from intramammary tumor implants and increased cure rate of SC implants. PL-DOX was significantly better than L-DOX or unencapsulated DOX	57
HSPC:Chol (L-DOX, L-EPI) HSPC:Chol:PEG-DSPE:Toc (PL-DOX, PL-EPI)	DOX EPI	C-26 (colon)	PL-DOX and PL-EPI were significantly more effective than L-DOX or L-EPI	35
HSPC/Chol/PEG-DSPE (PL-DOX)	DOX	MC2 (breast)	PL-DOX was significantly more effective than unencapsulated DOX	58
HSPC/Chol/PEG-DSPE (PL-DOX)	DOX	HEY (ovary)	PL-DOX was significantly more effective than unencapsulated DOX by both IV and IP routes. There was a significant reduction in toxicity associated with the IP route for PL-DOX	59
HSPC/Chol/Toc (L-DOX) HSP/Chol/PEG-DSPE/Toc (PL-DOX)	DOX	TL-1 (lung)	PL-DOX was significantly more active than either L-DOX or unencapsulated DOX	60
HSPC/Chol/PEG-DSPE (PL-DOX)	DOX	PC-3 (prostate)	PL-DOX was significantly more active than unencapsulated DOX	38
HSPC/Chol/PEG-DSPE (PL-DOX)	DOX	Malignant fibrous histiocytoma (sarcoma)	Treatment with PL-DOX significantly increased the life-span of animals compared with unencapsulated DOX	40
HSPC/Chol/PEG-DSPE (PL-DOX)	DOX	C3H/He mammary cancer (breast)	PL-DOX significantly reduced pulmonary metastases and increased survival compared with placebo	61
HSPC/Chol/PEG-DSPE (PL-DOX)	DOX	AsPC-1 (pancreas)	PL-DOX was significantly more active than unencapsulated DOX	39
HSPC/Chol/PEG-DSPE (PL-DOX)	DOX	J6456 (ascitic lymphoma)	PL-DOX significantly more active than unencapsulated DOX. For PL-DOX, the IV route was more active than the IP route. In contrast, for DOX, the IP route was more active than the IV route	62
HSPC/Chol/PEG-DSPE (PL-DOX)	DOX	KB (head and neck cancer)	Unencapsulated DOX was significantly more active than PL-DOX *in vitro* (IC50 12-fold lower for unencapsulated DOX). PL-DOX was significantly more active and better tolerated than unencapsulated DOX *in vivo*	63

* BHT, Butylated hydroxytoluene; Chol, cholesterol; DOX, doxorubicin; EPI, epirubicin; HSPC, hydrogenated soy phosphatidylcholine; IC_{50}, drug concentration which caused 50% cell survival; IP, intraperitoneal; IV, intravenous; L, liposomal; PC, phosphatidylcholine; PEG-DPPE, PEG-derivatized dipalmitoyl phosphatidylethanolamine; PEG-DSPE, PEG-derivatized distearoyl phosphatidylethanolamine; PG, phosphatidylglycerol; PL, pegylated liposomal; SC, subcutaneous; Toc, a-tocopherol.

Table 13.6 Preclinical *in vivo* therapeutic studies of non-anthracycline drugs encapsulated in sterically stabilized liposomes*

Liposomes	Agent	Tumor model	Outcome	Reference
HSPC:Chol:MPEG-DSPE (PL-VCR and PL-DOX)	VCR DOX	MC2 (breast)	PL-VCR was more effective than unencapsulated VCR. Combination therapy of PL-VCR and PL-DOX given simultaneously was less effective than either agent given as a single dose. Combination therapy of PL-VCR and PL-DOX given according to an alternating schedule was more effective than single dose treatment with either agent	58
PC:Chol PC:Chol:GM1 PC:Chol:PEG-PE DMPG:DMPC	NDDP	RIF-1 (sarcoma)	PEG-PE liposomal NDDP exhibited significantly greater cytotoxicity *in vitro* than GM1 liposomal NDDP. PEG-PE liposomal NDDP was significantly more effective *in vivo* than PC:Chol, DMPC:DMPG and GM1-liposomal NDDp	65
DSPC/Chol (L-MITO) DSPC/Chol/PEG-DPPE (PL-MITO)	MITO	IV L1210 (leukemia)	L-MITO and PL-MITO were significantly less toxic than unencapsulated MITO. L-MITO was as active as PL-MITO and each was more effective than unencapsulated MITO only at highest dose level	64
HSPC:Chol:MPEG-DSPE (PL-CDDP)	CDDP	HT29 (colon)O	PL-CDDP was significantly more effective than unencapsulated CDDP	66
HSP:Chol:MPEG-DSPE (PL-CDDP)	CDDP	Lewis lung tumor C26 (colon)	PL-CDDP was significantly more effective than unencapsulated CDDP. Equivalent levels of tumor control were achieved with a 50% dose reduction of PL-CDDP	
HSPC:Chol:MPEG-DSPE (PL-CDDP)	CDDP	BT474 (breast) MDA453 (breast)	Unencapsulated CDDP and PL-CDDP were both effective as single agents against xenograft tumors. At tolerable dose levels, PL-CDDP was superior to unencapsulated CDDP. Both agents enhanced the activity of the activity of a humanized monocloncal antibody directed against HER2 (Herceptin)	67
HSPC:Chol:MPEG-DSPE (PL-CDDP)	CDDP	KB (head and neck)	Unencapsulated CDDP was significantly more active than PL-CDDP *in vitro* (IC50 21-fold lower for CDDP). PL-CDDP displayed superior activity to unencapsulated CDDP *in vivo*, but only at the intermediate dose level. Toxicity was significantly reduced for PL-DOX	63

* CDDP, cis-dichlorodiammine platinum (II); Chol, cholesterol; DMPC, dimyristoyl phosphatidylcholine; DMPG, dimyristoyl phosphatidylglycerol; DOX, doxorubicin; DSPC, distearoyl phosphatidylcholine; GM1, monosialoganglioside; HSPC, hydrogenated soy phosphatidylcholine; L, liposomal MITO, mitoxantrone; MPEG-DSPE, PEG-derivatized distearoyl phosphatidylethanolamine; NDDP, cis-bis-neodecanoato trans-R, R-1,2 diaminocyclohexane platinum (II); PC, phosphatidylcholine; PEG-DPPE, PEG-derivatized dipalmitoyl phosphatidylethanolamine; PL, pegylated liposomal VCR, vincristine.

investigation in animal models. Of these, only a relatively small number have proceeded to the stage of formal clinical assessment. Initial clinical studies aimed to confirm the ability of liposomes to localize to tumor tissues in patients (Table 13.7). Such studies have continued to provide valuable information and will guide future application of liposomal agents in the clinic.

The liposomal formulation that has entered clinical studies as DaunoXome has been subjected to extensive evaluation. For these studies, neutral phospholipid liposomes were formulated from distearoyl phosphatidylcholine, cholesterol, and the ionophore A23187 in a ratio of 2:1:0.004. The liposomes had a median diameter of 77 nm and contained nitrilotriacetic acid, which was radiolabelled with ^{111}In prior to administration. Turner *et al.* injected such vesicles containing 18.5 MBq of liposome-encapsulated radioactivity into 24 patients with a variety of tumors (6 lung cancer, 5 breast cancer, 3 prostate cancer, 2 colorectal cancer, and 1 each of lymphoma, sarcoma, melanoma, renal cell cancer, cervix cancer, thyroid cancer, pancreatic cancer, and ovarian cancer). Pharmacokinetic analysis revealed approximately 50 per cent of the injected dose remaining in the circulation at 4 hours and 20 per cent at 24 hours. Gamma camera imaging at 24 and 48 hours demonstrated positive tumor images in 22 of the 24 patients. There was evidence of significant uptake in the liver (34 ± 19 per cent of the inject dose) and spleen (4.9 ± 3.4 per cent of the injected dose) from region of interest analysis (68, 69). In a further report dealing with the same group of patients, data were presented for two patients who underwent surgery at 7 and 10 days after the liposome infusion (70). Tumor to blood ratios between 6.5 and 18.3:1 were reported for the primary tumor and lymph node and liver metastases. Presant *et al.* (69) presented data on two patients with AIDS-related Kaposi's sarcoma and non-Hodgkin's lymphoma whose lesions were successfully imaged with the same ^{111}In-NTA-labeled liposomes, although no data relating to pharmacokinetic parameters or biodistribution were presented. A further study in 7 patients with solid cancers revealed positive tumor images in 4 patients (1/2 breast cancer, 2/2 colon cancer, 1/1 prostate cancer, 0/1 lung cancer, and 0/1 lymphoma). Analysis of the pharmacokinetic profile showed 23 ± 5 and 8.9 ± 7.5 per cent of the injected dose per liter of blood at 3 minutes and 4 hours, respectively (71). Prominent hepatic uptake was demonstrated with 32.6 ± 14.4 per cent and 34.8 ± 8.4 per cent of the injected dose in that

organ at 4 and 48 hours, respectively (72). The ability of the same ^{111}In-NTA-labeled liposomes to localize to recurrent high-grade gliomas has been reported with clear delineation of the tumor in 7 of the 8 patients (73). Approximately 1 per cent of the injected radioactivity was localized in the brain with a maximum tumor to normal tissue ratio of 1.4:1. Significant hepatic uptake was observed at levels of up to 50 per cent of the injected dose. In a similar study using liposomal daunorubicin (DaunoXome), 8 patients with heavily pretreated recurrent glioblastoma multiforme received 50 mg of DaunoXome 24 to 48 hours before undergoing tumor biopsy. Chromatographic analysis of various regions within the tumor demonstrated drug levels within a potentially therapeutic range at both time points (74).

In a similar fashion, the PEGylated liposomal formulation that is presently under clinical investigation as Caelyx/Doxil has been the subject of a number of studies. Gabizon *et al.* (75) assessed the pharmacokinetics of equivalent doses of unencapsulated and/or PEGylated liposomal doxorubicin in 7 patients. Another 9 patients received the liposomal drug alone. Plasma elimination of the PEGylated liposomal agent followed a biexponential curve with median $t_{1/2\alpha}$ and $t_{1/2\beta}$ of 2 and 45 hours, respectively. The drug detected in the plasma was exclusively in the liposomal form, confirming the stability of this agent *in vivo*. Both the plasma clearance (0.1 liters versus 45 liters/h) and the volume of distribution (4 versus 254 liters) were significantly lower for the liposomal compared to the unencapsulated drug. In a number of patients, the doxorubicin concentration in the fluid from malignant effusions was measured and was shown to be increased 4–16-fold for the liposomal agent, reaching a peak between 3 and 7 days after drug administration. Northfelt *et al.* (76) demonstrated the ability of Caelyx/Doxil to target cutaneous AIDS-related Kaposi's sarcoma lesions in 18 patients. The subjects were randomly allocated to receive either Caelyx/Doxil or unencapsulated doxorubicin and representative lesions were biopsied 72 hours later. The doxorubicin level in the Kaposi's sarcoma lesions was 5.2 to 11.4 times greater in those patients treated with the PEGylated liposomal form of the drug. Detailed pharmacokinetic analysis confirmed that the drug was essentially confined within the circulation with a volume of distribution of 2.2 to 4.4 liters/m^2. The $t_{1/2\alpha}$ and $t_{1/2\beta}$ were 3.8 and 41.3 hours, respectively. Data have also been reported from 2 patients who underwent surgical fixation of pathological femoral fractures

Table 13.7 Clinical studies assessing tumor localization of conventional and pegylated liposomes in patients with cancer*

Liposome	Tracer	No. of patients	Comments	Reference
Conventional DSPC/Chol	^{11}In-NTA	24	Patients with various tumors (5 breast, 6 lung, 3 prostate, 2 colorectal, 1 renal, 1 cervical, 1 thyroid, 1 pancreatic, 1 ovarian cancer, 1 lymphoma, 1 sarcoma, 1 melanoma). Rapid clearance of liposomes with blood levels of 50% and 20% of injected dose at 4 and 24 hours, respectively. Significant uptake of liposomes by the RES. Tumors seen on on gamma camera scans at 24 and 48 hours in 22 of 24 patients	68
Conventional DSPC/Chol	^{111}In-NTA	2	Report of positive tumor images by gamma camera scan in 2 patients with AIDS-related KS and NHL. No dosimetric data were presented	69
Conventional DSPC/Chol	^{111}In-NTA	24	Same group of patients as ref. 68. Additional data presented on 2 patients who underwent surgery after injection of liposomes. Tumor to blood ratios ranged between 6.5 to 18.3:1 for primary tumor and nodal and liver metastases	70
Conventional EPC/EPG/Chol	^{111}In-DF	9	Rapid clearance of radiolabeled liposomes by the RES. *In vivo* evidence of drug leakage from the liposome in the circulation. Only 1/9 tumors demonstrated weakly on gamma camera scan	71
Conventional DSPC/Chol	^{111}In-NTA	7	Patients with advanced tumors (2 breast, 2 colonic, 1 lung, 1 prostate cancer, 1 lymphoma). Rapid clearance of liposomes to a blood level of 45% of injected dose at 4 hours with significant RES uptake. Tumors seen on gamma camera scans at 24 and 48 hours in 4 of 7 patients	72
Pegylated HSPC/Chol /PEG-DSPE	DOX	16	Significantly prolonged half-life, reduced plasma clearance (0.1 vs. 45 liters/h), and volume of distribution (4 vs 254 liters) of PEGylated liposomal doxorubicin compared to unencapsulated drug. Levels of drug 4–16-fold greater in malignant effusions in patients treated with liposomal agent	75
Pegylated HSPC/Chol /PEG-DSPE	DOX	18	Biopsies of AIDS-related KS lesions after either PEGylated liposomal or unencapsulated drug. 5.2- to 11.4-fold increase in tumor drug levels after PEGylated liposomal, as compared to unencapsulated, doxorubicin	76
Conventional DSPC/Chol	^{111}In-NTA	8	Patients with recurrent high-grade gliomas. Tumors seen in 7 of 8 patients on gamma camera scans at 72 hours. Total tumor uptake 1% of injected dose (maximal tumor:normal brain tissue ratio 1.4:1). Significant uptake by the RES (mainly liver and spleen)	73
Conventional DSPC/Chol	DNR	8	Patients with recurrent high-grade gliomas. Tumor biopsies obtained 24–48 hours after DNR administration. Circulation half-life of 4.8 hours. Significant tumor accumulation of DNR in the range of anticipated cytotoxic activity	74
Pegylated HSP/Chol/ PEG-DSPE	DOX	2	Patients with metastatic breast cancer who underwent surgical fixation of femoral fracture 6 and 12 days after drug administration. The drug concentration was 10-fold greater in tumor than adjacent normal skeletal muscle	77
Pegylated HSPC/Chol/ PEG-DSPE	^{99m}TcO$_4$$^-$	30	Patients with NSCLC and SCCHN received radiolabeled PEGylated liposomes. Mean tumor to large blood vessel ratio of radioactivity was 1.01 ± 0.29 for NSCLC and 1.35 ± 0.39 for . SCCHN) Liposome uptake correlated with tumor response to liposomal doxorubicin	78

Table 13.7 Continued

Liposome	Tracer	No. of patients	Comments	Reference
Pegylated HSPC/Chol/ PEG-DSPE	$^{99m}TcO_4^-$	7	Patients with sarcoma received radiolabeled PEGylated liposomes. Intratumoral drug accumulation 2.8-fold higher than surrounding healthy tissue	79
Pegylated HSPC/Chol/ PEG-DSPE	$^{99m}TcO_4^-$	15	Patients with glioma and brain metastases received radiolabeled pegylated liposomes. Liposome accumulation 13–19-fold greater in glioma and 7–13-fold greater in metastatic lesions compared to normal brain	80
Pegylated HSPC/Chol/ PEG-DSPE	^{111}In-DTPA	20	Patients with locally advanced cancers (7 SCCHN, 4 NSCLC, 5 Breast, 1 cervix cancer, 2 glioma, 1 KS). Tumors seen on gamma camera imaging in 15 of 17 patients studied. Uptake on SCCHN 33.0 ± 5.7% i.d./kg, NSCLC 18.3 ± 5.7% i.d./kg, breast 5.3 ± 2.7% i.e./kg. Tumor uptake related to tumor size. Surgical study in 2 patients with SCCHN showed tumor to normal tissue ratios of 2–11-fold for a range of tissues	81

* % i.d./kg, percentage of injected dose per kilogram; AML, acute myeloblastic leukemia; Chol, cholesterol; DF, deferoxamine; DNR, daunorubicin; DOX, doxorubicin; DSPC, distearoyl phosphatidylcholine; EPC, egg phosphatidylcholine; EPG, egg phosphatidylglycerine; KS, Kaposi sarcoma; NHL, non-Hodgkin's lymphoma; NTA, nitrilotriacetic acid; PA, phosphatidic acid; PEG-DSPE, pegylated distearoyl phosphatidylethanolamine; PRV, polycythemia rubra vera; RES, reticuloendothelial system.

secondary to breast cancer 6 and 12 days after having received Caelyx/Doxil (77). Fragments of tumor obtained during these procedures revealed a 10-fold greater concentration of liposomal doxorubicin than in adjacent uninvolved muscle. Koukourakis *et al.* (78–80) have recently published three studies that demonstrate the accumulation of ^{99m}Tc-diethylenetri-aminepentaacetic acid radiolabeled liposomes in lung and head and neck cancers (78), sarcomas (79), and brain tumors (80). In the first study, high levels of intratumoral accumulation of the radiolabeled liposomes were documented for both tumor types. The tumor to blood ratios ranged from 0.6–1.6 (mean 1.01 ± 0.29) for the lung cancers and 0.8–1.85 (mean 1.35 ± 0.39) for head and neck cancers. Interestingly, where available, immunohistochemistry showed a strong association between tumor microvessel density and liposome uptake. In the second study of 7 patients with locally advanced or recurrent sarcoma, the level of radiolabeled liposome uptake was 2.8-fold greater in tumor compared to adjacent normal tissue. In a final study, when compared with the adjacent normal brain, the accumulation of radiolabeled PEGylated liposomes was 13–19-fold greater in 5 patients with glioblastoma multiforme and 7–13-fold greater in 10 patients with metastatic brain tumors. A detailed analysis of the biodistribution and pharmacokinetics of ^{111}In-DTPA-labeled PEGylated liposomes in 17 patients with locally advanced cancers has recently been published (81). The $t_{1/2\beta}$ of radiolabeled liposomes was 76.1 hours. Positive tumor images were obtained in 15 of 17 studies (4/5 breast cancer, 5/5 head and neck cancer, 3/4 lung cancer, 2/2 glioma, and 1/1 cervix cancer). The levels of tumor liposome uptake estimated from regions of interest on gamma camera images were approximately 0.5–3.5 per cent of the injected dose at 72 hours. The levels of tumor uptake were greatest in the patients with head and neck cancers, intermediate in the patients with lung cancers, and relatively low in the patients with breast cancers. Significantly, the liposomes uptake values were inversely correlated with the estimated tumor volumes of the various tumor types. In a further patient with extensive mucocutaneous AIDs-related Kaposi's sarcoma, prominent deposition of the radiolabeled liposomes was seen within the lesions. In two patients with resectable head and neck cancer, samples of the tumor and adjacent normal tissue were obtained at operation. The levels of tumor uptake exceeded those in adjacent normal tissues by 2.3–10.8-fold.

Clinical therapeutic trials of liposomal cytotoxic drugs

The initial large-scale clinical evaluations of liposomal cytotoxic drugs were carried out in patients with AIDS-related Kaposi's sarcoma. The impressive therapeutic results achieved in this group of patients without the occurrence of severe toxicity paved the way for subsequent studies in patients with solid tumors. The pace of this research has increased enormously in the last 3 years and, as yet, much of the available data has been published only in abstract form. In an attempt to provide a balanced account of the tumor types against which liposomal agents have been assessed, data from these non-peer-reviewed studies have been included in this review. However, it must be borne in mind that in many cases such data are rather incomplete. For ease of reference, some of the clinical studies that have been completed have been summarized in Tables 13.8 and 13.9.

Liposomal doxorubicin (TLC D-99, Evacet)

TLC D-99 (The Liposome Company, Princeton, New Jersey, USA) consists of doxorubicin encapsulated in liposomes composed of egg phosphatidylcholine and cholesterol (ratio 1.22:1). Pharmacokinetic, phase I, II, and III clinical trials have been conducted with this agent (82–90). Embree *et al.* (82) reported the pharmacokinetics of TLC D-99 at doses of 60 and 75 mg/m^2 in 12 patients with non-small cell lung cancer with no difference in the $t_{1/2\alpha}$ and $t_{1/2\beta}$ as compared to unencapsulated doxorubicin. In a phase I clinical study in which the drug was administered either at single doses of 20–90 mg/m^2 every 3 weeks or as daily doses of 20, 25, and 30 mg/m^2/day for 3 days (83), leukopenia was dose-limiting and defined the maximum tolerated dose at 90 mg/m^2 every 3 weeks or 25 mg/m^2/day for 3 days. In contrast to the unencapsulated drug, mucosal and gastrointestinal toxicity were minimal or absent and significant cardiac, hepatic, renal, or other organ toxicities did not occur. In a randomized phase II trial, 40 patients with AIDS-related Kaposi's sarcoma received either 10 mg/m^2 (19 patients) or 20 mg/m^2 (21 patients) of TLC D-99 every 2 weeks. There were partial responses in 15 per cent (6 of 40) of patients, and a further 65 per cent (26 of 40) achieved disease stabilization. Response to treatment was related to dose with 5 per cent (1 of 19) of patients in the low-

Table 13.8 Studies of single-agent PEGylated liposomal doxorubicin (Caelyx/Doxil) in patients with solid cancers*

Tumor	No. of patients	Dose schedule	Response rates	Reference
Ovary	35	40–50 mg/m^2 q3–4w	9 (26%) responses: 1 CR, 8 PR	114
Ovary	89	50 mg/m^2 q4w	82 pts with platinum-refractory disease. 15 (17%) responses: 1 CR, 14 PR	115
Ovary	49	40 mg/m^2 q4w	Platinum- and taxane-resistant disease. 4 (9%) PR in 44 evaluable pts	116
Ovary	118	50 mg/m^2 q4w	24 (20%) responses; 7 (12%) responses in 58 pts with platinum-refractory disease	117
FUGT	63	50 mg/m^2 q4w	48 pts with ovarian cancer. Response in 19% pts with measurable disease. Marker response in 59% with raised CA125	118
Breast	71	45–60 mg/m^2 q3–4w	20 (31%) responses in 64 evaluable pts: 4 CR, 16 PR	119
Breast	45	35–45 mg/m^2 q3w; 50–60 mg/m^2 q4w; 65 mg/m^2 q5w, 70 mg/m^2 q6w	9 (20%) PR, 20 (44%) MR or SD	120
SCCHN	24	30–50 mg/m^2 q3w	8 (33%) responses: 1 CR, 7 PR	121
SCCHN	20	40 mg/m^2 q3w	9 (50%) responses in 18 evaluable pts: 3 CR, 6 PR	122
CTCL	6	20 mg/m^2 q4w	5 (83%) responses: 4 CR, 1 PR	123
STS	25	30–50 mg/m^2 q3w	Previous anthracycline therapy. 3 (12%) PR (50 mg/m^2 q3w), 2 MR, 17 SD	125
HCC	30	50 mg/m^2 q4w	4 (13%) response: 1 CR, 3 PR, 11 pts with SD for up to 1 year	126
SCLC	19	50 mg/m^2 q4w	3 (30%) PR in 10 evaluable pts. 4 pts with SD	127
TCC	22	50 mg/m^2 q4w	3 (18%) PR in 14 evaluable pts. 7 pts with SD	128
Glioma	13	20 mg/m^2 q2w	1 (8%) PR, 5 pts with SD over 3 courses of treatment	129
NSCLC	28	50 mg/m^2 q4w or 12.5 mg/m^2 q1w	No responses in 19 evaluable pts. 3 pts with SD in 50 mg/m^2 q4w group	132
NSCLC	14	12.5 mg/m^2 q1w	Platinum-refractory disease. No responses in 14 pts	133
STS	13	50 mg/m^2 q4w	No responses in 13 evaluable pts	134
HCC	16	30–40 mg/m^2 q3w	No responses in 16 pts	136
SCLC	14	50 mg/m^2 q4w	No responses in 13 evaluable pts. 3 pts with SD	137

* CR, complete response; CTCL, cutaneous T-cell lymphoma; FUGT, female urogenital tract cancer; HCC, hepatocellular cancer; NSCLC, non-small cell lung cancer; PR, partial response; pts, patients; q1w, weekly; q3w, every 3 weeks; q4w, every 4 weeks; q5w, every 5 weeks; q6w, every 6 weeks; SCCHN, squamous cell cancer of the head and neck; SCLC, small cell lung cancer; SD, stable disease; STS, soft tissue sarcoma; TCC, transitional cell cancer.

Table 13.9 Studies of liposomal anthracyclines in combination regimens in patients with solid cancers*

Tumor	No.	Regimen	Response rates and/or toxicity	Reference
Breast	41	TL-99 60 mg/m^2 day 1, Cyclophosphamide 500 mg/m^2 day 1, 5FU 500 mg/m^2 day 1&8. Cycle = q3w	Response in 73% of pts. Median duration of response, 11 months. Median overall survival, 19 months. Cardiac toxicity in 3 (7%) pts	89
Various	NS	Caelyx 30–40 mg/m^2 day 1, Paclitaxel 110 mg/m^2 day 1 and 8 q4w or 90–150 mg/m^2 day 1 q3w	Caelyx 40 mg/m^2 plus Paclitaxel 110 mg/m^2 day 1 and 8 q4w not tolerated. Caelyx 30 mg/m^2 plus paclitaxel 135 mg/m^2 day 1 q3w well-tolerated	138
Various	16	Caelyx 30 mg/m^2 q3w or 60 mg/m^2 day q6w, Paclitaxel 175 mg/m^2 over 3 hours q3w	Caelyx not tolerated at 60 mg/m^2 dose. Caelyx 30 mg/m^2 and Paclitaxel 175 mg/m^2 q3w tolerated with PR in 14 evaluable pts	
Breast	23	Caelyx 30 mg/m^2, Paclitaxel 200 mg/m^2 vs Doxorubicin 60 mg/m^2, Paclitaxel 200 mg/m^2. Cycle = q3w	Responses in 9 of 13 pts treated with Caelyx/Paclitaxel vs 7 of 10 treated with Doxorubicin/Paclitaxel. Cardiac toxicity seen in 6 pts treated with Doxorubicin/Paclitaxel. Trial stopped early	140
Breast	21	Caelyx 20 mg/m^2 day 1, paclitaxel 100 mg/m^2 days 1 and 8. Cycle = q2w	Response seen in 10 pts (48%): 2 CR, 8 PR. Alopecia, cutaneous, neural, and hematological toxicity. No cardiac dysfunction	141
Various	28	Caelyx 30–35 mg/m^2 day 1, Paclitaxel 50–80 mg/m^2 day 1, 8 and 15. Cycle = q4w	No response data reported. Dose-limiting toxicity not reached. Caelyx 30 mg/m^2 plus Paclitaxel 80 mg/m^2 or Caelyx 35 mg/m^2 plus Paclitaxel 70 mg/m^2 safe for further evaluation	142
Breast	10	Caelyx 30–45 mg/m^2, Docetaxel 75 mg/m^2. G-CSF support. Cycle = q4w	Responses in 7 of 8 evaluable pts. MTD not established but Caelyx 40 mg/m^2, Docetaxel 75 mg/m^2 q4w judged to be safe with G-CSF support	143
Various	20	Caelyx 30 mg/m^2, Cisplatin 30–75 mg/m^2, q3w or Caelyx 40 mg/m^2, Cisplatin 40–50 mg/m^2, q4w	Responses in 5 of 20 pts. Toxicity mild	144
Various	22	Caelyx 50 mg/m^2 day 1, Vinorelbine 15 mg/m^2/d for 1, 2, or 3 days. Cycle = q4w	Responses seen in 3 of 8 pts with metastatic breast cancer and 1 pt with gastric cancer. G-CSF needed if Vinorelbine was given for more than 1 day	145
Breast	10	Caelyx 50 mg/m^2 day 1, Cyclophosphamide 100 mg/m^2 day 1–14. Cycle = q4w	Responses in 5 of 7 evaluable pts. Grade 3 or 4 neutropenia in 6 pts	147
Ovary	17	Caelyx 25–30 mg/m^2 day 1, Gemicitabine 650–80 mg/m^2 day 1&8. Cycle = q4w	Response in 6 of 14 evaluable pts. 5 CR, 1 PR, 5 SD. MTD established in Gemicitabine 650 mg/m^2 day 1&8 and Caelyx 30 mg/m^2 day 1	148
Various	15	Caelyx 30–40 mg/m^2, Temozolomide 500-1000 mg/m^2. Cycle = q4w	8 pts with melanoma, 7 with various other tumors. No responses but SD in 7 pts MTD established at Caelyx 40 mg/m^2, Temoxolomide 1000 mg/m^2	149
Myeloma	12	Caelyx 40 mg/m^2 day 1, Vincristine 2 mg day 1, dexamethasone 40 mg days 1–4. Cycle = q3–4	Complete hematological remission in 8 pts, PR in 3 pts. Toxicity mild	150

* CR, complete response; CTCL, cutaneous T-cell lymphoma; FUGT, female urogenital tract cancer, G-CSF, granulocyte colony-stimulating factor; HCC, hepatocellular cancer; MTD, maximum tolerated dose; NSCLC, non-small cell lung cancer; PR, partial response; pts, patients; q2w, every 2 weeks; q3w, every 3 weeks; q4w, every 4 weeks; SCCHN, squamous cell cancer of the head and neck; SCLC, small cell lung cancer; SD, stable disease; STS, soft tissue sarcoma; TCC, transitional cell cancer.

dose group achieving a response in comparison to 24 per cent (5 of 21) of patients in the high-dose group. The major toxicity was hematological, with neutropenia occurring in 68 and 81 per cent of patients in the low- and high-dose groups, respectively. Alopecia was reported in only 8 per cent of patients, and other non-hematological toxicities were mild (87). The preliminary results of a phase III evaluation of TLC D-99 versus unencapsulated doxorubicin (both administered at a dose of 75 mg/m^2 every 3 weeks) in 69 patients with metastatic breast cancer have been presented. The response rates were 33 and 29 per cent for TLC D-99 and unencapsulated doxorubicin, respectively, TLC D-99 was associated with less toxicity: nausea and vomiting (10 versus 25 per cent); stomatitis/mucositis (9 versus 16 per cent); and fever/infection (6 versus 11 per cent) (86). A significant reduction in the incidence of cardiotoxicity (16 versus 25 per cent) with TLC D-99, as manifest by reduced left ventricular ejection fraction, was reported separately (84). Similar findings have been reported in patients with treatment-naive breast cancer (90). In an attempt to increase these response rates, TLC D-99 was administered as a 135 mg/m^2 intravenous bolus every 3 weeks along with growth factor support in 52 patients with treatment-naive metastatic breast cancer. The overall response rate was 46 per cent but there was appreciable treatment-related toxicity (grade 4 neutropenia, thrombocytopenia, and mucositis in 92, 88, and 19 per cent of patients, respectively) (88).

TLC D-99 has also been administered as a component of combination chemotherapy regimens in patients with metastatic breast cancer (85, 89). Valero *et al.* (89) treated 41 patients with TLC D-99 60 mg/m^2 on day 1, cyclophosphamide 500 mg/m^2 on day 1, and 5-fluorouracil (5FU) 500 mg/m^2 on days 1 and 8 of a 3-week treatment cycle. A median of 10 cycles per patient were delivered to a median cumulative TLC D-99 dose of 528 mg/m^2. The regimen was highly active with an overall response rate of 73 per cent. The median duration of response was 11.2 months and the median overall survival was 19.4 months. A phase III study in which patients received cyclophosphamide 600 mg/m^2 plus 60 mg/m^2 of either TLC D-99 or doxorubicin has been presented in abstract form (85). Identical response rates (43 per cent) were reported for the two regimens but bone marrow suppression and cardiotoxicity were significantly reduced for the TLC D-99-containing combination. Therefore, it appears that this agent has promise as a component of combination chemotherapy regimens, although it remains to

be seen how it will perform in direct comparisons with other liposomal anthracyclines.

Liposomal daunorubicin (DaunoXome)

DaunoXome (NeXstar Pharmaceuticals Inc., San Dimas, USA) is a daunorubicin-containing small unilamellar vesicle of 50–80 nm diameter composed of distearoyl phosphatidylcholine and cholesterol in a molar ratio of 2:1. In a phase I/II pharmacokinetic and clinical analysis, this agent has been shown to alter the pharmacokinetic profile of the drug favorably when compared to that of the unencapsulated drug (91). At the 80 mg/m^2 dose level, the mean total body clearance (6.6 versus 233 ml/min) and volume of distribution (2.9 versus 1055 liters) were significantly lower for liposomal, as compared to unencapsulated, daunorubicin. Such data translate to a 36-fold increase in the area under the time: concentration curve for the liposomal agent. Initial phase II studies of DaunoXome were conducted in patients with AIDS-related Kaposi's sarcoma who were treated at doses ranging from 40 to 60 mg/m^2 every 2 weeks. Response rates on the order of 40–73 per cent were documented (91–95). In a subsequent phase III study 232 patients with AIDS-related Kaposi's sarcoma received either DaunoXome 40 mg/m^2 or standard combination chemotherapy (ABV—doxorubicin 10 mg/m^2, bleomycin 15 IU, vincristine 1 mg) every 2 weeks (96). Equivalent response rates were reported for the two treatment arms (25 and 28 per cent, respectively). DaunoXome caused significantly less neuropathy (13 versus 41 per cent) and alopecia (8 versus 36 per cent) than ABV but slightly more myelosuppression (grade 3 neutropenia 36 versus 36 per cent; grade 4 neutropenia 15 versus 5 per cent). The incidence of opportunistic infections was increased amongst the patients treated with DaunoXome (36 versus 26 per cent) but this did not reach statistical significance.

Thus far, there have been few studies of DaunoXome in patients with tumors other than Kaposi's sarcoma. A phase I study of three daily doses of 75–200 mg/m^2 of DaunoXome in 24 patients with refractory or relapsed acute myeloid leukemia or blast phase chronic myeloid leukemia has been reported (97). The dose-limiting toxicities were myelosuppression, requiring transfusional support, and mucositis. There were two complete responses to treatment. Steele *et al.* (98) conducted a phase I/II trial in 13 patients with malignant mesothelioma of the pleura. The maximum tolerated dose was 120 mg/m^2 every 3 weeks. There were no objective responses to treatment but 7 patients had stabilization of their disease during therapy. The activity of DaunoXome against hepatocellular carcinoma has been assessed in two separate phase I and II studies (99–100). Yeo *et al.* (99) administered doses of 100 mg/m^2 every 3 weeks but saw no objective tumor responses in 12 of 14 evaluable patients. In a phase I trial 11 patients with hepatocellular carcinoma complicating cirrhosis were enrolled on to a proposed dose escalation protocol starting at 80 mg/m^2. However, the occurrence of dose-limiting toxicity at the starting dose and subsequent reduced doses of 60 and 40 mg/m^2 resulted in premature termination of the study with no evidence of therapeutic activity (100).

Liposomal *cis*-bisneodecanoato *trans*-R, R-1,2-diaminocyclohexaneplatinum

A small number of phase I/II studies have been conducted with the lipophilic platinum derivative NDDP, encapsulated in conventional multilamellar vesicles composed of dimyristoyl phosphatidylcholine and dimyristoyl phosphatidylglycerol (7:3 molar ratio). An initial dose-escalation study was performed in 39 patients with a variety of malignant diagnoses who received intravenous infusions of liposomal NDDP every 4 weeks (101). Myelosuppression was dose-limiting and the maximum tolerated dose was 312.5 mg/m^2 every 4 weeks. Other toxicities included nausea, vomiting, and diarrhea but there was no evidence of nephrotoxicity or ototoxicity—side-effects that frequently occur in patients treated with unencapsulated cisplatin. Preclinical studies have demonstrated that this agent has favorable pharmacokinetics and is well-tolerated when given by the intraperitoneal route (34). As a result, clinical studies of locoregional administration of this agent have been carried out in patients with malignant effusions (102, 103). In the first of these studies, 21 patients with non-loculated pleural effusions due to lung cancer, ovarian cancer, and mesothelioma received escalating doses of intrapleural liposomal NDDP (102). Dose escalation was limited to 450 mg/m^2 by chest pain, which presumably occurred secondary to chemical pleuritis. Pharmacokinetic analysis revealed initial rapid systemic drug absorption within 2 hours of injection followed by stable blood levels between 6 and 24 hours. Significantly, the toxicities that were associated with intravenous administration were avoided by intrapleural infusion. This preparation had some activity with complete resolution or significant palliation of the pleural effusion in 6

patients. In a subsequent study, 20 patients with mesothelioma were treated with liposomal NDDP 450 mg/m^2 every 3 to 4 weeks (103). The intrapleural treatment route was associated with appreciable toxicity and two patients died soon after the first drug administration due to local complications. However, this drug schedule was very active against this very aggressive tumor, and there were f11 complete pathological responses in the 15 evaluable patient6s. However, despite these promising results there have been no further published reports of the clinical activity of this agent and its current state of development is rather unclear.

Liposomal vincristine (Onco-TCS)

A formulation of vincristine entrapped in 120 nm small unilamellar vesicles composed of distearoyl phosphatidylcholine and cholesterol has undergone limited clinical investigation (104, 105). Gelmon *et al.* (104) treated 25 patients with various malignancies with escalating doses of liposomal vincristine between 0.5 and 2.8 mg/m^2 every 3 weeks. The dose-limiting toxicities were pain and constipation defining a maximum tolerated dose of 2.4 mg/m^2. Other toxicities included fever, rigors, fatigue, myalgia, and peripheral neuropathy. One patient with pancreatic cancer achieved a partial response and minor responses were seen in two other patients. Subsequently, a phase II trial in 51 patients with relapsed and pretreated non-Hodgkin's lymphomas and acute lymphoblastic leukemia has also been completed (105). Patients received 2.0 mg/m^2 every 2 weeks up to a dose of 12 injections and responses were seen in 14 of 34 (41 per cent) evaluable patients. Severe (grade 3 or 4) motor or sensory neuropathy occurred in 11 patients and required cessation of therapy in five patients (all of whom had pre-existing neuropathy from previous treatment). From this limited clinical analysis it seems that this agent has promise, particularly in combination with other agents. Further clinical studies should provide useful information in this regard.

PEGylated liposomal doxorubicin (Caelyx/Doxil)

Very extensive clinical evaluation has been conducted with Caelyx/Doxil (Alza Corp., Mountain View, USA), which consists of doxorubicin encapsulated in a small unilamellar vesicle of mean diameter 96 nm. The liposome matrix is composed of hydrogenated soybean phosphatidylcholine (56.2 per cent), cholesterol (38.3 per cent), and N-(carbamoyl-methoxypolyethylene glycol 2000)-1, 2-distearoyl-*sn*-glycero-f3-phosphoethanolamine sodium salt (5.3 per cent). Initial evaluation of Caelyx/Doxil was performed in patients with AIDS-related Kaposi's sarcoma with response rates of 69–93 per cent (106–111). Subsequently, two large phase III studies were conducted comparing Caelyx/Doxil to standard combination chemotherapy (112, 113). In the first study, 241 patients received 6 cycles of either Caelyx/Doxil (20 mg/m^2) or bleomycin (15 IU/m^2) and vincristine (2 mg) every 3 weeks (112). The response rate for Caelyx/Doxil (59 per cent) was significantly greater than for bleomycin and vincristine (23 per cent). In addition, treatment with bleomycin and vincristine was significantly more toxic as measured by the need to discontinue treatment prematurely (27 versus 11 per cent) or the incidence of peripheral neuropathy (14 versus 3 per cent) and leukopenia (51 versus 72 per cent). In the second study, 258 patients received 6 cycles of either Caelyx/Doxil (20 mg/m^2), bleomycin (10 IU/m^2), and vincristine (1 mg) every 2 weeks (113). Caelyx/Doxil was significantly more effective than the combination regimen, with response rate of 45.9 and 24.8 per cent, respectively. Caelyx/Doxil was better tolerated than the combination in terms of alopecia (1 versus19 per cent), nausea and vomiting (15 versus 34 per cent), and neuropathy (6 versus 14 per cent), although there was no significant difference in grade 3 leukopenia (36 versus 42 per cent).

The reported efficacy of Caelyx/Doxil in patients with AIDS-related Kaposi's sarcoma resulted in a number of phase I/II studies being carried out in patients with solid cancers. The activity of this agent administered at doses of 40–50 mg/m^2 every 3–4 weeks against gynecological cancers, especially refractory ovarian cancer, has been extensively reported (114–118). The initial study reported a very promising response rate of 26 per cent in 35 patients with platinum- and taxane-resistant ovarian cancer (114). Subsequent studies confirmed the activity of Caelyx/Doxil in this setting but, as is often the case, the response rates were somewhat lower. Response rates of 17 per cent in 89 patients (115), 9 per cent in 44 patients (116), and 19 per cent in 63 patients (117) have been documented. It is noteworthy that toxicities were mainly mucocutaneous (see below) and generally manageable by dose adjustment in most patients. Drug-induced nausea, alopecia, and cardiomyopathy were either absent or uncommon. Caelyx/Doxil also possesses activity in patients with breast cancer (119, 120). Ranson *et al.* (119) reported the results of a phase I/II

trial of Caelyx/Doxil at a dose of 45–60 mg/m^2 every 3 to 4 weeks in 71 anthracycline-naïve women with stage IV disease. Cutaneous toxicity was excessive at doses beyond 45 mg/m^2 every 4 weeks. The objective response rate was 31 per cent, although a similar number of patients had stabilization of their disease during treatment. Lyass *et al.* (120) conducted a dose-finding and therapeutic study in 45 patients with previously treated metastatic disease. Six dose schedules were investigated (35 mg/m^2 every 3 weeks, 45 mg/m^2 every 3 weeks, 50 mg/m^2 every 4 weeks, 60 mg/m^2 every 4 weeks, 65 mg/m^2 every 5 weeks, and 70 mg/m^2 every 6 weeks) with a view to determining the effect of pharmacokinetic parameters on the incidence of treatment-related toxicities. Stomatitis and leukopenia were found to be dose-related and cutaneous toxicity was schedule-dependent with shorter dosing intervals associated with increased frequency and severity of skin manifestations. Objective responses were seen in 20 per cent (9 of 45) of patients with another 20 patients showing either minor response or disease stabilization. Caelyx/Doxil has been evaluated in patients with head and neck cancer (78, 121, 122). Caponigro *et al.* (121) treated 24 patients with relapsed or metastatic disease at doses of 30–50 mg/m^2 every 3 weeks. The maximum tolerated dose was 45 mg/m^2 every 3 weeks and a response rate of 33 per cent (8 of 24 patients) was reported. In addition, 20 patients with treatment-naïve head and neck cancer have been treated prior to commencing radical radiotherapy (122). Half the patients received 2 cycles of 40 mg/m^2 every 3 weeks and the others received a third escalating dose of 10 mg/m^2, 15 mg/m^2, or 20 mg/m^2 3 days before starting radiotherapy. Nine of 18 (50 per cent evaluate patients showed an objective response to treatment, despite the fact that the maximum cumulative dose before evaluation of chemotherapy response was only 80 mg/m^2. In a related approach, Koukourakis *et al.* (78) administered Caelyx/Doxil at doses of 10–25 mg/m^2 every 2 weeks concurrently with radiotherapy in patients with head and neck and lung cancers. It was impossible to comment on the independent efficacy of the chemotherapy. The treatment was generally well-tolerated but, as expected, dose-limiting exacerbation of mucosal toxicity occurred in the patients with head and neck cancer. There have been other isolated reports of the activity of Caelyx/Doxil in patients with cutaneous T-cell lymphoma (123), soft-tissue sarcoma (124, 125), hepatocellular carcinomas (126), small-cell lung cancer (127), transitional cell cancer (128), and glioma (129).

It is important to realize, however, that a number of studies have shown little or no activity of Caelyx/Doxil in patients with a variety of tumors including renal cell (130), pancreatic cancer (131), and non-small cell lung cancer (132, 133). Furthermore, in contrast to the positive data presented above (124–127), poor activity of this agent has been reported in patients with advanced soft-tissue sarcomas (134, 135) and hepatocellular (136) and small-cell lung cancer (137).

In addition, preliminary phase I and II studies have been conducted using Caelyx/Doxil in combination with other cytotoxic agents including paclitaxel (138–142), docetaxel (143), cisplatin (144), vinorelbine (145, 146), cyclophosphamide (147), gemcitabine (148), and temozolomide (149). A combination regimen of vincristine, Caelxy/Doxil, and dexamethasone has been shown to exert significant activity in 12 elderly patients with multiple myeloma (150) and offers the potential of avoiding the need for infusional doxorubicin therapy in such patients. Eight patients achieved complete hematological remission and three patients had a partial response. Treatment was given on an ambulatory basis and was well tolerated.

The ability of Caelyx/Doxil to ameliorate the familiar side-effects of unencapsulated doxorubicin has also been widely reported. Nausea and vomiting (110, 112, 114, 119, 120, 122, 141), alopecia (110, 112–115, 118, 119), local tissue vesicant activity (114, 151, 152), and doxorubicin-induced cardiomyopathy (153–155) are all significantly reduced by encapsulation of the drug in PEGylated liposomes. However, the administration of repeated doses of Caelyx/Doxil is associated with a novel toxicity, plantar–palmar erythrodysesthesia (PPE) or 'hand–foot' syndrome, which manifests as painful swelling and inflammation of the hands and feet, intertriginous areas, and sites of trauma (120, 152, 156). A similar mucosal toxicity associated with superficial mouth ulcers also occurs. As mentioned above, these mucocutaneous manifestations have been shown to be dose-limiting in many studies. A number of attempts have been made to define therapies to limit this toxicity, including the use of pyridoxine (157), ergotamine (158), topical dimethylsulfoxide (159), and amifostine (160). Such interventions offer the prospect of allowing large doses of Caelyx/Doxil to be administered safely but, as yet, none has been shown to be effective in a randomised study.

PEGylated liposomal cisplatin (SPI-077)

SPI-077 (Alza Corp, Mountain View, USA) is a small unilamellar vesicle with a mean diameter of 110 nm that contains cisplatin. Its lipid composition is as follows (values stated as per cent molar ratio): hydrogenated soybean phosphatidylcholine (51 per cent), cholesterol (44 per cent), and N-(carbamoyl-methoxy-polyethylene glycol 2000)-1, 2-distearoyl-*sn*-glycero-3-phospho-ethanolamine sodium salt (5 per cent). Promising preclinical data in a number of tumor models have been followed by pharmacokinetic and phase I/II studies. DeMario *et al.* (161) reported preliminary toxicity data in 14 patients who received escalating doses up to 120 mg/m^2 with no evidence of the expected adverse effects (nausea and vomiting, neurotoxicity, nephrotoxicity) of treatment with unencapsulated cisplatin. As with other PEGylated liposomal agents, the pharmacokinetic parameters were markedly altered such that they conformed to those of the liposomal vehicle. The volume of distribution was equal to plasma volume and the circulation half-life was approximately 60 hours. The liposome formulation was very stable in the circulation with no detectable free cisplatin in the plasma ultrafiltrate. A dose-escalation study of SPI-077 at doses up to 260 mg/m^2 in combination with paclitaxel has also been performed in patients with non-small cell lung cancer. There was no evidence of dose-limiting platinum-induced toxicity (162). In a subsequent phase I/II study, 18 patients with treatment-naive locally advanced head and neck cancer received two cycles of SPI-077 at doses of 200–260 mg/m^2 (163). As in previous studies, the treatment was very well-tolerated with no demonstrable platinum-related toxicities. However, there were only two partial responses in a group of patients who would have been expected to have a significant response rate to unencapsulated cisplatin. These data suggest that this agent has very limited promise for subsequent development as a cytotoxic agent

Conclusions

This chapter has detailed the slow process involved in the development of clinically relevant liposomal therapies and has shown that, after concerted effort, a number of formulations are entering routine clinical practice. In particular, liposomal anthracyclines have undergone extensive evaluation and are now approved as part of established patterns of care in a number of tumor types. In the near future, it is likely that more formulations of existing or novel cytotoxic agents will be developed. The next stage of the process is likely to involve the testing of liposomal agents in the context of combination drug regimens in patients with early-stage disease. In this way, it should be possible to assess the likely gains in therapeutic efficacy and amelioration of toxicity that will accrue from the use of liposomal chemotherapy. Therefore, in summary it is reasonable to expect that liposomes will gain increased prominence in the coming years and will make a significant contribution to the targeted treatment of cancer.

References

1. Bangham AD, Standish HM, Watkins JC. Diffusion of univalent ions across the lamellae of swollen phospholipids. J Mol Biol 1965, **13**, 238–52.
2. Sessa G, Weissmann G. Phospholipid spherules (liposomes) as a model for biological membranes. J Lipid Res 1968, 9, 310–18.
3. Gregoriades G, Swain CP, Wills EJ, Tavill AS. Drug-carrier potential of liposomes in cancer chemotherapy. Lancet 1974, **1**, 1313–16.
4. Gregoriadis G. The carrier potential of liposomes in biology and medicine [first of two parts]. New Engl J Med, 1976, **295**, 704–10.
5. Gregoriadis G. The carrier potential of liposomes in biology and medicine [second of two parts]. New Engl J Med 1976, **295**, 765–70.
6. Lasic DD, Papahadjopoulos D. Liposomes revisited. Science 1995, **267**, 1275–6.
7. Martin FJ. PEGylated liposomal doxorubicin: scientific rationale and preclinical pharmacology. Oncology 1997, **11** (suppl. 11), 11–20.
8. Adler-Moore J. AmBisome targeting to fungal infections. Bone Marrow Transplant 1994, **14** (suppl. 5), S3–S7.
9. Ng TT, Denning DW. Liposomal amphotericin B (AmBisome) therapy in invasive fungal infections. Evaluation of United Kingdom compassionate use data. Arch Intern Med 1995, **155**, 1093–8.
10. Russo R, Nigro LC, Minniti S. Visceral leishmaniasis in HIV infected patients: treatment with high dose liposomal amphotericin B (AmBisome). J Infect 1996, **32**, 133–7.
11. Prentice HG, Hann IM, Herbrecht R, *et al.* A randomised comparison of liposomal versus conventional amphotericin B for the treatment of pyrexia of unknown origin in neutropenic patients. Br J Haematol 1997, **98**, 711–18.
12. Durocher JR, Payne RC, Conrad ME. Role of sialic acid in erythrocyte survival. Blood 1975, **45**, 11–20.
13. Allen TM, Chonn A. Large unilamellar liposomes with low uptake by the reticuloendothelial system. FEBS Lett 1987, **223**, 42–6.
14. Gabizon A, Papahadjopoulos D. Liposome formulations with prolonged circulation time in blood and enhanced uptake in tumours. Proc Natl Acad Sci, USA 1988, **85**, 6949–53.
15. Klibanov AL, Maruyama K, Torchilin VP, Huang L. Amphipathic polyethyleneglycols effectively prolong the circulation times of liposomes. FEBS Lett 1990, **268**, 235–7.
16. Papahadjopoulos D, Allen TM, Gabizon A, *et al.* Sterically stabilised liposomes: improvements in pharmacokinetics and anti-tumour therapeutic efficacy. Proc Natl Acad Sci, USA 1991, 88, 11460–4.
17. Gabizon AA. Liposomal anthracyclines. Hematol Oncol Clin N America 1994, 8, 431–50.
18. Lasie DD. Doxorubicin in sterically stabilised liposomes. Nature 1996, **380**, 561–2.
19. Adlakha-Hutcheon G, Bally MB, Shew CR, Madden TD. Controlled destabilization of a liposomal drug delivery system enhances mitoxantrone antitumor activity. Nat Biotechnol 1999, **17**, 775–9.
20. Zalipsky S, Qazen M, Walker JA, Mullah N, Quinn YP, Huang SR. New detachable poly(ethylene glycol) conjugates: cysteine-cleavable lipopolymers regenerating natural phospholipid, diacyl phosphatidylethanolamine. Bioconjug Chem 1999, **10**,703–7.
21. Perez-Soler R. Liposomes as carriers of antitumour agents: toward a clinical reality. Cancer Treat Rev 1989, **16**, 67–82.
22. Leyland-Jones B. Targeted drug delivery. Sem Oncol 1993, 20, 12–17.
23. Gabizon A, Dagan A, Goren D, Barenholz Y, Fuks Z. Liposomes as *in vivo* carriers of adnamycin: reduced cardiac uptake and preserved antitumour activity in mice. Cancer Res 1982, **42**, 4734–9.
24. Gabizon A, Goren D, Fuks Z, Barenholz Y, Dagan A, Meshorer A. Enhancement of adriamycin delivery to liver metastatic cells with increased tumouricidal effect using liposomes as drug carriers. Cancer Res 1983, **43**, 4730–5.
25. Proffitt RT, Wiliams LE, Presant CA, *et al.* Tumour-imaging potential of liposomes loaded with In-111-NTA: biodistribution in mice. J Nucl Med 1983, **24**, 45–51.
26. Forssen EA, Coulter DM, Proffitt RT. Selective *in vivo* localisation of daunorubicin small unilamellar vesicles in solid tumours. Cancer Res 1992, **52**, 3255–61.
27. Forssen EA, Male-Brune R, Adler-Moore JP, *et al.* Fluorescence imaging studies for the disposition of daunorubicin liposomes (DaunoXome) within tumour tissue. Cancer Res 1996, **56**, 2066–75.
28. Ogihara-Umeda I, Sasaki T, Kojima S, Nishigori H. Optimal radiolabelled liposomes for tumour imaging. J Nucl Med 1996, **37**, 326–32.
29. Harasym TO, Cullis PR, Bally MB. Intratumour distribution of doxorubicin following i.v. administration of drug encapsulated in egg phosphatidylcholine/cholesterol liposomes. Cancer Chemother Pharmacol 1997, **40**, 309–17.
30. Mayer LD, Bally MB, Loughrey H, Masin D, Cullis PR. Liposomal vincristine preparations which exhibit decreased drugs toxicity and increased activity against murien L1210 and P388 tumors. Cancer Res 1990, **50**, 575–9.
31. Boman NL, Masin D, Mayer LD, Cullis PR, Bally MB. Liposomal vincristine which exhibits increased drug retention and increased circulation longevity cures mice bearing P388 tumors. Cancer Res 1994, **54**, 2830–3.
32. Webb MS, Harasym TO, Masin D, Bally MB, Mayer LD. Sphingomyelin-cholesterol liposomes significantly enhance the pharmacokinetic and therapeutic properties of vincristine in murine and human tumour models. Br J Cancer 1995, **72**, 896–904.

33. Khokhar AR, Wright K, Siddik ZH, Perez-Soler R. Organ distribution and tumour uptake of liposome entrapped cis-bis-neodecanoato trans-R, R-1, 2 diaminocyclohexane platinum (II) administered intravenously and into the proper hepatic artery. Cancer Chemother Pharmacol 1988, **22**, 223–7.

34. Vadiei K, Siddik ZH, Khokhar AR, al-Baker S, Sampedro F, Perez-Soler R. Pharmacokinetics of liposome-entrapped cis-bis-neodecanoato trans-R, R-1, 2 diaminocyclohexane platinum (II) and cisplatin given i.v. and i.p. in the rat. Cancer Chemother Pharmacol 1992, **30**, 365–9.

35. Huang SK, Mayhew E, Gilani S, Lasic DD, Martin FJ, Papahadjopoulos D. Pharmacokinetics and therapeutics of sterically stabilised liposomes in mice bearing C-26 colon carcinoma. Cancer Res 1992, **52**, 6774–81.

36. Huang SK, Lee K-D, Hong K. Friend DS, Papahadjopoulos D. Microscopic localisation of sterically stabilised liposomes in colon carcinoma-bearing mice. Cancer Res 1992, **52**, 5135–43.

37. Huang SK, Martin FJ, Jay G, Vogel J, Papahadjopoulos D, Friend DS. Extravasation and transcytosis of liposomes in Kaposi's sarcoma-like dermal lesions of transgenic mice bearing the HIV*tat* gene. Am J Pathol 1993, **143**, 1–14.

38. Vaage J, Barbera-Guillem E, Abra R, Huang A, Working P. Tissue distribution and therapeutic effect of intravenous free or encapsulated liposomal doxorubicin on human prostate carcinoma xenografts. Cancer 1994, **73**, 1478–84.

39. Vaage J, Donovan D, Uster P, Working P. Tumour uptake of doxorubicin in polyethylene glycol-coated liposomes and therapeutic effect against a xenografted human pancreatic carcinoma. Br J Cancer 1997, **75**, 482–6.

40. Siegal T, Horowitz A, Gabizon A. Doxorubicin encapsulated in sterically stabilised liposomes for the treatment of a brain tumour model: biodistribution and therapeutic efficacy. J Neurosurg 1995, **83**, 1029–37.

41. Newman MS, Colbern GT, Working PK, Engbers C, Amantea MA. Comparative pharmacokinetics, tissue distribution and therapeutic effectiveness of cisplatin encapsulated in long-circulating pegylated liposomes (SPI-077) in tumour-bearing mice. Cancer Chemother Pharmacol 1999, **43**, 1–7.

42. Harrington KJ, Rowlinson-Busza G, Syrigos KN, Uster PS, Abra RM, Stewart JS. Biodistribution and pharmacokinetics of IIIIn-DTPA-labelled pegylated liposomes in a human tumour xenograft model: implications for novel targeting strategies. Br J Cancer 2000, **83**, 232–8.

43. Harrinton KJ, Rowlinson-Busza G, Syrigos KN, *et al.* Influence of tumour size on uptake of ^{111}In-DTPA-labelled pegylated liposomes in a human tumour xenograft model. Br J Cancer 2000, **83**, 684–8.

44. Allen TM, Newman MS, Woodle MC, Mayhew E, Uster PS. Pharmacokinetics and anti-tumor activity of vincristine encapsulated in sterically stabilized liposomes. Int J Cancer 1995, **62**, 199–204.

45. Rahman A, Kessler A, More N, *et al.* Liposomal protection of adriamycin-induced cardiotoxicity in mice. Cancer Res 1980, **40**, 1532–7.

46. van Hoesel QGCM, Steerenberg PA, Crommelin DJA, *et al.* Reduced cardiotoxicity and nephrotoxicity with preservation of anti-tumour activity of doxorubicin entrapped in stable liposomes in the LIEU/M Wsl rat. Cancer Res 1984, **44**, 3698–703.

47. Gabizon A, Goren D, Fuks Z, Meshorer A, Barenholz Y. Superior therapeutic activity of liposome-associated adriamycin in a murine metastatic tumour model. Br J Cancer 1985, **51**, 681–9.

48. Forssen EA, Tokes ZA. Improved therapeutic benefits of doxorubicin by entrapment in anionic liposomes. Cancer Res 1983, **43**, 546–50.

49. Gabizon A, Meshorer A, Barenholz Y. Comparative long-term study of the toxicities of free and liposome-associated doxorubicin in mice after intravenous administration. J Natl Cancer Inst 1986, **77**, 459–69.

50. Mayhew EG, Goldrosen MH, Vaage J, Rustum YM. Effects of liposome-entrapped doxorubicin on liver metastases of mouse colon carcinomas 26 and 38. J Natl Cancer Inst 1987, **78**, 707–13.

51. Steerenberg PA, Storm G, de Groot G, *et al.* Liposomes as drug carrier system for cis-diamminedichloroplatinum (II). Antitumour activity *in vivo*, induction of drug resistance, nephrotoxicity and Pt distribution. Cancer Chemother Pharmacol 1988, **21**, 299–307.

52. Gondal JA, Preuss HG, Swartz R, Rahman A. Comparative pharmacological, toxicological and antitumoural evaluation of free and liposome-encapsulated cisplatin in rodents. Eur J Cancer 1993, **29A**, 1536–42.

53. Perez-Soler R, Khokhar AR, Lopez-Berenstein G. Treatment and prophylaxis of experimental liver metastases of M5076 reticulosarcoma with cis-bis-neodecanoato trans-R, R-1, 2 diaminocyclohexane platinum (II) entrapped in multilamellar vesicles. Cancer Res 1987, **47**, 6462–6.

54. Perez-Soler R, Young LY, Drewinko B, Lautersztain J, Khokhar AR. Increased cytoloxicity and reversal of resistance to cisplatin with entrapment of cis-bis-neodecanoato trans-R, R-1, 2 diaminocyclohexane platinum (II) in multilamellar vesicles. Cancer Res 1988, **48**, 4509–12.

55. Khokhar AR, al-Baker S, Krakoff IH, Perez-Soler R. Toxicity and antitumour activity of cis-bis-carboxylato(trans-R, R-1, 2-diaminocyclohexane) platinum (II) complexes entrapped in liposomes. Cancer Chemother Pharmacol 1989, **23**, 219–24.

56. Gabizon AA. Selective tumor localization and improved therapeutic index of anthracyclines encapsulated in long-circulating liposomes. Cancer Res 1992, **52**, 891–6.

57. Vaage J, Mayhew E, Lasic D, Martin F. Therapy of primary and metastatic mouse mammary carcinomas with doxorubicin encapsulated in long circulating liposomes. Int J Cancer 1992, **51**, 942–8.

58. Vaage J, Donovan D, Mayhew E, Uster P, Woodle M. Therapy of mouse mammary carcinomas with vincristine and doxorubicin encapsulated in sterically stabilised liposomes. Int J Cancer 1993, **54**, 959–64.

59. Vaage J, Donovan D, Mayhew E, Abra R, Huang A. Therapy of human ovarian carcinoma xenografts using doxorubicin encapsulated in sterically stabilised liposomes. Cancer 1993, **72**, 3671–5.

60. Williams SS, Alosco TR, Mayhew E, Lasic DD, Martin FJ, Bankert RB. Arrest of human lung tumour xenograft growth in severe combined immunodeficient mice using doxorubicin encapsulated in sterically stabilised liposomes. Cancer Res 1993, **53**, 3964–7.

61. Vaage J, Donovan D, Loftus T, Working P. Prevention of metastasis from mouse mammary carcinomas with liposomes carrying doxorubicin. Br J Cancer 1995, **72**, 1074–5.

62. Cabanes A, Tzemach D, Goren D, Horowitz AT, Gabizon A. Comparative study of the antitumor activity of free doxorubicin and polyethylene glycol-coated liposomal doxorubicin in a mouse lymphoma model. Clin Cancer Res 1998, **4**, 499–505.

63. Harrington KJ, Rowlinson-Busza G, Uster PS. Stewart JS. Pegylated liposome-encapsulated doxorubicin and cisplatin in the treatment of head and neck xenograft tumours. Cancer Chemother Pharmacol 2000, **46**, 10–18.

64. Chang CW, Barber L, Ouyang C, Masin D, Bally MB, Madden TD. Plasma clearance, biodistribution and therapeutic properties of mitoxantrone encapsulated in conventional and sterically stabilised liposomes after intravenous administration in BDF1 mice. Br J Cancer 1997, **75**, 169–77.

65. Mori A, Wu S-P, Han I, et al. In vivo antitumour activity of cis-bis-neodecanoato-trans-R, R-1, 2-diaminocyclohexane platinum (II) formulated in long-circulating liposomes. Cancer Chemother Pharmacol 1996, **37**, 435–44.

66. Vaage J, Donovan D, Wipff E, et al. Therapy of a xenografted human colonic carcinoma using cisplatin or doxorubicin encapsulated in long-circulating pegylated stealth liposomes. Int J Cancer 1999, **80**, 134–7.

67. Colbern GT, Hiller AJ, Musterer RS, Working PK, Henderson IC. Antitumor activity of Herceptin in combination with STEALTH liposomal cisplatin or nonliposomal cisplatin in a HER2 positive human breast cancer model. J Inorg Biochem 1999, **77**, 117–20.

68. Turner AF, Presant CA, Proffitt RT, et al. In-111-labelled liposomes: dosimetry and tumour depiction. Radiology 1988, **166**, 761–5.

69. Presant CA, Proffitt RT, Turner AF, et al. Successful imaging of human cancer with Indium-111-labelled phospholipid vesicles. Cancer 1988, **62**, 905–11.

70. Presant CA, Blayney D, Profitt RT, et al. Preliminary report: imaging of Kaposi sarcoma and lymphoma in AIDS with Indium-111-labelled liposomes. Lancet 1990, **335**, 1307–9.

71. Gabizon A, Chisin R, Amselem S, et al. Pharmacokinetic and imaging studies in patients receiving a formulation of liposome-associated adriamycin. Br J Cancer 1991, **64**, 1125–32.

72. Kubo A, Nakamura K, Sammiya T, et al. Indium-111-labelled liposomes: dosimetry and tumour detection in patients with cancer. Eur J Nucl Med 1993, **20**, 107–13.

73. Khalifa A, Dodds D, Rampling R, Paterson J, Murray T. Liposomal distribution in malignant glioma: possibilities for therapy. Nucl Med Commun 1997, **18**, 17–23.

74. Zucchetti M, Boiardi A, Silvani A, Parisi I, Piccolrovazzi S. D'Incalci M. Distribution of daunorubicin and daunorubicinol in human glioma tumours after administration of liposomal daunorubicin. Cancer Chemother Pharmacol 1999, **44**, 173–6.

75. Gabizon A, Catame R, Uziely B, et al. Prolonged circulation time and enhanced accumulation in malignant exudates of doxorubicin encapsulated in polethyleneglycol coated liposomes. Cancer Res 1994, **54**, 987–92.

76. Northfelt DW, Martin FJ, Working P, et al. Doxorubicin encapsulated in liposomes containing surface-bound polyethylene glycol: pharmacokinetics, tumour localisation, and safety in patients with AIDS-related Kaposi's sarcoma. J Clin Pharmacol 1996, **36**, 55–63.

77. Symon Z, Peyser A, Tzemach D, et al. Selective delivery of doxorubicin to patients with breast carcinoma metastases by stealth liposomes. Cancer 1999, **86**, 72–8.

78. Koukourakis MI, Koukouraki S, Giatromanolaki A, et al. Liposomal doxorubicin and conventionally fractionated radiotherapy in the treatment of locally advanced non-small-cell lung cancer and head and neck cancer. J Clin Oncol 1999, **17**, 3512–21.

79. Koukourakis MI, Koukouraki S, Giatromanolaki A, et al. High intratumoural accumulation of stealth liposomal doxorubicin in sarcomas–rationale for combination with radiotherapy. Acta Oncol 2000, **39**, 207–11.

80. Koukourakis MI, Koukouraki S, Fezoulidis I, et al. High intratumoural accumulation of stealth liposomal doxorubicin (Caelyx) in glioblastomas and in metastatic brain tumours. Br J Cancer 2000, **83**, 1281–6.

81. Harrington KJ, Mohammadtaghi S, Uster PS, et el. Effective targeting of solid tumours in patients with locally advanced cancers by radiolabelled pegylated liposomes. Clin Cancer Res 2001, **7**, 243–54.

82. Embree L, Gelmon KA, Lohr A. et al. Chromatographic analysis and pharmacokinetics of liposome-encapsulated doxorubicin in non small-cell lung cancer patients. J Pharm Sci 1993, **82**, 627–34.

83. Cowens JW, Creaven PJ, Greco WR, et al. Initial clinical (phase I) trial of TLC D-99 (doxorubicin encapsulated in liposomes). Cancer Res 1993, **53**, 2796–802.

84. Batist G, Winer E, Navari R, Rovira D, Azarnia N, and the TLC D-99 Study Group. Decreased cardiac toxicity by TLC D-99 (liposome encapsulated doxorubicin) vs. Doxorubicin in a randomised trial of metastatic breast carcinoma (MBC). Proc Am Soc Clin Oncol 1998, **17**, 115a (abstract 443).

85. Batist G, Rao SC, Ramakrishnan G, et al. Phase III study of liposome-encapsulated doxorubicin (TLC D-99) versus doxorubicin (DOX) in combination with cyclophosphamide (CPA) in patients with metastatic breast cancer (MBC). Proc Am Soc Clin Oncol 1999, **18**, 127a (abstract 486).

86. Harris L, Winer E, Batist G, et al. Phase III study of TLC D-99 (liposome encapsulated doxorubicin) vs. free doxorubicin (Dox) in patients with metastatic breast carcinoma (MBC). Proc Am Soc Clin Oncol 1998, **17**, 124a (abstract 474).

87. Cheung TW, Remick SC, Azarnia N, Proper JA, Barrueco JR, Dezube BJ. AIDS-related Karposi's sarcoma: a phase II study of liposomal doxorubicin. The TLC D-99 Study Group. Clin Cancer Res 1999, **5**, 3432–7.

88. Shapiro CL, Ervin T, Welles L, Azarnia N, Keating J, Hayes DF. Phase II trial of high-dose liposome-encapsulated doxorubicin with granulocyte colony-stimulating factor in metastatic breast cancer. TLC D-99 Study Group. J Clin Oncol 1999, 17, 1435–41.

89. Valero V, Buzdar AU, Theriault RL, *et al.* Phase II trial of liposome-encapsulated doxorubicin, cyclophosphamide, and fluorouracil as first-line therapy in patients with metastatic breast cancer. J Clin Oncol 1999, 17, 1425–34.

90. Winer E, Batist G, Belt R, Gutheil J, Park Y, Wells L. Reduced cardiotoxicity of liposome-encapsulated doxorubicin (TLC D-99) compared to free doxorubicin in first-line therapy of metastatic breast cancer in patients at increased risk for anthracycline-induced cardiac toxicity. Proc Am Soc Clin Oncol 2000, 19, 64a (abstract 323).

91. Gill PS, Espina BM, Muggia F. *et al.* Phase I/II clinical and pharmacokinetic evaluation of liposomal daunorubicin. J Clin Oncol 1995, 13, 996–1003.

92. Presant CA, Scolaro M, Kennedy P, *et al.* Liposomal daunorubicin treatment of HIV-associated Kaposi's sarcoma. Lancet 1993, 341, 1242–3.

93. Money-Kyrle JF, Bates F, Ready J, *et al.* Liposomal daunorubicin in advanced Kaposi's sarcoma: a phase II study. Clin Oncol (R Coll Radiol) 1993, 5, 367–71.

94. Uthayakumar S, Bower M, Money-Kyrle J, *et al.* Randomized cross-over comparison of liposomal daunorubicin versus observation for early Kaposi's sarcoma. AIDS 1996, 10, 515–19.

95. Girard PM, Bouchaud O, Goetschel A, *et al.* Phase II study of liposomal encapsulated daunorubicin in the treatment of AIDS-associated mucocutaneous Kaposi's sarcoma. AIDS 1996, 10, 753–7.

96. Gill PS, Wernz J, Scadden DT, *et al.* Randomised phase III trial of liposomal daunorubicin versus doxorubicin, bleomycin and vincristine in AIDS-related Kaposi's sarcoma. J Clin Oncol 1996, 14, 2353–64.

97. Cortes J, O'Brien S, Estey E. Giles F, Keating M, Kantarjian H. Phase I study of liposomal daunorubicin in patients with acute leukemia. Invest New Drugs 1999, 17, 81–7.

98. Steele JPC, O'Doherty CA, Evans M, *et al.* Phase I/II trial of liposomal daunorubicin in malignant mesothelioma. Proc Am Soc Clin Oncol 1998, 17, 502a (abstract 1933).

99. Yeo W, Chan KK, Mukwaya G, *et al.* Phase II studies with daunoxome in patients with non-resectable hepatocellular carcinoma clinical and pharmacokinetic outcomes. Cancer Chemother Pharmacol 1999, 44, 124–30.

100. Daniele B, De Vivo R, Perrone F, *et al.* Phase I clinical trial of liposomal daunorubicin in hepatocellular carcinoma complicating liver cirrhosis. Anticancer Res 2000, 20, 1249–51.

101. Perez-Soler R, Lopez-Berestein G, Lautersztain J, *et al.* Phase I clinical and pharmacology study of liposome-entrapped cis-bis-neodecanoato trans-R, R-1, 2 diaminocyclohexane platinum (II). Cancer Res 1990, 50, 4254–9.

102. Perez-Soler R, Shin DM, Siddik ZH, *et al.* Phase I clinical and pharmacological study of liposome-entrapped NDDP administered intrapleurally in patients with malignant pleural effusions. Clin Cancer Res 1997, 3, 373–9.

103. Perez-Soler R, Walsh GL, Swisher SG, *et al.* Phase II study of liposome-entrapped cisplatin-analog (L-NDDP) administered intrapleurally in patients with malignant pleural mesothelioma. Proc Am Soc Clin Oncol 1999, 18, 421a (abstract 1626).

104. Gelmon KA, Telcher A, Diab AR, *et al.* Phase I study of liposomal vincristine. J Clin Oncol 1999, 17, 697–705.

105. Sarris AH, Hagemeister F, Romaguera J, *et al.* Liposomal vincristine in relapsed non-Hodgkin's lymphomas: early results of an ongoing phase II trial. Ann Oncol 2000, 11, 69–72.

106. Hengge UR, Brockmeyer NH, Baumann M, Reimann G, Goos M. Liposomal doxorubicin in AIDS-related Kaposi's sarcoma. Lancet 1993, 343, 497.

107. Simpson JK, Miller RF, Spittle MF. Liposomal docorubicin for the treatment of AIDS-related Kaposi's sarcoma. Clin Oncol (R Coll Radiol) 1993, 5, 372–4.

108. Bogner JR, Kronawitter U, Rolinski B, Truebenach K, Goebel F-D. Liposomal doxorubicin in the treatment of advanced AIDS-related Kaposi's sarcoma. J AIDS 1994, 7, 463–8.

109. James ND, Coker RJ, Tomlinson D, *et al.* Liposomal doxorubicin (Doxil): an effective new treatment for Kaposi's sarcoma in AIDS. Clin Oncol (R Coll Radiol) 1994, 6, 294–6.

110. Harrison M, Tomlinson D, Stewart S. Liposomal entrapped doxorubicin: an active agent in AIDS-related Kaposi's sarcoma. J Clin Oncol 1995, 13, 914–20.

111. Goebel F-D, Goldstein D, Goos M, Jablonowski H, Stewart JS. Efficacy and safety of Stealth liposomal doxorubicin in AIDS-related Kaposi's sarcoma. Br J Cancer 1996, 73, 989–94.

112. Stewart JSW, Jablonowski H, Goebel F-D, *et al.* Randomised comparative trial of pegylated liposomal doxorubicin versus bleomycin and vincristine in the treatment of AIDS-related Kaposi's sarcoma: results of a randomised phase III clinical trial. J Clin Oncol 1998, 16, 2445–51.

114. Muggia FM, Hainsworth JD, Jeffers S, *et al.* Phase II study of liposomal doxorubicin in refractory ovarian cancer: antitumour activity and toxicity modification by liposomal encapsulation. J Clin Oncol 1997, 15, 987–93.

115. Gordon AN, Granai CO, Rose PG, *et al.* Phase II study of liposomal doxorubicin in platinum- and paclitaxel-refractory epithelial ovarian cancer. J Clin Oncol 2000, 18, 3093–100.

116. Markman M, Kennedy A, Webster K, Peterson G, Kulp B, Belinson J. Phase 2 trial of liposomal doxorubicin (40 mg/m^2) in platinum/paclitaxel-refractory ovarian and fallopian tube cancers and primary carcinoma of the peritoneum. Gynecol Oncol 2000, 78, 369–72.

117. Gordon AN, Fleagle JT, Guthrie D, *et al.* Interim analysis of a phase III randomized trial of Caelyx/Doxil (D) versus Topotecan (T) in the treatment of patients with relapsed ovarian cancer. Proc Am Soc Clin Oncol 2000, 19, 380a (abstract 1504).

118. Israel VP, Garcia AA, Roman L, *et al.* Phase II study of liposomal doxorubicin in advanced gynecologic cancers. Gynecol Oncol 2000, 78, 143–7.

119. Ranson MR, Carmichael J, O'Byrne K, Stewart S, Smith D, Howell A. Treatment of advanced breast cancer with sterically stabilized liposomal doxorubicin: results of a multicentre phase II trial. J Clin Oncol 1997, **15**, 3185–91.

120. Lyass O, Uziely B, Ben-Yosef R, *et al.* Correlation of toxicity with pharmacokinetics of pegylated liposomal doxorubicin (Doxil) in metastatic breast carcinoma. Cancer 2000, **89**, 1037–47.

121. Caponigro F, Comella P, Budillon A, *et al.* Phase I study of Caelyx (doxorubicin HCL, pegylated liposomal) in recurrent or metastatic head and neck cancer. Ann Oncol 2000, **11**, 339–42.

122. Harrington KJ, Lewanski CR, Northcote AD, *et al.* Phase II study of pegylated liposomal doxorubicin (Caelyx™) in patients with inoperable, locally advanced squamous cell cancer of the head and neck. Eur J Cancer 2001, **37**, 2015–22.

123. Wollina U, Graefe T, Karte K. Treatment of relapsing or recalcitrant cutaneous T-cell lymphoma with pegylated liposomal doxorubicin. J Am Acad Dermatol 2000, **42**, 40–6.

124. Judson I. Radford J, Blay J-Y, *et al.* A randomised phase II trial of Caelyx®/Doxil® versus doxorubicin in advanced or metastatic soft tissue sarcomas (STS)–an EORTC Soft Tissue and Bone Sarcoma (STBSG) trial. Proc Am Soc Clin Oncol 1999, **18**, 541 (abstract 2089).

125. Toma S, Tucci A, Villani G, Carteni G, Spadini N, Palumbo R. Liposomal doxorubicin (Caelyx) in advanced pretreated soft tissue sarcomas: a phase II study of the Italian Sarcoma Group (ISG).Anticancer Res 2000, **20**, 485–91.

126. Ruff P, Moodley SD, Rapoport BL, *et al.* Pegylated liposomal doxorubicin (Caelyx) in advanced hepatocellular carcinoma (HCC). Proc Am Soc Clin Oncol 2000, **19**, 268a (abstract 1044).

127. O'Brien M, Hickish T, Iveson T, *et al.* Phase II study of Caelyx® (Doxil®, doxorubicin HC1 pegylated liposomal) in the treatment of small cell lung cancer (SCLC). Proc Am Soc Clin Oncol 1998, **17**, 497 (abstract 1913).

128. Ernst DS, Winquist E, Moore M, Jonker D, Friel C. Activity of pegylated liposomal doxorubicin (Caelyx) in advanced transitional cell carcinoma (TCC). Proc Am Soc Clin Oncol 2000, **19**, 363a (abstract 1431).

129. Dietrich J, Fabel-Schulte K, Hau P, *et al.* Liposomal doxorubicin (Caelyx) in the treatment of recurrent high-grade glioma–a phase II/III study. Proc Am Soc Clin Oncol 2000, **19**, 170a (abstract 661).

130. Pennington K, Gordon M, Picus J. A phase II trial of liposomal doxorubicin (Doxil®) in the treatment of advanced renal cell cancer: a Hoosier Oncology Group (HOG) study. Proc Am Soc Clin Oncol 1998, **17**, 339a (abstract 1308).

131. Yip D, Halford S, Karapetis C, Steger A, Khawaja H, Harper P. A phase II trial of Caelyx™ (Liposomal Doxorubicin, Doxil™) in the treatment of advanced pancreatic cancer. Proc Am Soc Clin Oncol 1999, **18**, 306a (abstract 1177).

132. Koletsky A, Jahanzeb M, Radice P, *et al.* Pegylated liposomal doxorubicin (PEG-LD) as second line treatment of advanced non-small cell carcinoma (NSCLC) after platinum-based therapy: A randomised phase II trial. Proc Am Soc Clin Oncol 1999, **18**, 512a (abstract 1976).

133. Radice P, Jahanzeb M, Koletsky A, *et al.* Weekly pegylated liposomal doxorubicin is extremely well tolerated as second line chemotherapy. Proc Am Soc Clin Oncol 1999, **18**, 520a (abstract 2004).

134. Elson P, Chidiac T, Budd GT, *et al.* Phase II trial of Doxil in advanced soft tissue sarcomas (STS). Proc Am Soc Clin Oncol 1998, **17**, 513a (abstract 1979).

135. Skubitz KM. Early results of pegylated liposomal doxorubicin (Doxil®) in refractory sarcoma. Proc Am Soc Clin Oncol 1998, **17**, 524a (abstract 2013).

136. Halm U, Etzrodt G, Schiefke I, *et al.* A phase II study of pegylated liposomal doxorubicin for treatment of advanced hepatocellular carcinoma. Ann Oncol 2000, **11**, 113–14.

137. Samantas E, Kalofonos H, Linardou H, *et al.* Phase II study of pegylated liposomal doxorubicin: inactive in recurrent small-cell lung cancer. A Hellenic Cooperative Oncology Group Study. Ann Oncol 2000, **11**, 1395–7.

138. Israel VK, Jeffers S, Bernal G, *et al.* Phase 1 study of Doxil (liposomal doxorubicin) in combination with paclitaxel. Proc Am Soc Clin Oncol 1998, **17**, 245 (abstract 938).

139. Langley RE, Carmichael J, Woll PJ, Mason E, Welbank H. Phase II trial to evaluate the safety and tolerability of Caelyx® in combination with paclitaxel in the treatment of metastatic cancer. Proc Am Soc Clin Oncol 1998, **17**, 246a (abstract 943).

140. Moore MR, Srinivasiah J, Feinberg BA, *et al.* Phase II randomized trial of doxorubicin plus paclitaxel (AT) versus doxorubicin hcl liposome injection (Doxil®) plus paclitaxel (DT) in metastatic breast cancer. Proc Am Soc Clin Oncol 1998, **17**, 160a (abstract 614).

141. Schwonzen M, Kurbacher CM, Mallmann P. Liposomal doxorubicin and weekly paclitaxel in the treatment of metastatic breast cancer. Anticancer Drugs 2000, **11**,681–5

142. Tolis CF, Briasoulis EC, Tzamakou E, *et al.* Phase I trial and interaction pharmacokinetics of pegylated-liposomal doxorubicin (Caelyx: Doxil) and weekly Taxol. Proc Am Soc Clin Oncol 2000, **19**, 206a (abstract 803).

143. Malek UU, Sparano JA, Wolffe A. Phase I trial of liposomal doxorubicin (Doxil) and docetaxel (Taxotere) in patients (PTS) with advanced breast cancer (ABC). Proc Am Soc Clin Oncol 1998, **17**, 175a (abstract 672).

144. Klein P, Lyass O. Sorich J, *et al.* Doxil plus cisplatin: combined results of two phase I studies. Proc Am Soc Clin Oncol 1998, **17**, 246a (abstract 942).

145. Laufman LR, Spiridonidis CH, Jones JJ, Rhodes VA, Wallace K. Phase I trial of Doxil® plus vinorelbine (VNB) in patients (PTS) with advanced malignancies. Proc Am Soc Clin Oncol 1998, **17**, 246a (abstract 944).

146. Ramirez MR, Marcom PK, Sutton LM, *et al.* A phase I/II study of Doxil and vinorelbine in metastatic breast cancer patients. Proc Am Soc Clin Oncol 1998, **17**, 169a (abstract 650).

147. Holder L, Overmoyer B, Silverman P, Tripathy D, Marrs N, Teitelbaum AH. Doxil® and oral cyclophosphamide as first-line therapy for patients with metasta-

tic breast cancer (MBC): Preliminary results of a pilot trial. Proc Am Soc Clin Oncol 1998, **17**, 146a (abstract 556).

148. Tobias DH, Runowicz C, Mandeli J, *et al*. A phase I trial of gemcitabine and Doxil for recurrent epithelial ovarian cancer. Proc Am Soc Clin Oncol 2000, **19**, 392a (abstract 1551).

149. Volm M, Oratz R, Pavlick A, Farrell K, Lee J, Muggia F. A phase I study of liposomal doxorubicin and temozolomide in patients with advanced cancer. Proc Am Soc Clin Oncol 2000, **19**, 223a (abstract 872).

150. Tsiara SN, Kapsali E, Christou L, Panteli A, pritsivelis N, Bourantas KL. Administration of a modified chemotherapeutic regimen containing vincristine, liposomal doxorubicin and dexamethasone to multiple myeloma patients: preliminary data. Eur J Haematol 2000, **65**, 118–22.

151. Madhavan S, Northfelt DW. Lack of vesicant injury following extravasation of liposomal doxorubicin. J Natl Cancer Inst 1995, **87**, 1556–7.

152. Lotem M, Hubert A, Lyass O. *et al*. Skin toxic effects of polyethylene glycol-coated liposomal doxorubicin. Arch Dermatol 2000, **136**, 1475–80.

153. Berry G, Billingham M, Alderman E, *et al*. The use of cardiac biopsy to demonstrate reduced cardiotoxicity in AIDS Kaposi's sarcoma patients treated with pegylated liposomal doxorubicin. Ann Oncol 1998, **9**, 711–16.

154. Safra T, Muggia F, Jeffers S, *et al*. Pegylated liposomal doxorubicin (doxil): reduced clinical cardiotoxicity in patients reaching or exceeding cumulative doses of 500 mg/m², Ann Oncol 2000, **11**, 1029–33.

155. Speyer J, Wasserheit C. Strategies for reduction of anthracycline cardiac toxicity. Sem Oncol 1998, **25**, 525–37.

156. Gordon KB, Tajuddin A, Guitart J, Kuzel TM, Eramo LR, Von Roenn J. Hand–foot syndrome associated with liposome-encapsulated doxorubicin therapy. Cancer 1995, **75**, 2169–73.

157. Vail DM, Chun R, Thamm DH, Garrett LD, Cooley AJ, Obradovich JE. Efficacy of pyridoxine to ameliorate the cutaneous toxicity associated with doxorubicin containing pegylated (Stealth) liposomes: a randomized, double-blind clinical trial using a canine model. Clin Cancer Res 1998, **4**, 1567–71.

158. Colbern GT, Musterer R, Hiller AJ, *et al*. Treatment of palmar–plantar erythrodysaesthesia with pyridoxine or ergotamine: effect on efficacy of Doxil in Lewis lung carcinoma. Proc Am Soc Clin Oncol 1998, **17**, 238a (abstract 913).

159. Lopez AM, Wallace L, Dorr RT, Koff M, Hersh EM, Alberts DS. Topical DMSO treatment for pegylated liposomal doxorubicin-induced palmar-plantar erythrodysesthesia. Cancer Chemother Pharmacol 1999, **44**, 303–6.

160. Colbern GT, Steinmetz KL, Musterer R, *et al*. Amifostine reduces severity and incidence of Doxilinduced palmar/plantar erythrodysesthesis in rats but does not reduce Doxil antitumour efficacy or alter pharmacokinetics in mice. Proc Am Soc Clin Oncol 2000, **19**, 209a (abstract 815).

161. DeMario MD, Vogelzang NJ, Janish L, *et al*. A phase I study of liposome-formulated cisplatin (SPI-77®) given every 3 weeks in patients with advanced cancer. Proc Am Soc Clin Oncol 1998, **17**, 230a (abstract 883).

162. Devore RF, Johnson DH, Strupp J, *et al*. Phase I trial of SPI-077 plus paclitaxel in patients with refractory nonsmall cell lung cancer (NSCLC). Proc Am Soc Clin Oncol 1999, **18**, 488a (abstract 1881).

163. Harrington KJ, Lewanski CR, Northcote AD, *et al*. Phase I/II study of pegylated liposomal cisplatin (SPI-077™) in patients with inoperable head and neck cancer. Ann Oncol 2001, **12**, 493–6.

14 | *Targeting blood vessels* in vivo *by using phage display libraries*

Claudia Vidal, Marina Cardó-Vila, Johanna Lahdenranta, Wadih Arap, and Renata Pasqualini

Exploring vascular heterogeneity by in vivo *phage display*

We have recently identified a novel vascular address system, analogous to ZIP (postal) codes, that makes it possible to target organ-specific blood vessels and newly formed (angiogenic) blood vessels in tumors. Furthermore, we have isolated peptides that can home to normal blood vessels or sites of angiogenesis through the circulation via this vascular address system. Every normal or diseased organ appears to display a unique signature on its blood vessels that our probes can identify as a target. We have also developed complementary methods for assessing the distribution of probes targeted to the vasculature, the tissue-specificity of those probes, and their target cells (reviewed in reference 1).

We developed an *in vivo* phage display by selecting phage capable of homing to different vascular beds after administration of a phage display random peptide library (2). Screenings are based on the use of peptides that are expressed on the surface of bacteriophage (3, 4). Our extensive previous work (2, 5–11) has established that peptide libraries can be used to probe organ- and tumor-specific markers. In order to construct such libraries, random oligonucleotides are individually fused to cDNAs encoding a phage surface protein, and large collections of phage particles (10^9 individual clones) displaying unique peptides are produced. In the *in vivo* procedure, phage capable of homing to certain organs or tumors following an intravenous injection are selected from the libraries. The ability of individual peptides to target a tissue can also be analyzed by this method (2, 5–7). Furthermore, this system provides an innovative way of identifying endothelial cell surface markers expressed *in vivo* (6, 8, 9, 12). Thus, in addition to the isolation of novel tools for selective vascular targeting of therapies (13), vascu-

lar targeting *in vivo* will further our understanding of tumor endothelium specificity and define the role that endothelial cell markers play in angiogenesis. We have isolated several organ- and tumor-homing peptides by *in vivo* phage display. Each of these peptides binds to different receptors selectively expressed on the vasculature of target tissues (1). Some of these vascular markers are proteases that not only serve as receptors for circulating ligands but also modulate angiogenesis (6, 9, 14). Moreover, certain vascular receptors are also involved in tumor cell homing during the metastatic process (12; unpublished observations). Tumor-homing peptides bind to receptors that are upregulated in tumor angiogenic vasculature (5, 6, 8; reviewed in reference 1). Targeted delivery of cytotoxic chemotherapy (5), proapoptotic peptides (11), and cytokines (14) to receptors in the angiogenic vasculature has resulted in marked therapeutic efficacy in tumor-bearing mouse models. Initial steps towards the translation of these data into clinical applications are in progress.

Vascular targeting and relevance to cancer and other diseases with an angiogenesis component

The potential of an *in vivo* phage display to identify vascular targeting peptides has not yet been fully explored. It is currently of particular interest to target sites involved in cancer. These probes will be useful in peptide-guided therapy against tumors. We also hope to shed light on the vascular biology and heterogeneity of blood vessels in cancer metastasis.

Angiogenesis, the recruitment of new blood vessels, is a rate-limiting step in solid tumor growth (15–17). Angiogenic blood vessels express receptors that are either present at very low levels or entirely absent in normal blood vessels (10, 13, 17, 18). Tumor angiogenic markers include members of the receptor tyrosine kinase family (vascular endothelial growth factor receptor (VEGFR) and Tie; references 19–21) and αv integrins (18–22). Identification of cell surface markers characteristic of neovasculature activation should further our understanding of angiogenesis and lead to new therapeutic strategies. We have identified peptides that selectively target several proteases in angiogenic vasculature. Our results indicate that the vascular endothelium of tumors is modified in ways that allow differential targeting with peptide probes (5, 9–11).

Angiogenesis suppression and extracellular matrix degradation by targeted protease inhibitors

Tumor establishment, growth, and metastasis require alterations in cell adhesion to allow tumor-cell detachment from the primary tumor and degradation of the extracellular matrix (ECM) to facilitate migration, extravasation, and angiogenesis.

Metalloproteases (MMPs) are a family of enzymes (gelatinases) capable of degrading the constituents of the ECM. In cancer, MMP levels can be abnormally elevated, possibly enabling tumor cells to invade the extracellular matrix and promoting metastases at sites distant from the primary tumor. Indeed, high MMP levels are associated with poor prognosis in cancer patients. The formation of new capillaries by endothelial cells requires migration of endothelial cells and extensive remodeling of the tissue, a process that requires gelatinases and other proteinases (23, 24). In animal models, generic MMP inhibitors prevent tumor dissemination and formation of metastases. Anti-angiogenic properties of gelatinase inhibitors may contribute to this outcome (23). Because gelatinases and other MMPs are potential targets for therapeutic intervention in cancer, there is great interest in developing synthetic MMP inhibitors. MMPs are generally inhibited by compounds containing reactive zinc-chelating groups, such as thiol or hydroxamate. Despite extensive research, no inhibitors specific for gelatinases have been described until recently. The most potent gelatinase inhibitors also inhibit several other MMP family members and are highly toxic. The lack of inhibitors specific for the type-IV collagenase/gelatinase family of MMPs has thus far prevented selective targeting of MMP-2 (gelatinase A) and MMP-9 (gelatinase B) for therapeutic intervention in cancer.

We have recently described the isolation of specific gelatinase inhibitors from phage display peptide libraries (9). These inhibitors belong to a novel class of cyclic peptides that: (1) specifically inhibit MMP activity; (2) suppress migration of both tumor cells and endothelial cells *in vitro*; (3) home to tumor vasculature *in vivo*; (4) prevent the growth and invasion of tumors in mice. For example, the peptide CTTHWGFTLC inhibits only gelatinases and has minimal or no effect on several other MMP family members. Extensive work from our laboratory suggests that HWGF-derived peptidomimetics have great potential as anticancer agents. These novel gelatinase inhibitors have two levels of specificity. First, they specifically inhibit MMP-2 and MMP-9; second, they selectively target tumors because these enzymes are overexpressed in tumor cells and tumor vasculature, and, third, they are accessible for homing in the tumor vasculature. Treatment of tumor-bearing mice with the CTTHWGFTLC peptide results in delayed tumor growth and, ultimately, in increased survival of tumor-bearing mice. The combination of tumor-targeting, antiangiogenic, and anti-invasive properties of CTTHWGFTLC peptide makes it a potential lead compound for treatment of cancer.

CD13 is a pro-angiogenic peptidase and a vascular receptor for tumor-homing peptides

Selection of phage libraries in tumor-bearing mice yielded several peptide motifs capable of homing to tumor vasculature: an RGD embedded in a double-cyclic structure (CDCRGDCFC; termed RGD-4C), NGR (asparagine–glycine–arginine), and GSL (glycine–serine–leucine). The receptors for the RGD-4C peptide are αv integrins. The receptor for NGR is CD13/APN (25).

Despite its expression outside the vascular system in various epithelial and hemopoietic cells (26), APN/CD13 appears to be exposed to the circulation primarily in angiogenic blood vessels. We have shown that APN/CD13 is a receptor for tumor-homing NGR peptide ligands. This finding led us to study the expression and function of APN/CD13. We found that a selective expression pattern for APN/CD13 is observed in angiogenic vasculature associated with tumors, increased cytokine activity, and oxygen deprivation. We also found that antagonists of APN/CD13 activity block angiogenesis and inhibit tumor growth (25).

Cell-surface CD13/APN enzymatic activity can be blocked by bestatin and *o*-phenatroline (27, 28). Studies involving these inhibitors have contributed to the understanding of how this enzyme functions. For example, bestatin has been shown to possess immunomodulatory effects (27, 29). It has also been reported that administration of high doses of bestatin suppresses experimental or spontaneous metastasis and inhibits tumor cell invasion (28). However, specific targets for CD13/APN remain unknown. Although it is expressed outside the vascular system in normal tissues, CD13/APN may be exposed to the circulation only in tumor vessels, as suggested by our *in vivo* screening and immunohistochemistry results.

Based on our *in vivo* studies involving both tumor targeting with NGR-phage and blocking of blood vessel formation with CD13/APN antagonists, we have established that CD13/APN is a key regulator in angiogenesis. Recent work focusing on the transcriptional regulation of CD13 shows that the expression of this peptidase is modulated during angiogenesis. Upregulation of CD13 is observed in endothelial cells following stimulation with angiogenic growth factors and hypoxia (30). Thus, CD13 is not only a pro-angiogenic molecule that can be targeted in proliferating blood vessels, but transcriptional regulatory proteins that inhibit CD13 expression could also be exploited as targeted anti-angiogenic agents.

Targeting chemotherapy, proapoptotic peptides, and cytokines to vascular receptors

In vivo selection of phage display libraries was used to isolate peptides that home specifically into tumor blood vessels. When coupled to the anticancer drug doxorubicin, two of these peptides—one containing an αv integrin-binding RGD motif and the other an NGR motif—enhanced the efficacy of the drug against human tumor xenografts in nude mice and reduced its toxicity. These results indicate that it may be possible to develop strategies for targeting therapy based on selective expression of receptors in tumor vasculature (1). We have also designed short peptides composed of two functional domains—one a tumor blood vessel homing motif and the other a programed cell death-inducing sequence—and synthesized them by simple peptide chemistry. The homing domain is designed to guide the peptide to targeted cells and allow its internalization. The proapoptotic domain is designed to be nontoxic outside of cells, but toxic when internalized into targeted cells. Although these prototypes contain only 21 and 26 residues, respectively, they are selectively toxic to angiogenic endothelial cells and have antitumor and anti-metastatic activity in mice (11).

To improve the therapeutic index (toxicity and efficacy) of tumor necrosis factor (TNF)α, Curnis *et al.* (14) have coupled murine TNFα to CNGRC, an

Fig. 14.1 (a) Vascular targeting *in vivo* using phage peptide libraries. *In vivo* screening of phage display libraries allows for the selection of specific peptide ligands that bind to different vascular beds. Phage display libraries contain up to 10^9 random peptides. Three to five copies of a peptide are expressed on the fd-bacteriophage surface as a fusion to its capsid protein pIII. In general, 10^{10} to 10^{11} transforming units of phage are injected intravenously into a deeply anesthetized mouse via the tail vein, and phage are allowed to circulate for 5–10 minutes. The mouse is then perfused with medium (Dulbecco's modified Eagle's medium; DMEM) through a catheter inserted in the left ventricle and bled through a small incision in the right atrial chamber. After perfusion, the desired organs are recovered and weighed. Organs are then processed with a Dounce homogenizer and washed. Phage are recovered from the tissue by infecting log-phase *Escherichia coli* bacteria with the homogenate. After infection, serial dilutions of bacteria are plated in LB/agar plates containing the appropriate antibiotics, and the rest of the bacterial culture is grown overnight. The next day, the selective binding of the phage pool is quantified by calculating the number of recovered phage from each organ. The amplified phage is precipitated from the bacterial culture and used for another round of *in vivo* selection. Generally, three rounds of *in vivo* selection are sufficient to select for specific organ- and tumor-homing phage. Peptide sequences (obtained based on the insert within the phage DNA) are compared to identify enriched peptides or peptide motifs. It is a very common observation that the binding motif of a targeting peptide is a tripeptide motif appearing several times in different sequence contexts. The selectivity of individual clones is then validated by comparing homing to the target organ versus control organs, and also the relative enrichment given compared to a control phage that displays no peptide, or displays an unrelated peptide. Further validation is obtained by inhibiting phage homing upon co-injection of the corresponding synthetic peptide or recombinant protein containing the peptide. These reagents can then be used to identify the receptor that mediates selective homing of the peptide to a particular organ or tissue. (b) Targeted therapies based on peptides derived from *in vivo* phage display. A schematic illustration of a peptide isolated by *in vivo* phage display coupled to a therapeutic agent. (See also 'Plates' section.)

aminopeptidase N (CD13) ligand that homes to activated blood vessels in tumors (25). The *in vivo* cytotoxic activity of this conjugate (NGR–TNFα) was dramatically reduced when compared to similar doses of untargeted TNFα. However, the antitumor activity *in vivo* was 10–15 times greater than that of TNFα, as evaluated by comparing tumor burden, animal survival, and weight loss after treatment. The antitumor activity of NGR–TNFα was partially inhibited by co-administration of CNGRC or an anti-CD13 monoclonal antibody, supporting the hypothesis that cells expressing CD13 are targeted. Evidence for the induction of protective immunity by NGR–TNFα was also obtained. Targeting of TNFα to tumor markers of activated blood vessels may represent a major improvement in selective delivery of cytokines to tumors.

Preclinical evidence (14) strongly suggests that redirecting cytokines to the site of interest might enhance

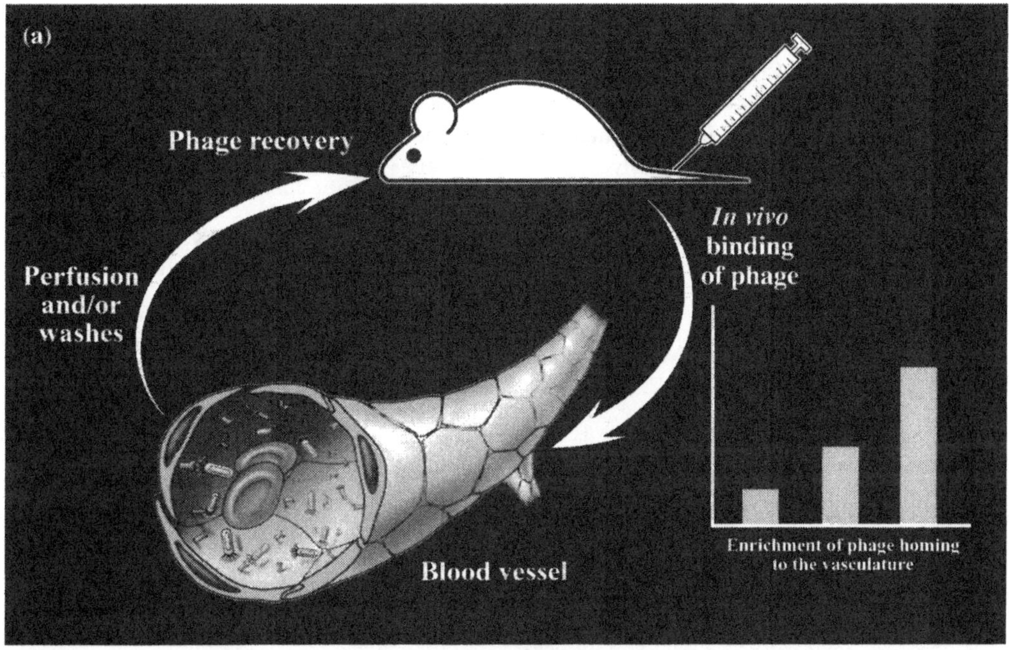

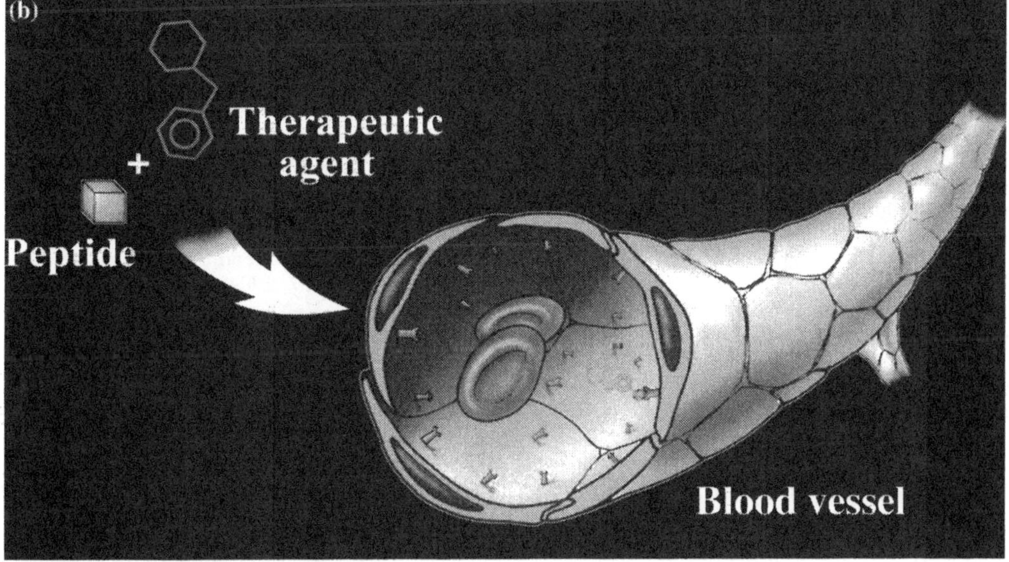

therapeutic effects. We and others have explored TNFα as a potential agent against primary and metastatic tumors (reviewed in reference 31). However, the systemic side-effects secondary to TNFα administration have thus far precluded its clinical application. Thus, targeting TNFα might be useful in developing a therapy (14). Efforts undertaken to this end have used bispecific conjugates or genetically modified antibodies (32). Bispecific conjugates were used to target TNFα to angiogenic vasculature. TNFα re-targeting was also demonstrated using antibodies (31, 32). The two major limitations of these approaches are that the receptors targeted: (1) are not restricted to specific tissues; and (2) are not—or not selectively—expressed on the luminal surface of endothelial cells, a requirement for therapies that are to be delivered intravenously.

Targeting the vasculature of normal or diseased organs may enable us to establish the foundation of a new pharmacology and lead ultimately to targeted medicine.

References

1. Kolonin MG, Pasqualini R, Arap W. Molecular addresses in blood vessels as targets for therapy. Curr Opin Chem Biol 2001, **5**, 308–13.
2. Pasqualini R, Ruoslahti E. Organ targeting *in vivo* using phage display peptide libraries. Nature 1996, **380**, 364–6.
3. Smith GP. Filamentous fusion phage: novel expression vectors that display cloned antigens on the virion surface. Science 1985, **228**, 1315–17.
4. Smith GP, Scott JK. Libraries of peptides and proteins displayed on filamentous phage. Methods Enzymol 1993, **217**, 228–57.
5. Arap W, Pasqualini R, Ruoslahti E. Cancer treatment by targeted drug delivery to tumor vasculature in a mouse model. Science 1998, **279**, 377–80.
6. Pasqualini R. Vascular targeting with phage peptide libraries. Quart J Nucl Med 1999, **43**, 159–62.
7. Rajotte D, Arap W, Hagedorn M, Koivunen E, Pasqualini R, Ruoslahti E. Molecular heterogeneity of the vascular endothelium revealed by *in vivo* phage display. J Clin Invest 1998, **102**, 430–7.
8. Burg MA, Pasqualini R, Arap W, Ruoslahti E, Stallcup WB. NG2 proteoglycan-binding peptides target tumor neovasculature. Cancer Res 1999, **59**, 2869–74.
9. Koivunen E, Arap W, Valtanen H, *et al.* Tumor targeting with a selective gelatinase inhibitor. Nat Biotechnol 1999, **17**, 768–74.
10. Arap W, Pasqualini R, Ruoslahti E. Chemotherapy targeted to tumor vasculature. Curr Opin Oncol 1998, **10**, 560–5.
11. Ellerby HM, Arap W, Ellerby LM, *et al.* Anti-cancer activity of targeted pro-apoptotic peptides. Nat Med 1999, **5**, 1032–8.
12. Rajotte D, Ruoslahti E. Membrane dipeptidase is the receptor for a lung-targeting peptide identified by *in vivo* phage display. J Biol Chem 1999, **274**, 11593–8.
13. Burrows FJ, Thorpe PE. Vascular targeting—a new approach to the therapy of solid tumors. Pharmacol Ther 1994, **64**, 155–74.
14. Curnis F, Sacchi A, Borgna L, Magni F, Gasparri A, Corti A. Enhancement of tumor necrosis factor alpha antitumor immunotherapeutic properties by targeted delivery to aminopeptidase N (CD13). Nat Biotechnol 2000, **18**, 1185–90.
15. Folkman J. Angiogenesis in cancer, vascular, rheumatoid and other disease. Nat Med 1995, **1**, 27–31.
16. Rak JW, St Croix BD, Kerbel RS. Consequences of angiogenesis for tumor progression, metastasis and cancer therapy. Anticancer Drugs 1995, **6**, 3–18.
17. Zetter BR. Angiogenesis and tumor metastasis. Annu Rev Med 1998, **49**, 407–24.
18. Brooks PC, Clark RA, Cheresh DA. Requirement of vascular integrin alpha v beta 3 for angiogenesis. Science 1994, **264**, 569–71.
19. Korpelainen EI, Alitalo K. Signaling angiogenesis and lymphangiogenesis. Curr Opin Cell Biol 1998, **10**, 159–64.
20. Brekken RA, Huang X, King SW, Thorpe PE. Vascular endothelial growth factor as a marker of tumor endothelium. Cancer Res 1998, **58**, 1952–9.
21. Peters KG, Coogan A, Berry D, *et al.* Expression of Tie2/Tek in breast tumour vasculature provides a new marker for evaluation of tumour angiogenesis. Br J Cancer 1998, **77**, 51–6.
22. Hammes HP, Brownlee M, Jonczyk A, Sutter A, Preissner KT. Subcutaneous injection of a cyclic peptide antagonist of vitronectin receptor-type integrins inhibits retinal neovascularization. Nat Med 1996, **2**, 529–33.
23. Folkman J. Addressing tumor blood vessels. Nat Biotechnol 1997, **15**, 510.
24. Bussolino F, Mantovani A, Persico G. Molecular mechanisms of blood vessel formation. Trends Biochem Sci 1997, **22**, 251–6.
25. Pasqualini R, Koivunen E, Kain R, *et al.* Aminopeptidase N is a receptor for tumor-homing peptides and a target for inhibiting angiogenesis. Cancer Res 2000, **60**, 722–7.
26. Look AT, Ashmun RA, Shapiro LH, Peiper SC. Human myeloid plasma membrane glycoprotein CD13 (gp150) is identical to aminopeptidase N. J Clin Invest 1989, **83**, 1299–307.
27. Taylor A. Aminopeptidases: structure and function. FASEB J 1993, **7**, 290–8.
28. Saiki I, Fujii H, Yoneda J, *et al.* Role of aminopeptidase N (CD13) in tumor-cell invasion and extracellular matrix degradation. Int J Cancer 1993, **54**, 137–43.
29. Talmadge JE, Lenz BF, Pennington R, *et al.* Immunomodulatory and therapeutic properties of bestatin in mice. Cancer Res 1986, **46**, 4505–10.
30. Bhagwat SV, Lahdenranta J, Giordano R, Arap W, Pasqualini R, Shapiro L. CD13/APN is activated by angiogenic signals and is essential for capillary tube formation. Blood 2001, **97**, 652–9.

31. Dellabona P, Moro M, Crosti MC, Casorati G, Corti A. Vascular attack and immunotherapy: a 'two hits' approach to improve biological treatment of cancer. Gene Ther 1999, **6**, 153–4.

32. Gasparri A, Moro M, Curnis F, *et al*. Tumor pretargeting with avidin improves the therapeutic index of biotinylated tumor necrosis factor alpha in mouse models. Cancer Res 1999, **59**, 2917–23.

Section IV

15 | *Photodynamic therapy*

Michael R. Hamblin

Introduction

Photodynamic therapy (PDT) can be defined as the administration of a nontoxic drug known as a photosensitizer (PS) either topically, locally, or systemically to a patient bearing a lesion (generally but not always cancer), followed after some time by the illumination of the lesion with visible light (usually long-wavelength red light), which, in the presence of oxygen, leads to the generation of cytotoxic species and tissue destruction. A schematic representation is shown in Fig. 15.1.

The concept dates from the early days of this century when workers used dyes such as eosin together with light to treat skin cancer (1). Hematoporphyrin (HP) was also first used at this time (2) and sporadic reports (3) of both selective localization of porphyrins in tumors and regression after exposure to visible light appeared until the 1960s. The modern explosion of interest in PDT dates from the discovery of hematoporphyrin deriva-

tive (HPD) by Lipson and Baldes in 1960 (4), and was fueled by pioneering studies in both basic science and clinical application (5–8) by Dougherty *et al.* (notable among many groups). A semi-purified preparation of HPD known as Photofrin® (PF) was the first PS to gain regulatory approval for treatment of various cancers in many countries throughout the world, including the USA. After experience of treating tumors with HPD-PDT was accumulated, it was realized that this compound had disadvantages, including prolonged skin sensitivity necessitating the avoidance of sunlight for many weeks (9), suboptimal tumor selectivity (10), poor tumor penetration due to the relatively short wavelength used (630 nm) (11), and the fact that it was a complex mixture of uncertain structure (12). In recent times much work has been done on developing new PSs (13, 14), novel targeting strategies for delivering PSs to tumors (15), and new light sources including user-friendly lasers (16).

One of the chief attractions of PDT as a cancer therapy is the concept of dual selectivity. Collateral damage to normal tissue can be minimized by increasing the selective accumulation of the PS in the tumor, and by delivering the light in a spatially confined and focused manner. However, the use of light delivery to increase selectivity may not be possible when the intention is to treat multifocal or disseminated disease in a body cavity such as the urinary bladder or the peritoneal cavity. For these applications it may be necessary to achieve higher tumor selectivity by targeting the PS.

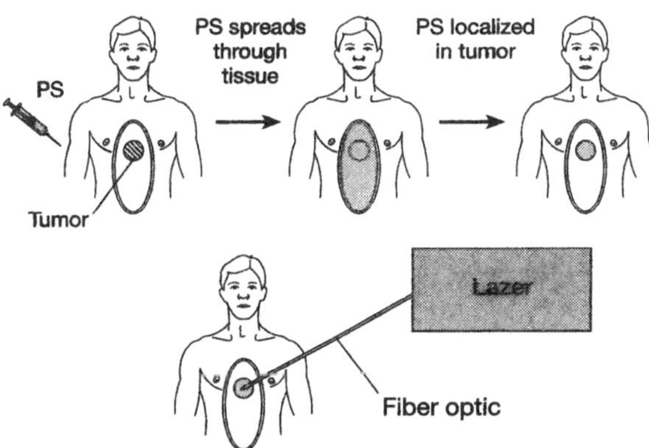

Fig. 15.1 Cartoon illustrating PDT for cancer. PS is injected intravenously and spreads throughout the tissues. After a predetermined time the PS selectively localizes in the tumor, whereupon activating light of the appropriate wavelength is delivered to the tumor via a flexible fiber optic.

PDT components

PDT requires the simultaneous presence of three components to be effective: (1) the photosensitizer; (2) light of the correct wavelength; (3) oxygen. Each will be dealt with below.

Photosensitizer

The majority of PSs used both clinically and experimentally, are derived from the tetrapyrrole aromatic nucleus found in many naturally occurring pigments such as heme and chlorophyll. They can be divided into several structural groups including porphyrins, chlorins, phthalocyanines, purpurins, and texaphyrins. Examples of these groups that are undergoing clinical or preclinical testing are given in Fig. 15.2. These compounds generally have low levels of dark toxicity to both humans and experimental animals, and have relatively high absorption bands in the red wavelengths of visible light (600–750 nm). The tetrapyrrole nucleus frequently holds a coordinated metal atom, but it has been found that only diamagnetic metals such as Al, Zn, Sn, and Lu allow the tetrapyrrole to retains its photosensitizing ability, while paramagnetic metals such as Fe, Cu, and Gd do not (17). Many of these compounds are lipophilic and some are even insoluble in water. These compounds must either be delivered in an emulsion or else incorporated in liposomes (see later). Although much research has been undertaken, the structural features of the molecule necessary to make the ideal PS, that is, one with both a high selectivity for tumors and a high level of phototoxicity towards tumors, are still unknown.

Light

As the second component for PDT tumor treatment it is necessary to bring light of the correct wavelength to activate the PS to the target tissue. Light fluence in tissue decreases exponentially with the distance; the effective penetration depth is inversely proportional to the effective attenuation coefficient. The latter is influenced by the optical absorption (due to endogenous tissue chromophores, mainly hemoglobin) and by optical scattering within the tissue. Both of these parameters differ from tissue to tissue, with liver, for example, affording especially poor light penetration due to its high hemoglobin content, and brain tissue being particularly light-scattering. On the average, however, the effective depth is about 1–3 mm at 630 nm, the wave length used for clinical treatment with PII, while penetration is approximately twice that at 700–850 nm (18, 19). The increased penetration depth of longer wavelength light is a major incentive for the development of PSs absorbing at such wavelengths, and a naphthalocyanine (776 nm) (20) and bacteriochlorin (780 nm) (21) fall into this category.

The absorption of light by the PS itself can limit tissue light penetration. This phenomenon has been termed 'self-shielding' and is particularly pronounced with PSs that absorb very strongly at the treatment wavelength (22). Many sensitizers are prone to photodestruction during light exposure—a process called 'photobleaching' (23). This may have beneficial effects regarding treatment differential. These are based on the following considerations. There exists a threshold PDT dose to produce tissue necrosis (24). If photobleaching occurs (which does not have such a threshold) before this threshold is achieved, no tissue damage is incurred. This is desirable for normal tissue exposed to therapeutic light but not for the tumor tissue to be treated. Thus, the net result is that one can achieve greater depth of tumor necrosis while sparing the normal skin.

Oxygen

In type II photoprocesses the PS triplet state is quenched by oxygen, which is then consumed in undergoing the photodynamic process. It has been shown that, when all the available oxygen has been consumed, the tumoricidal efficacy is reduced. This is likely to happen *in vivo* because oxygen must diffuse at a certain rate from the capillaries into the tumor parenchyma and, if the concentration of PS and intensity of light are sufficiently high, the consumption of oxygen will exceed its supply. The rate of oxygen consumption during PF-PDT can be sufficient to consume the majority of oxygen present in the tumor tissue, outpacing the rate of oxygen diffusion from the capillaries, and shrinking the radius of oxygenated tissue volume around them (25). In this case it has been shown that, if the light is delivered at a lower fluence rate (26) or in a cycled manner (30 seconds on and 30 seconds off) (27), the tumoricidal effect is improved. Another way in which the supply of oxygen to parts of the tumor can be limited is through the microvascular shutdown, which is a common occurrence in PDT of tumors (28).

Mechanisms of action

Photophysics and photochemistry

The mechanism by which illumination of the PS with light can lead to cytotoxic species is schematically illustrated in Fig. 15.3. Light of the correct wavelength to be absorbed by the ground-state PS excites the molecule to the excited singlet state, which, if it does not

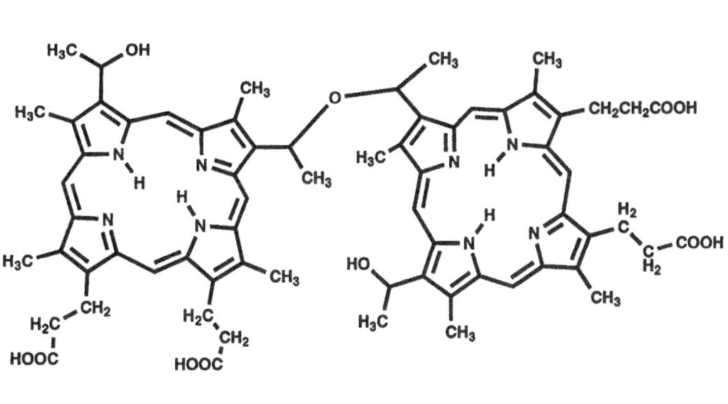

Fig. 15.2 Chemical structures of six PSs with regulatory approval or undergoing clinical trials for PDT of cancer. 1, Dihematoporphyrin ether, Photofrin®; 2, benzoporphyrin derivative mono acid ring A, Verteporfin®; 3, tin etiopurpurin, Purlytin®; 4, meta-tetrahydroxyphenylchlorin, Foscan®; 5, zinc phthalocyanine; 6, lutetium texaphyrin, Lutex®.

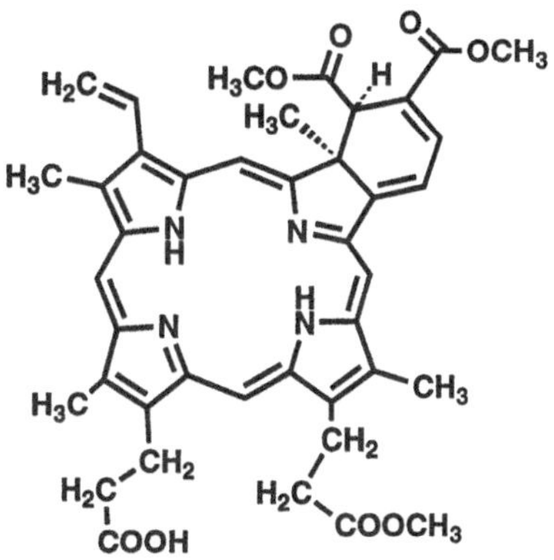

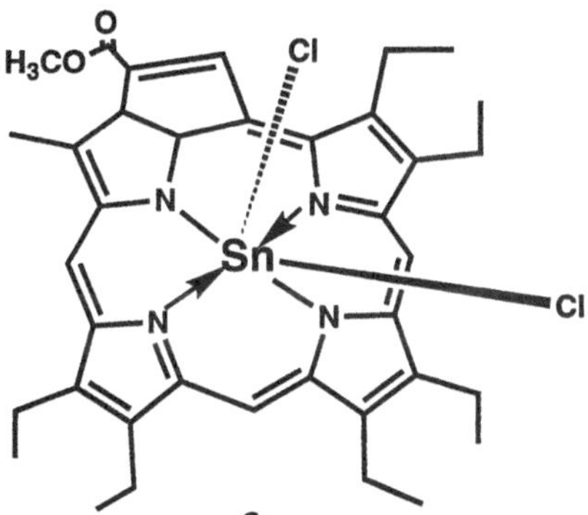

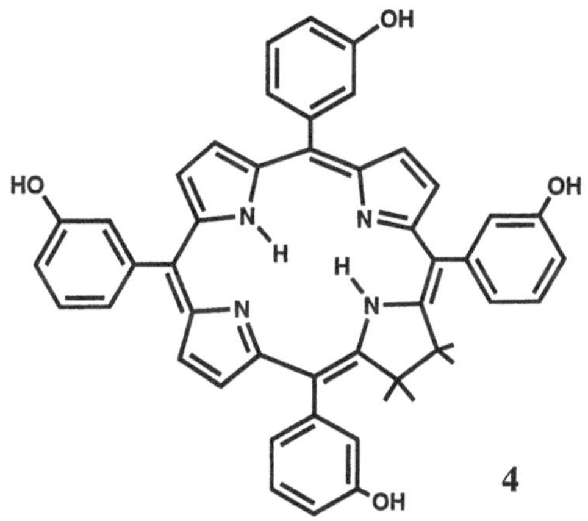

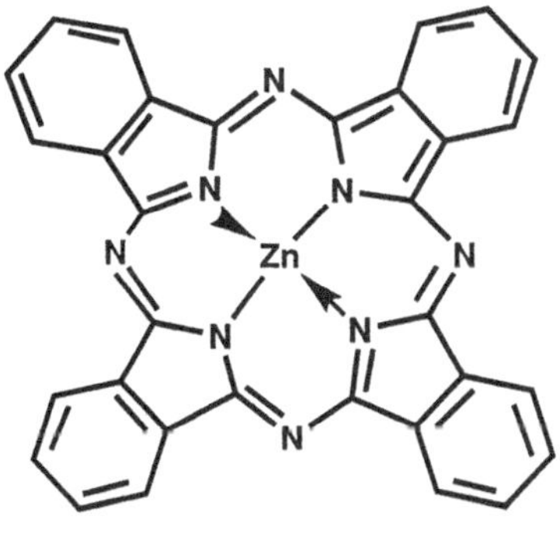

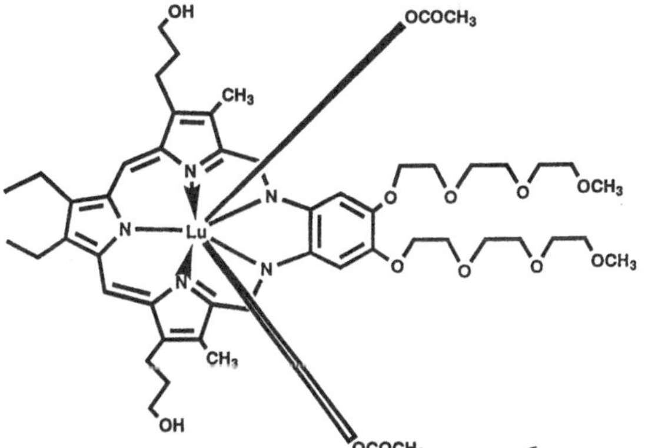

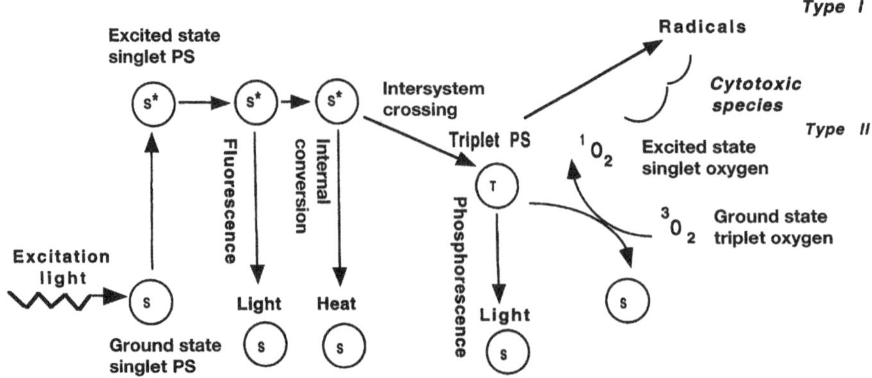

Fig. 15.3   Photophysical/photochemical mechanisms underlying PDT. Light is absorbed by the ground-state PS, which then moves to the first singlet excited state, from where it can lose energy by fluorescence or internal conversion and return to the ground state. Alternatively, the excited singlet-state PS can undergo intersystem crossing to the excited triplet state, which, in addition to losing energy by phosphorescence, can transfer its energy to the ground state of molecular oxygen, which is also a triplet. This results in the PS returning to the ground singlet state, and the oxygen rising to the excited singlet state (type II). Alternatively, the triplet PS may undergo reactions with substrates leading to free radicals (type I). Both these pathways lead to highly cytotoxic species by reacting with proteins, nucleic acids, and lipids in cells.

lose energy by fluorescence or as heat by internal conversion, may undergo intersystem crossing to the somewhat lower energy triplet state. If this PS triplet state has a sufficiently long lifetime, and a sufficiently high energy level, it may undergo further reaction to produce reactive and cytotoxic species. These species can arise from the PS triplet by two distinct mechanisms. The first mechanism (known as type I process) involves electron transfer reactions that produce PS radicals or radical ions, which usually react quickly with other molecules such as oxygen or biological substrates to produce a mixture of reactive and cytotoxic molecules known as reactive oxygen species (ROS). These consist of the very reactive hydroxyl radical, less reactive alkoxy radicals, superoxide, and hydrogen peroxide. The second mechanism (known as type II process) involves the transfer of energy from the PS triplet state to ground-state oxygen (which is also a triplet) producing the excited state singlet oxygen, which is also a reactive oxidant. Both singlet oxygen and type I radicals (or superoxide) can oxidize important biomolecules such as lipids (unsaturated fatty acids), proteins (histidine, tryptophan, and cysteine residues), and nucleic acids (guanosine residues). Even though type I processes frequently involve oxygen, the degree of oxygen dependence is much less than for type II processes. Since both type I and II processes depend on the PS triplet state, it is clear that those PSs with a high triplet yield and a long triplet lifetime will be most active in PDT (29). There is a considerable debate in the literature (30) on the relative contributions of type I

and II processes to the PDT-mediated destruction of tumors observed both in experimental animal models and clinically in patients.

In vitro cellular mechanisms

Many investigations into PDT mechanisms *in vitro* have focused on: (1) subcellular distribution of PSs; (2) PDT-mediated cellular damage; (3) the biochemical effects of PDT. It is thought that approximately 108 active species (each one produced by the interaction of a molecule of PS with a photon and a molecule of oxygen) are needed to kill each cell.

Subcellular distribution of PSs

Intracellular distributions in cultured cells have been determined for a range of PSs with widely differing structures. The important structural features are: (1) the net ionic charge, which can range from −4 (anionic) to +4 cationic; (2) the degree of hydrophobicity expressed as the logarithm of the octanol/water partition coefficient; (3) the degree of asymmetry present in the molecule. PSs that are hydrophobic and have two or less negative charges can diffuse across the plasma membrane, and then relocate to other intracellular membranes such as those of the mitochondria, lysosomes, Golgi apparatus, and endoplasmic reticulum. These PSs also tend to have the greatest uptakes into cells *in vitro*, especially when present in relatively low concentrations in the medium (< 1 μM). Those PSs that are less hydrophobic and have ε 2 negative charges tend to be too polar to diffuse across the plasma membrane, and are therefore taken up by endocytosis, and are routed to endosomes and lysosomes. PSs with cationic charges and which are also hydrophobic can localize in mitochondria (31); this is thought to be due to the influence of the mitochondrial membrane potential as well as the lipid bilayer of the membrane (32).

Confocal laser scanning fluorescence microscopy has made the determination of intracellular location of PSs much easier, and gives more sensitivity and better spatial resolution than earlier non-confocal techniques. Co-localization of subcellular organelle-specific probes with differing fluorescence emission maxima to that of the PS can be used to more closely identify the site of localization (33), and these probes can also be used to identify sites of damage after illumination (34). Woodburn *et al.* (35) studied the intracellular localization, in V79 Chinese hamster lung fibroblasts and C6 glioma cells, of a series of porphyrins derived from hemato- and protoporphyrin IX with side chains chemically modified to give hydrophobic and anionic or cationic residues at physiological pH. Compounds were selected to represent all combinations of these characteristics, and it was found that those with a net cationic character localized in mitochondria, while those with net anionic character localized in lysosomes. As the anionic porphyrins all bore two negative charges, these results are in accord with previous work suggesting that sensitizers with a net charge of −2 or greater accumulate in lysosomes.

The intracellular localization of PSs may redistribute due to photodynamic action after only a small amount of light has been delivered. It was found that exposure of cells pre-incubated with anionic porphyrins to light doses that inactivated 20 per cent of the cells resulted in relocalization of the sensitizers from the lysosomes to the cytoplasm in general, and, more specifically, the nucleus (36, 37). This behavior was attributed to photodynamic permeabilization of the lysosomal membrane, thus allowing small molecules, including the PSs to leak out into the cytoplasm.

PDT-mediated cellular damage

The most striking and immediate cellular *in vitro* response observed following PDT is damage to membranes, particularly the plasma membrane. Within hours of treatment, visible damage is characterized by cessation of normal cellular movement and formation of multiple membrane blebs. The blebs, which are often as large as the cell itself, develop as balloon-like structures protruding from the cell membrane and indicate severe membrane damage (38). After cell blebbing, there is no longer cell division, and cell lysis follows. Other experimental indications of membrane dysfunction after PDT are leakage of cellular constituents from intact cells. Other cellular membranes, in addition to the plasma membrane, may be at risk, including those of the nucleus, mitochondria, lysosome, Golgi apparatus, and endoplasmic reticulum (39).

In recent years it has been reported that PDT (in common with many other cancer therapies) can produce cell death with the characteristic features of apoptosis. Apoptosis is a mechanism whereby organisms initiate cellular death via a process that is normally part of the genetic apparatus (40). The end result is fragmentation of nuclear DNA and the changing of the cell into membrane-bound particles that are engulfed by adjoining cells and macrophages, minimizing release of inflammatory products. The time required for initiation of apoptosis after application of a specific toxic insult varies widely. Many apoptosis-inducing agents first induce cells to enter a latency period, variable in duration, which usually results in the death of greater than 80 per cent of a cell population in 1–3 days. A novel feature of apoptosis after PDT is the rapidity of execution, as judged by the appearance of DNA ladders as early as 30 minutes after photodamage (41). The mechanism of apoptosis after PDT has been investigated and has been shown to involve mitochondrial photodamage (42), cytochrome c release into the cytoplasm (43), and activation of caspases leading to the final cleavage of DNA (42). PSs that localize in mitochondria have been found to be especially likely to cause PDT-mediated apoptosis (34). It has also been found that higher doses of PDT that cause concurrent membrane photodamage can delay apoptosis, possibly by damaging essential components of the apoptotic pathway (44).

Biochemical effects of PDT

Biochemical studies performed over the past 15 years have provided much information on subcellular targets involving PDT-mediated cytotoxicity. Molecular biology procedures are playing an integral role in current research designed to examine the relevance of cell-signaling events induced by PDT-mediated oxidative stress. The downstream effector molecules of signal transduction pathways are often proteins encoded for by early response genes. These proteins function as transcription factors and act by regulating the expression of a variety of genes via specific regulatory domains. PDT-mediated oxidative stress induces a transient increase in the downstream early response genes c-fos, c-jun, c-myc, and egr- I (45). PDT induces a strong dose- and time-dependent activation of stress-activated protein kinase and a high-osmolarity glycerol (HOG)-I protein kinase in keratinocytes (46). Tyrosine phosphorylation of a non-receptor-type protein (HSI) has also been observed in PDT-treated mouse lymphoma cells and concomitantly shown to correlate with protection of cells from PDT lethality (47). Multiple genes encoding for stress-induced proteins can be activated following PDT. PDT induces increased expression of glucose-regulated proteins and the translation of these proteins appears to play a role in modulating the cytotoxic effects of oxidative stress (48). Heat shock proteins are also overexpressed following PDT when examined at either the *in vitro* or *in vivo* level (49).

Tumor destruction mechanisms—*in vivo*

Three distinct (but possibly interrelated) mechanisms have been identified that contribute to the observed shrinkage (and frequent disappearance) of tumors when treated with PDT.

Tumor-specific mechanism

Exposure of tumors to PDT *in vivo* can reduce the number of clonogenic tumor cells through direct photodamage; however, this is thought to be insufficient for tumor cure. Studies (50, 51) in rodent tumor systems employing curative procedures with several PSs showed direct photodynamic tumor cell kill to be less than 2 logs and in most cases less than 1 log, that is, far short of the 8-log reduction required for tumor cure, if tumor cell killing were the only mechanism operating. The *in vitro* illumination of tumor cells isolated from photosensitized tumors *in vivo* predicts that total eradication is feasible with a sufficiently high light dose with some PSs (51). But limitations appear to exist that do not allow the eradication to be realized for *in vivo* PDT treatment. Inhomogeneous PS distribution within the tumor might be one of these limitations. Korbelik and Krosl (52) have also shown that both PS accumulation and tumor cell kill decrease with the distance of tumor cells from the vascular supply. Another parameter that can limit direct tumor cell kill is the

availability of oxygen within the tissue undergoing PDT treatment. The rates of singlet oxygen generation and therefore tissue oxygen consumption/depletion are high when both tissue PS levels and the fluence rate of light are high (25). An important parameter influencing the rate of tissue oxygen consumption is photobleaching of the sensitizer because the reduction of sensitizer levels also reduces the rate of photochemical oxygen consumption (53). Since all of these parameters can impose limits on the direct photodestruction of tumor cells, other mechanisms must operate to account for the demonstrable success of the treatment.

Vascular mechanisms

The first additional mechanism shown to operate is the vascular effect in which vascular damage, occurring after completion of the PDT treatment, contributes to long-term tumor control. Microvascular collapse can be readily observed following PDT (54, 55) and can lead to severe and persistent post-PDT tumor hypoxia (55). The mechanisms underlying the vascular effects of PDT differ greatly with different PSs. PF-PDT leads to vessel constriction, macromolecular vessel leakage, leukocyte adhesion, and thrombus formation, all apparently linked to platelet activation and release of thromboxane (56). PDT with certain phthalocyanine derivatives causes primarily vascular leakage (57), and PDT with mono-L-aspartyl chlorin e6 results in blood flow stasis, primarily because of platelet aggregation (58). All of these effects may include components related to damage of the vascular endothelium. PDT may also lead to vessel constriction via inhibition of the production or release of nitric oxide by the endothelium (59). In preclinical experiments, the microvascular PDT responses can be partially or completely inhibited by the administration of agents that affect eicosanoid generation, such as indomethacin (60), and this inhibition can markedly diminish the tumor response. Much of the above information was obtained from studies on normal microvasculature. Damage to the tumor-supplying normal vasculature may greatly affect tumor curability by PDT as demonstrated by the lack of tumor cures when the normal tissue surrounding the tumor was shielded from PDT light (60).

Immune response

There are two aspects to this effect: (1) antitumor activity of inflammatory cells; (2) generation of an antitumor immune response. These effects can be elicited by phototoxic damage that is not necessarily lethal to all tumor cells and bears an inflammatory impact. Photodynamically induced changes in the plasma membrane and membranes of cellular organelles can prompt a rapid activation of membranous phospholipases (61) leading to accelerated phospholipid degradation with a massive release of powerful inflammatory mediators (62). Other cytokines and growth factors that are potent immunodulators have been found to be strongly enhanced in PDT-treated mouse tumors (63, 64).

The inflammatory signaling after PDT initiates a massive regulated invasion of neutrophils, mast cells, and monocytes/macrophages (65) that may outnumber resident cancer cells. Most notable is a rapid accumulation of large numbers of neutrophils, which have been shown to have a profound impact on PDT-mediated destruction of tumors, and it has been shown that depletion of neutrophils in tumor-bearing mice decreased the PDT-mediated tumor cure rate (66). Another class of nonspecific immune effector cells whose activation substantially contributes to the antitumor effects of PDT is monocytes/macrophages. The tumoricidal activity of these cells was found to be potentiated by PDT *in vivo* and *in vitro* (67). Adjuvant treatment with a selective vitamin D_3-binding protein macrophage-activating factor was shown to potentiate the cures of PDT-treated tumors (68).

There have been substantial advances in the understanding of the PDT-induced tumor-specific immune reaction. This effect may not be relevant to the initial tumor ablation, but may be decisive in attaining long-term tumor control. Anticancer immunity elicited by PDT has the attributes of an inflammation-primed immune development process (66) and bears similarities to the immune reaction induced by tumor inflammation caused by bacterial vaccines or some cytokines. Macrophages phagocytose large numbers of cancer cells killed or damaged by the cytotoxic effects of PDT. Directed by powerful inflammation-associated signaling, the antigen-presenting cells will process tumor-specific peptides and present them on their membranes in the context of major histocompatibility class (MHC) II molecules. Presentation of tumor peptides, accompanied by intense accessory signals, creates conditions for the recognition of tumor antigens by helper T lymphocytes. These lymphocytes become activated and in turn sensitize cytotoxic T cells to tumor-specific epitopes. The activity of tumor-sensitized lymphocytes is not limited to the original PDT-treated site but can include disseminated and metastatic lesions

of the same cancer. Thus, although the PDT treatment is localized to the tumor site, its effect can have systemic attributes due to the induction of an immune reaction. PDT-generated tumor-sensitized lymphocytes can be recovered from distant lymphoid tissues (spleen, lymph nodes) at protracted times after light treatment (69).

Photosensitizer targeting

We shall consider four strategies in which PSs can be targeted to tumors: (1) the original tumor-localizing effect of PSs mentioned above; (2) the use of noncovalent complexes between PSs and various delivery vehicles; (3) the preparation of covalent conjugates between PSs and passive macromolecular targeting vehicles designed to increase the accumulation of PSs in the tumor; (4) the use of conjugates of PSs with active targeting vehicles that employ the interaction between specific ligands, and receptors or antigens overexpressed on tumor cells or other components of tumors.

Tumor-localizing PSs

Since the observation of the tumor-localizing ability of HPD, many workers have investigated the mechanism of this tendency of PSs to preferentially localize in tumors and other specific organs and anatomical sites (13, 70, 71). The precise definition of tumor to normal tissue ratio has also been subject to debate. Some investigators working with subcutaneous (SC) tumors in experimental animals use the ratio between the tumor and peritumoral muscle or skin, while others use distant muscle and skin In addition, there has been much effort made to determine which factors in the chemical structures of the PS are optimal for maximizing the selectivity for the tumor over normal tissue and organs. This has proved quite complicated because the pharmacokinetics can vary dramatically. For instance, one PS can have its best tumor to normal tissue ratio at a relatively early time point after administration such as 3 hours, while with another this can be at 7 days after injection. One of the particular properties of these tetrapyrrole compounds relevant to their tumor-localizing ability is their tendency to bind strongly to serum proteins and to each other. This means that most PSs when injected into the bloodstream behave as macromolecules either because they are more or less firmly bound to large protein molecules or because they have formed intermolecular aggregates of similar size. Many workers have reported (72–74) on the distribution of PS between the various classes of serum proteins when mixed with serum *in vitro*. These proteins are usually divided into four classes: albumin and other heavy proteins; high-density lipoprotein (HDL); low-density lipoprotein (LDL); and very low-density lipoprotein (VLDL). However, even this study has been complicated by the fact that the most lipophilic PSs are insoluble in aqueous media and need to be delivered in a solvent mixture that may alter the serum protein distribution of the PS. It has been found that the more lipophilic compounds generally bind preferentially to LDLs and VLDLs, while those of moderate lipophilicity bind to HDLs, and those of more hydrophilic character bind to albumin and other heavy proteins (globulins). It has been argued that PSs that preferentially bind to LDLs are better tumor localizers (see below) (71), but this is by no means always the case (75).

It is useful to make a distinction between selective accumulation and selective retention. The tumor-localizing ability of the PSs with the faster pharmacokinetics is probably due to selective accumulation in the tumor, while the localization of PSs with slower-acting pharmacokinetics is more likely to be due to selective retention. In the selective accumulation model it is thought that the increased vascular permeability to macromolecules typical of tumor neovasculature is chiefly responsible for the preferential extravasation of the PSs. These quick-acting PSs frequently bind to albumin which is of ideal size and Stokes radius to pass through the 'pores' in the endothelium of the tumor microvessels (76). The selective retention of PSs in tumors has been the subject of much speculation. As mentioned above, a popular theory maintains that the binding of the PSs to LDLs is of major importance (71). In this theory, it is proposed that cancer cells overexpress the LDL (apoB/E) receptor. Upregulation of the expression of LDL receptors is one way in which rapidly growing malignant cells gain cholesterol needed for the biosynthesis of lipids needed for the rapid turnover of cellular membranes. There is experimental evidence both for and against this theory (75, 77). Other theories have been proposed to account for the selective retention of PS in tumor tissue. One is that tumors have poorly developed lymphatic drainage, and that macromolecules, which extravasate from the hyperpermeable tumor neovasculature, are retained in the extravascular space (78). Another involves the macrophages, which infiltrate solid tumors to varying extents (70). These tumor-associated macrophages have been shown to accumulate up to 13 times the amount of some PSs compared to cancer cells (79). The explanation for this has been proposed to be either the phagocytosis of aggregates of PSs (80), or the preferential uptake by macrophages of lipoproteins that have been altered by the binding of porphyrins (70). Another theory proposes that the low pH commonly found in tumors has the effect of trapping some of the anionic PSs, which are ionized at normal physiological pH. These PSs then become neutrally charged, and hence more lipophilic, when they encounter the lowered pH in the tumor environment (81).

Recently, there has been much interest in a different approach where, instead of being administered in a presynthesized form, a PS precursor is administered and the PS is synthesized *in situ* in tumors (82). This is the case with 5-aminolevulinic acid (ALA). Almost all types of cells of the human body, with the exception of mature red blood cells, are equipped with the biosynthetic machinery to synthesize heme (Fig. 15.4). In the first step of the heme biosynthetic pathway ALA is formed from glycine and succinyl CoA. The synthesis of ALA by ALA-synthetase is under feedback regulation by the amount of heme in the cell. The last step in the formation of heme is rate-limiting and is the incorporation of iron into protoporphyrin (PPIX), catalyzed by the enzyme, ferrochelatase. By adding exogenous ALA, the feedback inhibition is bypassed, and PPIX will accumulate because of the limited capacity of ferrochelatase to transform PPIX to heme. PPIX is formed in the mitochondria of cells, but rapidly diffuses to other intracellular membrane sites. *In vivo* the ALA may be administered orally (83), intravenously (84), or topically (85). The reasons why cancer cells tend to synthesize more PPIX than normal cells have been much investigated. Hypotheses include greater expression of heme biosynthesis enzymes, porphobilinogen deaminase (86), coproporphyrinogen oxidase (87), or reduced expression of ferrochelatase (88), but increased delivery of ALA to the tumor may play a role especially in topical application (89). Recent attempts to increase the efficacy of ALA-mediated PDT include the use of iron chelators to decrease the amount of PPIX converted to heme by ferrochelatase (90), and the administration of ALA as the alkyl ester in order to increase cellular uptake by making the molecule more lipophilic (91).

Noncovalent complexes

As mentioned above, many of the most effective PSs are too hydrophobic to dissolve in aqueous solvents, and this necessitates the use of a delivery vehicle to

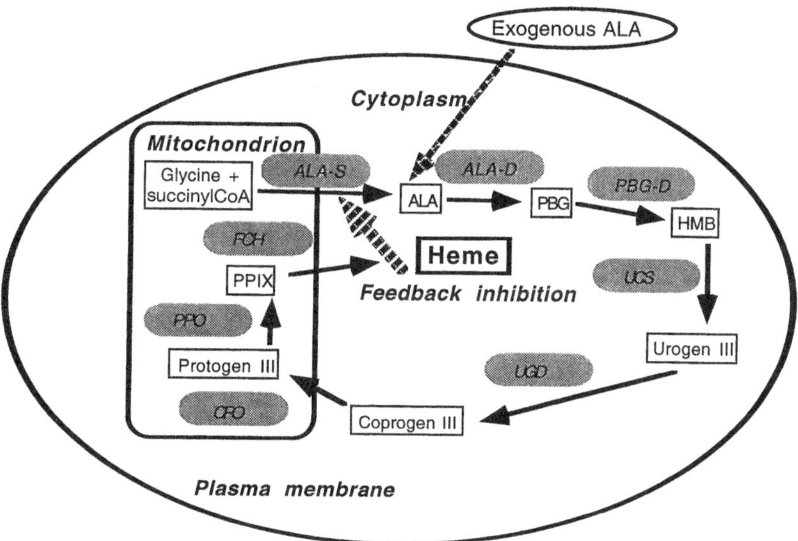

Fig. 15.4 Biosynthetic pathway from ALA to PPIX. ALA, 5-Aminolevulanic acid; PBG, porphobilinogen; HMB, hydroxymethylbilane; Urogen III, uroporphyrinogen III; Coprogen III, coproporphyrinogen III; Protogen III, protoporphyrinogen III; PPIX, protoporphyrin IX; *ALA-S*, ALA synthetase; *ALA-D*, ALA dehydratase; *PBG-D*, porphobilinogen deaminase; *UCS*, uroporphyrinogen cosynthase; *UGD*, uroporphyrinogen decarboxylase; *CPO*, coproporphyrinogen oxidase; *PPO*, protoporphyrinogen oxidase; *FCH*, ferrochelatase.

keep the molecules in a sufficiently disaggregated state to be able to travel in the blood vessels and to extravasate into tumors. It has been found that the choice of delivery vehicle can influence the tumor selectivity of the PS (92). The castor oil derivative Cremophor EL has been used as a delivery vehicle, but Kessel and colleagues have shown that its use actually changes the lipoprotein profile (93) and can affect the biodistribution of PS and the efficacy of the tumor treatment (94). An alternative method of PS delivery is encapsulation in liposomes. It has been suggested that, when liposomal PSs are administered to animals, the PS is more efficiently transferred to LDL than an aqueous formulation (95). *In vivo* liposomal delivery has been shown to give advantages in either biodistribution or tumor destruction compared to non-liposomal delivery for Photofrin (96), benzoporphyrin derivative (BPD) (97), and zinc phthalocyanine (Zn-PC) (98). Other workers have used polyethylene-glycol-coated poly-(lactic acid) nanoparticles (99) or albumin microspheres (100) to deliver PSs.

Some workers have investigated the pre-complexing with various serum proteins. The protein most frequently investigated has been LDL for two reasons. Firstly the hydrophobic core of the LDL particle can act as a solubilizing medium for hydrophobic PSs in a similar way to liposomes or Cremophor and, secondly,

it was proposed to increase tumor targeting by taking advantage of receptor-mediated endocytosis of the complex by the LDL receptor, which has been reported to be overexpressed on cancer cells (see above). Barel *et al.* (101), used HP pre-complexed to lipoproteins to target a murine fibrosarcoma. An increased delivery of HP to the mouse tumor was reported with the HP–LDL complex compared to HP complexes of HDL, VLDL, or free HP. Similarly, pre-complexing of BPD with LDL led to a greater accumulation of the PS in tumors as compared to BPD administration of an aqueous solution at 3 h. (77). Some authors have suggested that PS delivery with various macromolecular systems may lead to differing mechanisms of tumor destruction as PSs are delivered to different sites. For example, although albumin and globulins are believed to deliver PSs mainly to the vascular stroma of tumors (102), HDL apparently deliver PSs to cells via a nonspecific exchange with the plasma membrane. LDL probably delivers a large fraction of the PSs via an active receptor-mediated pathway (103). Zhou *et al.* (104) have suggested that aqueous solutions of HP lead to predominantly vascular damage, while LDL-mediated PDT leads predominantly to damage of neoplastic cells. However, this is not always true. In a study of PDT of ocular melanoma in a rabbit model, LDL complexed to BPD was used. Despite the use of

LDL as a carrier, early damage to the vasculature was demonstrated by light and electron microscopy (105). Larroque *et al.* (106) showed that the insoluble Zn-PC could be formulated for intravenous (IV) administration as a complex with serum albumin, after which it redistributed primarily to HDLs.

Conjugates with passive macromolecular tumor-targeting vehicles

In recent years much progress has been made in the use of conjugates between cytotoxic drugs and polymeric carriers to increase the therapeutic ratio of tumor treatment, that is, to increase tumor selectivity while simultaneously reducing toxicity to normal organs (107). Similar arguments have been made in favor of the use of polymeric PS conjugates to increase the targeting ability of PSs. Many of the synthetic schemes for preparing polymer–PS conjugates have arisen from work on conjugates between monoclonal antibodies (mAbs) and PSs (see later). These polymers may be either natural polymers such as dextran (108) and polyamino-acids (109, 110), or synthetic polymers such as *N*-(2-hydroxypropyl)-methacrylamide (111) and polyvinyl alcohol (112). The preparation of conjugates between tetrapyrrole PSs and polymers poses special challenges. They may aggregate to a greater or lesser extent due to the amphiphilic nature of hydrophobic tetrapyrroles joined to hydrophilic polymer chains. Water-soluble PS–polymer conjugates must be relatively hydrophilic, but may bear net cationic, anionic, or neutral charges. Soukos *et al.* (109) showed that the cationic conjugate had the highest cellular uptake, but that the neutral conjugate was considerably more phototoxic. Conjugates may also be prepared with varying size distributions according to the molecular weight range of the original polymer. A recent study by Hamblin *et al.* (113) showed that poly-l-lysine chlorin e6 conjugates that had been succinylated to give them an overall anionic charge were able to extravasate from tumor vasculature faster than conjugates with a cationic charge, and that the molecular weight of the polymers also had a remarkable effect.

Ris and co-workers have studied the effects of covalent attachment of polyethylene glycol (PEG)ylation) on the PS *meta*-tetrahydroxyphenylchlorin (mTHPC) (114, 115). The PS molecule was modified by the covalent attachment of 4 PEG chains in order to make it water-soluble and improve its tumor targeting and PDT properties. It was found that the PEGylated molecule was less phototoxic *in vitro* (even on an equimolar basis) than the native molecule, but that *in vivo* this may have benefits in reducing phototoxicity to normal tissue. Recently, Hornung *et al.* (116) used IV administered PEG-mTHPC and intraperitoneal (IP) light to treat ovarian cancer in the rat and found a significant survival advantage. There has been a report (117) on both PEG and polyvinylalcohol being axially attached to aluminum phthalocyanine. Improved water solubility and longer serum half-lives in mice were found, and some indication of improved tumor control after illumination. Bachor *et al.* (118) prepared conjugates between chlorin e6 and 1 μm diameter microspheres and found they gave a distinct increase in phototoxicity compared to unconjugated PS. They showed that some cancer cells take up several times more PS than nonmalignant cells, due to increased rates of phagocytosis.

Conjugates with active macromolecular tumor-targeting vehicles

Monoclonal antibody–PS conjugates (or photoimmunoconjugates)

The emergence in recent years of mAbs that recognize tumor-associated antibodies and are available in reasonable quantities has led to their being investigated for targeted delivery of PSs, in addition to being well known targeting vehicles for toxins and radioisotopes. The advantages claimed for this approach include those specific to mAbs (high specificity and affinity for their target antigens) and those specific for PSs (nontoxic to normal organs that do not receive light). Because relatively large quantities of immunoconjugates can accumulate in organs such as liver and kidneys, there can be toxicity to normal organs when the cytotoxic moiety is a radioisotope or a protein toxin, but this is avoided if these organs do not receive light. It was thought that, in contrast to immunoconjugates with toxin molecules and cytotoxic drugs, photoimmunoconjugates (PICs) could be active if they bound to the plasma membranes of tumor cells, since the reactive species generated upon illumination could diffuse into the cells and produce fatal damage. However, it is now thought that PICs will kill cells more efficiently if they are internalized (119). In contrast to mAb–toxin or mAb–radionuclide conjugates, photoimmunotargeting requires conjugates with high PS-to-mAb ratios, which makes the synthesis and purification complicated. The goal of any such synthesis should be to retain features essential for both PS and antibody activities and at the same time allow maximal PS incorporation.

Two basic approaches for the synthesis of PICs have been used: (1) PSs are linked chemically to mAbs directly, (2) PSs are linked to mAbs via polymers. The PS is bound to polymeric carriers in the first step, and the carriers are attached to the mAb in a second step. This method allows for a high PS:mAb ratio with only a small number of attachment sites on the mAb itself and, therefore, in principle, minimal losses in the immunoreactivity of the mAb. A variety of PS-carrying polymers have been used. These include dextrans (120), polyglutamic acid (PGA) (121), polyvinyl alcohols (PVA) (122), and poly[*N*-(2-hydroxypropyl) methacrylamide] (123) and poly-L-lysines (124). Since the antigen-binding capabilities of antibodies largely reside in the Fab portion of the antibodies, conjugation at sites removed from these antigen recognition sites are most desirable, and such site-specific syntheses have recently been developed (121, 122, 124). In the first study of mAb–PS conjugates (125), HP was coupled directly to an mAb directed against the DBA/2J myosarcoma, M-1. Modestly increased photosensitized inhibition of tumor growth in mice treated with these conjugates and light was demonstrated, compared with controls treated with HP, mAb, or light alone. A different approach to photoimmunotargeting was exemplified in a study by Steele *et al.* (126) in which immune stimulation was demonstrated by targeting T-suppressor cells using an mAb (B16G)–HP conjugate directed against an epitope on T-suppressor cells in DBA/2J mice. Photosensitized tumor regression, reported in 10–40 per cent of the mice, was correlated with an increase in the killing activity of specific cytotoxic T lymphocytes against the target tumor cells. Hasan and collaborators have developed this approach as a potential application for treating the disseminated intraperitoneal spread of ovarian cancer (127, 128). It is hoped that the intraperitoneal administration of the conjugate will avoid the twin difficulties posed by high liver uptake and restricted transport of large macromolecules from the capillaries to the tumor (129). Light can be administered laparoscopically via a fiber optic into the peritoneal cavity where a diffusing liquid will allow fairly uniform illumination of all the surfaces (130). Schmidt *et al.* (131, 132) have used a similar approach to target ovarian cancer and, in addition to showing selective phototoxicity to target cells *in vitro* and *in vivo* in a tumor-bearing nude rat model, they treated three patients with advanced ovarian cancer by

IP administration of 1 mg mAb–phthalocyanine conjugate. At laparotomy 72 h later, after removal of gross tumor the peritoneum was irradiated with 50 J/cm² 670-nm light and histological evidence of tumor cell death was obtained.

Hamblin and co-workers have shown (124) that the overall charge conferred on the immunoconjugate by the polymer–PS moiety can produce major differences in both the phototoxicity towards cells, and also in the biodistribution in tumor-bearing mice (129). Recently, such a positively charged conjugate targeted against human ovarian cancer was shown to combine well with cisplatin in *ex vivo* primary cultures, and it was found that pre-treatment with photoimmunotherapy had the potential to reverse platinum resistance, which frequently presents a major problem in ovarian cancer therapy (133). A recent report (119) describes the preparation of immunoconjugates using mTHPC and an anti-head and neck cancer mAb. Biodistribution studies showed greater tumor selectivity than that of unconjugated PS in a nude mouse xenograft model. A slightly different approach (134) uses polymeric linkers that bear both a PS and a cytotoxic drug (adriamycin) attached to anti-ovarian cancer mAbs. These conjugates showed dark toxicity, which could be significantly increased after illumination, and which could also be competed by unconjugated mAb.

Conjugates targeted towards other receptors on cancer cells

Malignant cells have both faster growth rates and faster metabolic rates than normal cells, and consequently have a much higher demand for many of the nutrients and building blocks that are delivered to normal cells by well regulated pathways. Cancer cells satisfy this increased demand by upregulating the expression of many of the membrane receptors that are responsible for supplying cells with these necessary molecules by receptor-mediated endocytosis. There are two approaches for taking advantage of this selective overexpression for tumor targeting of PSs. The approach of attaching PSs to mAbs that recognize the extracellular portion of these membrane receptors has been discussed above. An alternative approach, however, is to attach the PS to the natural ligand of these receptors, which may have advantages in that the maximum cellular uptake may be higher, and the intracellular location may be more sensitive due to normal intracellular processing.

As discussed above, LDLs may be a tumor-targeting delivery vehicle for PSs and the formation of covalent conjugates with the apolipoprotein may serve to obviate the possibility of the PSs exchanging between LDLs and cellular membranes. Schmidt-Erfurth *et al.* (135) showed that retinoblastoma cells took up four times as much PS when delivered as a covalent conjugate with LDL compared to a complex with LDL, and the uptake could be partly competed by added native LDL, while Hamblin and Newman (136) reported that an LDL–HP conjugate, although recognized by the LDL receptor on colon cancer cells and fibroblasts, was also recognized by a scavenger receptor on macrophages.

Transferrin receptors are also overexpressed on many types of cancer cell that can have an increased demand for iron, and have been used as targets to deliver various cytotoxic moieties by both mAb- and transferrin-conjugates. Hamblin and Newman (137) found that a conjugate between holotransferrin and HP was recognized by transferrin receptors on a colorectal cancer cell line, as demonstrated by the observation that both uptake and phototoxicity could be competed by addition of native transferrin. Gijsins and de Witte (138) used epidermal growth factor (EGF) attached to a polymer–PS carrier to target EGF receptors, which are known to be frequently upregulated in malignant cells. A small effect of the EGF ligand was observed together with a larger effect depending on the nature of the carrier. Akhlynina and co-workers have used insulin–PS conjugates to produce receptor-mediated endocytosis via insulin receptors (139), and in addition have shown that a nuclear localization signal from simian virus 40 (SV40) large T antigen increases photo-toxicity by directing the PS to the cell nucleus (140).

Conclusions

The outlook for PDT as a part of the cancer treatment armamentarium appears to be promising. At the present time its most suitable roles are to treat early superficial lesions of mucosal surfaces, to palliate advanced obstructive lesions, and as an adjuvant intra-operative treatment to destroy remaining tumor deposits or tumor cells spilled during surgery. The more demanding applications are to destroy dissemi-nated metastatic disease, for example, in body cavities, which may require better tumor to normal tissue ratios of PS than are presently available. It is expected that advances in basic research will reveal the mechanisms behind the tumor-localizing effect of various PSs, and

that this knowledge will allow rational decisions to be made concerning the usefulness of PS-targeting vehi-cles. Covalent attachment of the PS to targeting macro-molecules may have effects on its photophysical properties and/or its intracellular localization and these effects should be studied. Most successful cancer therapy is likely to involve a combination of two or more modalities. PDT has been found to combine well with hyperthermia, but the precise way in which PDT interacts with systemic chemotherapy or radiation therapy is uncertain. Research is necessary to determine which combinations can be favorable, and in which order they should be administered. When the role of the immune system is understood in the PDT response, it may play a role in treating disseminated cancer by helping to generate a systemic antitumor immune response.

References

1. Jesionek A, von Tappenier H. Zur Behandlung der Hautcarcinoma mit fluorescierenden Stoffen. Muench Med Wochenschr 1903, 47, 2042.
2. Hausman W. Die sensibilisierende wirkung des hemato-porphyrins. Biochem Z 1911, 30, 276.
3. Figge FH, Weiland GS, Manganiello LO. Affinity of neoplastic, embryonic and traumatized tissues for por-phyrins and metalloporphyrins. Proc Soc Exp Biol Med 1948, 68, 640.
4. Lipson RL, Baldes EJ. The photodynamic properties of a particular hematoporphyin derivative. Arch Dermatol 1960, 82, 508.
5. Dougherty TJ. Activated dyes as antitumor agents. J Natl Cancer Inst 1974, 52, 1333–6.
6. Dougherty TJ, Kaufman JE, Goldfarb A, *et al.* Photoradiation therapy for the treatment of malignant tumors. Cancer Res 1978, 38, 2628–35.
7. Dougherty T. J, Lawrence G, Kaufman J. H, *et al.* Photoradiation in the treatment of recurrent breast car-cinoma. J Natl Cancer Inst 1979, 62, 231–237.
8. Dougherty, TJ. Photoradiation therapy for bron-chogenic cancer. Chest 1982, 81, 265–6.
9. Baas P, van Mansom I, van Tinteren H, *et al.* Effect of N-acetylcysteine on Photofrin-induced skin photosensi-tivity in patients. Lasers Surg Med 1995, 16, 359–67.
10. Orenstein A, Kostenich G, Roitman L, *et al.* A compar-ative study of tissue distribution and photodynamic therapy selectivity of chlorin e6, Photofrin II and ALA-induced protoporphyrin IX in a colon carcinoma model. Br J Cancer 1996, 73, 937–44.
11. Spikes JD. Chlorins as photosensitizers in biology and medicine. J Photochem Photobiol B 1990, 6, 259–74.
12. Kessel D, Thompson P. Purification and analysis of hematoporphyrin and hematoporphyrin derivative by gel exclusion and reverse-phase chromatography. Photochem Photobiol 1987, 46, 1023–5.

13. Boyle RW, Dolphin D. Structure and biodistribution relationships of photodynamic sensitizers. Photochem Photobiol 1996, **64**, 469–85.

14. Gomer CJ. Preclinical examination of first and second generation photosensitizers used in photodynamic therapy. Photochem Photobiol 1991, **54**, 1093–107.

15. Hasan T. Photosensitizer delivery mediated by macromolecular carrier systems. In: Photodynamic therapy: basic principles and clinical applications (ed. B Henderson and T Dougherty). Marcel Dekker, New York, 1992, 187–200.

16. Hammer-Wilson MJ, Sun CH, Ghahramanlou M, *et al. In vitro* and *in vivo* comparison of argon-pumped and diode lasers for photodynamic therapy using second-generation photosensitizers. Lasers Surg Med 1998, **23**, 274–80.

17. Rosenthal I, Murali Krishna C, Riesz P, *et al.* The role of molecular oxygen in the photodynamic effect of phthalocyanines. Radiat Res 1986, **107**, 136–42.

18. Svaasand LO. Optical dosimetry for direct and interstitial photoradiation therapy of malignant tumors. Prog Clin Biol Res 1984, **170**, 91–114.

19. Wilson BC, Jeeves WP, Lowe DM. *In vivo* and post mortem measurements of the attenuation spectra of light in mammalian tissues. Photochem Photobiol 1985, **42**, 153–62.

20. Firey PA, Rodgers MA. Photo-properties of a silicon naphthalocyanine: a potential photosensitizer for photodynamic therapy. Photochem Photobiol 1987, **45**, 535–8.

21. van Leengoed HL, Schuitmaker JJ, van der Veen N, *et al.* Fluorescence and photodynamic effects of bacteriochlorin a observed *in vivo* in 'sandwich' observation chambers. Br J Cancer 1993, **67**, 898–903.

22. Dougherty TJ, Potter WR. Of what value is a highly absorbing photosensitizer in PDT? J Photochem Photobiol B 1991, **8**, 223–5.

23. Spikes JD, Bommer JC. Photobleaching of mono-L-aspartyl chlorin e6 (NPe6): a candidate sensitizer for the photodynamic therapy of tumors. Photochem Photobiol 1993, **58**, 346–50.

24. Fingar VH, Henderson BW. Drug and light dose dependence of photodynamic therapy: a study of tumor and normal tissue response. Photochem Photobiol 1987, **46**, 837–41.

25. Foster TH, Murant RS, Bryant RG, *et al.* Oxygen consumption and diffusion effects in photodynamic therapy. Radiat Res 1991, **126**, 296–303.

26. Sitnik TM, Henderson BW. The effect of fluence rate on tumor and normal tissue responses to photodynamic therapy. Photochem Photobiol 1998, **67**, 462–6.

27. van Geel IP, Oppelaar H, Marijnissen JP, *et al.* Influence of fractionation and fluence rate in photodynamic therapy with Photofrin or mTHPC. Radiat Res 1996, **145**, 602–9.

28. Fingar VH, Wieman TJ, Wiehle SA, *et al.* The role of microvascular damage in photodynamic therapy: the effect of treatment on vessel constriction, permeability, and leukocyte adhesion. Cancer Res 1992, **52**, 4914–21.

29. Ando T, Irie K, Koshimizu K, *et al.* Photocytotoxicity of water-soluble metalloporphyrin derivatives. Photochem Photobiol 1993, **57**, 629–33.

30. Ochsner M. Photophysical and photobiological processes in the photodynamic therapy of tumours. J Photochem Photobiol B 1997, **39**, 1–18.

31. Dummin H, Cernay T, Zimmermann HW. Selective photosensitization of mitochondria in HeLa cells by cationic Zn (II) phthalocyanines with lipophilic side-chains. J Photochem Photobiol B 1997, **37**, 219–29.

32. Rashid F, Horobin RW. Interaction of molecular probes with living cells and tissues. Part 2. A structure–activity analysis of mitochondrial staining by cationic probes and a discussion of the synergistic nature of image-based and biochemical approaches. Histochemistry 1990, **94**, 303–8.

33. Wilson BC, Olivo M, Singh G. Subcellular localization of Photofrin and aminolevulinic acid and photodynamic cross-resistance *in vitro* in radiation-induced fibrosarcoma cells sensitive or resistant to photofrin-mediated photodynamic therapy. Photochem Photobiol 1997, **65**, 166–76.

34. Kessel D, Luo Y, Deng Y, *et al.* The role of subcellular localization in initiation of apoptosis by photodynamic therapy. Photochem Photobiol 1997, **65**, 422–6.

35. Woodburn KW, Vardaxis NJ, Hill JS, *et al.* Subcellular localization of porphyrins using confocal laser scanning microscopy. Photochem Photobiol 1991, **54**, 725–32.

36. Berg K, Madslien K, Bommer JC, *et al.* Light induced relocalization of sulfonated meso-tetraphenylporphines in NHIK 3025 cells and effects of dose fractionation. Photochem Photobiol 1991, **53**, 203–10.

37. Peng Q, Farrants GW, Madslien K, *et al.* Subcellular localization, redistribution and photobleaching of sulfonated aluminum phthalocyanines in a human melanoma cell line. Int J Cancer 1991, **49**, 290–5.

38. Moan J, Pettersen EO, Christensen T. The mechanism of photodynamic inactivation of human cells *in vitro* in the presence of haematoporphyrin. Br J Cancer 1979, **39**, 398–407.

39. Kessel D, Morgan A, Garbo GM. Sites and efficacy of photodamage by tin etiopurpurin *in vitro* using different delivery systems. Photochem Photobiol 1991, **54**, 193–6.

40. Dixon SC, Soriano BJ, Lush RM, *et al.* Apoptosis: its role in the development of malignancies and its potential as a novel therapeutic target. Ann Pharmacother 1997, **31**, 76–82.

41. Luo Y, Chang CK, Kessel D. Rapid initiation of apoptosis by photodynamic therapy. Photochem Photobiol 1996, **63**, 528–34.

42. Kessel D, Luo Y. Photodynamic therapy: a mitochondrial inducer of apoptosis. Cell Death Differ 1999, **6**, 28–35.

43. Granville DJ, Carthy CM, Jiang H, *et al.* Rapid cytochrome c release, activation of caspases 3, 6, 7 and 8 followed by Bap31 cleavage in HeLa cells treated with photodynamic therapy. FEBS Lett 1998, **437**, 5–10.

44. Kessel D, Luo Y. Mitochondrial photodamage and PDT-induced apoptosis. J Photochem Photobiol B 1998, **42**, 89–95.

45. Luna MC, Wong S, Gomer CJ. Photodynamic therapy mediated induction of early response genes. Cancer Res 1994, **54**, 1374–80.

46. Tao J, Sanghera JS, Pelech SL, *et al.* Stimulation of stress-activated protein kinase and p38 HOG1 kinase in murine keratinocytes following photodynamic therapy with benzoporphyrin derivative. J Biol Chem 1996, **271**, 27107–15.

47. Xue LY, He J, Oleinick NL. Rapid tyrosine phosphorylation of HS1 in the response of mouse lymphoma L5178Y-R cells to photodynamic treatment sensitized by the phthalocyanine Pc 4, Photochem Photobiol 1997, **66**, 105–13.

48. Gomer CJ, Luna M, Ferrario A, *et al.* Increased transcription and translation of heme oxygenase in Chinese hamster fibroblasts following photodynamic stress or Photofrin II incubation. Photochem Photobiol 1991, **53**, 275–9.

49. Gomer CJ, Ryter SW, Ferrario A, *et al.* Photodynamic therapy-mediated oxidative stress can induce expression of heat shock proteins. Cancer Res 1996, **56**, 2355–60.

50. Chan W. S, Brasseur N, La Madeleine C, *et al.* Evidence for different mechanisms of EMT-6 tumor necrosis by photodynamic therapy with disulfonated aluminum phthalocyanine or photofrin: tumor cell survival and blood flow. Anticancer Res 1996, **16**, 1887–92.

51. Henderson B. W, Waldow S. M, Mang T. S, *et al.* Tumor destruction and kinetics of tumor cell death in two experimental mouse tumors following photodynamic therapy. Cancer Res 1985, **45**, 572–6.

52. Korbelik M, Krosl G. Cellular levels of photosensitisers in tumours: the role of proximity to the blood supply. Br J Cancer 1994, **70**, 604–10.

53. Georgakoudi I, Nichols MG, Foster TH. The mechanism of Photofrin photobleaching and its consequences for photodynamic dosimetry. Photochem Photobiol 1997, **65**, 135–44.

54. Star WM, Marijnissen HP, van den Berg-Blok AE, *et al.* Destruction of rat mammary tumor and normal tissue microcirculation by hematoporphyrin derivative photoradiation observed *in vivo* in sandwich observation chambers. Cancer Res 1986, **46**, 2532–40.

55. Henderson BW, Fingar VH. Relationship of tumor hypoxia and response to photodynamic treatment in an experimental mouse tumor. Cancer Res 1987, **47**, 3110–14.

56. Fingar VH, Siegel KA, Wieman TJ, *et al.* The effects of thromboxane inhibitors on the microvascular and tumor response to photodynamic therapy. Photochem Photobiol 1993, **58**, 393–9.

57. Fingar VH, Wieman TJ, Karavolos PS. *et al.* The effects of photodynamic therapy using differently substituted zinc phthalocyanines on vessel constriction, vessel leakage and tumor response. Photochem Photobiol 1993, **58**, 251–8.

58. McMahon KS, Wieman TJ, Moore PH, *et al.* Effects of photodynamic therapy using mono-L-aspartyl chlorin e6 on vessel constriction, vessel leakage, and tumor response. Cancer Res 1994, **54**, 5374–9.

59. Gilissen MJ, van de Merbel-de Wit LE, Star WM, *et al.* Effect of photodynamic therapy on the endothelium-dependent relaxation of isolated rat aortas. Cancer Res 1993, **53**, 2548–52.

60. Fingar VH, Wieman TJ, Doak KW. Role of thromboxane and prostacyclin release on photodynamic therapy-induced tumor destruction. Cancer Res 1990, **50**, 2599–603.

61. Agarwal ML, Larkin HE, Zaidi SI, *et al.* Phospholipase activation triggers apoptosis in photosensitized mouse lymphoma cells. Cancer Res 1993, **53**, 5897–902.

62. Yamamoto N, Homma S, Sery TW, *et al.* Photodynamic immunopotentiation: *in vitro* activation of macrophages by treatment of mouse peritoneal cells with haematoporphyrin derivative and light. Eur J Cancer 1991, **27**, 467–71.

63. Herman S, Kalechman Y, Gafter U, *et al.* Photofrin II induces cytokine secretion by mouse spleen cells and human peripheral mononuclear cells. Immunopharmacology 1996, **31**, 195–204.

64. Gollnick SO, Liu X, Owczarczak B, *et al.* Altered expression of interleukin 6 and interleukin 10 as a result of photodynamic therapy *in vivo*. Cancer Res 1997, **57**, 3904–9.

65. Krosl G, Korbelik M, Dougherty GJ. Induction of immune cell infiltration into murine SCCVII tumour by photofrin-based photodynamic therapy. Br J Cancer 1995, **71**, 549–55.

66. Korbelik M. Induction of tumor immunity by photodynamic therapy. J Clin Laser Med Surg 1996, **14**, 329–34.

67. Yamamoto N, Hoober JK, Yamamoto N, *et al.* Tumoricidal capacities of macrophages photodynamically activated with hematoporphyrin derivative. Photochem Photobiol 1992, **56**, 245–50.

68. Korbelik M, Naraparaju VR, Yamamoto N. Macrophage-directed immunotherapy as adjuvant to photodynamic therapy of cancer. Br J Cancer 1997, **75**, 202–7.

69. Korbelik M, Dougherty GJ. Photodynamic therapy-mediated immune response against subcutaneous mouse tumors. Cancer Res 1999, **59**, 1941–6.

70. Hamblin MR, Newman EL. On the mechanism of the tumour-localising effect in photodynamic therapy. J Photochem Photobiol B 1994, **23**, 3–8.

71. Jori G, Reddi E. The role of lipoproteins in the delivery of tumour-targeting photosensitizers. Int J Biochem 1993, **25**, 1369–75.

72. Maziere JC, Santus R, Morliere P, *et al.* Cellular uptake and photosensitizing properties of anticancer porphyrins in cell membranes and low and high density lipoproteins. J Photochem Photobiol B 1990, **6**, 61–8.

73. Kessel D, Dougherty TJ, Chang CK. Photosensitization by synthetic diporphyrins and dichlorins *in vivo* and *in vitro*. Photochem Photobiol 1991, **53**, 475–9.

74. Kongshaug M, Moan J, Brown SB. The distribution of porphyrins with different tumour localising ability among human plasma proteins. Br J Cancer 1989, **59**, 184–8.

75. Korbelik M. Low density lipoprotein receptor pathway in the delivery of Photofrin: how much is it relevant for selective accumulation of the photosensitizer in tumors? J Photochem Photobiol B 1992, **12**, 107–9.

76. Yuan F, Leunig M, Berk DA, *et al.* Microvascular permeability of albumin, vascular surface area, and vascu-

lar volume measured in human adenocarcinoma LS174T using dorsal chamber in SCID mice. Microvasc Res 1993, **45**, 269–89.

77. Allison BA, Pritchard PH, Levy JG. Evidence for low-density lipoprotein receptor-mediated uptake of benzoporphyrin derivative [published erratum appears in Br J Cancer 1995, **71** (1), 214]. Br J Cancer 1994, **69**, 833–9.

78. Roberts WG, Hasan T. Role of neovasculature and vascular permeability on the tumor retention of photodynamic agents. Cancer Res 1992, **52**, 924–30.

79. Korbelik M, Krosl G. Photofrin accumulation in malignant and host cell populations of a murine fibrosarcoma. Photochem Photobiol 1995, **62**, 162–8.

80. Korbelik M, Krosl G, Chaplin DJ. Photofrin uptake by murine macrophages. Cancer Res 1991, **51**, 2251–5.

81. Pottier R, Kennedy JC. The possible role of ionic species in selective biodistribution of photochemotherapeutic agents toward neoplastic tissue. J Photochem Photobiol B 1990, **8**, 1–16.

82. Peng Q, Warloe T, Berg K, *et al.* 5-Aminolevulinic acid-based photodynamic therapy. Clinical research and future challenges. Cancer 1997, **79**, 2282–308.

83. van den Boogert J, van Hillegersberg R, de Rooij F. W, *et al.* 5-Aminolaevulinic acid-induced protoporphyrin IX accumulation in tissues: pharmacokinetics after oral or intravenous administration. J Photochem Photobiol B 1998, **44**, 29–38.

84. Svanberg K, Liu DL, Wang I, *et al.* Photodynamic therapy using intravenous delta-aminolaevulinic acid-induced protoporphyrin IX sensitisation in experimental hepatic tumours in rats. Br J Cancer 1996, **74**, 1526–33.

85. Calzavara-Pinton PG. Repetitive photodynamic therapy with topical delta-aminolaevulinic acid as an appropriate approach to the routine treatment of superficial non-melanoma skin tumours. J Photochem Photobiol B 1995, **29**, 53–7.

86. Gibson SL, Cupriks DJ, Havens JJ, *et al.* A regulatory role for porphobilinogen deaminase (PBGD) in delta-aminolaevulinic acid (delta-ALA)-induced photosensitization? Br J Cancer 1998, **77**, 235–43.

87. Ortel B, Chen N, Brissette J, *et al.* Differentiation-specific increase in ALA-induced protoporphyrin IX accumulation in primary mouse keratinocytes. Br J Cancer 1998, **77**, 1744–51.

88. Van Hillegersberg R, Van den Berg JW, Kort WJ, *et al.* Selective accumulation of endogenously produced porphyrins in a liver metastasis model in rats. Gastroenterology 1992, **103**, 647–51.

89. Szeimies RM, Sassy T, Landthaler M. Penetration potency of topical applied delta-aminolevulinic acid for photodynamic therapy of basal cell carcinoma. Photochem Photobiol 1994, **59**, 73–6.

90. Curnow A, McIlroy BW, Postle-Hacon MJ, *et al.* Enhancement of 5-aminolaevulinic acid-induced photodynamic therapy in normal rat colon using hydroxypyridinone iron-chelating agents. Br J Cancer 1998, **78**, 1278–82.

91. Kloek J, Akkermans W, Beijersbergen van Henegouwen GM. Derivatives of 5-aminolevulinic acid for photodynamic therapy: enzymatic conversion into protoporphyrin. Photochem Photobiol 1998, **67**, 150–4.

92. Reddi E. Role of delivery vehicles for photosensitizers in the photodynamic therapy of tumours. J Photochem Photobiol B 1997, **37**, 189–95.

93. Woodburn K, Sykes E, Kessel D. Interactions of Solutol HS 15 and Cremophor EL with plasma lipoproteins. Int J Biochem Cell Biol 1995, **27**, 693–9.

94. Woodburn K, Chang CK, Lee S, *et al.* Biodistribution and PDT efficacy of a ketochlorin photosensitizer as a function of the delivery vehicle. Photochem Photobiol 1994, **60**, 154–9.

95. Ginevra F, Biffanti S, Pagnan A, *et al.* Delivery of the tumour photosensitizer zinc(II)-phthalocyanine to serum proteins by different liposomes: studies *in vitro* and *in vivo*. Cancer Lett 1990, **49**, 59–65.

96. Jiang F, Lilge L, Logie B, *et al.* Photodynamic therapy of 9L gliosarcoma with liposome-delivered photofrin. Photochem Photobiol 1997, **65**, 701–6.

97. Richter AM, Waterfield E, Jain AK, *et al.* Liposomal delivery of a photosensitizer, benzoporphyrin derivative monoacid ring A (BPD), to tumor tissue in a mouse tumor model. Photochem Photobiol 1993, **57**, 1000–6.

98. Polo L, Segalla A, Jori G, *et al.* Liposome-delivered 131I-labelled Zn(II)-phthalocyanine as a radiodiagnostic agent for tumours. Cancer Lett 1996, **109**, 57–61.

99. Allemann E, Rousseau J, Brasseur N, *et al.* Photodynamic therapy of tumours with hexadecafluoro zinc phthalocynine formulated in PEG-coated poly(lactic acid) nanoparticles. Int J Cancer 1996, **66**, 821–4.

100. Margalit R, Silbiger E. Albumin microspheres as delivery systems for photodynamic drugs: physico-chemical studies and their implications for *in vivo* situations. J Microencapsul 1985, **2**, 183–96.

101. Barel A, Jori G, Perin A, *et al.* Role of high-, low- and very low-density lipoproteins in the transport and tumor-delivery of hematoporphyrin *in vivo*. Cancer Lett. 1986, **32**, 145–50.

102. Jori G. *In vivo* transport and pharmacokinetic behavior of tumour photosensitizers. Ciba Found Symp 1989, **146**, 78–86.

103. Morliere P, Kohen E, Reyftmann JP, *et al.* Photosensitization by porphyrins delivered to L cell fibroblasts by human serum low density lipoproteins. A microspectrofluorometric study. Photochem Photobiol 1987, **46**, 183–91.

104. Zhou CN, Milanesi C, Jori G. An ultrastructural comparative evaluation of tumors photosensitized by porphyrins administered in aqueous solution, bound to liposomes or to lipoproteins. Photochem Photobiol 1988, **48**, 487–92.

105. Schmidt-Erfurth U, Bauman W, Gragoudas E, *et al.* Photodynamic therapy of experimental choroidal melanoma using lipoprotein-delivered benzoporphyrin. Ophthalmology 1994, **101**, 89–99.

106. Larroque C, Pelegrin A, Van Lier JE. Serum albumin as a vehicle for zinc phthalocyanine: photodynamic activities in solid tumour models. Br J Cancer 1996, **74**, 1886–90.

107. Duncan R, Spreafico F. Polymer conjugates. Pharmacokinetic considerations for design and development. Clin Pharmacokinet 1994, **27**, 290–306.

108. Rakestraw SL, Tompkins RG, Yarmush ML. Preparation and characterization of immunoconjugates for antibody-targeted photolysis. Bioconjug Chem 1990, **1**, 212–21.

109. Soukos NS, Hamblin MR, Hasan T. The effect of charge on cellular uptake and phototoxicity of polylysine chlorin(e6) conjugates. Photochem Photobiol 1997, **65**, 723–9.

110. Goff BA, Bamberg M, Hasan T. Photoimmunotherapy of human ovarian carcinoma cells *ex vivo*. Cancer Res 1991, **51**, 4762–7.

111. Krinick NL, Sun Y, Joyner D, *et al.* A polymeric drug delivery system for the simultaneous delivery of drugs activatable by enzymes and/or light. J Biomater Sci Polym Ed 1994, **5**, 303–24.

112. Davis N, Liu D, Jain AK, *et al.* Modified polyvinyl alcohol–benzoporphyrin derivative conjugates as phototoxic agents. Photochem Photobiol 1993, **57**, 641–7.

113. Hamblin MR, Rajadhyaksha M, Momma T, *et al. In vivo* fluorescence imaging of the transport of charged chlorin e6 conjugates in a rat orthotopic prostate tumour. Br J Cancer 1999, **81**, 261–8.

114. Ris HB, Im Hof V, Stewart CM, *et al.* Endobronchial photodynamic therapy: comparison of mTHPC and polyethylene glycol-derived mTHPC on human tumor xenografts and tumor-free bronchi of minipigs. Lasers Surg Med 1998, **23**, 25–32.

115. Ris HB, Krueger T, Giger A, *et al.* Photodynamic therapy with mTHPC and polyethylene glycol-derived mTHPC: a comparative study on human tumour xenografts. Br J Cancer 1999, **79**, 1061–6.

116. Hornung R, Fehr M.K, Monti-Frayne J, *et al.* Minimally-invasive debulking of ovarian cancer in the rat pelvis by means of photodynamic therapy using the pegylated photosensitizer PEG-mTHPC. Br J Cancer 1999, **81**, 631–7.

117. Brasseur N, Ouellet R, La Madeleine C, *et al.* Water-soluble aluminium phthalocyanine–polymer conjugates for PDT: photodynamic activities and pharmacokinetics in tumour-bearing mice. Br J Cancer 1999, **80**, 1533–41.

118. Bachor R, Shea CR, Gillies R, *et al.* Photosensitized destruction of human bladder carcinoma cells treated with chlorin e6-conjugated microspheres. Proc Natl Acad Sci, USA 1991, **88**, 1580–4.

119. Vrouenraets MB, Visser GW, Stewart FA, *et al.* Development of meta-tetrahydroxyphenylchlorin-monoclonal antibody conjugates for photoimmunotherapy. Cancer Res 1999, **59**, 1505–13.

120. Oseroff AR, Ohuoha D, Hasan T, *et al.* Antibody-targeted photolysis: selective photodestruction of human T-cell leukemia cells using monoclonal antibody-chlorin e6 conjugates. Proc Natl Acad Sci, USA 1986, **83**, 8744–8.

121. Hasan T, Lin A, Yarmush D, *et al.* Monoclonal antibody–chromophore conjugates as selective phototoxins. J Controlled Release 1989, **10**, 107–17.

122. Jiang FN, Jiang S, Liu D, *et al.* Development of technology for linking photosensitizers to a model monoclonal antibody. J Immunol Methods 1990, **134**, 139–49.

123. Omelyanenko V, Kopeckova P, Gentry C, *et al.* HPMA copolymer-anticancer drug-OV-TL16 antibody conjugates. 1. Influence of the method of synthesis on the binding affinity to OVCAR-3 ovarian carcinoma cells *in vitro*. J Drug Target 1996, **3**, 357–73.

124. Hamblin MR, Miller JL, Hasan T. Effect of charge on the interaction of site-specific photoimmunoconjugates with human ovarian cancer cells. Cancer Res 1996, **56**, 5205–10.

125. Mew D, Wat CK, Towers GH, *et al.* Photoimmunotherapy: treatment of animal tumors with tumor-specific monoclonal antibody-hematoporphyrin conjugates. J Immunol 1983, **130**, 1473–7.

126. Steele JK, Liu D, Stammers AT, *et al.* Suppressor deletion therapy: selective elimination of T suppressor cells *in vivo* using a hematoporphyrin conjugated monoclonal antibody permits animals to reject syngeneic tumor cells. Cancer Immunol Immunother 1988, **26**, 125–31.

127. Goff BA, Hermanto U, Rumbaugh J, *et al.* Photoimmunotherapy and biodistribution with an OC125-chlorin immunoconjugate in an *in vivo* murine ovarian cancer model. Br J Cancer 1994, **70**, 474–80.

128. Goff BA, Blake J, Bamberg MP, *et al.* Treatment of ovarian cancer with photodynamic therapy and immunoconjugates in a murine ovarian cancer model .Br J Cancer 1996, **74**, 1194–8.

129. Duska LR, Hamblin MR, Bamberg MP, *et al.* Biodistribution of charged F(ab')$_2$ photoimmunoconjugates in a xenograft model of ovarian cancer. Br J Cancer 1997, **75**, 837–44.

130. Lilge L, Molpus K, Hasan T, *et al.* Light dosimetry for intraperitoneal photodynamic therapy in a murine xenograft model of human epithelial ovarian carcinoma. Photochem Photobiol 1998, **68**, 281–8.

131. Schmidt S, Wagner U, Oehr P, *et al.* Clinical use of photodynamic therapy in gynecologic tumor patients—antibody-targeted photodynamic laser therapy as a new oncologic treatment procedure. Zentralbl Gynakol 1992, **114**, 307–11.

132. Schmidt S, Wagner U, Schultes B, *et al.* Photodynamic laser therapy with antibody-bound dyes. A new procedure in therapy of gynecologic malignancies. Fortschr Med 1992, **110**, 298–301.

133. Duska LR, Hamblin MR, Miller JL, *et al.* Combination photoimmunotherapy and cisplatin: effects on human ovarian cancer *ex vivo*. J Natl Cancer Inst 1999, **91**, 1557–63.

134. Omelyanenko V, Gentry C, Kopeckova P, *et al.* HPMA copolymer-anticancer drug-OV-TL16 antibody conjugates. II. Processing in epithelial ovarian carcinoma cells *in vitro*. Int J Cancer 1998, **75**, 600–8.

135. Schmidt-Erfurth U, Diddens H, Birngruber R, *et al.* Photodynamic targeting of human retinoblastoma cells using covalent low-density lipoprotein conjugates. Br J Cancer 1997, **75**, 54–61.

136. Hamblin MR, Newman EL. Photosensitizer targeting in photodynamic therapy. II. Conjugates of haematoporphyrin with serum lipoproteins. J Photochem Photobiol B 1994, **26**, 147–57.

137. Hamblin MR, Newman EL. Photosensitizer targeting in photodynamic therapy. I. Conjugates of haematoporphyrin with albumin and transferrin. J Photochem Photobiol B 1994, **26**, 45–56.

138. Gijsens A, De Witte P. Photocytotoxic action of EGF-PVA-Sn(IV)chlorine and EGF–dextran–Sn(IV)chlorine internalizable conjugates on A431 cells. Int J Oncol 1998, **13**, 1171–7.

139. Akhlynina TV, Rosenkranz AA, Jans DA, *et al*. Insulin-mediated intracellular targeting enhances the photodynamic activity of chlorine. Cancer Res 1995, **55**, 1014–19.

140. Akhlynina TV, Jans DA, Rosenkranz AA, *et al*. Nuclear targeting of chlorine enhances its photosensitizing activity. J Biol Chem 1997, **272**, 20328–31.

16 | *Boron neutron capture therapy: a chemically targeted radiation modality*

Gerard M. Morris and Jeffrey A. Coderre

Introduction

An inherent limitation of conventional radiotherapeutic modalities is specific targeting of neoplastic tissue. Even with the recent advances in conformal radiotherapy, tumor metastatic spread cannot be adequately targeted due to considerations related to normal tissue tolerance. However, an emerging radiotherapeutic modality, boron neutron capture therapy (BNCT), offers considerably higher levels of radiation targeting than conventional radiotherapy. BNCT is a binary approach: a tumor-specific compound labeled with boron-10 (^{10}B) is administered and, after a time interval governed by the pharmacokinetic/biodistribution profile of that compound, the target tumor is irradiated with a beam of thermal or epithermal neutrons (which become thermalized at depth in tissues). The minor stable isotope of boron, ^{10}B, interacts with low-energy (thermal) neutrons with the resultant fission reaction producing highly energetic, short-range disintegration products (1). Of itself, the thermal neutron component of this therapy has no significant effect on normal or neoplastic tissue, due to insufficient energy (< 0.4 eV). It is primarily the high linear energy transfer (LET) radiation released after boron neutron capture (^{10}B + ^{1}n $\rightarrow$ [^{11}B] $\rightarrow$ ^{7}Li + ^{4}He + 2.79 MeV) that is responsible for cell kill or sterilization. The short travel distance of the particles produced by the neutron capture reaction (< 10 μm) essentially limits the radiation damage to cells containing ^{10}B. In practice, epithermal beams are contaminated with gamma rays and fast neutrons, but these have a limited effect, providing that relatively high levels of ^{10}B can be maintained in the tumor relative to the surrounding normal tissue. The therapeutic ratio in BNCT is primarily governed by the tumor-targeting capacity of the boron delivery agent.

This chapter reviews: (1) boron delivery agents; (2) neutron beams; (3) the radiobiology of BNCT; (4) BNCT clinical studies; and (5) future developments.

Boron delivery agents

As a minimum requirement, it is generally recognized that a boron delivery agent must achieve 30 mg ^{10}B/g in the tumor with tumor to normal tissue boron concentration ratios appreciably higher than unity. Toxicity must also be low.

The sulfhydryl borane Na$_2$B$_{12}$H$_{11}$SH (BSH) has been used in clinical BNCT for over 30 years (Fig. 16.1). BSH does not cross the intact blood–brain barrier in the normal brain (2), but accumulates in brain tumors, due to the fact that the blood vessels in intracranial tumors do not have a fully functional blood–brain barrier. BSH has been demonstrated to be carried in the blood as a disulfide complex with serum albumin (3). Biodistribution data from studies using animal tumor models have indicated that the tumor:blood boron concentration ratios are in the range 0.5:1 to 1:1 (2, 4–6). Comparable clinical data for glioblastoma indicated tumor:blood ratios ranging from 1.3:1 to 2:1 (7, 8). These relatively low tumor-to-blood ratios suggest that the primary mode of accumulation of BSH in tumor is passive diffusion from the blood. Although BSH does

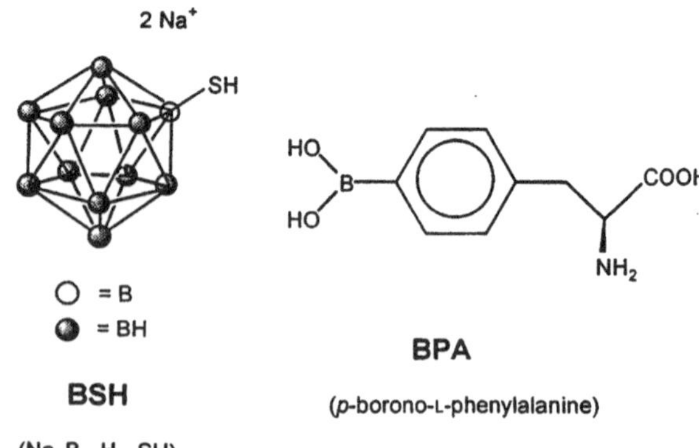

Fig. 16.1 The chemical structures of *p*-boronophenylalanine (BPA) and the sulfhydryl borane Na$_2$B$_{12}$H$_{11}$SH (BSH).

not cross the intact blood–brain barrier, it readily penetrates tumor vasculature. However, Ceberg *et al.* (9) noted that, in the RG2 rat glioma model, BSH was taken up by distant metastases. It was postulated by these authors that BSH targeted the tumor through the disrupted blood–brain barrier and diffused along the same white matter tracts as the infiltrating tumor cells (9). *In vitro*, boron from BSH has been detected in both the cytoplasm and the nucleus. Chandra *et al.* (10) reported a relatively uniform distribution of boron in glioblastoma cells, whereas Zha *et al.* (11) found that the nuclear boron content was lower than the cytoplasmic content in various tissue culture systems. In human glioblastoma tissue, Otersen *et al.* (12) reported boron from BSH to be in both the cytoplasm and the nucleus.

The amino acid analog *p*-(dihydroxyboryl)-phenylalanine (BPA) was synthesized in the late 1950s (13). The structure is shown in Fig. 16.1. BPA was demonstrated to accumulate selectively in B16 melanoma cells both *in vitro* and *in vivo*. BNCT of BPA-loaded tumors resulted in high levels of tumor control (14). Based on encouraging preclinical data, Mishima began a clinical BNCT program in 1987 for the treatment of malignant cutaneous melanoma using BPA as the boron delivery agent.

The utilization of BPA in experimental brain tumor therapy studies (15, 16) followed reports indicating its preferential accumulation in a rat gliosarcoma, a human glioma xenograft, and a murine mammary adeocarcinoma (17). In contrast to BSH, BPA is transported across the blood–brain barrier into the normal brain. In both experimental animals and patients, the average concentration of boron in the normal brain approximates to that in the blood; but the average concentration of boron in tumor (melanoma and glioma) is 2–4 times higher than in blood and brain (for example, see references 17–20). The biochemical rationale for the uptake of BPA in tumor appears to be related to an elevated rate of amino acid transport across the tumor cell membrane. A pharmacokinetic study with either melanoma or glioblastoma involving ^{18}F-labelled BPA indicated that the net incorporation rate for tumor was about four times that for normal brain (21–22). Recent ion microscopy studies have revealed that, after exposure of cells either to BPA *in vitro* or in normal and neoplastic tissue from rats administered BPA, boron was distributed uniformly across the cytoplasm and the nucleus (23). BPA has also been shown, using ion microscopy, to accumulate preferentially in rat 9L gliosarcoma cells infiltrating the brain away from the main tumor mass, although the boron content in these

cells was about half that measured in cells in the main tumor mass (24). For highly infiltrative brain tumors, such as glioblastoma multiforme, the ability of the boron carrier to cross the blood–brain barrier is probably essential for effective BNCT. Compromising the blood–brain barrier with mannitol has been demonstrated to enhance the uptake of BPA and BSH by the F98 rat glioma (6).

Many additional candidate boron delivery agents are currently under evaluation. These were recently reviewed in detail by Soloway *et al.* (25). Most prominent among these compounds are liposomes and porphyrins. Compounds from both of these classes can be loaded with relatively large amounts of boron. The *in vivo* uptake of boron delivered to subcutaneous EMT-6 murine mammary tumors using a unilamellar synthetic liposome has been demonstrated (26, 27). The tumor boron content of ~ 35 μg ^{10}B/g achieved using this delivery modality was encouraging. Potentially therapeutic levels of boron have been reported in a murine mammary carcinoma using a range of boronated porphyrins (28). However, the ability of these carriers to effectively target gliomas and their metastatic spread have yet to be evaluated. An extensive review of boron compounds is beyond the scope of this chapter.

Low-energy neutron beams

The neutron energies involved in BNCT are much lower than those that have been used in fast-neutron therapy. Thermal neutron beams were used in the early BNCT trials in the USA and continue to be used clinically in Japan (7, 14, 18). Thermal neutrons are attenuated exponentially as a function of depth in tissue,

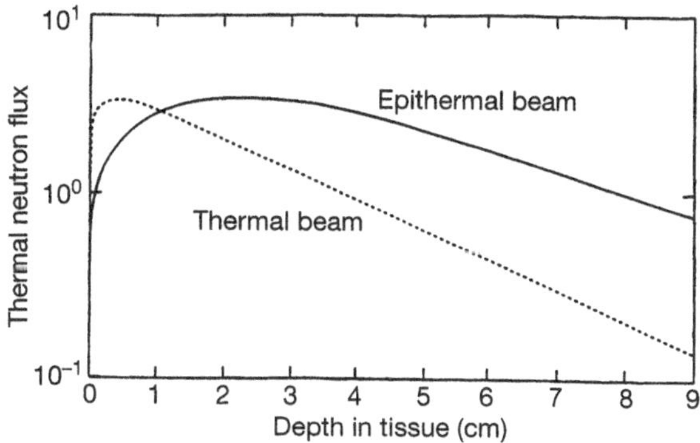

Fig. 16.2 Variation of the thermal neutron fluence with tissue depth using a thermal or epithermal neutron beam.

primarily by capture in hydrogen. Thermal neutron scattering and diffusion in tissue make it impossible to collimate or limit the beam to the tumor region. As a consequence of this limitation, higher-energy epithermal neutron beams were developed by moderation and filtration of nuclear-reactor-generated neutrons (29, 30). The fission process in the core of a reactor produces neutrons that range in energy from thermal (< 0.4 eV), followed by epithermal (0.4 eV to 10 keV), to high-energy or fast (10 keV to 14 MeV). Fast neutrons have considerable penetration depths in tissue but can induce considerable damage along their path length. While a thermal neutron beam is at its highest intensity (fluence) in the skin, an epithermal beam is progressively moderated by tissue hydrogen to produce thermal neutrons with a peak fluence at a depth of 2 to 3 cm (Fig. 16.2). There are currently four fully operational clinical epithermal neutron beams (Table 16.1). In addition, there are numerous nuclear reactors around the world in the process of conversion to clinical epithermal beam facilities for BNCT. The production of an epithermal beam entails the positioning of a moderator and filter between the reactor core and the beam port. Moderators attenuate the energy of the fast neutrons down to the epithermal range, and filters absorb higher-energy neutrons and gamma rays. A representation of the epithermal beam facility at the Brookhaven Medical Research Reactor (BMRR) is given in Fig. 16.3.

Dosimetric characteristics of the mixed radiation field during BNCT

The predominant component of the radiation dose delivered to neoplastic tissue in BNCT is derived from

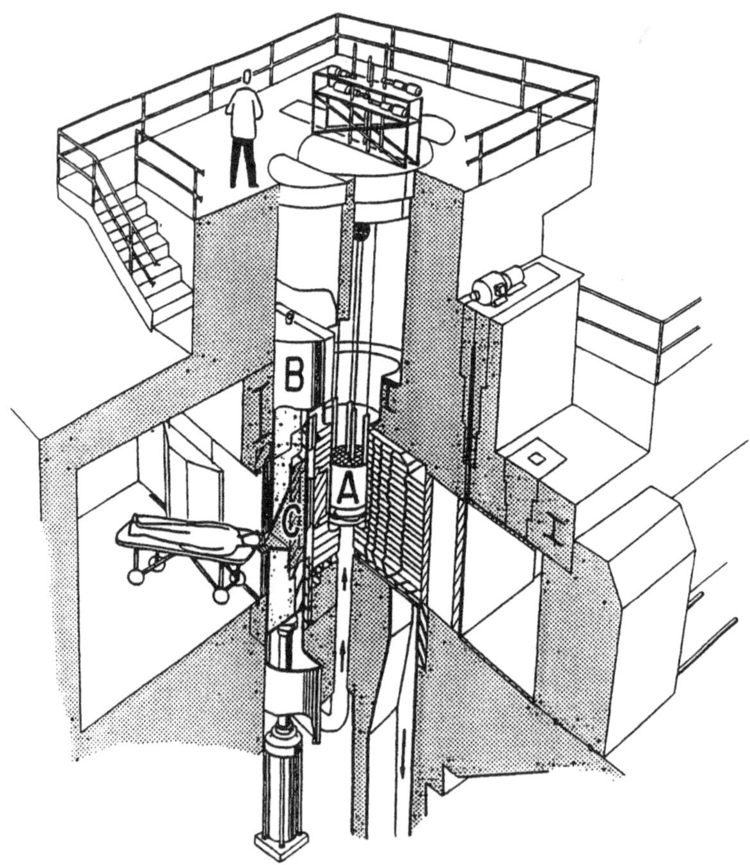

Fig. 16.3 Diagrammatic representation of the clinical BNCT facility at the BMRR. A, Reactor core; B, epithermal beam shutter; C, beam filter. A patient is shown undergoing epithermal neutron irradiation.

Table 16.1 Clinical epithermal neutron beams

Reactor facility*	Epithermal neutron flux ($\times 10^8$ n/cm^2/s)	Dose per epithermal neutron ($\times 10^{-11}$ cGy/cm^2/n)	
		Fast neutron dose	Gamma dose
BMRR	18.0	4.3	1.4
MITR	2.1	9.3	14.1
HFR-Petten	3.3	8.6	10.0
FIR 1	10.0	2.5	< 3

* BMRR, Brookhaven Medical Research Reactor; MITR, Massachusetts Institue of Technology Reactor; HFR-Petten, High Flux Reactor, Petten; FIR 1, Finnish Research Reactor.

the capture of thermal neutrons (^{1}n$_{th}$) by boron-10, with the resultant fission reaction yielding high-LET alpha particles (^{4}He) and recoiling lithium-7 (^{7}Li) nuclei: ^{10}B + ^{1}n$_{th}$ → [^{11}B] → ^{4}He + ^{7}Li + 2.8 MeV. The radiation field in tissue during BNCT consists of a mixture of radiation types with differing LET characteristics. In addition to the high-LET products of the ^{10}B(n, α)^{7}Li reaction, the interaction of the neutron beam with the nuclei of hydrogen and nitrogen in tissue delivers a mixture of high- and low-LET radiation components. Thermal neutron capture by hydrogen releases a gamma ray due to the ^{1}H(n, γ)^{2}H reaction, whilst the capture of thermal neutrons by nitrogen, through the ^{14}N(n, p)^{14}C reaction, releases a high-LET proton with an energy of 590 keV. Contaminating fast neutrons (> 10 keV), present in all the current epithermal beams, produce high-LET recoil protons, with similar average energy to those produced by the ^{14}N(n, p) ^{14}C reaction, through collisions with hydrogen nuclei (^{1}H(n, n з)p reaction) in tissue. The dose resulting from fast neutrons is highest at the skin surface and decreases exponentially with depth. Both tumor and surrounding normal tissues are present in the radiation field. As a consequence, there will be an unavoidable, nonspecific background dose to normal tissues. This will be primarily from the neutron beam, provided that the boron is selectively localized in the tumor. In clinical practice, using either BPA or BSH, reaction products from boron neutron capture reactions contribute to the background dose due to a low level of boron present in the normal tissues.

To illustrate the complexity of BNCT dosimetry, Fig. 16.4 details the various radiation components of the epithermal beam at the BMRR along the beam axis, as a function of depth in tissue. The dose components shown are all physical doses (Gy). Each of the high-LET components must be multiplied by an experimentally determined factor for biological effectiveness in order to express the total dose in photon-equivalent units. The derivation of these factors is the subject of

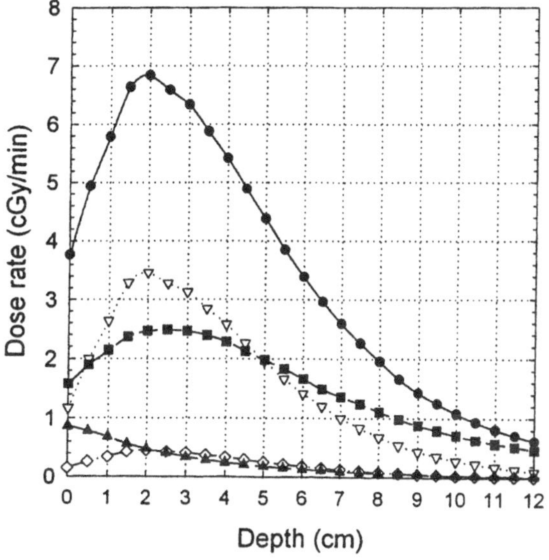

Fig. 16.4 The various components of the epithermal neutron beam at the Brookhaven Medical Research reactor (BMRR) along the beam axis as a function of depth in tissue. The boron dose was calculated assuming 13 ppm ^{10}B in the blood. Circle, Total dose; white inverted triangle; ^{10}B dose; square, total gamma dose; diamond, nitrogen capture dose; black triangle, fast neutron dose.

the next section. The treatment planning software in use for clinical BNCT must take into consideration these dose components, the variation of each component as a function of depth, and the relevant biological effectiveness factors (31).

Biological effectiveness of the components of the mixed irradiation field

It has been estimated that the minimum requirement for BNCT is ~ 10^9 atoms of ^{10}B distributed uniformly throughout a tumor cell (32). The microdistribution of ^{10}B relative to the cell nucleus is of critical significance due to the short ranges of the two particles produced by ^{10}B neutron capture. These particle ranges are 9 and 5 μm for the 1.47 MeV α particle and the 0.84 MeV Li^7 nucleus, respectively. Using Monte Carlo simulations, it has been demonstrated that ^{10}B located in the cell nucleus is more effective than ^{10}B distributed in the cytoplasm, which is in turn more effective than ^{10}B attached to the cell membrane (33). The dependence of the biological effect on the microdistribution of ^{10}B warrants the use of a more appropriate terminology than relative biological effectiveness (RBE) in defining the biological effectiveness of the ^{10}B(n, α)^{7}Li reaction. Measured biological effectiveness factors for the component of dose from the ^{10}B(n, α)^{7}Li reaction have been termed compound factor or, more frequently, compound biological effectiveness (CBE) factor (34). This factor is calculated according to the following formalism:

CBE factor = ([X-ray ED$_{50}$] – [Beam component of ED$_{50}$][Beam RBE])/[^{10}B(n,α)^{7}Li component of ED$_{50}$]

where ED$_{50}$ is the median effective dose.

The mode of compound administration, the boron distribution pattern within the cell and within the tissue, the dose per fraction, and even the size of the nucleus in the target cell population will influence the experimental determination of a CBE factor. It is critical that experimental determinations of CBE factors be carried out under conditions that approximate the clinical situation as closely as possible. The discussion in the following sections on the skin and central nervous system illustrates the dependence of the measured CBE factor on experimental conditions.

Normal tissue tolerance

There have been relatively few reports on skin tolerance to BNCT irradiation modalities (Table 16.2). RBE values in the range of 2.7–3.9 have been estimated for pig and rabbit skin using thermal neutron beams (35, 36). CBE factor estimates for BPA in the range 1.9–3.7 have been determined for rodent and human skin using moist desquamation as the end point (18, 34). Analogous estimates for BSH, using the same end point, were considerably lower at ~ 0.5 (34, 37). Determination of the CBE factor, using dermal necrosis as the endpoint has only been undertaken in rat skin (34). The values obtained were 0.73 ± 0.42 for BPA and 0.86 ± 0.08 for BSH. These studies indicate that the microdistribution of these two compounds had a profound effect on the CBE factors. It has recently been demonstrated (Morris *et al.*, unpublished), using high-resolution neutron autoradiography, that BPA accumulates preferentially in the epidermis, whereas BSH does not. This would account for the relatively high CBE factor for moist desquamation observed for BPA. For the dermal necrosis endpoint, the CBE factors for BPA and BSH were comparable. This is consistent with neutron autoradiography data for the dermis, which indicates a comparable microdistribution for BPA and BSH. Similar observations have been made for the oral mucosa of the rat (38). Using an alternative technique, ion microscopy, for the analysis of boron microdistribution, it was determined that BPA and BSH had similar distribution profiles to those observed in skin. This was reflected in the calculated CBE factors (tongue ulceration endpoint), which were 4.9 for BPA and 0.3 for BSH.

Selective damage to the vasculature after BSH-mediated BNCT irradiation has been demonstrated to duplicate the pathology of necrosis seen after conventional irradiation modalities such as X-rays (39). This underlines the crucial role played by the vasculature in the radiation pathogenesis of the central nervous system (CNS). Capillaries in the CNS have a lower limit to their diameter of about 8 μm. Mathematical modeling has indicated that the dose delivered to the endothelial cell is 1/3 to 1/5 that delivered to an infinite pool of blood, depending on the diameter of the vessel (40).

Table 16.2 Relative biological effectiveness (RBE) and compound biological effectiveness (CBE) factor values calculated for skin after single-dose neutron capture irradiation

Irradiation	Tissue*	RBE	CBE factor	First author (ref. no.)
Thermal beam	Pig skin (MD)	3.9	—	Archambeau (35)
BSH + epithermal beam	Dog skin	—	0.52	Gavin (37)
BPA + thermal beam	Rat skin (MD)	—	3.7 ± 0.7	Morris (34)
BPA + thermal beam	Rat skin (DN)	—	0.73 ± 0.42	Morris (34)
BPA + thermal beam	Human skin (MD)	—	2.5	Fukuda (18)

* MD, Moist desquamation; DN, dermal necrosis.

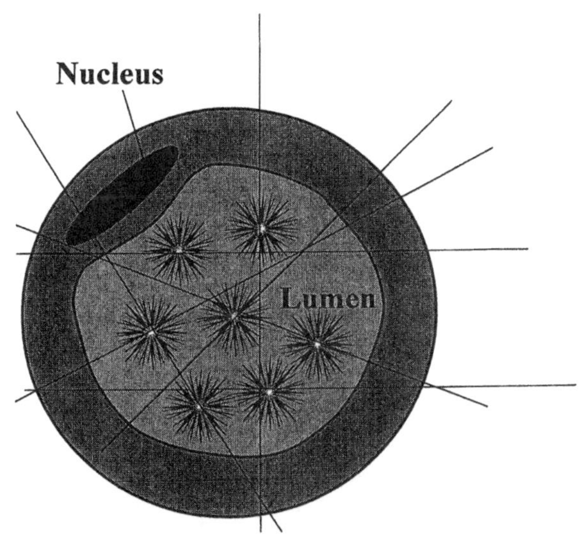

Fig. 16.5 Diagrammatic representation of the attenuation of dose delivery to the endothelial cell nucleus from the products of the ^{10}B(n, α)^{7}Li neutron capture reaction in a small blood vessel.

This is due to the fact that the travel distance of the particles from the ^{10}B(n, α) ^{7}Li reaction is ≤ 9 μm. Thus, a significant proportion of particles will deposit their energy outside of the vessel and will not target the endothelial cell nucleus (Fig. 16.5). The differing distribution patterns of BPA and BSH have a significant effect on the radiation response of the CNS (Table 16.3). With BSH, which does not cross the BBB and distribute in the CNS parenchyma, damage to the vascular endothelium is due primarily to high-LET particles produced by the neutron capture reactions in the lumen of the vessel. The parenchymal tissue elements of the CNS receive a relatively small dose of radiation due to the limited range of these particles. The predominant exclusion of BSH from the CNS parenchyma and the attenuation of the ^{10}B(n, α) ^{7}Li dose in the blood vessel lumen are the major factors responsible for the low CBE factor for BSH in the CNS. This has been estimated at ~ 0.4–0.5 using the rat spinal cord and dog brain models (37, 41). In the case of BPA, where the ^{10}B concentrations in the vessel lumen and surrounding CNS parenchyma are similar, there are contributions to the total dose received by the endothelial cell nucleus from both the ^{10}B within the endothelial cell and from ^{10}B in the adjacent parenchyma. This is reflected in an increase in the CBE factor, which has been estimated at ~ 1.1–1.3 (37, 42–44).

BNCT is generally administered clinically in a single fraction, although a four-fraction protocol is now in use in the clinical trial for glioblastoma at the High Flux Reactor, Petten, The Netherlands. It was concluded from studies using rat spinal cord and dog brain models that fractionation of BNCT results in a minor sparing of the CNS, typical of that seen after conventional high-LET irradiation (37, 44, 45; see Table 16.3).

Table 16.3 Relative biological effectiveness (RBE) and compound biological effectiveness (CBE) factor values calculated for the central nervous system after single-dose or fractionated neutron capture irradiation. Fractionated exposures were equal in size and spaced 24 hours apart. Errors indicate ± SE

Irradiation	Tissue (endpoint*)	RBE	CBE factor	First author (ref. no.)
Single-dose studies				
Thermal beam proton component	Rat spinal cord (MY)	1.80	—	Morris (42)
Epithermal beam proton component	Dog brain (BN)	4.40	—	Gavin (37)
BSH + epithermal beam	Dog brain (MRI)	—	0.27–0.49	Gavin (37)
BSH + epithermal beam	Dog brain (BN)	—	0.37–0.55	Gavin (37)
BPA + epithermal beam	Dog brain (MRI/BN)	—	1.10	Gavin (37)
Thermal beam	Rat spinal cord (MY)	1.40 ± 0.04	—	Morris (42)
BSH + thermal beam	Rat spinal cord (MY)	—	0.53 ± 0.03	Morris (45)
BPA + thermal beam	Rat spinal cord (MY)	—	1.33 ± 0.16	Morris (42)
BPA + thermal beam	Rat spinal cord (MY)	—	1.34 ± 0.13	Coderre (44)
Fractionated studies: 2 fractions				
Thermal beam	Rat spinal cord (MY)	1.76 ± 0.03	—	Coderre (44)
BSH + thermal beam	Rat spinal cord (MY)	—	0.60 ± 0.04	Morris (45)
BPA + thermal beam	Rat spinal cord (MY)	—	1.70 ± 0.20	Coderre (44)
Fractionated studies: 4 fractions				
Thermal beam	Rat spinal cord	2.46 ± 0.10	—	Coderre (44)
BSH + thermal beam	Rat spinal cord	—	0.81 ± 0.06	Morris (45)
BPA + thermal beam	Rat spinal cord	—	2.46 ± 0.29	Coderre (44)

* Endpoints: magnetic resonance imaging changes (MRI); brain necrosis (BN); myeloparesis (MY).

These results indicate that the rationale for fractionation of BNCT should not be the sparing of normal tissue damage. However, retargeting of boron through repeated administration of the delivery agent during a fractionation protocol merits further investigation.

Experimental boron neutron capture therapy

A variety of animal tumor models have been used in experimental therapeutic studies related to BNCT. BPA-based BNCT has been shown to inhibit the growth of melanoma with a high percentage of cures, in mice, hamsters, and pigs (14, 46). BPA has also proven effective in BNCT studies on hamster melanoma xenografts in the rabbit eye (47). The first successful treatments of an experimental brain tumor (rat 9L gliosarcoma) were carried out by Joel *et al.* in the late 1980s (48) using the dimeric form of BSH in combination with thermal neutrons at the BMRR. This was followed in 1992 by another study involving the first treatment of the rat 9L gliosarcoma with BPA-mediated BNCT (49). These experiments were repeated in 1994, employing an improved BPA delivery system that resulted in long-term survival levels approaching 100 per cent (15). Additional work by Saris *et al.* (16) using the murine GL 261 glioma and by Matalka *et al.* (50) using a human melanoma cell line (MRA 27) implanted in the brain of nude rats also demonstrated the efficacy of BPA-mediated BNCT. More recently, the preferential uptake of BPA and BSH by the rat F98 glioma has been considerably enhanced by disruption of the blood–brain barrier with intracarotid injection of mannitol (6). Dramatic improvements in F98 tumor growth inhibition were observed in subsequent BNCT studies, using either BPA or BSH, when combined with blood–brain barrier disruption (6).

The CBE factors for use in estimating the photon-equivalent dose to tumor are much less certain than those for the CNS for both BPA and BSH. With BPA, a CBE factor value of 3.8 (range 3.6–4.0 for survival fractions of 10, 1, and 0.1 per cent, respectively) was derived in the 9L rat gliosarcoma model, using an *in-vivo/in-vitro* clonogenic assay (51). A CBE factor value using the 9L gliosarcoma of 1.2 for BSH is based primarily on the published value for the oxidized dimeric form of BSH (BSSB). Ideally, CBE factors for BPA and BSH should be derived using survival data, but this has been difficult with the intracranial 9L gliosarcoma due

to the normal tissue complications resulting from the large single fractions of X-rays needed to control this tumor.

Clinical BNCT

Although the clinical potential of BNCT was recognized in the 1930s, it was not until the 1950s that the first clinical trials were initiated. The US BNCT trials at Brookhaven National Laboratory (BNL) and at Massachusetts Institute of Technology (MIT) were halted in 1961. The disappointing outcomes of these trials were attributed to two primary factors: (1) inadequate tumor specificity of the boron compounds employed; (2) insufficient penetration of thermal neutrons. The high boron concentrations in blood and brain tissue resulted in excessive damage to the normal brain (52, 53).

BNCT clinical studies were resumed in Japan in the late 1960s using a thermal beam and BSH as the delivery agent. A 19.3 per cent 5-year survival rate was achieved in a group of 38 patients with grade III or grade IV glioblastoma (7). Of these patients, 12 had tumors within 6 cm of the cortical surface. The 5- and 10-year survival rates in this subset of patients were 58.3 and 29.2 per cent, respectively. These survival data compare with a median survival of 9 to 10 months following conventional postoperative radiotherapy for glioblastoma and of approximately 28 months for lower grade malignant gliomas (54). Although encouraging, the Japanese clinical data must be viewed with caution. The influences of the different age distributions and of the different genetic backgrounds of Japanese versus American patients in the interpretation of these comparisons have yet to be assessed. Additionally, histopathological information to validate the diagnosis of high-grade glioma in the Japanese patients is not readily available. The clinical outcome of 14 American glioblastoma patients treated with BSH-mediated BNCT in Japan was evaluated by Laramore and Spence (55). The survival times of these patients were found to be no better than for those receiving conventional radiotherapy. However, no information was provided on the size of the tumors in the American patients. The Japanese BNCT treatment appeared to be more effective for smaller superficially located brain tumors.

More recently, there have been improvements in low-energy neutron beam technology and considerably more is now known about the radiation biology of BNCT. Several BNCT clinical trials have recently been started to take advantage of these improvements: at BNL in 1994 for glioblastoma (56, 57); at MIT in 1994 for cutaneous melanoma (58); at MIT in 1996 for intracerebral melanoma or glioblastoma (59); and at the High Flux Reactor, Petten, The Netherlands in 1997 for glioblastoma (60).

Initial BNCT clinical studies using epithermal neutrons are primarily safety- and dose-ranging trials. In these trials, a BNCT dose to a specific volume or critical region of the normal brain is prescribed. As the dose escalation trials have progressed, the treatments have changed from single field irradiations (BNL) or parallel opposed irradiations (MIT and Petten), to multiple non-coplanar irradiation fields arranged so as to maximize the dose to the tumor. A consequence of this approach is concomitant increase in the average doses to the normal brain. The current BNCT clinical trials at BNL and the MIT in the USA, involve the use of the boron delivery agent BPA and epithermal neutron beams. The clinical trial in Europe is based at the epithermal beam facility at the Petten, The Netherlands and utilizes BSH as the delivery agent. The European trial uses four fractions of BNCT administered on sequential days.

The calculation of photon-equivalent (Gy-Eq) BNCT doses requires a number of assumptions about RBEs, CBE factors, and the boron concentrations in various tissues, which are based on the available human or experimental data. The approach used for the BNCT trial at BNL is reviewed here as an example of the clinical approach (56, 57). An RBE of 3.2 is used in all tissues for the high-LET components of the beam: protons resulting from thermal neutron capture in nitrogen, and the recoil proton resulting from the collision of a fast neutron with hydrogen. Table 16.4 summarizes the assumptions made in various tissues for calculation of the Gy-Eq doses resulting from the $^{10}B(n, \alpha)$ ^7Li reaction during BPA-based BNCT. The $^{10}B(n, \alpha)$ ^7Li component of the dose to the normal brain is estimated from the measured boron concentration in the blood at the time of BNCT using a CBE factor of 1.3 (42). The $^{10}B(n, \alpha)$ ^7Li component of the dose to the scalp is based on the measured boron concentration in the blood at the time of BNCT, assuming a blood/scalp boron concentration ratio of 1.5:1 (18, 56, 61) and a CBE factor for BPA in skin of 2.5 (18). The $^{10}B(n, \alpha)$ ^7Li component of the dose to tumor is based on the measured boron concentration in the blood at the time of BNCT, a tumor/blood boron concentration ratio of 3.5:1 (62), and a CBE factor for BPA in tumor of 3.8 (51). It must be stressed that the tissue distribution of the boron compound in humans must be similar to that in the experimental animal model in order to use the experimentally derived values for estimation of Gy-Eq doses in the clinical situation.

Follow-up on 38 patients treated in the BNL trial has recently been reported (57). These patients all had a gross or subtotal tumor resection at 3–5 weeks prior to BNCT. BPA–fructose was infused over 2 hours at doses in the range of 250–290 mg/kg. Epithermal neutron irradiation commenced at approximately 45 min after the end of the infusion and lasted for 38–65 min. The maximum radiation dose to 1 cm^3 of normal brain ranged from 8.9 to 14.8 Gy-Eq. The average doses to the entire brain volume ranged from 1.9–6.0 Gy-Eq. No treatment-related toxicities (grade 3 or 4) were observed. The median time to tumor progression was ~ 32 weeks, and the median survival time from diagnosis was 13 months. The conclusion from this series of patients was that the palliation afforded by a single session of BNCT was comparable to the palliation provided by conventional fractionated radiotherapy. The results indicate that further dose escalation to the limit of brain tolerance is warranted, and that implementation of a fractionation study to evaluate the potential benefits of BPA tumor retargeting is justified.

Table 16.4 Assumptions used in the clinical trial of BPA-based BNCT at Brookhaven National Laboratory for calculation of the $^{10}B(n, \alpha)$$^7Li$ component of the Gy-Eq dose in various tissues

Tissue	Boron concentration (ref.)	CBE factor (ref.)
Blood	Measure directly	
Brain	1.0 × blood (56, 61)	1.3 (42)
Scalp/skin	1.5 × blood (18, 56, 61)	2.5 (18)
Tumor	3.5 × blood (62)	3.8 (ref. 51)

Optimization of clinical BNCT

The most effective way to optimize BNCT is to maximize the preferential delivery of boron to the target tumor. Increasing the neutron exposure will increase the nonspecific background dose to the normal tissues and produce no net gain in the therapeutic ratio. A boron compound with a high degree of tumor specificity, long retention in the tumor, and complete clearance from blood and normal tissues would be optimal for BNCT, producing very substantial therapeutic ratios. In reality, compounds like BPA, capable of producing tumor-to-normal tissue boron concentration ratios of between 3:1 and 4:1, may be sufficient to prove the principle of BNCT. Any modality that can improve the tumor-to-normal tissue boron concentration ratios will improve the therapeutic gain significantly. Even if the tumor/blood boron concentration ratio remains fixed, the therapeutic ratio improves as more boron compound is administered and higher absolute boron concentrations are produced in both tumor and normal tissues. It is more important to have higher ^{10}B levels in the tumor at a fixed tumor-to-normal tissue ratio than lesser amounts of ^{10}B in the tumor (below the effective threshold) but very high tumor-to-normal-tissue ratios (39, 49). This is because the beam alone produces background doses in the normal tissues.

Future developments

Improved reactor-based epithermal neutron beams

Programs are underway at BNL and at MIT to significantly boost the epithermal neutron output of the existing clinical epithermal neutron beams. This will be achieved using a fission plate converter (FPC), which will have the effect of moving the source of fission neutrons closer to the moderator. Calculations indicate that the new epithermal beam with an FPC source will increase the epithermal flux of the present BMRR beam by a factor of 6 to 7 and reduce the fast neutron contaminants by ~30 per cent (per epithermal neutron). This will have a number of clinical benefits that include a reduction in treatment time (from 30–45 min to ~ 5 min), greatly improved depth–dose distribution, and a considerable reduction in beam contaminants.

Accelerator-based epithermal neutron beams

Research and development is progressing on non-reactor-based epithermal beams that can be deployed at hospital sites. Most attention is currently focused on proton beams of one or more milliamperes intensity, with lithium or beryllium as target materials for the generation of the epithermal neutron beam. The development of accelerator-based neutron beams for BNCT applications is an active area of research that is beyond the scope of this review. The interested reader is directed to the proceedings of a recent conference on this topic (63). A working, but relatively low-intensity, accelerator-based neutron facility is in place at MIT (64, 65).

New boron compounds

An optimal boron delivery agent needs to exhibit a range of key characteristics. These include low toxicity, high levels of accumulation in tumor and metastases (ideally in cell nuclei), and a lengthy tumor retention time to facilitate clearance from the blood and normal tissues. The objective of new boron compound development is to approach this ideal. A variety of boronated analogs of biomolecules have been synthesized as potential boron delivery agents, including amino acids, peptides, nucleic acid bases, nucleosides, carbohydrates, liposomes, low-density lipoproteins, porphyrins, monoclonal antibodies, and epidermal growth factors. The limited availability of many of these potentially interesting compounds has restricted detailed evaluation.

Optimization of boron delivery modalities

In experimental studies using a rat intracranial brain tumor model, it has been demonstrated that temporary disruption of the blood–brain barrier, using mannitol, can appreciably enhance the delivery of BPA to both the main tumor mass and the metastatic spread as well as improve the therapeutic efficacy of BNCT (6). More recently, similar effects have been reported after administration of the bradykinin analog RMP-7 (66). At the present time, both BSH and BPA are administered clinically (for BNCT of glioma) using intravenous infusion (7, 56, 57, 61, 67). Although this is the easiest route of delivery, it is not necessarily the most effective. Alternative approaches being investigated include intracarotid infusion, direct intratumoral injection, implantation of sustained release polymers, and convection-enhanced delivery (67).

Expansion of BNCT to other tumor types

It is probable that the remit of BNCT will be extended from glioma and melanoma to other types of neoplasm. These could include breast cancer, lung carcinomas, soft-tissue sarcomas, head and neck tumors, and primary hepatoma. However, future expansion of this therapeutic modality will depend upon the ability of existing or newly developed boron compounds to selectively target such tumors.

Acknowledgements

G.M.M. is supported by the UK Cancer Research Campaign. J.A.C. is supported by the Office of Biological and Environmental Research, US Department of Energy, under contract number DE-AC02-98CH10886.

References

1. Taylor HJ, Goldhaber M. Detection of nuclear disintegration in a photographic emulsion. Nature 1935, **135**, 341.

2. Soloway AH, Hatanaka H, Davis MA. Penetration of brain and brain tumor. VII. Tumor-binding sulfhydryl boron compounds. J Med Chem 1967, **10**, 714–17.

3. Bauer WF, Bradshaw KN, Richards TL. Interaction between boron containing compounds and serum albumin observed by nuclear magnetic resonance. In: Progress in neutron capture therapy for cancer (ed. BJ Allen, DE Moore, and BV Harrington). Plenum Press, New York, 1992, 339–43.

4. Soloway AL, Wright RL, Messer JR. Evaluation of boron compounds for use in neutron capture therapy of brain tumors. 1. Animal investigations. J Pharmacol Exp Therapeut 1961, **134**, 117–22.

5. Kraft SL, Gavin PR, DeHaan CE, et al. Borocaptate sodium—a potential boron delivery compound for boron neutron capture therapy evaluated in dogs with spontaneous intracranial tumors. Proc Natl Acad Sci, USA 1992, **89**, 11973–7.

6. Barth RF, Yang WL, Rotaru JH, et al. Boron neutron-capture therapy of brain tumors. Enhanced survival following intracarotid injection of either sodium borocaptate or boronophenylalanine with or without blood–brain-barrier disruption. Cancer Res 1997, **57**, 1129–36.

7. Hatanaka H, Nakagawa Y. Clinical results of long-surviving brain tumor patients who underwent boron neutron capture therapy. Int J Radiat Oncol Biol Phys 1994, **28**, 1061–6.

8. Gabel D, Preusse D, Haritz, D, et al. Pharmacokinetics of $Na_2B_{12}H_{11}SH$ (BSH) in patients with malignant brain tumors as prerequisite for a phase I clinical trial of boron neutron capture therapy. Acta Neurochir 1997, **139**, 606–12.

9. Ceberg CP, Brun A, Kahl SB, et al. A comparative study on the pharmacokinetics and biodistribution of boronated porphyrin (BOPP) and sulfhydryl boron hydride (BSH) in the RG2 rat glioma model. J Neurosurg 1995, **83**, 86–92.

10. Chandra S, Lorey DR, Lessig SL, et al. Quantitative imaging of boron from BPA and BSH in glioblastoma cells with ion microscopy. In: Advances in neutron capture therapy. Volume II, Chemistry and biology (ed. B. Larsson, J. Crawford, and R. Weinreich). Elsevier Science B.V., Lausanne, 1997, 315–20.

11. Zha X, Ausser WA, Morrison GH. Quantitative imaging of a radiotherapeutic drug, $Na_2B_{12}H_{11}SH$, at subcellular resolution in tissue cultures using ion microscopy. Cancer Res 1992, **52**, 5219–22.

12. Otersen B, Haritz D, Grochulla F, et al. Binding and distribution of $Na_2B_{12}H_{11}SH$ on cellular and subcellular level in tumor tissue of glioma patients in boron neutron capture therapy. J Neuro-Oncol 1997, **33**, 131–9.

13. Snyder HR, Reedy AH, Lennarz W. Synthesis of aromatic boronic acids. Aldehydo boronic acids and a boronic acid analog of tyrosine. J Am Chem Soc 1958, **80**, 835–8.

14. Mishima Y, Ichihashi M, Nakanishi T, et al. Cure of malignant melanoma by single thermal neutron capture treatment using melanoma seeking compounds:10-B/melanogenesis interaction to in vitro/in vivo radiobiological analysis to preclinical studies. In: Proceedings of the First International Symposium on Neutron Capture Therapy (ed. RG Fairchild and G Brownell). Brookhaven National Laboratory, Upton, 1983, 355–64.

15. Coderre JA, Joel DD, Micca PL, et al. Control of intracerebral gliosarcomas in rats by boron neutron capture therapy with p-boronophenylalanine. Radiat Res 1992, **129**, 290–6.

16. Saris SC, Solares GR, Wazer DE, et al. Boron neutron capture therapy for murine malignant gliomas. Cancer Res 1992, **52**, 4672–7.

17. Coderre JA, Glass JD, Fairchild RG, et al. Selective delivery of boron by the melanin precursor analog p-boronophenylalanine to tumors other than melanoma. Cancer Res 1990, **50**, 138–41.

18. Fukuda H, Hiratsuka J, Honda C, et al. Boron neutron capture therapy of malignant melanoma using ^{10}B-paraboronophenylalanine with special reference to evaluation of radiation dose and damage to the skin. Radiat Res 1994, **138**, 435–42.

19. Coderre JA, Glass JD, Fairchild RG, et al. Selective targeting of boronophenylalanine to melanoma for neutron capture therapy. Cancer Res 1987, **47**, 6377–83.

20. Coderre JA. A Phase 1 biodistribution study of p-boronophenylalanine. In: Boron neutron capture therapy: towards clinical trials of glioma with BNCT (ed. R. Moss and D. Gabel). Plenum Press, New York, 1992, 111–21.

21. Kabalka GW, Smith, GT, Dyke, JP, et al. Evaluation of fluorine-18-BPA-fructose for boron neutron capture treatment planning. J Nucl Med 1997, **38**, 1762–7.

22. Imahori Y, Ueda S, Ohmori Y, et al. Fluorine-18-labeled fluoroboronophenylalanine PET in patients with glioma. J Nucl Med 1998, **39**, 325–33.

23. Bennett BD, Mumford-Zisk J, Coderre JA, et al. Subcellular localization of p-boronophenylalanine-delivered boron-10 in the rat 9L gliosarcoma: cryogenic preparation in vitro and in vivo. Radiat Res 1994, **140**, 72–8.

24. Smith DR, Chandra S, Coderre JA, *et al.* Ion microscopy imaging of [10]B from *p*-boronophenylalanine in a brain tumor model for boron neutron capture therapy. Cancer Res 1996, **56**, 4302–6.

25. Soloway AH, Tjarks W, Barnum BA, *et al.* The chemistry of neutron capture therapy. Chem Rev 1998, **98**, 1515–62.

26. Feakes DA, Shelly K, Hawthorne MF. Selective boron delivery to murine tumors by lipophilic species incorporated in the membranes of unilamellar liposomes. Proc Natl Acad Sci, USA 1995, **92**, 1367–70.

27. Shelly K, Georgiev EM, Watson-Clark R, *et al.* Boron delivery to tumors for BNCT: recent murine results with liposomes. In: Advances in neutron capture therapy. Volume II, Chemistry and biology (ed. B. Larsson, J. Crawford, and R. Weinreich). Elsevier Science B.V., Lausanne, 1997, 357–61.

28. Miura M, Micca PL, Fisher CD, *et al.* Evaluation of carborane-containing porphyrins as tumor targeting agents for boron neutron capture therapy. Br J Radiol 1998, **71**, 773–81.

29. Moss RL, Aizawa O, Beynon D, *et al.* The requirements and development of neutron beams for neutron capture therapy of brain cancer. J Neuro-Oncol 1997, **33**, 27–40.

30. Liu H, Brugger R, Rorer D. Enhancement of the epithermal neutron beam at the Brookhaven Medical Research Reactor. In: Advances in neutron capture therapy (ed. A.H. Soloway, R.F. Barth, and D.E. Carpenter). Plenum Press, New York, 1993, 75–9.

31. Nigg DW, Wheeler FJ, Wessol DE, *et al.* Computational dosimetry and treatment planning for boron neutron capture therapy. J Neuro-Oncol 1997, **33**, 93–103.

32. Fairchild RG, Bond VP. Current status of [10]B boron neutron capture therapy: enhancement of tumor dose via beam filtration and dose rate, and the effects of these parameters on minimum boron content: a theoretical evaluation. Int J Radiat Oncol Biol Phys 1985, **11**, 831–40.

33. Verrijk R, Huiskamp R, Begg AC, *et al.* A comprehensive pc-based computer model for microdosimetry of BNCT. Int J Radiat Biol 1994, **65**, 241–53.

34. Morris GM, Coderre JA, Hopewell JW, *et al.* Response of rat skin to boron neutron capture therapy with *p*-boronophenylalanine or borocaptate sodium. Radiother Oncol 1994, **32**, 144–53.

35. Archambeau JO. The effect of increasing exposures of the[10]B(n,α) [7]Li reaction on the skin of man. Radiology 1970, **94**, 179–87.

36. Yamamoto YL. The biological effectiveness of thermal neutrons and of the heavy particles from the [10]B(n,α) [7]Li reaction for the rabbits ear and its utilization for neutron capture therapy. Yokohama Med Bull 1961, **12**, 4–22.

37. Gavin PR, Kraft SL, Huiskamp R, *et al.* A review: CNS effects and normal tissue tolerance in dogs. J Neuro-Oncol 1997, **33**, 71–80.

38. Morris GM, Smith DR, Patel H, *et al.* Boron microlocalization in oral mucosal tissue: implications for boron neutron capture therapy. Br J Cancer 2000, **82**, 1764–71.

39. Coderre JA, Morris GM. The radiation biology of boron neutron capture therapy. Radiat Res 1999, **151**, 1–18.

40. Rydin RA, Deutsch OL, Murray BW. The effect of geometry on capillary wall dose for boron neutron capture therapy. Phys Med Biol 1976, **21**, 134–8.

41. Morris GM, Coderre JA, Hopewell JW, *et al.* Boron neutron capture irradiation of the rat spinal cord: effects of variable doses of borocaptate sodium. Radiother Oncol 1996, **39**, 253–9.

42. Morris GM, Coderre JA, Hopewell JW, *et al.* Response of the central nervous system to boron neutron capture irradiation: evaluation using rat spinal cord model. Radiother Oncol 1994, **32**, 249–55.

43. Morris GM, Coderre JA, Micca, PL, *et al.* Central nervous system tolerance to boron neutron capture therapy with *p*-boronophenylalanine. Br J Cancer 1997, **76**, 1623–9.

44. Coderre JA, Morris GM, Micca PL, *et al.* Comparative assessment of single-dose and fractionated boron neutron capture therapy. Radiat Res 1995, **144**, 310–17.

45. Morris GM, Coderre JA, Hopewell JW, *et al.* Response of the central nervous system to fractionated boron neutron capture irradiation: studies with borocaptate sodium. Int J Radiat Biol 1997, **71**, 185–92.

46. Coderre JA, Slatkin, Micca PL, *et al.* Boron neutron capture therapy of a murine melanoma with para-boronophenylalanine: Dose response analysis using a morbidity index. Radiat Res 1991, **128**, 177–85.

47. Packer S, Coderre J, Saraf S, *et al.* Boron neutron capture therapy of anterior chamber melanoma with *p*-boronophenylalanine. Invest Ophthalmol Vis Sci 1992, **33**, 395–403.

48. Joel DD, Fairchild RG, Laissue JA, *et al.* Boron neutron capture therapy of intracerebral rat gliosarcomas. Proc Natl Acad Sci, USA 1990, **87**, 9808–12.

49. Coderre JA, Button TM, Micca PL, *et al.* Neutron capture therapy of the 9L rat gliosarcoma using the *p*-boronophenylalanine–fructose complex. Int J Radiat Oncol Biol Phys 1994, **30**, 643–52.

50. Matalka KZ, Bailey MQ, Barth RF, *et al.* Boron neutron capture therapy of intracerebral melanoma using boronophenylalanine as a capture agent. Cancer Res 1993, **53**, 3308–13.

51. Coderre JA, Makar MS, Micca PL, *et al.* Derivations of relative biological effectiveness for the high-LET radiations produced during boron neutron capture irradiations of the 9L rat gliosarcoma *in vitro* and *in vivo*. Int J Radiat Oncol Biol Phys 1993, **27**, 1121–9.

52. Farr LE, Sweet WH, Robertson JS, *et al.* Neutron capture therapy with boron in the treatment of glioblastoma multiforme. Am J Roentgenol 1954, **71**, 279–91.

53. Slatkin DN. A history of boron neutron capture therapy of brain tumors—postulation of a brain radiation dose tolerance limit. Brain 1991, **114**, 1609–29.

54. Curran WJ, Scott CB, Horton J, *et al.* Recursive partition analysis of prognostic factors in three radiation oncology group malignant glioma trials. J Natl Canc Inst 1993, **85**, 704–10.

55. Laramore GE, Spence AM. Boron neutron-capture therapy (BNCT) for high-grade gliomas of the brain—a cautionary note. Int J Radiat Oncol Biol Phys 1996, **36**, 241–6.

56. Coderre JA, Elowitz EE, Chadha M, *et al*. Boron neutron capture therapy of glioblastoma multiforme using the *p*-boronophenylalanine–fructose complex and epithermal neutrons: trial design and early clinical results. J Neuro-Oncol 1997, **33**, 141–52.

57. Chanana AD, Capala J, Chada M, *et al*. Boron neutron capture therapy for glioblastoma multiforme: interim results from the phase I/II dose-escalation studies. Neurosurgery 1999, **44**, 1–12.

58. Busse, PM., Zamenhof, RG , Madoc-Jones H, *et al*. Clinical follow-up of patients with melanoma of the extremity treated in a phase I boron neutron capture therapy protocol. In: Advances in neutron capture therapy. Vol. I, Medicine and physics (ed. B Larsson, J Crawford, and R Weinreich). Elsevier Science B.V., Amsterdam, 1997, 60–4.

59. Busse PM, Kaplan I, Zamenhof RG, *et al*. BNCT for glioblastoma multiforme and intracranial metastatic melanoma: clinical results of the Harvard–Massachusetts Institute of Technology (MIT) phase I trial. In: Proceedings of the Eighth International Symposium on Neutron Capture Therapy (ed. MF Hawthorne and K Shelly). Plenum, New York, in press.

60. Hideghety K, Sauerwein W, Haselsberger K, *et al*. Postoperative treatment of glioblastoma with BNCT at the Petten irradiation facility (EORTC protocol 11,961). Strahlenther Onkol 1999, **175** (suppl. 2), 111–14.

61. Elowitz EH, Bergland RM, Coderre JA,, *et al*. Biodistribution of *p*-boronophenylalanine (BPA) in patients with glioblastoma multiforme for use in boron neutron capture therapy. Neurosurgery 1998, **42**, 463–9.

62. Coderre JA, Chanana AD, Joel DD, *et al*. Biodistribution of boronophenylalanine in patients with glioblastoma multiforme: boron concentration correlates with tumor cellularity. Radiat Res 1998, **149**, 163–70.

63. Nigg DW. Proceedings of the First International Workshop on Accelerator-Based Neutron Sources for Boron Neutron Capture Therapy. Idaho National Engineering Laboratory, Report # CONF-940976, 1995.

64. Blackburn BW, Yanch JC, Klinkowstein RE. Development of a high-power water cooled beryllium target for use in accelerator-based boron neutron capture therapy. Med Phys 1998, **25**, 1967–74.

65. Klinkowstein RE, Shefer RE, Yanch JC, *et al*. Operation of a high current tandem electrostatic accelerator for boron neutron capture therapy. In: Advances in neutron capture therapy. Vol. I, Medicine and physics (ed. B Larsson, J Crawford, and R Weinreich). Elsevier Science B.V., Amsterdam, 1997, 522–7.

66. Barth RF, Yang W, Bartus RT, *et al*. Enhanced delivery of boronophenylalanine for neutron capture therapy of brain tumors using the bradykinin analog cereport (receptor-mediated permeabiliser-7). Neurosurgery 1999, **44**, 351–9.

67. Barth RF, Soloway AH, Goodman JH, *et al*. Boron neutron capture therapy of brain tumors: an emerging therapeutic modality. Neurosurgery 1999, **44**, 433–51.

Section V

17 | *Cancer immunotherapy directed at growth factor receptor: the erbB/HER network as a prototype*

Michael Sela, Bilha Schecheter, and Yosef Yarden

Introduction

Growth factors and their transmembrane receptors with intrinsic tyrosine kinase activity play a central role in the regulation of cell growth, migration, and interactions with neighboring cells. Because of their genetic alterations in human cancer and accessibility to extracellular manipulations, receptors of the erbB/HER family are attractive targets for cancer therapy. Here we concentrate on two erbB proteins, erbB-1 (epidermal growth factor receptor, EGFR) and erbB-2 (also called HER2), and review the current status of immunotherapeutic attempts to block cancers of various types by targeting signaling downstream to these receptors. Lessons gained in clinical applications of antibodies or their derivatives, as well as insights from experimental model systems, are expected to yield a new generation of cancer drugs whose targets and mechanisms of action are well defined at the molecular level.

Growth factors in cancer

The role played by growth factors in human cancer may be considered in light of their function in embryonic development as carriers of inductive interactions between juxtaposed cells of different origins. Often, these interactions culminate in cell cycle alterations and concomitant differentiation. An example relevant to carcinomas is the determination of epithelial identity b the underlying mesenchyme through the action of mesenchyme-derived growth factors (1). While in embryonic development most inductive interactions are paracrine, that is, the inductive (secreting) cell and the responding cell are daughters of different cell lineages. Autocrine mechanisms widely occur in tumors (2). In addition, tumor cells may express genetically altered versions of specific components of the signaling pathways activated by growth factors. For example, cells infected by oncogenic strains of retroviruses not only express constitutively active forms of signaling proteins such as receptors, adaptors, and transcription factors, but they are also endowed with potent autocrine loops (3).

One family of growth factors that has been repeatedly implicated in cancer is the EGF/neuregulin group. First described as part of the EGF precursor, this 50–60 amino acid long motif that includes six cysteine residues characterizes all growth factors of the family. Mammalian members of the family are usually processed from a transmembrane precursor (4) and travel a relatively short distance before they meet an erbB receptor at the surface of a responsive cell (*Note.* The terms HER and erbB are synonymous. Likewise, erbB-1 and erbB-2 are also called EGFR and Neu, respectively.) Beside EGF and the four neuregulins and their multiple isoforms, the family includes also transforming growth factor alpha (TGFα), betacellulin, epiregulin, and the heparin-binding EGF-like growth factor (HB-EGF). Expression of the latter ligand is higher in malignant cells relative to the surrounding tissues (5). Likewise, tumors of several origins overexpress TGFα (6), a ligand whose promoter is activated by several oncogenic viruses. Consistent with a role in gynecological and other cancers, expression of this ligand in certain tumors correlates with short patient survival and increased tumor size (7). Similar observations were reported in tumors of the pancreas, colon, ovary, and lung (reviewed in reference 8), but less information is available on other members of the EGF/neuregulin family.

Signal transduction by erbB proteins

All members of the EGF/neuregulin family bind to receptors of the erbB family, but each ligand displays specificity to one or more erbB proteins (9). The four erbB proteins share a transmembrane structure. The extracellular domain includes two stretches of cysteine-rich sequences that stabilize a ligand-binding site, whereas the cytoplasmic domain carries a large catalytic region that function as a tyrosine kinase. A juxtamembrane regulatory region and a hydrophilic carboxy terminus containing several tyrosine autophosphorylation sites flank the kinase domain. As is the case with other receptor tyrosine kinases, ligand binding to the extracellular domain of an erbB protein is followed by receptor dimerization and subsequent autophosphorylation (10). Phosphorylated tyrosine residues serve as reversible docking sites for cytoplasmic proteins containing a phosphotyrosine-binding motif (reviewed in reference 11). Once recruited to an active receptor, the signaling protein transforms to an active state and initiates a signaling cascade, resulting in a cellular output. Examples of such cascades include the mitogen-activated protein kinase (MAPK) pathway and the phosphatidyl inositol 3-kinase (PI3K) pathway, which control both cell survival and proliferation.

Although erbB-3 includes a tyrosine kinase domain, this function is catalytically inactive (12). On the other hand, erbB-2 seems to bind no known ligand with high affinity (13). Instead, this highly oncogenic protein acts as a shared signaling subunit of the other receptors (14). Thus, neither erbB-3 nor erbB-2 can function in isolation. However, when either receptor is engaged in ligand-promoted heterodimers, it initiates potent mitogenic signals (15). Heterodimerization is not limited to erbB-2 and erbB-3; all ten possible combinations of the four erbB proteins may exist, but erbB-2-containing heterodimers are preferred over other dimers (16, 17). As a result of ligand-induced dimerization and recruitment of different sets of signaling proteins to each o the nine functional receptor combinations, a richly interactive network is functional in erbB-expressing cells. The network configuration, as opposed to linear signaling pathways, offers large potential for diversification and tuning of the biochemical and cellular outputs (18).

erbB proteins in cancer

erbB-1

Cloning of the erbB-1 transcript from a vulval carcinoma cell line revealed dramatic overexpression, gene amplification, and genetic aberrations (19). *In vitro* studies and experiments performed in animals attributed to an overexpressed erbB-1 the ability to transform cells in culture, but co-expression of a ligand seemed essential (20, 21). In addition, overexpression of erbB-1 in murine cells grown in animals confers to them resistance to radiotherapy (22). The original observation made with a vulval cell line has later been extended to a number of solid tumors, including head and neck, gastric, ovarian, renal and bladder, prostate, esophageal, and pancreatic cancer (reviewed in reference 8). In advanced breast cancer, overexpression of erbB-1 can predict overall patient survival (23). Similarly, erbB-1 is overexpressed in more than 50 per cent of renal cell carcinoma, and overexpression correlates with poor clinical outcome. One study correlated co-overexpression of erbB-1 and erbB-2 with tumor grade, a dedifferentiated phenotype, and metastasis (24). Other tumors in which erbB-1 may serve as a prognostic marker are those of the bladder, prostate, kidney, and lung. However, although overexpression of erbB-1 is frequent in many types of carcinomas and in some cases correlates with overexpression of one of its ligands, namely TGFα, association with an aggressive tumor behavior is not always clear. For example, analysis of 57 non-small cell lung cancers (NSCLC) revealed no correlation between overexpression of erbB-1, or two of its ligands, with tumor stage or overall survival (25). The majority of studies indicate that erbB-1 can provide valuable prognostic information in ovarian, cervical, and possibly head and neck cancer. Significant associations between the status of erbB-1 and recurrence-free survival and overall survival were observed in these tumors. However, in another class of tumors, which includes breast, endometrial, bladder, and colorectal cancer, the prognostic value of erbB-1 is less clear.

Amplification of the erbB-1 gene occurs in 40 per cent of gliomas (26) and overexpression of the receptor correlates with higher tumor grade and higher cell proliferation. Mutations frequently associate with the amplified gene. A relatively minor class of mutations affects the 3′ portion of the transcript (27). As a result, internal deletions remove a portion of the carboxy terminus involved in negative regulation of the receptor (28), including a c-Cbl association site (29). The most frequently observed mutation (type III) deletes amino acids 6–276 of the extracellular domain (30) and enhances tumorigenicity (31). This mutation is frequent not only in gliomas but also in breast carcinomas, lung tumors, and ovarian cancers (32). Although the mutant receptor is defective in ligand binding, its kinase function is hyperactive, presumably due to constitutive dimerization. Thus, the oncogenic fusion protein, which encodes a tumor-specific sequence, is an attractive target for immunotherapy (33).

erbB-2

As in the case of erbB-1, an oncogenic mutant of erbB-2 has been identified in rodents (34). The point mutation affects a transmembrane residue and results in constitutive activation of the tyrosine kinase (35). No similar mutation has been found in human cancer, but overexpression of the erbB-2 gene, primarily as a result of gene amplification, is frequently observed in human carcinomas (reviewed in reference 36 and 37). Examples include breast, ovarian, and lung cancer, tumors of the pancreas, colon, esophagus, prostate, endometrium, and cervix. Ubiquitous, but low, expression of erbB-2 characterizes all types of epithelia, and in most cases the major partners of erbB-2, namely, erbB-3 and erbB-1, are co-expressed. Although several types of cancers present high expression of erbB-2, only in a few cases has an association between overexpression and poor prognosis been demonstrated. A significant fraction of ovarian cancers overexpresses erbB-2, and in some studies this has been associated with p21-Ras, p53, and worse prognosis (38). The association of erbB-2 expression with disease parameters is by far better studied in the case of breast cancers (for a recent review see reference 37). The protein is overexpressed as a result of gene amplification in 15–30 per cent of invasive ductal cancers. The incidence is higher in the relatively aggressive inflammatory breast cancer (39) and, in ductal carcinoma *in situ* (DCIS) of the comedo type, overexpression is detected in up to 90 per cent of cases (40). Paget's disease, an aggressive type of DCIS, often overexpresses erbB-2, but overexpression is significantly lower in infiltrating ductal cancer, the probable outcome of DCIS. These observations and the association of overexpression

with tumor size, lymph node status, high grade, high percentage of S-phase cells, aneuploidy, and lack of steroid hormone receptors imply that erbB-2 confers to tumor cells primarily a proliferative, rather than an invasive advantage. The prognostic value of erbB-2 has been a matter of some controversy. Following the first evidence of an association between overexpression and poor prognosis of breast cancer patients (41), it became clear that the prognostic value of erbB-2 is more significant in patients whose cancer cells metastasized to the lymph nodes. Association with shorter disease-free survival, overall patient survival, and even shorter time to relapse was noted when relatively large (> 200 patients) and randomized groups of patients were analyzed (for an example see reference 42). The prognostic value of erbB-2 in node-negative patients is less clear. However, careful analyses of overexpression by using fluorescence *in situ* hybridization (FISH) and large patient populations support the prognostic value of gene amplification in node-negative patients and its ability to predict recurrence (43).

Several studies have shown that erbB-2 overexpression is associated with resistance of cancer patients to anti-estrogen therapy, even in steroid hormone-positive cases. The majority of erbB-2-overexpressing tumors do not express the estrogen and progesterone receptors, indicating inverse relationships between the steroid axis and signaling by the erbB network. Clinically, this cross-talk may be critical: patients treated in the adjuvant setting with or without an anti-estrogen drug (tamoxifen) had worse outcome of the drug if their tumors overexpressed erbB-2 (reviewed in reference 44). The prospect that erbB-2 overexpression can predict patient response to specific chemotherapeutic drugs may have a great clinical impact. Several retrospective studies of breast cancer patients treated with specific drugs (for example, doxorubicin and taxol) and recent applications of combined immunotherapy–chemotherapy protocols demonstrate the importance of the issue. Unlike erbB-2 non-overexpressing patients, treatment of overexpressors with a high dose of doxorubicin, and two other drugs, almost doubled their overall survival relative to patients treated with a low dose (45). The conclusion that erbB-2 overexpression confers sensitivity to high-dose doxorubicin was supported by studies that managed to isolate the effect of doxorubicin and used a long follow-up (46, 47). The mechanism underlying these clinical observations is unknown, but an indirect mechanism involving topoisomerase II, an intracellular target of doxorubicin, has been proposed (48). Less studied are the associations between erbB-2 overexpression in metastatic breast cancer and relatively high response to taxanes (49) and lower response to methotrexate. In the case of taxanes, *in vitro* studies point to an opposite effect: overexpression conferred resistance to taxol (50) through an effect of erbB-2 on p21-WAF (51).

erbB-3 and erbB-4

Unlike erbB-4, whose expression in human carcinomas is limited and relatively low, the catalytically inactive member of the erbB family, erbB-3, is abundantly expressed in several carcinomas (for example, breast, colon, and gastric tumors). Although no mutants of erbB-3 or erbB-4 have been reported in cancers, it is of relevance that alternative splicing generates several types of the erbB-4 protein. Splicing affects the extracellular domain, a site of proteolysis by an ecto-kinase (52, 53), as well as the cytoplasmic domain. The latter differentially affects of docking site for PI3K and confers cell migration in response to a ligand of erbB-4 (54). Overexpression of erbB-3 in oral squamous cell cancer has been correlated with lymph node involvement and patient survival (55), and a recent study found that co-expression of erbB-2 with erbB-1 or erbB-3 can improve the clinical predicting power (56). A paracrine loop involving erbB-3 has been noted in prostate cancer (57). The function of the other neuregulin receptor seems to be different, and perhaps more associated with differentiation. Thus, when expressed in PC12 cells and stimulated with NRG1, erbB-4 promoted cellular differentiation (58). An association between erbB-4 expression and a relatively differentiated histological phenotype has been reported in breast cancers (59). However, co-expression of erbB-4 with erbB-2 has a prognostic value in childhood medulloblastomas (60). Clearly, more studies on the relevance of the two neuregulin receptors to human cancers are needed.

Immunotherapy with unarmed antibodies directed at erbB proteins

The targeting properties of the immune system offer an attractive approach for improving the selectivity of antitumor therapies. The immune system is capable of exquisite sensitivity ad specificity, and these properties could be harnessed with therapeutic benefits. In principle, patients could be immunized against tumor antigens and antibodies could be used to directly modulate tumor functions, to promote tumor lysis by immune effector cells, and to deliver radionuclides and toxins, as well as chemotherapeutic drugs. The apparent correlation between erbB expression and human cancer has attracted attention to these molecules as potential targets for the development of therapeutic modalities. Being mostly correlated to aggressiveness and poor prognosis of epithelial cancers, erbB-2 has been the focus of most of the attempts, utilizing strategies directed to inhibit its activity, including the promotion of specific immunity (61, 62).

Antibodies directed at erbB-1

Antibodies that can block the biological activities of growth factor receptors are expected to alter autocrine and paracrine loops. The rationale that inhibition of specific ligand–receptor interactions can decrease the mitogenic signaling of erbB receptors led to the development of several types of antibodies adequate and beneficial for human treatment (63). Monoclonal antibodies (mAbs) to erbB-1 were shown to bind to several solid tumors to a much higher extent than to normal cells. A radiolabeled mAb 108.4, raised against the extracellular domain of EGFR, was bound to xenografts of human oral epidermoid carcinoma (KB) cells in athymic nude mice (64). These anti-EGFR antibodies interfered with clonal growth *in vitro*, but the addition of the 108.4 mAb resulted in an 80 per cent decrease in the number of colonies. Antitumor activity of an antibody against erbB-1 expressed in KB tumors was demonstrated by several criteria: retardation of tumor growth when xenografted subcutaneously into athymic mice; prolongation of the life span of animals carrying intraperitoneal tumors; and reduction in the number and size of tumors in an experimental lung metastasis model (64). The antitumor effect persisted when mice were treated with the F(ab')$_2$ fragment of the antibody, although it was less efficient. The monovalent Fab fragment of the antibody, which conserved its ability to bind to the cell-associated receptor, did not affect the growth of the tumor. Activity manifested by the F(ab')$_2$ fragment of the anti-EGF receptor antibodies suggested that the antitumor effect was not due to immune mechanisms requiring the Fc portion of the antibody.

The most extensively studied mAbs to erbB-1 are 528-IgG2a and 225-IgG1 (65, 66). Comparison of their activities *in vitro* and in animals implied that 528-IgG recruited immunological mechanisms more efficiently than the 225-IgG, which seems to directly alter erbB-1 functions (67). This murine mAb was chimerized for use in cancer patients. The anti-erbB-1 binding region was linked to the constant region of human IgG1 in order to increase its clinical adequacy by decreasing the potential for generation of human anti-mouse antibodies. This chimeric antibody, termed C225, which is apparently well tolerated in patients receiving repeated administrations, was shown to exert a significant antitumor activity against a variety of cultured and xenografted cancer cell lines (68). It could successfully target primary lung cancers and metastasis (69), and was found effective in the treatment of human prostate carcinoma xenografts in athymic mice (68). Other erbB-1-specific mAbs were assessed in phase I clinical studies for their safety and efficient binding in patients suffering from malignant gliomas (70), NSCLC (71), and head and neck cancer (72). In a series of studies by Mendelsohn and his colleagues, where the C225 antibodies were investigated in a model of A431 tumor xenografted in athymic mice, it was found that the chimeric C225 counterpart was more effective than the murine 225 mAb (73). It was suggested that the increased capacity of chimeric C225 (cetuximab) to compete with ligands for binding to erbB-1 was responsible for its enhanced *in vivo* antitumor effect. However, comparison of the *in vitro* effects of bivalent and monovalent fragments of antibody 225 failed to correlate inhibition of ligand-binding with a capacity to inhibit cell growth (74). Instead, the ability of the antibody to dimerize erbB-1 and thereby increase its downregulation seems essential for the growth inhibitory effect.

erbB-1-directed therapy could also exert its effect by impairing angiogenesis and production of angiogenic factors associated with tumor growth and metastasis, as shown for human transitional cell carcinoma (TCC) of the bladder (75). *In vitro* treatment with a chimeric C225 antibody inhibited mRNA and protein synthesis of the vascular endothelial growth factor (VEGF), interleukin 8 (IL-8), and basic fibroblast growth factor (bFGF) by the TCC cells in a dose-dependent manner. Likewise, intraperitoneal treatment of established tumors with the chimeric C225 mAb resulted in inhibition of growth and metastasis accompanied by a decrease in VEGF, IL-8, and bFGF expression. The downregulation of these angiogenic factors preceded the involution of blood vessels. It thus seems that the antitumor effect of the chimeric C225 may be partially

due to inhibition of angiogenesis. This finding was substantiated by a study showing that the chimeric C225 inhibited pancreatic carcinoma growth and metastasis in an orthotopic athymic mouse model via tumor-mediated angiogenesis. This effect was potentiated by gemcitabine, resulting in additive cytotoxic effects that increased with increasing gemcitabine concentrations (76).

A fully human IgG2 kappa mAb, E7.6.3, specific to the human erbB-1, was generated from human antibody-producing Xeno mouse strains. These strains were engineered to be deficient in mouse antibody production and contain the majority of the human antibody gene repertoire on megabase-sized fragments from the human heavy and kappa light chain loci (77). The antibody could completely prevent the formation of human epidermoid carcinoma xenografts in athymic mice. Moreover, the administration of E7.6.3 without concomitant chemotherapy resulted in complete eradication of established tumors. Being a fully human antibody, E7.6.3 is expected to exhibit minimal immunogenicity and longer half-life as compared with mouse or mouse-derived antibodies.

It has been shown that antibodies specific to a mutated erbB-1 are effective in the central nervous system (33). As discussed above, erbB-1 is often amplified and rearranged in malignant gliomas and in some carcinomas. The most common mutation in brain tumors, EGFRvIII, is characterized by an in-frame deletion of 801 base pairs, resulting in the generation of a novel tumor-specific epitope at the fusion junction. A murine homolog of the human EGFRvIII mutation was prepared, and an IgG2a murine mAb Y10 was generated that recognizes the human and murine equivalents of this tumor-specific antigen. *In vitro*, Y10 was found to inhibit DNA synthesis and cellular proliferation, and to induce autonomous, complement-mediated, and antibody-dependent cell-mediated cytotoxicity. Intraperitoneal treatment with Y10 of subcutaneous B16 melanoma, transfected to express stably the murine EGFRvIII, led to long-term survival. The same treatment failed to increase survival of mice with EGFRvIII-expressing B16 melanomas in the brain, but treatment with a single intratumoral injection increased median survival by almost fourfold with 26 per cent long-term survivors.

Lastly, overexpression of erbB-1 and erbB-2 may both contribute to the growth of human cancer. The anti-erbB-1 chimeric C225 and a humanized anti-erbB-2 antibody 4D5 were examined for concurrent treatment of human ovarian cancer cells (78). The combination treatment resulted in additive anti-proliferative effects leading to growth arrest at the G_1 phase of the cell cycle. Concomitantly, the authors reported elevated expression of the p27 inhibitor and its association with cyclin-dependent kinases, CGK2, CDK4, and CDK6, and a greater decrease in the activities of these CDKs.

Antibodies directed at erbB-2

Among the members of the erbB receptor family, erbB-2 undoubtedly plays a paramount role, notwithstanding the fact that it is an orphan receptor and is capable of acting only upon heterodimerizing with another erbB receptor (erbB-1, erbB-3, or erbB-4). Antibodies directed to the rat ortholog of erbB-2, namely, Neu, effectively inhibited tumorigenicity of cells expressing the oncogenic mutant of Neu (79, 80) and thus opened the way for the generation of several antibodies specific to the human protein. Successful inhibition of tumor growth has been accomplished by the use of mAbs that specifically recognize erbB-2 in either a conventional athymic murine system or in a transgenic animal model of breast cancer (81). The immunological approach has been extended to patients. A phase II clinical trial revealed that a humanized antibody was clinically active in patients with erbB-2-overexpressing metastatic breast cancers (82). Following clinical testing of an anti-erbB-2 antibody as a single agent, several studies examined its effect in combination with cisplatin, paclitaxel, or anthracyclines. These studies have led to the approval in 1998 of one antibody, Herceptin/trastuzumab, for treatment of breast cancer patients, and by the end of 2000 close to 30 000 women had been treated with the recombinant drug.

Mechanisms underlying tumor inhibition

Possible mechanisms underlying the antitumorigenic effect are constantly challenged. Different antibodies directed against the extracellular domain of the receptor have been shown to both decrease and increase receptor phosphorylation (83), implying that simple inhibition of an evoked signaling cascade cannot explain the outcome. Indeed, opposing *in vivo* effects were observed with a panel of mAbs specific to the extracellular portion of the erbB-2 protein (83). Although some antibodies almost completely inhibited the growth of transfected murine fibroblasts that overexpress erbB-2, other antibodies either accelerated tumor growth or resulted in intermediate response. Of particular interest is the capability of inhibitory antibodies to downregulate the receptor from the cell surface (84). When human tumor cells (grown as xenografts in athymic mice) were incubated with three different radiolabeled antibodies, it was found that all three tumor-inhibitory antibodies rapidly disappeared from the cell surface, that is, became inaccessible to acidic dissociation due to their endocytosis. However, a tumor-stimulatory antibody remained accessible to extracellular acidic treatment, indicating that endocytosis did not take place. In addition, intracellular fragments of the inhibitory mAbs, but not of the stimulatory antibodies, were identified, indicating proteolytic degradation of the receptor following internalization. Electron microscopy of colloidal gold–antibody conjugates confirmed the absence of endocytosis of the stimulatory antibody but detected endocytic vesicles containing the inhibitory antibody (84). Consistent with an endocytic mechanism, combinations of mAbs that better arrest tumor growth were found to be relatively effective in degrading the oncoprotein (85). An alternative explanation of a decreased signaling capacity may be due to destabilization of heterodimeric complexes (86). One group of tumor-inhibitory antibodies that was elicited against the most antigenic site of erbB-2 inhibited in *trans* binding of neuregulins and EGF to their direct receptors. The inhibitory effect was due to acceleration of ligand dissociation and resulted in reduced ability of erbB-2 to transactivate the mitogenic signals of the ligands. These results identify two potential mechanisms of antibody-induced therapy: acceleration of erbB-2 endocytosis by homodimerization and blocking of heterodimerization between erbB-2 and the other growth factor receptors.

To get a better insight into the mechanism underlying receptor downregulation by anti-erbB-2 antibodies, Klapper *et al.* (87) studied the antibody- and EGF-induced degradation of erbB-2, showing that enhanced degradation is preceded by polyubiquitination of erbB-2. This process necessitates recruitment of the c-Cb1 ubiquitin ligase (29, 88) to tyrosine 1112 of erbB-2. Consequently, mutagenesis of this site retards antibody-induced degradation. Thus, the therapeutic potential of certain antibodies may be due to their ability to direct erbB-2 to a c-Cb1-regulated proteolytic pathway. It was previously shown that c-Cb1 undergoes rapid and sustained phosphorylation of tyrosine residues upon stimulation of fibroblast and epithelial cell lines with ligands of erbB-1, but not by neuregulin activation of erbB-3 or erbB-4 (89).

Recently, it was established that c-Cb1 is a suppressor of the rat *neu* oncogene (90). The oncogenic form of Neu is constitutively associated with the product of the c-Cb1 proto-oncogene, and is part of a large complex that includes the phosphoinositide 3 kinase and Shc. Ectopic expression of c-Cb1 caused rapid removal of the Neu protein from the cell surface and severely reduced signaling downstream of oncogenic *neu*. c-Cb1-induced downregulation of Neu involves covalent attachment of ubiquitin molecules and requires the carboxy terminal domain of Neu. In an *in vivo* model, infection of a Neu-transformed neuroblastoma with a c-Cb1-encoding retrovirus caused enhanced downregulation of Neu and correlated with tumor retardation (90).

Anti-erbB-2 antibodies have also been shown to affect the progression of the cell cycle, wither by inducing differentiation (91, 92) or by driving cells towards apoptosis (93). To understand the cellular mechanisms underlying antibody-induced tumor inhibition, the effect of the mAb was tested on various cultured human breast cancer cells (94). The tumor-inhibitory antibodies specifically induced phenotypic cellular differentiation, which included growth arrest at late S or early G_2, marked alterations of cytoplasm and nuclear morphology, synthesis and secretion of milk components (casein and lipids), and translocation of the erbB-2 protein to cytoplasmic and perinuclear sites (92). The extent of cellular differentiation by various antibodies could be correlated with their tumor-inhibitory potential, whereas a tumor-stimulatory mAb and control immunoglobulins were completely inactive with respect to cellular differentiation. Other *in vitro* effects of anti-erbB-2 antibodies include reversed cytokine resistance, restored cadherin expression levels, and reduced VEGF production (94).

Modification of naked antibodies with PEG

In order to facilitate the activity of anti-erbB-2 mAbs and to evaluate the possibility of using Fab fragments of the antibody, poly (ethylene glycol) (PEG) modification was introduced. PEGylation of substances was reported to improve their pharmacokinetic properties, due to prolongation of *in vivo* half-life, decreased immunogenic properties, enhanced penetration into growing solid tumors, and extended antitumor effects. Accordingly, PEG was introduced as a modifier to two types of mAbs specific to the erbB-2 (HER-2) oncoprotein that suppress the growth of tumors overexpressing erbB-2 (for example, N87

human gastric tumor cells) (95). The effect of PEG on their antitumor activity was evaluated. A branched *N*-hydroxysuccinimide-activated PEG (PEG2), conjugated through amino groups of the protein, was used for binding to the whole antibody (Ab) or to its monomeric Fab' fragment. When tested against N87 cells *in vitro*, the binding activity and antitumor cytotoxic effects of Ab–PEG2 were mostly preserved. PEG2 modification did not seem to alter the tumor-inhibitory activity of the antibodies *in vivo*, and the same pattern of tumor development was observed during the first few weeks following administration. However, the stimulating effects of PEG were manifested at later stages of tumor growth, since tumor development was either slowed down or completely arrested. Furthermore, a second tumor implanted into the same mice during this later stage was significantly or completely inhibited as compared to those in mice treated with the unmodified antibody. The Fab'–PEG2 monomeric derivative was also shown to be effective in inhibiting the growth of a second tumor. The extended and prolonged enhancing effect of PEG on the antitumor activity of antibodies or Fab' fragments directed against erbB-2 may be of importance in the development of treatment modalities based on erbB-2-overexpressing neoplasms.

Vaccination against erbB-2

Patients with erbB-2-positive cancers have been occasionally shown to develop an immune response against the protein (96), suggesting that antireceptor vaccines could be successful in evoking an anticancer response. The high expression of erbB-2 on cancer cells, in comparison to that on normal tissues, suggests that such a response could be preferentially directed against malignancies with no or negligible autoimmune toxicity. Originally, murine tumors overexpressing the rat oncogenic *neu* were successfully treated by immunization with a vaccinia virus recombinant of the protein's extracellular domain (97). Peptides from both intracellular (98, 99) and extracellular (100) portions of the receptor can elicit in cancer patients a specific response of cytotoxic T lymphocytes (CTL). Tolerance to self-proteins has been suggested to depend upon dominant epitopes allowing the promotion of an immune response to such molecules, mainly by the exposure of subdominant epitopes (101). Accordingly, immunizing rats with peptides derived from the self-antigen, namely, rat Neu, but not with the whole protein, can promote antibody and T-cell responses against the native protein (102). Similar peptides, derived from the murine erbB-2, could induce CTL activity resulting in the suppression of growth of receptor-overexpressing cells in syngeneic hosts (103).

In order to confer erbB-2 recognition to T cells without the need for antigen processing, while circumventing MHC restriction, chimeric antibodies against erbB-2 fused to the signaling subunit of the T cell receptor were designed (104). Adoptive transfer of the CTLs could markedly inhibit the growth of erbB-2 transformed cells in athymic mice (105) and in a syngeneic immunocompetent model 106). erbB-2-specific targeting and activation of T cells could also be achieved by fusing an antibody specific for erbB-2 to a sequence encoding the extracellular domain of the B7-1 (107) or B7-2 (108) T-cell co-stimulatory proteins. A similar methodology is utilized to attract and activate additional arms of the immunological response, including monocytes and macrophages. A bispecific antibody, directed against erbB-2 and the Fc-gamma-RIII receptor, and systematically administered to severe combined immunodeficiency (SCID) mice bearing ovarian cancer, significantly improved survival, while associated with no observed toxicity (109). This encouraged a phase I clinical trial and future studies are contemplated (110). Similarly, antibodies directed against Fc-gamma-RI receptor and erbB-2 or erbB-1 were evaluated in phase II clinical trials for treatment of a variety of neoplasms (111), showing a promising range of responses as expressed by a reduction in metastasis and serum markers. A phase I study of a bispecific antibody to erbB-2 and the granulocyte colony-stimulating factor in patients with metastatic breast cancer that overexpresses erbB-2 has been reported (112). A total of 23 patients were treated, and several variables were quantified. No objective clinical responses were seen in this group of heavily pre-treated patients.

Antigenic epitopes of erbB-2

Epitopes on erbB-2 that lead to mAb generation appear to be conformation- and not amino acid sequence-dependent. In order to obtain peptides of specificity similar to that of conformation-dependent epitopes, recourse was made to phage display libraries. A phage clone was isolated that competes with the binding of an anti erbB-2 mAb to tumor cells overexpressing erbB-2 (112). In another study, a free peptide, deduced from the sequence of the isolated phage clones, was synthesized (113). The isolated mimotope specifically inhibited the binding of mAb L26 to erbB-2-overexpressing cells. These results open the possibility of active immu-

nization with conformation-mimicking peptides against erbB-2-overexpressing tumors. Another approach was to look for a small peptide mimetic that could replace the complete anti-erbB-2 antibody (114). Using a structure-based approach, a small exocyclic anti-erbB-2 peptide mimic of Herceptin that specifically binds to erbB-2 with high affinity, has been identified. This resulted in inhibition of proliferation of erbB-2-overexpressing tumor cells, inhibition of colony formation, and retardation of erbB-2-expressing tumors in athymic mice.

Antibodies to an active erbB-2

An interesting study introduced the PN2A mAb, which recognizes Neu only in the phosphorylated and, therefore, actively signaling state (115). Immunohistochemistry using PN2A demonstrated that Neu actively signals in the tumors of Neu transgenic mice and that the expression of Neu is always accompanied by co-overexpression of the endogenous erbB-1. Similar results were found in mammary tumors from mice bitransgenic for *neu* and TGFα (both driven by the mouse mammary tumor virus promoter). Early mammary lesions demonstrated distinctive patterns of Neu activation relative to expression levels. Overexpression and activation were separable both temporally and spatially. These results refine the multi-step model for the role of Neu in mammary neoplasia and establish phosphorylation-state-specific antibodies as a powerful tool for investigating tumor progression.

Intracellular antibodies to erbB-2

Several studies were directed towards making use of single-chain Fv (scFv) fragments of antibodies. In order to enhance the specific retention of scFv in tumors, mutants of the human anti-erbB-2 scFv were generated by site-directed mutagenesis (116). *In vitro*, the dissociation constant, K_d, of each scFv closely correlated with the duration of its retention on the surface of human ovarian carcinoma SK-OV-3 cells overexpressing erbB-2. In biodistribution studies performed in SCID mice bearing established SK-OV-3 tumors, the degree and specificity of tumor localization increased significantly with increasing affinity. Since rapid renal clearance of scFv may blunt the impact of improved affinity on tumor targeting, the distributions were also assayed in the absence of renal clearance. In this model, the peak tumor retention of the two higher-affinity scFv molecules approximated that reported previously for IgG targeting the same SK-OV-3 tumors in SCID mice with intact kidneys. In contrast, the mutant with the lowest affinity for erbB-2 failed to accumulate in the tumor, indicating the presence of an affinity threshold that must be exceeded for active *in vivo* tumor uptake and specific retention of the scFv molecules. In another study (117) the same scFv molecules were dimerized to yield 'diabodies'. These had greater affinity and significantly prolonged association with the antigen on the surface of SK-OV-3 tumors in SCID mice.

To shed more light on the mechanism by which erbB-2 mediates tumor proliferation, the receptor was functionally inactivated using an intracellularly expressed scFv (118). Inducible expression of scFv-5R in the erbB-2-overexpressing SKBr-3 breast tumor cell line led to loss of plasma-membrane-localized erbB-2 (119). Simultaneously, activity of erbB-3, MAP kinase, and PKB/Akt decreased dramatically, suggesting that active erbB-2/erbB-3 dimers are necessary for sustained activity of these kinases. Loss of functional erbB-2 caused the SKBr-3 tumor cells to accumulate in the G_1 phase of the cell cycle. The scFv-5R was also expressed in the erbB-2-overexpressing ovarian carcinoma SK-OV-3 cell line with prominent suppression of the c-erbB-2 gene product and decreased transformation abilities, but no decrease in proliferation and secretion of proteases (120). It was concluded that the expression of the oncogene product offers a strong growth advantage, since, in contrast to the parental SK-OV-3 cells, the growth of the scFv-5R-expressing clones was impaired.

Preclinical and clinical testing of Herceptin

The mouse mAb 4D5, directed against the extracellular region of HER2, was found to be a potent inhibitor of the growth of human breast cancer cells that express HER2 (121). Unfortunately, administration of mouse antibodies in humans is limited due tot their immunogenicity. To allow the use of this antibody in human clinical investigation, 4D5 was humanized by inserting its murine erbB-2 antigen-binding regions into the framework of a human immunoglobulin molecule (122). The resulting recombinant humanized anti-erbB-2 antibody, termed Herceptin/Trastuzumab, exhibited higher affinity for erbB-2 than the mouse 4D5 antibody and a similar growth-inhibitory activity. The administration of Herceptin prolongs the survival of mice carrying erbB-2-expressing tumors. To increase the therapeutic potential of Herceptin, clinical strategies that combine the antibody therapeutic potential with

chemotherapeutic agents have been employed. In preclinical studies, both *in vitro* and in xenografted tumors, Herceptin markedly potentiated the antitumor effects of several chemotherapeutic agents, including cisplatin, doxorubicin, and paclitaxel, without an apparent increase in toxicity (123). In most cases, the effects of the antibody and the cytotoxic agent were at least additive. Data from these studies suggest that anti-erbB-2 antibodies can interfere with DNA repair mechanisms in cells that overexpress the oncoprotein (124).

The first phase II trial that examined Herceptin recruited 46 patients with erbB-2-overexpressing breast metastases, most having received prior therapy (82). Objective response was observed in 5 cases, and minor response or stable disease was observed in 16 patients. Two larger studies (125, 126) that tested Herceptin as a single agent and used a similar design reported 15 and 23 per cent response rates, respectively. However, these three initial studies uncovered two limitations. First, some patients displayed high levels of circulating erbB-2. This correlated with decreased half-life of the antibody and abolished clinical response. Second, although toxicity was mild, a minority of patients experienced cardiac toxicity. The reason for a possible effect of Herceptin on heart function is unknown, but it may relate to prior chemotherapeutic treatment of the patients involved. Additional successful trials with Herceptin, including combinations with chemotherapy (127), led to the approval in September, 1998 of Herceptin (Trastuzumab; Genentech, San Franciso, CA) by the United States Food and Drug Administration for the treatment of erbB-2-positive metastatic breast cancer as first-line therapy in combination with paclitaxel, and as a single agent for patients who have received one or more chemotherapy regimens for metastatic disease. Herceptin is the first biological agent to show favorable clinical results in slowing the progression of breast cancer. The achievements of Herceptin offer a new prospect for a class of more specific, less toxic therapies for the treatment of cancer.

Circulating erbB-2 and antibodies

Despite the fact that erbB-2 is a normal unmutated self-antigen, significant antibody responses have been observed in association with breast cancer. Disis *et al.* showed titers greater than 1:100 in 20 per cent of erbB-2-expressing breast carcinoma patients(128), with several of the patients having titers greater than 1:5000. As mentioned above, tumors expressing erbB-2 were found to release a soluble factor that corresponds to the extracellular domain of erbB-2 (129, 130). Circulating erbB-2 itself, at serum levels greater than 120 fmol/ml, was shown to serve as a negative prognostic factor for disease-free survival (131), poor prognosis in breast or ovarian cancer (132–139), and was correlated with larger tumor size and nodal status (138, 139) was well as decreased response to hormonal treatment (133). Yet, in many of the studies cited, this was independent of the detection of erbB-2 on tumor specimens themselves by immunohistochemistry.

Antibodies directed at the neuregulin receptors erbB-3 and erbB-4

As mentioned earlier, the group of subtype I receptor tyrosine kinases includes the epidermal growth factor (EGF) receptor (erbB-1), an orphan receptor (erbB-2), and two receptors for neuregulins, namely, erbB-4, mAbs to erbB-3 and erbB-4, generated through immunization with recombinant ectodomains of the receptors fused to immunoglobulin molecules, activated the catalytic site and induced downregulation of Erb-4 but not of erbB-3 (140). Apparently, the inability to stimulate and downregulate erbB-3 is a result of the inactive kinase function of erbB-3 and a defect in lysosomal targeting after endocytosis (141). By using these antibodies it was found that the effect of neuregulin-1 on differentiation of breast tumor cells can be mimicked by anti-erbB-4 antibodies, but not by mAbs to erbB-3. By contrast, another group has reported that an anti-erbB-3 antibody can modestly but significantly stimulate the anchorage-independent cloning efficiency of breast tumor cells expressing erbB-3 (142). Clearly, more studies on the cellular effects of antibodies to erbB-3 and erbB-4 are needed. It is relevant, however, that chimeric toxins composed of neuregulin-1 and the *Pseudomonas* exotoxin preserved the ability to elevate tyrosine phosphorylation (143). The fusion proteins were highly cytotoxin against cells expressing the erbB-4 receptor, alone or together with other members of the erbB family. Because toxin-induced cytotoxicity requires penetration into the cell, it seems that the potential of the kinase-defective neuregulin receptor, erbB-3, to mediate toxin- or antibody-induced cellular effects is limited.

Antibody–drug conjugates and combinations

Chemotherapy plays a major role in the treatment of cancer, with certain advantages in comparison to surgery and radiotherapy, since chemotherapy can be used effectively against disseminated as well as localized cancer. A major limitation is that cytotoxic agents effective in killing neoplastic cells are often toxic to proliferating normal cells and, as a result, cancer chemotherapy is ultimately dose-limited. Efficient targeting of chemotherapeutic drugs to malignant tissues could offer a major improvement in the treatment of cancer, and antibodies have been a natural choice for such targeting. The more attachment of a low-molecular-weight drug to a macromolecular carrier, while preserving its pharmacological activity, may render the drug more effective in low doses due to facilitation of slow and continuous release, better stability, and, possibly, a different pattern of distribution in the body. When the carrier is a specific antitumor antibody, the selective delivery becomes an additional advantage. Studies up to 1986 have been summarized (144). More recent investigations on the use of mAb–drug conjugates in the treatment of cancer (145) include the use of mAbs, their fragments, and also hormones and growth factors to deliver to tumors not only drugs and toxins, but also radionuclides, enzymes, photosensitizers, and cytokines. Here we describe the use of antibodies to growth factor receptors as 'guided missiles' for chemotherapeutic drugs. A major additional advantage in this case is that the antibodies are often not inert delivery vehicles but rather exert antitumor activity by themselves. It is, therefore, of interest to elucidate their possible synergistic effects with chemotherapeutic drugs, whether as separate entities or in the conjugated form.

A study investigating a covalent conjugate of a chemotherapeutic drug, doxorubicin, with an mAb against a growth factor receptor, namely, erbB-1, has been described (146). An antibody that recognizes the extracellular domain of erbB-1 (mAb108) was conjugated with doxorubicin through a dextran bridge that enables drug activity. Several antibody–drug conjugates, containing different amounts of doxorubicin, retained binding capacity to human epidermoid carcinoma (KB) cells overexpressing EGFR. Most of the drug's cytoxicity was preserved as seen in *in vitro* tests, by determining either inhibition of DNA synthesis or reduction in number and size of KB-cell colonies. When tested against KB tumor xenografted into athymic mice, the anti-erbB-1 drug conjugates with high drug-substitution levels were significantly more effective than free doxorubicin, antibody alone, a mixture of dextran–doxorubicin and antibody, or drug conjugated to a control nonspecific antibody. When the labile covalent bonds linking the antibody–dextran–drug were stabilized by reduction, the therapeutic efficacy of the conjugate was markedly decreased. These results showed that antibodies against the extracellular domain of the erbB-1 can deliver doxorubicin specifically and efficiently to tumor sites that express high receptor levels, thus exerting a specific antitumor effect. In a study utilizing the avidin–biotin system (147), cisplatin was complexed to a carboxymethyl dextran–avidin conjugate and the resulting composite was targeted 24 hours following the administration of biotinyl–mAb108. The treatment was specifically effective in suppressing the growth of established KB tumor xenografts, or in inhibiting the development of lung metastasis in athymic mice.

As mentioned earlier in this review, the anti-EGFR mAb108 was shown to exhibit antitumor activity by itself (64). It was, therefore, of interest to find out whether this antibody can act synergistically with chemotherapeutic drugs. Indeed, when mice were treated with an antibody to erbB-1 in combination with cisplatin, the antitumor effect was greatly enhanced, suggesting that the toxic activity of these agents is synergistic. In accord with the study of possible synergistic effects between anti-erbB-1 and cisplatin, different anti-erbB antibodies were later examined for enhanced cytotoxicity in combinations with various chemotherapeutic drugs. Augmented activity of ciplatin was observed when breast and ovarian cells overexpressing erbB-2 were concomitantly exposed to an anti-erbB-2 antibody (124, 148). Further analysis showed a reduction in both DNA synthesis and repair of cisplatin–DNA adducts in the presence of the antibody, suggesting an elevated chemosensitivity as a result of antibody treatment. Enhanced cisplatin sensitivity in the presence of anti-erbB-2 mAbs has been shown to depend on agonistic properties of the antibody (149). Tyrphostin 50864-2, a low-molecular-weight tyrosine kinase inhibitor, can abrogate the elevated drug-mediated cell killing induced by an anti-erbB-2 antibody. Moreover, the enhancement of cisplatin toxicity was not observed with an anti-erbB-2 mAb that does not induce cell sig-

naling. Induction of signal transduction thus seems to amplify the ability of cisplatin to interact with DNA. A similar sensitization effect was achieved for the treatment with the anti-estrogen drug, tamoxifen (150), as well as with TNF (151), showing an enhanced inhibitory effect *in vitro* in the presence of an anti-erbB-2 antibody.

Mendelsohn and his colleagues have shown that the anti-erbB-1 mAb 225 exhibits an antitumor effect when administered either with cisplatin (152) or with doxorubicin (153). Slamon and his colleagues (154) extended their studies to the synergistic effect of cisplatin and anti-erbB-2 antibodies. A phase II, open-label, multicenter clinical trial for patients with erbB-2 overexpressing metastatic breast cancer was performed in order to determine the toxicity, pharmacokinetics, response rate, and response duration of intravenous administration of Herceptin plus ciplatin. Objective clinical response rates were observed, higher than those reported previously for cisplatin alone or recombinant humanized antibody alone. In addition, the combination resulted in no apparent increase in toxicity. These results formed the basis for an ongoing phase III clinical trial for evaluating combinations of the above recombinant humanized antibody with doxorubicin plus cyclophosphamide or paclitaxel in previously untreated patients with erbB-2-overexpressing metastatic breast cancer (154).

The same group investigated the inhibitory effects of combinations of the anti-erbB-2 antibody and various chemotherapeutic agents for the treatment of human breast cancer (155). Synergistic interactions at clinically relevant drug concentrations were observed for the recombinant humanized mAb in combination with cisplatin, thiotepa, and etoposide. Additive cytotoxin effects were observed with doxorubicin, paclitaxel, methotrexate, and vinblastine. One drug, 5-fluorouracil, was found to be antagonistic with the antibody *in vitro*. Thus, rational combinations were found suitable for testing in human clinical trials. Finally, the results of the phase III clinical trial evaluating Herceptin in combination with chemotherapy (anthracycline and cyclophosphamide or paclitaxel) have become available. A group of 469 erbB-2-expressing breast cancer patients was randomized to receive chemotherapy with or without Herceptin as first-time therapy for metastatic disease (see references 156, 157). The study showed that patients who received Herceptin plus chemotherapy did better than those receiving chemotherapy alone. The overall response rate with chemotherapy alone was 29 per cent, whereas the combination of chemotherapy with Herceptin produced a 45 per cent response rate. The Herceptin arm of the trial had a statistically significant improvement in median duration of response and in time to progression compared with chemotherapy alone.

Sterically stabilized anti-erbB-2 immunoliposomes were designed, making use of Fab' fragments, and targeted to human breast cancer cells *in vitro* (158). The immunoliposomes, showing high levels of selective internalization by erbB-2-overexpressing breast cancer cells, were loaded with doxorubicin and, when administered *in vivo*, exhibited prolonged circulation (159). In multiple HER-2-overexpressing human breast tumor xenograft models, treatment with doxorubicin-loaded immunoliposomes produced significantly increased antitumor cytotoxicity as compared to free doxorubicin or doxorubicin-loaded non-targeted liposomes (160). In another study (161), the synergistic effect of Herceptin and cisplatin was compared with that of Herceptin and liposome-incorporated cisplatin. Non-liposomal and liposomal cisplatin were both effective antitumor agents but, at tolerable dose levels, liposomal cisplatin was superior.

The chimeric C225 anti erbB-1 antibody (IMC-C225), already in phase II clinical trials, was evaluated in human ovarian, breast, and colon cancer lines, in combination with topotecan, a cytotoxic drug that specifically inhibits topoisomerase I and that has antitumor activity against these malignancies (162). An almost complete tumor regression was observed in all mice treated with the two agents, thus providing a rationale for evaluating this combination in clinical trials. In a report of phase I studies of the chimeric antibody, administered either alone or in combination with cisplatin, it was found that antibody doses that achieve saturation of systemic clearance are well tolerated, and that the chimeric C225 antibody given in combination with cisplatin is biologically active at pharmacologically relevant doses (163).

An appealing approach is that of prodrugs. Antibody–enzyme conjugates targeted to tumors, were used for the activation of anticancer prodrugs administered systemically (reviewed in reference 164). Until now, with one exception (165), no such conjugates have been reported making use of antibodies to growth factor receptors, even though this approach is certainly worth investigating. The humanized anti-HER2 antibody was used as a building block to engineer a disulfide-linked Fv beta-lactamase fusion protein for use in antibody-dependent enzyme-mediated prodrug therapy using cephalosporin-based prodrugs (165).

Antibody–toxin conjugates

Antibodies directed to growth factor receptors can serve as useful vehicles for the targeting of therapeutic agents such as toxins. Since most toxins require an internalization step for their intracellular action, anti-receptor antibodies are appropriate for use as immuno-toxins (conjugates of antibodies with toxins) due to their ability to specifically interact with the cell, internalize together with the surface receptor, and introduce the toxic agent into the cell. Conjugates of mAbs and toxins have been used in preclinical trials as antitumor agents (166). Several immunotoxins have been constructed using various anti-erbB-2 antibodies coupled to Lys-PE40, a recombinant form of the *Pseudomonas* exotoxin lacking its cell-binding domain (167). An anti-erbB-2 exotoxin successfully inhibited the growth of Schwannoma cells in athymic mice (168) and several agents have similarly been targeted, including ricin (169) and enzyme prodrugs (169), all presenting specific cell-inhibitory effects. A bispecific single-chain antibody–toxin specific to both erbB-2 and erbB-1 inhibited the growth of cancer cells *in vivo* (170), probably by the induction of heterodimeric complexes and subsequent internalization of the toxin. A prolonged tumor-localized supply of an erbB-2-specific toxin has been elegantly achieved by the development of a new class of tumor-specific killer lymphocytes. These cells produce and secrete an antibody-targeted toxin in the vicinity of the tumor, overcoming depletion by clearance and resulting in high cytotoxicity toward tumors in an athymic murine model (171).

An original approach to immunotoxins has been taken in a study making use of the streptavidin–biotin system (172). Biotin was linked to ricin via a disulfide-containing reagent and the product, biotinyl-S, S-ricin (b-ricin), was shown to retain most of its *in vitro* cytotoxic activity against human epidermoid carcinoma (KB) cells. Complexing b-ricin to streptavidin resulted in > 99 per cent loss of its cellular toxicity, which is associated with loss of cell-binding activity. The streptavidin–b-ricin complex could, however, be targeted to KB cells via the biotinylated mAb 108 specific to EGFR overexpressed on KB cells. The complex did not regain its activity if the specific antibody was not biotinylated or if the biotinylated antibody was of a different specificity. Streptavidin is thus used to block b-ricin, presumably due to a steric restraint of the streptavidin on the ricin B-chain. Avidin could not replace streptavidin in this system since a complex between b-ricin and avidin retained a major part (60 per cent) of ricin cytotoxic activity. This was attributed to the non-specific binding of avidin to cells *in vitro*, including KB cells. It is suggested that b-ricin is blocked by both streptavidin and avidin but, once the complex gains specific access to the cell surface, its cytotoxic activity is specifically retrieved (172).

Another immunotoxin was prepared in which a modified version of *Pseudomonas* exotoxin-A was conjugated to a mAb against a deletion mutant erbB-1, which is frequently expressed in malignant glioblastomas (173). The immunotoxin was specifically targeted to the mutant receptor and showed little or no cytotoxicity to cells expressing high levels of the normal receptor. An increase in affinity and cytotoxic activity was observed by using random complementarity determining region (CDR) mutagenesis to obtain mutants of the Fv portion of the antibody with increased affinity for the mutated erbB-1 molecules (174). In another study, suppression of metastasis formation was achieved by using a recombinant single-chain antibody–*Pseudomonas* toxin specific to both the full-length erbB-1 protein and the oncogenic variant EGFRvIII (175).

The ribosome-inhibiting plant toxin gelonin was coupled to two antibodies, namely, to erbB-2, a murine antibody, and to a human chimeric antibody. The authors reported clear correlation between erbB-2 expression levels and the toxicity of the cytoimmunotoxin (176). The immunotoxin, which was concentrated 2–10-fold higher in tumors than in normal tissues, slowed tumor growth by over 90 per cent and lengthened the median survival by 40 per cent. Using mAbs genetically fused to a truncated *Pseudomonas* exotoxin, it was suggested that erbB-1- and erbB-2-specific immunotoxins may become valuable therapeutic reagents for the treatment of squamous cell carcinomas of the head and neck (177).

Not only antibodies, but also growth factors themselves could target toxins to their specific receptors. Ligands interacting with erbB proteins could serve as beneficial carriers, utilizing their high binding affinity to the respective receptors. Heparin-binding EGF binds to erbB-1 with high affinity, and recombinant fusion proteins consisting of mature human heparin-binding EGF fused to the plant ribosome-inactivating protein saporin were expressed in *Escherichia coli*. The conjugate inhibited protein synthesis in a cell-free assay and competed with EGF for binding to receptors on intact cells (178). A fusion toxin of NRG1 with exotoxin-A induced complete regression of human breast cancer xenografts in athymic mice (179). A betacellulin–*Pseudomonas* toxin fusion protein was effective against cells expressing erbB-1, but not cells expressing erbB-4, probably due to a limited internalizing capacity of the latter receptor (180).

Immunotoxins have also been constructed with antibodies to growth factor receptors other than those of the erbB family. Mesothelin, also known as megakaryocyte potentiating factor (115), is a differentiation antigen present on the surface of ovarian cancers, mesotheliomas, and several other types of human cancers. Since among normal tissues mesothelin is present only on mesothelial cells, it represents a potential target for antibody-mediated delivery of cytotoxic agents. Mice were immunized with an eukaryotic expression vector coding for mesothelin and, when high serum antibody titers were obtained, a phage display library was made from the splenic mRNA of these mice (181). After three rounds of panning on recombinant mesothelin, a single-chain Fv (scFv)-displaying phage was selected that bound specifically to recombinant mesothelin and mesothelin-positive cells. The scFv was used to construct an immunotoxin by genetically fusing it with a truncated mutant of *Pseudomonas* exotoxin-A. The purified immunotoxin binds mesothelin with high affinity (K_d = 11 nM), is stable for over 40 at 37°C and is highly hours cytotoxic to cells expressing mesothelin. It also resulted in regression of tumors expressing mesothelin (181). The combination of high and selective cytotoxicity makes the immunotoxins attractive candidates for development as therapeutic agents.

Two immunotoxins specific for the low-affinity receptor for NGF (nerve growth factor), namely, p75, were compared, one in which the antibody was coupled to saporin and the other to trichosanthin (182). Both immunotoxins were potent as lesion inducers. Immunotoxins were also prepared by using antibodies to endoglin, the proliferation-associated antigen on endothelial cells. An immunotoxin composed of a murine IgM mAb that recognizes endoglin coupled to deglycosylated ricin A was potent in specifically inhibiting protein synthesis (183). Two other immunotoxins, made of anti-endoglin mAbs fused to ricin A lacking sugar residues, displayed weak, but specific cytotoxic activity against murine endothelial cells *in vitro* (184). The conjugates were highly therapeutic relative to control molecules, and tumor regression persisted without further therapy for a long as the mice were followed. High activity against endothelial cells was shown also with a recombinant immunotoxin comprised of diphtheria toxin and VEGF (185). The fusion protein was highly toxic to proliferating endothelial cells, but not to vascular smooth muscle cells ad it retarded the growth of Kaposi's sarcoma tumors in mice.

Radioimmunoconjugates and the effect of antibodies on radiotherapy

Antibodies to erbB-1

Radioconjugates of antitumor antibodies may be of value both for localization of tumors and for directed radiotherapy. In addition, non-radiotagged antibodies may have a synergistic or additive value when given together with conventional radiotherapy. Several studies were concerned with radioactive anti-erbB-1 antibodies. mAbs specific for EGFRvIII were radiolabeled by using *N*-sucinimidyl 5-iodo-3-pyridine-carboxylate, a reagent of higher intracellular retention because of the positive charge of its pyridine ring (186). Technetium-labeled antibodies to erbB-1 were tested for biodistribution and dosimetry in patients with epithelial tumors. The authors concluded that the radiolabeled antibody may permit regional radioimmunotherapy (187–189).

An imaging study of brain tumors reported on the ability of peptidergic radiopharmaceuticals to reach cancer cells by penetrating through the blood–brain barrier (BBB) (190). Present-day imaging of brain tumors requires a disrupted BBB. However, the BBB is intact in the early stages of brain tumor growth, when diagnosis is most critical. Relative to normal brain, brain tumor cells frequently overexpress receptors, such as erbB-1. Readiolabeled erbB-1 ligands could be used to image early brain tumors, should these radiopharmaceuticals be made transportable through the BBB. A bifunctional molecule was prepared that contains an EGF molecule radiolabeled with ^{111}In and an anti-transferrin receptor mAb that undergoes transcytosis through the BBB via the endogenous transferrin transport system. The two domains of the bifunctional conjugates were fused by a PEG linker, which releases steric hindrance and allows the conjugate to bind to both the EGF-receptor for brain imaging, and to the transferrin receptor, to enable transport through the BBB. Successful imaging of experimental brain tumors was demonstrated in nude rats bearing cerebral implants of human glioma cells.

Antibodies to erbB-2

The feasibility of targeting radioactive antibodies to erbB-2 was investigated in athymic mice grafted subcutaneously with NIH-3T3 cells overexpressing erbB-2 (191). The authors reached the conclusion that, while the radioiodinated antibodies are attractive agents for radioimmunodiagnosis and radioimmunotherapy, effective strategies for retarding intratumoral catabolism may be necessary to optimize their clinical utility. In a later study (192), the murine 4D5 antibody and the respective humanized antibody to erbB-2 (Herceptin) were radiolabeled with ^{125}I, ^{131}I, or ^{186}Re. Superior retention of physical and biological characteristics of ^{186}Re-labeled antibodies compared with their ^{131}I-labeled counterparts suggests the potential for their use as radioimaging and radioimmunotherapeutic agents in the treatment of erbB-2-overexpressing tumors. Additional investigations were reported on the best methods for radioiodination of anti-erbB-2 antibodies, for improved uptake in tumors compared with antibody labeled by direct iodination, and for lower whole-body retention (193). Similarly, binding affinity, internalization, and degradation rates were determined (194).

The specificity, toxicity, and efficacy of lead (^{212}Pb) radioimmunotherapy were evaluated in athymic mice bearing the SK-OV-3 human ovarian tumor cells overexpressing erbB-2 (195). The authors concluded that linking the isotope to the antibody through an AE1-DOTA linker is of only modest value in the therapy of bulky solid tumors due to the short physical half-life of ^{212}Pb and the time required to achieve a useful tumor-to-normal tissue ratio of radionuclide after administration. However, the radiolabeled mAb may be useful in therapy of tumors in the adjuvant setting. Furthermore, ^{212}Pb may be of value in selected situations, including treatment of leukemia, intercavitary therapy, or strategies that target vascular endothelial cells of tumors.

Another study on the biodistribution and radioimmunotherapy of human breast cancer xenografts with radiometal-labeled DOTA-conjugated antibody 4D5 to erbB-2 has recently been reported (196). The conjugate was labeled either with ^{111}In or with ^{90}Y, and antibody distribution and therapy tested in athymic mice bearing xenografts of a human breast cancer line transfected with the erbB-2 gene. ^{111}In-labeled 4D5 antibody gave superior antibody uptake in tumors. In the therapy study, treatment of athymic mice bearing the xenografts caused a threefold reduction of tumor growth compared to that in untreated controls.

Radiotherapy combined with immunotherapy

In analogy to the additive effects of antibodies and chemotherapy, a similar effect exists with radiotherapy. Enhanced efficacy was observed when athymic mice bearing established xenografts of human squamous cell carcinoma of the head and neck were treated with a combination of radioactive rhenium and an anti-erbB-1 antibody (197). In another study performed in mice, a combination of antibody C225 to erbB-1 and radiotherapy yielded enhanced tumor regression and prolongation of animal survival (198). Similarly, in a study investigating whether treatment with an anti-erbB-1 antibody would improve the response of human epidermoid tumors to radiotherapy, it was found that the antibody dramatically improved the efficacy of local tumor irradiation, particularly upon multiple injections of the antibody (199).

Other studies attempting to increase the efficiency of radiotherapy by using mAbs to erbB-2 were described. Plasmid and adenoviral vectors were developed, expressing an anti-erbB-2 single-chain antibody directed to the endoplasmic reticulum of target cells, that is, cytotoxic to tumor cells overexpressing erbB-2 through induction of apoptosis. When the single-chain antibody was tested in athymic mice on human ovarian cancer cells with or without radiotherapy, it was found that the regression rates of irradiated tumors were significantly higher, and they also displayed a longer delay of re-growth, relative to animals with tumors that were irradiated in the absence of antibodies (200).

Along with the prognostic value of erbB-2 and its ability to predict responses to adjuvant chemotherapy, a recent study correlated amplification of the gene with the risk for local relapse in patients treated with conservative surgery and radiation (201). *In vitro* lines of evidence confirm the possibility that the oncoprotein plays a role, along with other growth factor receptors (202), in conferring a radiation-resistant phenotype to tumor cells. In line with this notion, erbB-2-overexpressing cells are relatively resistant to ionic irradiation, and blocking erbB-2 by using an mAb dramatically promotes the ability of irradiation to induce remission of human breast cancer xenografts

(203). Apparently, an overexpressed erbB-2 enhances DNA repair following radiation-indcued DNA damage, and its removal from the cell surface sensitizes a cell to the deleterious effect of ionizing radiation. Radiation treatment is known to promote cell cycle arrest predominantly at G_1 with low S-phase fractions but, in the presence of an erbB-2-specific antibody, radiation elicited a similar reduction in S phase at 24 hours, but a significant reversal of this arrest appeared 48 hours after exposure to radiation (203). The level of S-phase fraction at 48 hours was significantly greater than that found at 24 hours with the combined antibody–radiation therapy, suggesting that early escape from cell cycle arrest in the presence of an anti-receptor antibody may not allow sufficient time for completion of DNA repair, thus enhancing radiosensitivity of the erbB-2-overexpressing cells.

Vascular endothelial growth factor (VEGF) expression is induced in Lewis lung carcinoma, both *in vitro* and *in vivo*, after exposure to ionizing radiation, and in several human tumor cell lines this induction was observed *in vitro* (204). Treatment of tumor-bearing mice with a neutralizing anti-VEGF antibody before irradiation was associated with a greater than additive antitumor effect. *In vitro*, the addition of VEGF decreases radiation-induced killing of human umbilical vein endothelial cells, whereas blocking of the growth factor by using antibodies can potentiate radiation-induced lethality. These findings support a model by which induction of VEGF by radiation contributes to the protection of tumor blood vessels from radiation-mediated cytotoxicity and thereby to tumor radioresistance.

Lessons from immunotherapy directed at other growth factor receptors

Tumor-derived VEGFs play an important role in neovascularization and the development of tumor stroma. Furthermore, VEGF receptors are frequently overexpressed in the endothelial cells of the tumor vasculature and almost undetectable in the vascular endothelium of adjoining normal tissues. VEGF regulates angiogenesis by binding to its cognate receptors, VEGFR-1 (flt-1) and VEGFR-2 (flk-1, fetal liver kinase 1), endothelial cell-specific transmembrane tyrosine kinases that are important for vascular endothelial cell development. The importance of angiogenesis in malignant tumor growth and invasion emphasizes the role of VEGFRs as potential targets for innovative anticancer therapy.

Anti-angiogenic therapy has been proposed as a new strategy for the treatment of solid tumors. mAb DC101 directed against VEGFR-2 was shown to disrupt ongoing angiogenesis and prevent invasion of malignant keratinocytes, without reducing tumor cell proliferation, thus reverting a malignant tumor into a benign phenotype (205). The same mAb was shown to potently inhibit VEGF binding and consequent signaling. Treatment with mAb DC101 significantly suppressed the growth of primary lung, mammary, and melanocytic tumors, and completely inhibited the growth of established epidermoid, glioblastoma, pancreatic, and renal human tumor xenografts. Histological examination showed evidence of decreased microvessel density and tumor cell proliferation, as well as increased cell apoptosis and extensive tumor necrosis (206, 207). The mAb also inhibited the growth of transitional cell carcinoma (TCC) of the bladder in athymic mice, and inhibition was augmented by paclitaxel (208). The growth of neuroblastoma tumors could be inhibited by the DC101 mAb, but this effect was most remarkable in combination with low-dose vinblastine, with full and sustained regression of large established tumors (209).

Another study related to angiogenesis was directed to therapy via erbB-1. It was suggested that (proto)–oncogenes such as EGFR may regulate critical survival functions, including angiogenesis. mAb C225, a chimerized antibody to erbB-1, inhibited human epidermoid carcinoma A431 (210), TCC (211), and pancreatic carcinoma (76) due in part to inhibition of angiogenesis that resulted from downregulation of the angiogenic factors VEGF, IL-8, and fibroblast growth factor (211). Likewise, several humanized antibodies to VEGF itself were described, reporting on their pharmacokinetics, interspecies and tissue distribution (212), preclinical safety (213), and antitumor activity in preclinical models (214). Another strategy made use of recombinant VEGF linked to a truncated form of diphtheria toxin (215). The fusion protein was selectively toxic to endothelial cell lines and inhibited experimental neovascularization of chick chorioallantoic membrane. The VEGF–toxin conjugate caused hemorrhagic necrosis consistent with a vascular-mediated injury, and it displayed a significant inhibition of established subcutaneous tumors without apparent toxicity. Two other VEGF–diphtheria toxin fusion proteins significantly inhibited the growth of Kaposi's sarcoma tumors in mice (185). In conclusion, antibodies to angiogenic factors and their receptors, or conjugates of the growth factors themselves may allow future treatment of a variety of solid tumors.

The membrane protein endoglin is part of the transforming growth factor beta-1 receptor complex, and it serves as an endothelial marker of angiogenesis in cervical cancer tissues (216). Endoglin levels were significantly increased in patients who developed distant metastasis compared with disease-free patients (217). Murine mAbs against endoglin were prepared, and used for targeting cytotoxic agents to the tumor vasculature (183), as well as for *in vivo* imaging of tumors (218). Additional anti-endoglin antibodies were generated and used for treating distinct performed solid tumors (184).

Other strategies to inhibit growth factor receptors: potential facilitators of immunotherapy

Tyrphostins and other low-molecular-weight tyrosine kinase inhibitors

In an attempt to inhibit the mitogenic signaling of receptor tyrosine kinases, many chemical compounds have been designed and synthesized to interfere with the enzymatic activity (219–222). Tyrosine phosphorylation may be the primary, or even the exclusive, indicator of signal transduction of multicellular organisms. The receptor tyrosine kinases participate in transmembrane signaling, whereas the intracellular tyrosine kinases take part in signal transduction within the cell. Levitzki and his colleagues, as well as several other laboratories, have developed a large family of tyrosine kinase inhibitors, denoted tyrphostins (tyrosine phosphorylation inhibitors). Such tyrphostins have been developed to bear selective specificities toward the ATP-binding sites of erbB-1 and erbB-2, resulting in inhibition of proliferation of cells expressing the respective receptors (223).

Tyrphostins specific for the erbB-1 receptor can inhibit primary glioblastoma cells from invading brain aggregates (224), and prostate cancer from proliferation (225). A similar compound, capable of inhibiting activation of erbB receptors, is a potent *in vivo* inhibitor of various xenografts expressing erbB proteins (226). In the last decade many highly potent and selective tyrosine kinase inhibitors were generated, mostly by semirational drug design (221). One of the most surprising findings on the selectivity of inhibitors discovered so far is that adenosine 5′-triphosphate (ATP)-competitive inhibitors can be highly selective. Especially attractive is a class of new irreversible inhibitors that selectively bind to the catalytic domain of the epidermal growth factor receptor with a 1:1 stoichiometry and alkylate a nearby cysteine residue essential for catalysis (227). AG825, a specific inhibitor of the erbB-2 tyrosine kinase, sensitizes receptor-overexpressing cells to chemotherapy including doxorubicin, etoposide, and cisplatin (228), suggesting the involvement of erbB-2 signaling in resistance toward chemotherapy. Thus, low-molecular-weight compounds capable of selective inhibition of the catalytic activity of specific erbB proteins, either alone or in combination with other drugs, are potential future cancer therapeutic agents. Because of the key role that vascular endothelial growth factor receptor (VEGFR) plays in angiogenesis, inhibitors of the receptor that show efficacy *in vivo* have been synthesized (229). Clinical trials making use of VEGFR kinase inhibitors have recently started, and low-molecular-weight angiogenesis inhibitors could possibly become universal anti-cancer agents.

Tyrphostin AG1295 and its close analog AG1296 (both are quinoxalines) have been shown to selectively block the kinase of the platelet-derived growth factor receptor (PDGFR) with insignificant inhibitory effects on erbB-1, Src, Flk-1, erbB-2, and the insulin-like growth factor receptor (IGF-1R). These tyrphostins reverse the transformed phenotype of sis-transformed fibroblasts (229), and slow C6 glioma-induced tumors in athymic mice. In experiments in pigs, AG 1295 was shown to block balloon injury-induced stenosis in the femoral artery (230). The finding that PDGFR kinase-directed tyrphostins block ~ 60 per cent stenosis strongly suggests that other signaling pathways should be targeted in order to block other proliferative signals, including those elicited by fibroblast and transforming growth factors. Since accelerated atherosclerosis in the transplanted heart is the major cause of death of patients who undergo heart transplantation, the use of AG1295 and its analogs may extend from cancer therapy to the treatment of atherosclerosis.

In a recent study on the involvement of erbB-1 in epithelial repair in asthma (231), it was shown that EGF accelerated repair of scrape-wounded monolayers and that the EGFR-selective inhibitors, the AG1478 quinazoline, inhibited both EGF-stimulated and basal wound closure. In looking for an effect of a neutralizing anti-erbB-1 antibody on wound closure, results were inconclusive as the antibody appeared to activate erbB-1 by direct cross-linking (231). In another recent study it was shown that AG1478 delayed breast tumor formation in a bigenic mouse model carrying transgenes of the mammary tumor virus (MMTV)/Neu and MMTV/TGFα (232). This inhibitor can induce formation of inactive, unphosphorylated erbB-1•erbB-2 heterodimers, thereby sequestering erbB-2 from signaling interactions with other erbB co-receptors (233). AG1478 inhibits erbB-1 as well as erbB-2 signaling and alters the natural history of MMTV/Neu + TGFα breast tumors, most likely by modulating downstream kinases that regulate molecules involved in G_1/S traverse, thereby inducing cell cycle arrest (232).

Gene therapy

Several gene-based strategies to block the biochemical action of the erbB network or to interfere with the transcription, translation, or maturation of erbB proteins are currently at different stages of preclinical research, or at more advanced stages. Potentially, such approaches will lead in the future to combinatorial therapies targeting the network at more than one critical component. Because the network may require Ras (234), Raf1, P13K, and Src for signaling, specific inhibitors of these targets (235) are expected to enhance the efficacy of erbB-directed therapies. The most advanced gene-based strategy is the one that makes use of the adenovirus *E1A* gene (236). Apparently, the product of the viral *E1A* gene can downregulate transcription from the *erbB-2* promoter. This strategy has been tested in mice carrying human breast cancer xenografts and resulted in tumor inhibition and prolongation of survival (237). Phase I trials in patients with ovarian or breast cancer currently test delivery of E1A, and a report on the ability of E1A to sensitize erbB-2-overexpressing cells to chemotherapy suggests a potential for clinical application (238). A different approach is to use the promoter of *erbB-2* to selectively express suicide genes in erbB-2-overexpressing tumors (239, 240). Alternatively, the Ets protein PEA3, which downregulates erbB-2 expression by binding to the promoter of the oncoprotein, may become a target for gene therapy (241).

Alternative methods to block the expression of erbB-2 make use of triplex-formation (242) and hammerhead ribozymes, expressed under the control of a tetracycline-regulated promoter (243). Introduction of the erbB-2-specific ribozyme into tumor cells almost completely abrogated their tumorigenic growth in athymic mice, and withdrawal of tetracycline led to tumor regression. The use of antisense cDNA constructs is another way to destabilize the transcript of erbB-2 (244–246). On the other hand, deletion constructs and kinase-defective mutants of erbB proteins are candidates for gene delivery, because in model systems they seem to be recruited into inactive dimeric receptor complexes (247, 248). Finally, specific intracellular single-chain antibodies (sFvs) can effectively inhibit receptor transfer from the endoplasmic reticulum to the plasma membrane, and thereby reduce signaling (249, 250). A human protocol for the treatment of erbB-2-positive ovarian cancer has been developed following demonstration of selectivity and phenotypic effects *in vitro* (251).

Concluding remarks

Immunotherapy emerges as a major route of targeted cancer therapy. Unlike conventional drug therapy, the targeted strategies are based upon comprehensive understanding of biochemical processes and their connections. The identification of the erbB/HER network as a target for cancer therapy is one of the first fruits of an in depth understanding of signaling mechanisms gained through the molecular biological revolution. Integration of biochemical, molecular, and embryological studies with experiments in invertebrates implies that the erbB family of growth factor receptors evolved through the last billion years to function in inductive processes that control cell lineage determination. These are most critical in the very heterogeneous epithelial system and, due to the rapid rate of proliferation and shedding of the epithelium, the epithelium serves as a target for oncogenic mutations in human. To what extent the network plays a role also in the process of cell migration (metastasis) and endothel formation (and hence angiogenesis) is currently an open question.

Due to its accessibility and prognostic significance, the erbB network can serve as a target for several distinct approaches of pharmacological intervention. While the use of antibodies is currently the only approach that is widely used in the clinics, low-molecular-weight inhibitors of tyrosine kinases, antagonists of small guanosine 5′-triphosphate (GTP)-binding proteins, and specific blockers of transcriptional events are expected to reach the clinic in the next few years. Other promising approaches are gene delivery and intervention of chaperones and specific proteins

responsible for delivery and stabilization of erbBs at the basolateral membrane. Perhaps most appealing is the potential of combined therapy. Combinations of tyrphostins, gene therapy, and angiogenesis blockers are expected to enhance the therapeutic value of anti-erbB antibodies. Likewise, the combination of chemotherapy or radiotherapy with-targeted strategies is already a useful therapeutic protocol. Future research will explore the potential of each route of advanced therapy alone, as well as in combination with conventional approaches. Moreover, the erbB network may become a model for future translational research that can yield effective drugs to eradicate cancer.

References

1. Birchmeyer C, Birchmeyer W. Molecular aspects of mesenchymal–epithelial interactions. Ann Rev Cell Biol 1993, 9, 511–40.
2. Aaronson SA, Rubin JS, Finch PW, *et al.* Growth factor-regulated pathways in epithelial cell proliferation. Am Rev Respir Dis 1990, **142**, S7–10.
3. Miller WE, Raab-Traub N. The EGFR as a target for viral oncoproteins. Trends Microbiol 1999, 7, 453–8.
4. Massague J, Pandiella A. Membrane-anchored growth factors. Ann Rev Biochem 1993, **62**, 515–41.
5. Raab G, Klagsbrun M. Heparin-binding EGF-like growth factor. Biochem Biophys Acta 1997, **1333**, 179–99.
6. Derynck R, Goeddel DV, Ullrich A, *et al.* Synthesis of messenger RNAs for transforming growth factors alpha and beta and the epidermal-growth-factor-receptor by human tumors. Cancer Res 1987, 47, 707–12.
7. Ebert AD, Wechselberger C, Martinez-Lacaci I, *et al.* Expression and function of EGF-related peptides and their receptors in gynecological cancer—from basic science to therapy. J Recept Signal Transduct Res 2000, **20**, 1–46.
8. Salomon DS, Brandt R, Ciardiello F, *et al.* Epidermal growth factor-related peptides and their receptors in human malignancies. Crit Rev Oncol Hematol 1995, **19**, 183–232.
9. Riese DJ, 2nd, Stern DF. Specificity within the EGF family/erbB receptor family signaling network. Bioessays 1998, **20**, 41–8.
10. Yarden Y, Schlessinger J. Epidermal growth factor induce rapid, reversible aggregation of purified epidermal growth factor receptor. Biochemistry 1987, **26**, 1443–5.
11. van der Geer P, Hunter T, Lindberg RA. Receptor protein-tyrosine kinases and their signal transduction pathways. Ann Rev Cell Biol 1994, **10**, 251–37.
12. Guy PM, Platko JV, Cantley LC *et al.* Insect cell-expressed p180erbB3 possesses an impaired tyrosine kinase activity. Proc Natl Acad Sci, USA 1994, **91**, 8132–6.

13. Klapper LN, Glathe S, Vaisman N, *et al.* The erbB-2/HER2 oncoprotein of human carcinomas may function solely as a shared coreceptor for multiple stroma-derived growth factors. Proc Natl Acad Sci, USA 1999, **96**, 4995–5000.

14. Tzahar E, Yarden Y. The erbB-2/HER2 oncogenic receptor of adenocarcinomas: from orphanhood to multiple stromal ligands. BBA Rev Cancer 1998, **1377**, M25–M37.

15. Pinkas-Kramarski R, Soussan L, Waterman H, *et al.* Diversification of Neu differentiation factor and epidermal growth factor signaling by combinatorial receptor interactions. EMBO J 1996, **15**, 2452–67.

16. Tzahar E, Waterman H, Chen X, *et al.* A hierarchical network of interreceptor interactions determines signal transduction by Neu differentiation factor/neuregulin and epidermal growth factor. Mol Cell Biol 1996, **16**, 5276–87.

17. Graus Porta D, Beerli RR, Daly JM, *et al.* erbB-2, the preferred heterodimerization partner of all erbB receptors, is a mediator of lateral signaling. EMBO J 1997, **16**, 1647–55.

18. Alroy I, Yarden Y. The erbB signaling network in embryogenesis and oncogenesis: signal diversification through combinatorial ligand–receptor interactions. FEBS Lett 1997, **410**, 83–6.

19. Llrich A, Coussens L, Hayflick JS, *et al.* Human epidermal growth factor receptor cDNA sequence and aberrant expression of the amplified gene in A431 epidermoid carcinoma cells. Nature 1984, **309**, 418–425.

20. Rosenthal A, Lindquist PB, Bringman TS, *et al.* Expression in rat fibroblasts of a human transforming growth factor-alpha cDNA results in transformation. Cell 1986, **46**, 301–9.

21. Di Fiore PP, Pierce JH, Kraus MH, *et al.* erbB-2 is a potent oncogene when overexpressed in NIH/3T3 cells. Science 1987, **237**, 178–82.

22. Akimoto T, Hunter NR, Buchmiller L, *et al.* Inverse relationship between epidermal growth factor receptor expression and radiocurability of murine carcinomas. Clin Cancer Res 1999, **5**, 2884–90.

23. Archer SG, Eliopoulos A, Spandidos D, *et al.* Expression of ras p21, p53 and c-erbB-2 in advanced breast cancer and response to first line hormonal therapy. Br J Cancer 1995, **72**, 1259–66.

24. Stumm G, Eberwein S, Rostock Wolf S, *et al.* Concomitant overexpression of the EGFR and erbB-2 genes in renal cell carcinoma (RCC) is correlated with dedifferentiation and metastasis. Int J Cancer 1996, **69**, 17–22.

25. Rusch V, Baselga J, Cordon-Cardo C, *et al.* Differential expression of the epidermal growth factor receptor and its ligands in primary non-small cell lung cancers and adjacent benign lung. Cancer Res 1993, **53**, 2379–85.

26. Wikstrand CJ, Reist CJ, Archer GE, *et al.* The class III variant of the epidermal growth factor receptor (EGFRvIII): characterization and utilization as an immunotherapeutic target. J Neurovirol 1998, **4**, 148–58.

27. Ekstrand AJ, Sugawa N, James CD, *et al.* Amplified and rearranged epidermal growth factor receptor genes in human glioblastomas reveal deletions of sequences encoding portions of the N- and/or C-terminal tails. Proc Natl Acad Sci, USA 1992, **89**, 4309–13.

28. Chen WS, Lazar CS, Lund KA, *et al.* Functional independence of the epidermal growth factor receptor from a domain required for ligand-induced internalization and calcium regulation. Cell 1989, **59**, 33–43.

29. Levkowitz G, Waterman H, Ettenberg SA, *et al.* Ubiquitin ligase activity and tyrosine phosphorylation underlie suppression of growth factor signaling by c-Cb1/Sli-1. Mol Cell 1999, **4**, 1029–40.

30. Wong AJ, Ruppert JM, Bigner SH, *et al.* Structural alterations of the epidermal growth factor receptor gene in human gliomas. Proc Natl Acad Sci, USA 1992, **89**, 2965–9.

31. Batra SK, Castelino-Prabhu S, Wikstrand CJ, *et al.* Epidermal growth factor ligand-independent, unregulated, cell-transforming potential of a naturally occurring human mutant EGFRvIII gene. Cell Growth Differ 1995, **6**, 1251–9.

32. Moscatello DK, Holgado-Madruga M, Godwin AK, *et al.* Frequent expression of a mutant epidermal growth factor receptor in multiple human tumors. Cancer Res 1995, **55**, 5536–9.

33. Sampson JH, Crotty LE, Lee S, *et al.* Unarmed, tumor-specific monoclonal antibody effectively treats brain tumors. Proc Natl Acad Sci, USA 2000, **97**, 7503–8.

34. Bargmann CI, Hung MC, Weinberg RA. Multiple independent activations of the *neu* oncogene by a point mutation altering the transmembrane domain of p185. Cell 1986, **45**, 649–57.

35. Weiner DB, Liu J, Cohen JA, *et al.* A point mutation in the *neu* oncogene mimics ligand induction of receptor aggregation. Nature 1989, **339**, 230–1.

36. Hynes NE and Stern DF. The biology of erbB-2/neu/HER-2 and its role in cancer. Biochem Biophys Acta 1994, **1198**, 165–84.

37. Klapper LN, Kirschbaum MH, Sela M, *et al.* Biochemical and clinical implications of the erbB/HER signaling network of growth factor receptors. Adv Cancer Res 2000, **77**, 25–79.

38. Katsaros D, Theillet C, Zola P, *et al.* Concurrent abnormal expression of erbB-2 myc and ras genes is associated with poor outcome of ovarian cancer patients. Anticancer Res 1995, **15**, 1501–10.

39. Charpin C, Bonnier P, Khouzami A, *et al.* Inflammatory breast carcinoma: an immunohistochemical study using monoclonal anti-pHER-2/*neu*, pS2, cathepsin, ER and PR. Anticancer Res 1992, **12**, 591–7.

40. Barnes DM, Lammie GA, Millis RR, *et al.* An immunohistochemical evaluation of c-*erb*B-2 expression in human breast carcinoma. J Cancer 1988, **58**, 448–52.

41. Slamon DJ, Clark GM, Wong SG, *et al.* Human breast cancer: correlation of relapse and survival with amplification of the HER-2/*neu* oncogene. Science 1987, **235**, 177–82.

42. Anbazhagan R, Gelber RD, Bettelheim R, *et al.* Association of c-erbB-2 expression and S-phase fraction in the prognosis of node positive breast cancer. Ann Oncol 1991, **2**, 47–53.

43. Press MF, Bernstein L, Thomas PA, *et al.* HER-2/*neu* gene amplification characterized by fluorescence *in situ*

hybridization: poor prognosis in node-negative breast carcinomas. J Clin Oncol 1997, **15**, 2894–904.

44. Menard S, Tagliabue E, Campiglio M, *et al.* Role of HER2 gene overexpression in breast carcinoma. J Cell Physiol 2000, **182**, 150–62.

45. Muss HB, Thorr AD, Berry DA, *et al.* c-cerbB-2 expression and response to adjuvant therapy in women with node-positive early breast cancer [published erratum appears in New Engl J Med 1994, **331** (3), 211]. New Engl J Med 1994, **330**, 1260–6.

46. Paik S, Bryant J, Park C, *et al.* erbB-2 and response to doxorubicin in patients with axillary lymph node-positive, hormone receptor-negative breast cancer. J Natl Cancer Inst 1998, **90**, 1361–70.

47. Thor AD, Berry DA, Budman DR, *et al.* erbB-2, p53, and efficacy of adjuvant therapy in lymph node-positive breast cancer. J Natl Cancer Inst 1998, **90**, 1346–60.

48. Jarvinen TA, Tanner M, Rantanen V, *et al.* Amplification and deletion of topoisomerase Iialpha associate with erbB-2 amplification and affect sensitivity to topoisomerase II inhibitor doxorubicin in breast cancer. Am J Pathol 2000, **156**, 839–47.

49. Baselga, J, Seidman AD, Rosen PP, *et al.* HER2 overexpression and paclitaxel sensitivity in breast cancer: therapeutic implications. Oncology 1997, **11**, 43–8.

50. Yu D, Liu B, Tan M, *et al.* Overexpression of c-erbB-2/neu in breast cancer cells confers increased resistance to Taxol via mdr-1-independent mechanisms. Oncogene 1996, **13**, 1359–65.

51. Yu D, Hung MC. The erbB2 gene as a cancer therapeutic target and the tumor- and metastasis-suppressing function of E1A. Cancer Metastasis Rev 1998, **17**, 195–202.

52. Vecchi M, Baulida J, Carpenter G. Selective cleavage of the heregulin receptor erbB-4 by protein kinase C activation. J Biol Chem 1996, **271**, 18989–95.

53. Vecchi M, Carpenter G. Constitutive proteolysis of the erbB-4 receptor tyrosine kinase by a unique, sequential mechanism. J Cell Biol 1997, **139**, 995–1003.

54. Elenius K, Choi CJ, Paul S, *et al.* Characterization of a naturally occurring erbB4 isoform that does not bind or activate phosphatidyl inositol 3-kinase. Oncogene 1999, **18**, 2607–15.

55. Shintani S, Funayama T, Yoshihama Y, *et al.* Prognostic significance of ERBB3 overexpression in oral squamous cell carcinoma. Cancer Lett 1995, **95**, 79–83.

56. Xia W, Lau YK, Zhang HZ, *et al.* Combination of EGFR, HER-2/neu, and HER-3 is a stronger predictor for the outcome of oral squamous cell carcinoma than any individual family members. Clin Cancer Res 1999, **5**, 4164–74.

57. Lyne JC, Melhem MF, Finley GG, *et al.* Tissue expression of neu differentiation factor/heregulin and its receptor complex in prostate cancer and its biologic effects on prostate cancer cells *in vitro*. Cancer J Sci Am 1997, **3**, 21–30.

58. Vaskovsky A, Lupowitz Z, Erlich S, *et al.* erbB-4 activation promotes neurite outgrowth in PC12 cells. J Neurochem 2000, **74**, 979–87.

59. Kew TY, Bell JA, Pinder SE, *et al.* c-erbB-4 protein expression in human breast cancer. Br J Cancer 2000, **82**, 1163–70.

60. Gilbertson RJ, Perry RH, Kelly PJ, *et al.* Prognostic significance of HER2 and HER4-coexpression in childhood medulloblastoma. Cancer-Res 1997, **57**, 3272–80.

61. Weiner LM. An overview of monoclonal antibody therapy of cancer. Sem Oncol 1999, **26**, 41–50.

62. Disis ML, Cheever MA. HER-2/neu protein: a target for antigen-specific immunotherapy of human cancer. Adv Cancer Res 1998, **71**, 344–71.

63. Fan Z, Mendelsohn J. Therapeutic application of anti-growth factor receptor antibodies. Curr Opin Oncol 1998, **10**, 67–73.

64. Aboud Pirak E, Hurwitz E, Pirak ME, *et al.* Efficacy of antibodies to epidermal growth factor receptor against KB carcinoma *in vitro* and in nude mice. J Natl Cancer Inst 1988, **80**, 1605–11.

65. Gill GN, Kawamoto T, Cochet C, *et al.* Monoclonal anti-epidermal growth factor receptor antibodies which are inhibitors of epidermal growth factor binding and antagonists of epidermal growth factor binding and antagonists of epidermal growth factor-stimulated tyrosine protein kinase activity. J Biol Chem 1984, **259**, 7755–60.

66. Masui H, Kawamoto T, Sato JD, *et al.* Growth inhibition of human tumor cells in athymic mice by anti-epidermal growth factor receptor monoclonal antibodies. Cancer Res 1984, **44**, 1002–7.

67. Masui H, Moroyoma T, Mendelsohn J. Mechanism of anti-tumor activity in mice for anti-epidermal growth factor receptor monoclonal antibodies with different isotypes. Cancer Res 1986, **46**, 5592–8.

68. Prewett M, Rockwell P, Rockwell RF, *et al.* The biologic effects of C225, a chimeric monoclonal antibody to the EGFR, on human prostate carcinoma. J Immunother Emphasis Tumor Immunol 1996, **19**, 419–27.

69. Divgi CR, Welt S, Kris M, *et al.* Phase I and imaging trial of indium 111-labeled anti-epidermal growth factor receptor monoclonal antibody 225 in patients with squamous cell lung carcinoma. J Natl Cancer Inst 1991, **83**, 97–104.

70. Faillot T, Magdelenat H, Mady E, *et al.* A phase I study of an anti-epidermal growth factor receptor monoclonal antibody for the treatment of malignant gliomas. *Neuro*surgery 1996, **39**, 478–83.

71. Perez-Soler R, Donato NJ, Shin DM, *et al.* Tumor epidermal growth factor receptor studies in patients with non-small-cell lung cancer or head and neck cancer treated with monoclonal antibody RG 83852 [published erratum appears in J Clin Oncol 1994, **12** (7), 1526]. J Clin Oncol 1994, **12**, 730–9.

72. Modjtahedi H, Hickish T, Nicolson M, *et al.* Phase I trial and tumour localisation of the anti-EGFR monoclonal antibody ICR62 in head and neck or lung cancer. Br J Cancer 1996, **73**, 228–35.

73. Goldstein NI, Prewett M, Zuklys K, *et al.* Biological efficacy of a chimeric antibody to the epidermal growth factor receptor in a human tumor xenograft model. Clin Cancer Res 1995, **1**, 1311–18.

74. Fan Z, Lu Y, We X, *et al.* Antibody-induced epidermal growth factor receptor dimerization mediates inhibition of autocrine proliferation of A431 squamous carcinoma cells. J Biol Chem 1994, **269**, 27595–602.

75. Baselga J, Pfister D, Cooper MR, *et al*. Phase I studies of anti-epidermal growth factor receptor chimeric antibody C225 alone and in combination with cisplatin. J Clin Oncol 2000, **18**, 904–14.

76. Bruns CJ, Harbison MT, Davis DW, *et al*. Epidermal growth factor receptor blockade with C225 plus gemcitabine results in regression of human pancreatic carcinoma growing orthotopically in nude mice by antiangiogenic mechanisms. Clin Cancer Res 2000, **6**, 1936–48.

77. Yang XD, Jia XC, Corvalan JR, *et al*. Eradication of established tumors by a fully human monoclonal antibody to the epidermal growth factor receptor without concomitant chemotherapy. Cancer Res 1999, **59**, 1236–43.

78. Ye D, Mendelsohn J, Fan Z. Augmentation of a humanized anti-HER2 mAb 4D5 induced growth inhibition by a human-mouse chimeric anti-EGF receptor mAb C225. Oncogene 1999, **18**, 731–8.

79. Drebin JA, Stern DF, Link VC, *et al*. Monoclonal antibodies identify a cell-surface antigen associated with an activated cellular oncogene. Nature 1984, **312**, 579–88.

80. Drebin JA, Link VC, Greene MI. Monoclonal antibodies specific for the *neu* oncogene product directly mediate anti-tumor effects *in vivo*. Oncogene 1988, **2**, 387–94.

81. Katsumata M, Okudaira T, Samanta A, *et al*. Prevention of breast tumour development in vivo by downregulation of the p185neu receptor. Nat Med 1995, **1**, 644–8.

82. Baselga J, Tripathy D, Mendelsohn J, *et al*. Phase II study of weekly intravenous recombinant humanized anti-p185HER2 monoclonal antibody in patients with HER2/neu-overexpressing metastatic breast cancer. J Clin Oncol 1996, **14**, 737–44.

83. Stancovski I, Hurwitz E, Leitner O, *et al*. Mechanistic aspects of the opposing effects of monoclonal antibodies to the ERBB2 receptor on tumor growth. Proc Natl Acad Sci, USA 1991, **88**, 8691–5.

84. Hurwitz E, Stancovski I, Sela M, *et al*. Suppression and promotion of tumor growth by monoclonal antibodies to erbB-2 differentially correlate with cellular uptake. Proc Nat Acad Sci, USA 1995, **92**, 3353–7.

85. Kasprzyk PG, Song SU, Di Fiore PP, *et al*. Therapy of an animal model of human gastric cancer using a combination of anti-erbB-2 monoclonal antibodies. Cancer Res 1992, **52**, 2771–6.

86. Klapper LN, Vaisman N, Hurwitz E, *et al*. A subclass of tumor-inhibitory monoclonal antibodies to erbB-2/HER2 blocks crosstalk with growth factor receptors. Oncogene 1997, **14**, 2099–109.

87. Klapper LN, Waterman H, Sela M, *et al*. Tumor-inhibitory antibodies to HER-2/erbB 2 may act by recruiting c-Cb1 and enhancing ubiquitination of HER-2. Cancer Res 2000, **60**, 3384–8.

88. Joazeiro CA, Wing SS, Huang H, *et al*. The tyrosine kinase negative regulator c-Cb1 as a RING-type, E2-dependent ubiquitin-protein ligase. Science 1999, **286**, 309–12.

89. Levkowitz G, Klapper LN, Tzahar E, *et al*. Coupling of the c-Cb1 protooncogene product to erbB-1/EGF-receptor but not to other erbB proteins. Oncogene 1996, **12**, 1117–25.

90. Levkowitz G, Oved S, Klapper LN, *et al*. c-Cb1 is a suppressor of the neu oncogene. J Biol Chem 2000, **275**, 35522–g.

91. Bacus SS, Huberman E, Chin D, *et al*. A ligand for the erbB-2 oncogenic product (gp30) induces differentiation of human breast cancer cells. Cell Growth Diff 1992, **3**, 401–11.

92. Bacus SS, Stancovski I, Huberman E, *et al*. Tumor-inhibitory monoclonal antibodies to the HER-2/Neu receptor induce differentiation of human breast cancer cells. Cancer Res 1992, **52**, 2580–9.

93. Kita Y, Tseng J, Horan T, *et al*. erbB receptor activation, cell morphology changes, and apoptosis induced by anti-Her2 monoclonal antibodies. Biochem Biophys Res Commun 1996, **226**, 59–69.

94. Sliwkowski MX, Lofgren JA, Lewis GD, *et al*. Nonclinical studies addressing the mechanism of action of trastuzumab (Herceptin). Sem Oncol 1999, **26**, 60–70.

95. Hurwitz E, Klapper LN, Wilchek M, *et al*. Inhibition of tumor growth by poly(ethylene glycol) derivatives of anti-erbB2 antibodies. Cancer Immunol mmunother 2000, **49**, 226–34.

96. Fisk B, Blevins TL, Wharton JT, *et al*. Identification of an immunodominant peptide of HER-2/neu protooncogene recognized by ovarian tumor-specific cytotoxic T lymphocyte lines. J Exp Med 1995, **181**, 2109–17.

97. Bernards R, Destree A, McKenzie S, *et al*. Effective tumor immunotherapy directed against an oncogene-encoded product using a vaccinia virus vector. Proc Natl Acad Sci, USA 1987, **84**, 6854–8.

98. Peiper M, Goedegebuure PS, Linehan DC, *et al*. The HER2/neu-derived peptide p654-662 is a tumor-associated antigen in human pancreatic cancer recognized by cytotoxic T lymphocytes. Eur J Immunol 1997, **27**, 1115–23.

99. Ioannides CG, Ioannides MG, O'Brian CA. T-cell recognition of oncogene products: a new strategy for immunotherapy. Mol Carcinog 1992, **6**, 77–82.

100. Fisk B, Blevins TL, Wharton JT, *et al*. Identification of an immunodominant peptide of HER-2/neu protooncogene recognized by ovarian tumor-specific cytotoxic T lymphocyte lines, J Exp Med 1995, **181**, 2109–17.

101. Sercarz EE, Lehmann PV, Ametani A, *et al*. Dominance and crypticity of T cell antigenic determinants. Annu Rev Immunol 1993, **11**, 729–66.

102. Disis MJ, Gralow JR, Bernhard H, *et al*. Peptide-based, but not whole protein, vaccines elicit immunity to HER-2/neu, oncogenic self-protein. J Immunol 1996, **156**, 3151–8.

103. Nagata Y, Furugen R, Hiasa A, *et al*. Peptides derived from wild type murine proto-oncogene c-erbB-2/HER2/neu can induce CTL and tumor suppression in syngeneic hosts. J Immunol 1997, **159**, 1336–43.

104. Stancovski I, Schindler DG, Waks T, *et al*. Targeting of T lymphocytes to Neu/HER2-expressing cells using chimeric single chain Fv receptors. J Immunol 1993, **151**, 6577–82.

105. Moritz D, Wels W, Mattern J, *et al*. Cytotoxic T lymphocytes with a grafted recognition specificity for

ERBB2-expressing tumor cells. Proc Natl Acad Sci, USA 1994, **91**, 4318–22.

106. Altenschmidt U, Klundt E, Groner B. Adoptive transfer of *in vitro*-targeted, activated T lymphocytes results in total tumor regression. J Immunol 1997, **159**, 5509–15.

107. Challita Eid PM, Penichet ML, Shin SU, *et al.* A B7.1-antibody fusion protein retains antibody specificity and ability to activate via the T cell costimulatory pathway. J Immunol 1998, **160**, 3419–26.

108. Gerstmayer B, Altenschmidt U, Hoffmann M, *et al.* Costimulation of T cell proliferation by a chimeric B7-2 antibody fusion protein specifically targeted to cells expressing the erbB2 proto-oncogene. J Immunol 1997, **158**, 4584–90.

109. Weiner LM, Clark JI, Davey M, *et al.* Phase I trial of 2B1, a bispecific monoclonal antibody targeting c-erbB-2 and Fc gamma RIII. Cancer Res 1995, **55**, 4586–93.

110. Curnow RT. Clinical experience with CD64-directed immunotherapy. An overview. Cancer Immunol Immunother 1997, **45**, 210–15.

111. van-Ojik HH, Repp R, Groenewegen G, *et al.* Clinical evaluation of the bispecific antibody MDX-H210 (anti-Fc gamma RI × anti-HER-2/neu) in combination with granulocyte-colony-stimulating factor (filgrastim) for treatment of advanced breast cancer. Cancer Immunol Immunother 1997, **45**, 207–9.

112. Orlandi R, Formantici C, Menard S, *et al.* A linear region of a monoclonal antibody conformational epitope mapped on p185HER2 oncoprotein. Biol Chem 1997, **378**, 1387–92.

113. Vaisman N, Nissim A, Klapper LN, *et al.* Specific inhibition of the reaction between tumor-inhibitory antibody and the erbB-2 receptor by a mimotope derived from a phage display library. Immunol Lett 2000, **75**, 61–7.

114. Park BW, Zhang HT, Wu C, *et al.* Rationally designed anti-HER2/neu peptide mimetic disables P185HER2/neu tyrosine kinases *in vitro* and *in vivo*. Nat Biotechnol 2000, **18**, 194–8.

115. DiGiovanna MP, Lerman MA, Coffey RJ, *et al.* Active signaling by Neu in transgenic mice. Oncogene 1998, **17**, 1877–84.

116. Adams GP, Schier R, Marshall K, *et al.* Increased affinity leads to improved selective tumor delivery of single-chain Fv antibodies. Cancer Res 1998, **58**, 485–90.

117. Adams GP, Schier R, McCall AM, *et al.* Prolonged *in vivo* tumour retention of a human diabody targeting the extracellular domain of human GER2/neu. Br J Cancer 1998, **77**, 1405–12.

118. Beerli RR, Wels W, Hynes NE. Intracellular expression of single chain antibodies reverts erbB-2 transformation. J Biol Chem 1994, **269**, 23931–6.

119. Neve RM, Sutterluty H, Pullen N, *et al.* Effects of oncogenic erbB2 on G1 cell cycle regulators in breast tumour cells. Oncogene 2000, **19**, 1647–56.

120. Wiechen K, Karaaslan S, Turzynski A, *et al.* Suppression of the c-erbB-2 gene product decreases transformation abilities but not the proliferation and secretion of proteases of SK-OV-3 ovarian cancer cells. Br J Cancer 1999, **81**, 790–5.

121. Lewis GD, Figari I, Fendly B, *et al.* Differential responses of human tumor cell lines to anti-p185HER2 monoclonal antibodies. Cancer Immunol Immunother 1993, **37**, 255–63.

122. Carter P, Presta L, Gorman CM, *et al.* Humanization of an anti-p185HER2 antibody for human cancer therapy. Proc Natl Acad Sci, USA 1992, **89**, 4285–9.

123. Baselga j, Norton L, Albanell J, *et al.* Recombinant humanized anti-HER2 antibody (Herceptin) enhances the antitumor activity of paclitaxel and doxorubicin against HER2/neu overexpressing human breast cancer xenografts. Cancer Res 1998, **58**, 2825–31.

124. Pietras RJ, Fendly BM, Chazin VR, *et al.* Antibody to HER-2/neu receptor blocks DNA repair after cisplatin in human breast and ovarian cancer cells. Oncogene 1994, **9**, 1829–38.

125. Cobleigh M, Vogel CL, Tripathy D, *et al.* Efficacy and safety of Herceptin (humanized anti-HER2 antibody) as a single agent in 222 women with HER2 overexpression who relapsed following chemotherapy for metastatic breast cancer [abstract]. Proc Am Soc Clin Oncol 1998, **17**, 376.

126. Vogel C. First-line, non-hormonal treatment of women with HER2 overexpressing metastatic breast cancer with Herceptin (Trastuzumab, humanized anti-HER2 antibody). Proc Am Soc Clin Oncol 2000, **19**, 275.

127. Slamon DJ, Leyland-Jones B, Shak S, *et al.* Addition of Herceptin (humanized Anti-HER2 antibody) to first line chemotherapy for HER2 overexpressing metastatic breast cancer (HER2+/MBC) markedly increases anti-cancer activity: a randomized, multinational controlled phase III trial. Proc Am Soc Clin Oncol 1998, **17**, 98a [abstract 377].

128. Disis ML, Pupa SM, Gralow JR, *et al.* High-titer HER-2/neu protein-specific antibody can be detected in patients with early-stage breast cancer. J Clin Oncol 1997, **15**, 3363–7.

129. Langton BC, Crenshaw MC, Chao LA, *et al.* An antigen immunologically related to the external domain of gp185 is shed from nude mouse tumors overexpressing the c-*erbB*-2 (HER-2/*neu*) oncogene. Cancer Res 1991, **51**, 2593–8.

130. Lin YZ, Clinton GM. A soluble protein related to the HER-2 proto-oncogene product is released from human breast carcinoma cells. Oncogene 1991, **6**, 639–43.

131. Fehm T, Maimonis P, Weitz S, *et al.* Influence of circulating c-erbB-2 serum protein on response to adjuvant chemotherapy in node-positive breast cancer patients. Breast Cancer Res Treat 1997, **43**, 87–95.

132. Kandl H, Seymour L, Bezwoda WR. Soluble c-erbB-2 fragment in serum correlates with disease stage and predicts for shortened survival in patients with early-stage and advanced breast cancer. Br J Cancer 1994, **70**, 739–42.

133. Leitzel K, Teramoto Y, Konrad K, *et al.* Elevated serum c-erbB-2 antigen levels and decreased response to hormone therapy of breast cancer. J Clin Oncol 1995, **13**, 1129–35.

134. Mansour OA, Zekri AR, Harvey J, *et al.* Tissue and serum c-erbB-2 and tissue EGFR in breast carcinoma: three years follow-up. Anticancer Res 1997, **17**, 3101–6.

135. Meden H, Marx D, Schauer A, *et al.* Prognostic significance of p105 (c-erbB-2 HER2/neu) serum levels in patients with ovarian cancer. Anticancer Res 1997, **17**, 757–60.

136. Molina R, Jo J, Filella X, *et al.* C-erbB-2 oncoprotein in the sera and tissue of patients with breast cancer. Utility in prognosis. Anticancer Res 1996, **16**, 2295–300.

137. Molina R, Jo J, Filella X, *et al.* Serum levels of C0erbB-2 (HER-2/neu) in patients with malignant and non-malignant diseases. Tumour Biol 1997, **18**, 188–96.

138. Fontana X, Ferrari P, Namer M, *et al.* C-erb-B2 gene amplification and serum level of c-erb-B2 oncoprotein at primary breast cancer diagnosis. Anticancer-Res 1994, **14**, 2099–104.

139. Krainer M, Brodowicz T, Zeillinger R, *et al.* Tissue expression and serum levels of HER-2/neu in patients with breast cancer. Oncology 1997, **54**, 475–81.

140. Chen X, Levkowitz G, Tzahar E, *et al.* An immunological approach reveals biological differences between the two NDF/heregulin receptors, erbB-3 and erbB-4. J Biol Chem 1996, **271**, 7620–9.

141. Waterman H, Sabanai I, Geiger B, *et al.* Alternative intracellular routing of erbB receptors may determine signaling potency. J Biol Chem 1998, **273**, 13819–27.

142. Rajkumar T, Gullick WJ. A monoclonal antibody to the human c-erbB3 protein stimulates the anchorage-independent growth of breast cancer cell lines. Br J Cancer 1994, **70**, 459–65.

143. Yang D, Kuan CT, Payne J, *et al.* Recombinant heregulin-*Pseudomonas* exotoxin fusion proteins: interactions with the heregulin receptors and antitumor activity *in vivo.* Clin Cancer Res 1998, **4**, 993–1004.

144. Hurwitz E, Sela M. Conjugates of antibodies with cytotoxin drugs. In: Immunoconjugates (ed. CW Vogel). Oxford University Press, New York, 1987, 189–216.

145. Trail PA, Bianchi AB. Monoclonal antibody drug conjugates in the treatment of cancer. Curr Opin Immunol 1999, **11**, 584–8.

146. Aboud-Pirak E, Hurwitz E, Bellot F, *et al.* Inhibition of human tumor growth in nude mice by a conjugate of doxorubicin with monoclonal antibodies to epidermal growth factor receptor. Proc Natl Acad Sci, USA 1989, **86**, 3778–81.

147. Schechter B, Arnon R, Wilchek M, *et al.* Indirect immunotargeting of cis-Pt to human epidermoid carcinoma KB using the avidin–biotin system. Int J Cancer 1991, **48**, 167–72.

148. Hancock MC, Langton BC, Chan T, *et al.* A monoclonal antibody against the c-erbB-2 protein enhances the cytotoxicity of cis-diamminedichloroplatinum against human breast and ovarian tumor cell lines. Cancer Res 1991, **51**, 4575–80.

149. Arteaga CL, Winnier AR, Poirier MC, *et al.* p185c-erbB-2 signal enhances cisplatin-induced cytotoxicity in human breast carcinoma cells: association between an oncogenic receptor tyrosine kinase and drug-induced DNA repair. Cancer Res 1994, **54**, 3758–65.

150. Witters LM, Kumar R, Chinchilli VM, *et al.* Enhanced anti-proliferative activity of the combination of tamoxifen plus HER-2-neu antibody. Breast Cancer Res Treat 1997, **42**, 1–5.

151. Hudziak RM, Lewis GD, Winget M, *et al.* p185HER2 monoclonal antibody has antiproliferative effects *in vitro* and sensitizes human breast tumor cells to tumor necrosis factor. Mol Cell Biol 1989, **9**, 1165–72.

152. Fan Z, Baselga J, Masui H, *et al.* Antitumor effect of anti-epidermal growth factor receptor monoclonal antibodies plus cis-diamminedichloroplatinum on well established A431 cell xenografts. Cancer Res 1993, **53**, 4637–42.

153. Baselga J, Norton L, Masui H, *et al.* Antitumor effects of doxorubicin in combination with anti-epidermal growth factor receptor monoclonal antibodies. J Natl Cancer Inst 1993, **85**, 1327–33.

154. Pegram MD, Lipton A, Hayes DF, *et al.* Phase II study of receptor-enhanced chemosensitivity using recombinant humanized anti-p185HER2/neu monoclonal antibody plus cisplatin in patients with HER2/ neu-overexpressing metastatic breast cancer refractory to chemotherapy treatment. J Clin Oncol 1998, **16**, 2659–71.

155. Pegram M, Hsu S, Lewis G, *et al.* Inhibitory effects of combinations of HER-2/neu antibody and chemotherapeutic agents used for treatment of human breast cancers. Oncogene 1999, **18**, 2241–51.

156. Pegram M and Slamon D. Biological rationale for HER2/neu (c-erbB2) as a target for monoclonal antibody therapy. Sem Oncol 2000, **27**, 13–19.

157. Pegram MD, Konecny G, Slamon DJ. The molecular and cellular biology of HER2/neu gene amplification/ overexpression and the clinical development of herceptin (trastuzumab) therapy for breast cancer. Cancer Treat Res 2000, **103**, 57–75.

158. Kirpotin D, Park JW, Hong K, *et al.* Sterically stabilized anti-HER2 immunoliposomes: design and targeting to human breast cancer cells *in vitro.* Biochemistry 1997, **36**, 66–75.

159. Park JW, Hong K, Kirpotin DB, *et al.* Anti-HER2 immunoliposomes for targeted therapy of human tumors. Cancer Lett 1997, **118**, 153–60.

160. Senter PD, Svensson HP. A summary of monoclonal antibody–enzyme/prodrug combination. Adv Drug Delivery Rev 1996, **22**, 341–9.

161. Colbern GT, Hiller AJ, Musterer RS, *et al.* Antitumor activity of Herceptin in combination with STEALTH liposomal cisplatin or nonliposomal cisplatin in a HER2 positive human breast cancer model. J Inorg Biochem 1999, **77**, 117–20.

162. Ciardiello F, Bianco R, Damiano V, *et al.* Antitumor activity of sequential treatment with topotecan and anti-epidermal growth factor receptor monoclonal antibody C225. Clin Cancer Res 1999, **5**, 909–16.

163. Baselga, J, Pfister D, Cooper MR, *et al.* Phase I studies of anti-epidermal growth factor receptor chimeric antibody C225 alone and in combination with cisplatin. J Clin Oncol 2000, **18**, 904.

164. Melton RG, Sherwood RF. Antibody–enzyme conjugates for cancer therapy. J Natl Cancer Inst 1996, **88**, 153–65.

165. Rodrigues ML, Presta LG, Kotts CE, *et al.* Development of a humanized disulfide-stabilized anti-p185HER2 Fv-beta-lactamase fusion protein for activation of a cephalosporin doxorubicin prodrug. Cancer Res 1995, **55**, 63–70.

166. Pastan I, FitzGerald D. Recombinant toxins for cancer treatment. Science 1991, **254**, 1173–7.

167. Batra JK, Kasprzyk PG, Bird RE. Recombinant anti-erbB-2 immunotoxins containing *Pseudomonas* exotoxin. Proc Natl Acad Sci, USA 1992, **89**, 5867–71.

168. Altenschmidt U, Schmidt M, Groner B, *et al.* Targeted therapy of schwannoma cells in immunocompetent rats with an erbB2-specific antibody-toxin. Int J Cancer 1997, **73**, 117–24.

169. Rodriguez GC, Boente MP, Berchuck A, *et al.* The effect of antibodies and immunotoxins reactive with HER-2/neu on growth of ovarian and breast cancer cell lines. Am J Obstet Gynecol 1993, **168**, 228–32.

170. Schmidt M, Hynes NE, Groner B, *et al.* A bivalent single-chain antibody-toxin specific for erbB-2 and the EGF receptor. Int J Cancer 1996, **65**, 538–46.

171. Chen SY, Yang AG, Chen JD, *et al.* Potent antitumour activity of a new class of tumour-specific killer cells. Nature 1997, **385**, 78–80.

172. Schechter B, Arnon R, Wilchek M. Cytotoxicity of streptavidin-blocked biotinyl-ricin is retrieved by *in vitro* immunotargeting via biotinyl monoclonal antibody. Cancer Res 1992, **52**, 4448–52.

173. Lorimer IA, Wikstrand CJ, Batra SK, *et al.* Immunotoxins that target an oncogenic mutant epidermal growth factor receptor expressed in human tumours. Clin Cancer Res 1995, **1**, 859–64.

174. Beers R, Chowdhury P, Bigner D, *et al.* Immunotoxins with increased activity against epidermal growth factor receptor vIII-expressing cells produced by antibody phage display. Clin Cancer Res 2000, **6**, 2835–43.

175. Schmidt M, Maurer-Gebhard M, Groner B, *et al.* Suppression of metastasis formation by a recombinant single chain antibody-toxin targeted to full-length and oncogenic variant EGF receptors. Oncogene 1999, **18**, 1711–21.

176. Rosenblum MG, Shawver LK, Marks JW, *et al.* Recombinant immunotoxins directed against the c-erb-2/HER2/neu oncogene product: *in vitro* cytotoxicity, pharmacokinetics, and *in vivo* efficacy studies in xenograft models. Clin Cancer Res 1999, **5**, 865–74.

177. Azemar M, Schmidt M, Arlt F, *et al.* Recombinant antibody toxins specific for erbB2 and EGF receptor inhibit the *in vitro* growth of human head and neck cancer cells and cause rapid tumor regression *in vivo*. Int J Cancer 2000, **86**, 269–75.

178. Chandler LA, Sosnowski BA, McDonald JR, *et al.* Targeting tumor cells via EGF receptors: selective toxicity of an HBEGF–toxin fusion protein. Int J Cancer 1998, **78**, 106–11.

179. Groner B, Wick B, Jeschke M, *et al.* Intra-tumoral application of a heregulin–exotoxin—a fusion protein causes rapid tumor regression without adverse systemic or local effects. Int J Cancer 1997, **70**, 682–7.

180. Mixan B, Cohen BD, Bacus SS, *et al.* Betacellulin–*Pseudomonas* toxin fusion proteins bind but are not cytotoxic to cells expressing HER4; correlation of EGFR for cytotoxic activity. Oncogene 198, **16**, 1209–15.

181. Chowdhury PS, Viner JL, Beers R, *et al.* Isolation of a high-affinity stable single-chain FV specific for mesothe-lin from DNA-immunized mice by phage display and construction of a recombinant immunotoxin with anti-tumor activity. Proc Natl Acad Sci, USA 1998, **95**, 669–74.

182. Kwok KH, Law KB, Wong RN, *et al.* Immunolesioning of glutamate receptor GluR1-containing neurons in the rat neostriatum using a novel immunotoxin. Cell Mol Neurobiol 2000, **20**, 483–96.

183. Burrows FJ, Derbyshire EJ, Tazzari PL, *et al.* Up-regulation of endoglin on vascular endothelial cells in human solid tumors: implications for diagnosis and therapy. Clin Cancer Res 1995, **1**, 1623–34.

184. Matsuno F, Haruta Y, Kondo M, *et al.* Induction of lasting complete regression of preformed distinct solid tumors by targeting the tumor vasculature using two new anti-endoglin monoclonal antibodies. Clin Cancer Res 1999, **5**, 371–82.

185. Arora N, Masood R, Zheng T, *et al.* Vascular endothelial growth factor chimeric toxin is highly active against endothelial cells. Cancer Res 1999, **59**, 183–8.

186. Reist CJ, Garg PK, Alston KL, *et al.* Radioiodination of internalizing monoclonal antibodies using *N*-succinimidyl 5-iodo-3-pyridinecarboxylate. Cancer Res 1996, **56**, 4970–7.

187. Iznaga-Escobar N, Torres Arocha LA, Morales Morales A, *et al.* Technetium-99m-antiepidermal growth factor-receptor antibody in patients with tumors of epithelial origin: part II. Pharmacokinetics and clearances. J Nucl Med 1998, **39**, 1918–27.

188. Morales AA, Crespo FZ, Gandolff GN, *et al.* Technetium-99m direct radiolabeling of monoclonal antibody ior egf/r3. Nucl Med Biol 1998, **25**, 25–30.

189. Iznaga Escobar N, Morales AM, Duconge J, *et al.* Pharmacokinetics, biodistribution and dosimetry of 99mTc-labeled anti-human epidermal growth factor receptor humanized monoclonal antibody R3 in rats. Nucl Med Biol 1998, **25**, 17–23.

190. Kurihara A, Pardridge WM. Imaging brain tumors by targeting peptide radiopharmaceuticals through the blood–brain barrier. Cancer Res 1999, **59**, 6159–63.

191. De Santes K, Slamon D, Anderson SK, *et al.* Radiolabeled antibody targeting of the HER-2/*neu* oncoprotein. Cancer Res 1992, **52**, 1916–23.

192. Kotts CE, Su FM, Leddy C, *et al.* 186Re-labeled antibodies to p185HER2 as HER2-targeted radioimmunopharmaceutical agents: comparison of physical and biological characteristics with 125I and 131I-labeled counterparts. Cancer Biother Radiopharm 1996, **11**, 133–44.

193. Smellie WJ, Dean CJ, Sacks NP, *et al.* Radioimmunotherapy of breast cancer xenografts with monoclonal antibody ICR12 against c-erbB2 p185: comparison of iodogen and N-succinimidyl 4-methyl-3-(tri-*n*-butylstannyl)benzoate radioiodination methods. Cancer Res 1995, **55**, 5842s–6s.

194. Xu FJ, Yu YH, Bae DS, *et al.* Radioiodinated antibody targeting of the HER-2/neu oncoprotein. Nucl Med Biol 1997, **24**, 451–9.

195. Horak E, Hartmann F, Garmestani K, *et al.* Radioimmunotherapy targeting of HER2/neu oncoprotein on ovarian tumor using lead-212-DOTA-AE1. J Nucl Med 1997, **38**, 1944–50.

196. Tsai SW, Sun Y, Williams LE, *et al.* Biodistribution and radioimmunotherapy of human breast cancer xenografts with radiometal-labeled DOTA conjugated anti-HER2/neu antibody 4D5. Bioconjug Chem 2000, **11**, 327–34.

197. van Gog FB, Brakenhoff RH, Stigter-van Walsum M, *et al.* Perspectives of combined radioimmunotherapy and anti-EGFR antibody therapy for the treatment of residual head and neck cancer. Int J Cancer 1998, **77**, 13–18.

198. Saleh MN, Raisch KP, Stackhouse MA, *et al.* Combined modality therapy of A431 human epidermoid cancer using anti-EGFr antibody C225 and radiation. Cancer Biother Radiopharm 1999, **14**, 451–63.

199. Milas L, Mason K, Hunter N, *et al. In vivo* enhancement of tumor radioresponse by C225 antiepidermal growth factor receptor antibody. Clin Cancer Res 2000, **6**, 701–8.

200. Stackhouse MA, Buchsbaum DJ, Grizzle WE, *et al.* Radiosensitization mediated by a transfected anti-erbB-2 single-chain antibody *in vitro* and *in vivo*. Int J Radiat Oncol Biol Phys 1998, **42**, 817–22.

201. Haffty BG, Brown F, Carter D, *et al.* Evaluation of HER-2 neu oncoprotein expression as a prognostic indicator of local recurrence in conservatively treated breast cancer: a case-control study. Int J Radiat Oncol Biol Phys 1996, **35**, 751–7.

202. Pirollo KF, Hao Z, Rait A, *et al.* Evidence supporting a signal transduction pathway leading to the radiation-resistant phenotype in human tumor cells. Biochem Biophys Res Commun 1997, **230**, 196–201.

203. Pietras RJ, Poen JC, Gallardo D, *et al.* Monoclonal antibody to HER-2/neureceptor modulates repair of radiation-induced DNA damage and enhances radiosensitivity of human breast cancer cells overexpressing this oncogene. Cancer Res 1999, **59**, 1347–55.

204. Gorski DH, Beckett MA, Jaskowiak NT, *et al.* Blockage of the vascular endothelial growth factor stress response increases the antitumor effects of ionizing radiation. Cancer Res 1999, **59**, 3374–8.

205. Skobe M, Rockwell P, Goldstein N, *et al.* Halting angiogenesis suppresses carcinoma cell invasion. Nat Med 1997, **3**, 1222–7.

206. Prewett M, Huber J, Li Y, *et al.* Antivascular endothelial growth factor receptor (fetal liver kinase 1) monoclonal antibody inhibits tumor angiogenesis and growth of several mouse and human tumors. Cancer Res 1999, **59**, 5209–18.

207. Witte L, Hicklin DJ, Zhu Z, *et al.* Monoclonal antibodies targeting the VEGF receptor-2 (Flk1/KDR) as an anti-angiogenic therapeutic strategy. Cancer Metastasis Rev 1998, **17**, 155–61.

208. Inoue K, Slaton JW, Davis DW, *et al.* Treatment of human metastatic transitional cell carcinoma of the bladder in a murine model with the anti-vascular endothelial growth factor receptor monoclonal antibody DC101 and paclitaxel. Clin Cancer Res 2000, **6**, 2635–43.

209. Klement G, Baruchel S, Rak J, *et al.* Continuous low-dose therapy with vinblastine and VEGF receptor-2 antibody induces sustained tumor regression without overt toxicity. J Clin Invest 2000, **105**, R15–24.

210. Petit AM, Rak J, Hung MC, *et al.* Neutralizing antibodies against epidermal growth factor and erbB-2/neu receptor tyrosine kinases down-regulate vascular endothelial growth factor production by tumor cells *in vitro* and *in vivo*: angiogenic implications for signal transduction therapy of solid tumors. Am J Pathol 1997, **151**, 1523–30.

211. Perrotte P, Matsumoto T, Inoue K, *et al.* Anti-epidermal growth factor receptor antibody C225 inhibits angiogenesis in human transitional cell carcinoma growing orthotopically in nude mice. Clin Cancer Res 1999, **5**, 257–65.

212. Lin YS, Nguyen C, Mendoza JL, *et al.* Preclinical pharmacokinetics interspecies scaling, and tissue distribution of a humanized monoclonal antibody against vascular endothelial growth factor. J Pharmacol Exp Ther 1999, **288**, 371–8.

213. Ryan AM, Eppler DB, Hagler KE, *et al.* Preclinical safety evaluation of rhuMAbVEGF, an antiangiogenic humanized monoclonal antibody. Toxicol Pathol 1999. **27**, 78–86.

214. Presta LG, Chen H, O'Connor SJ, *et al.* Humanization of an anti-vascular endothelial growth factor monoclonal antibody for the therapy of solid tumors and other disorders. Cancer Res 1997, **57**, 4593–9.

215. Olson TA, Mohanraj D, Roy S, *et al.* Targeting the tumor vasculature: inhibition of tumor growth by a vascular endothelial growth factor–toxin conjugate. Int J Cancer 1997, **73**, 865–70.

216. Brewer CA, Setterdahl JJ, Li MJ, *et al.* Endoglin expression as a measure of microvessel density in cervical cancer. Obstet Gynecol 2000, **96**, 224–8.

217. Li C, Guo B, Wilson PB, *et al.* Plasma levels of solubleCD105 correlate with metastasis in patients with breast cancer. Int J Cancer 2000, **89**, 122–6.

218. Fonsatti E, Jekunen AP, Kairemo KJ, *et al.* Endoglin is a suitable target for efficient imaging of solid tumors: *in vivo* evidence in a canine mammary carcinoma model. Clin Cancer Res 2000, **6**, 2037–43.

219. Peles E, Yarden Y. Inhibitors of protein tyrosine kinases. In: Design of enzyme inhibitors as drugs, Vol. 2 (ed. M. Sandler and J. Smith). Oxford University Press, Oxford, 1993.

220. Levitzki A, Gazit A. Tyrosine kinase inhibition: an approach to drug development. Science 1995, **267**, 1782–8.

221. Levitzki A. Protein tyrosine kinase inhibitors as novel therapeutic agents. Pharmacol Ther 1999, **82**, 231–9.

222. Klohs WD, Fry DW, Kraker AJ. Inhibitors of tyrosine kinase. Curr Opin Oncol 1997, **9**, 562–8.

223. Osherov N, Gazit A, Gilon C, *et al.* Selective inhibition of the epidermal growth factor and HER2/neu receptors by tyrphostins. J Biol Chem 1993, **268**, 11134–42.

224. Penar PL, Khoshyomn S, Bhushan A, *et al.* Inhibition of epidermal growth factor receptor-associated tyrosine kinase blocks glioblastoma invasion of the brain. Neurosurgery 1997, **40**, 141–51.

225. Kondapaka BS, Reddy KB. Tyrosine kinase inhibitor as a novel signal transduction and antiproliferative agent: prostate cancer. Mol Cell Endocrinol 1996, **117**, 53–8.

226. Rewcastle GW, Murray DK, Elliott WL, *et al.* Tryosine kinase inhibitors. 14. Structure–activity relationships for

methylamino-substituted derivatives of 4-[(3-bro-mophenyl)amino]-6-(methylamino)-pyrido[3,4-d]pyrimidine (PD 158780), a potent and specific inhibitor of the tyrosine kinase activity of receptors for the EGF family of growth factors. J Med Chem 1998, **41**, 742–51.

227. Fry DW, Bridges AJ, Denny WA, *et al*. Specific, irreversible inactivation of the epidermal growth factor receptor and erbB2, by a new class of tyrosine kinase inhibitor. Proc Natl Acad Sci USA 1998, **95**, 12022–7.

228. Tsai CM, Levitzki A, Wu LH, *et al*. Enhancement of chemosensitivity by tyrphostin AG825 in high-p185(neu) expressing non-small cell lung cancer cells. Cancer Res 1996, **56**, 1068–74.

229. Kovalenko M, Ronnstrand L, Heldin CH, *et al*. Phosphorylation site-specific inhibition of platelet-derived growth factor beta-receptor autophosphorylation by the receptor blocking tyrphostin AG1296. Biochemistry 1997, **36**, 6260–9.

230. Banai S, Wolf Y, Golomb G, *et al*. PDGF-receptor tyrosine kinase blocker AG1295 selectively attenuates smooth muscle cell growth *in vitro* and reduces neointimal formation after balloon angioplasty in swine. Circulation 1998, **97**, 1960–9.

231. Puddicombe SM, Polosa R, Richter A, *et al*. Involvement of the epidermal growth factor receptor in epithelial repair in asthma. FASEB J 2000, **14**, 1362–74.

232. Lenferink AE, Simpson JF, Shawver LK, *et al*. Blockade of the epidermal growth factor receptor tyrosine kinase suppresses tumorigenesis in MMTV/Neu + MMTV/TGF-alpha bigenic mice. Proc Natl Acad Sci, USA 2000, **97**, 9609–14.

233. Arteaga CL, Ramsey TT, Shawver LK, *et al*. Unliganded epidermal growth factor receptor dimerization induced by direct interaction of quinazolines with the ATP binding site. J Biol Chem 1997, **272**, 23247–54.

234. Ben-Levy R, Peles E, Goldman Michael R, *et al*. An oncogenic point mutation confers high affinity ligand binding to the neu receptor. Implications for the generation of site heterogeneity. J Biol Chem 1992, **267**, 17304–13.

235. Brugge JS. New intracellular targets for drug design. Science 1993, **260**, 918–19.

236. Hung MC, Matin A, Zhang Y, *et al*. HER-2/neu-targeting gene therapy—a review. Gene 1995, **159**, 65–71.

237. Chang JY, Xia W, Shao R, *et al*. Inhibition of intratracheal lung cancer development by systemic delivery of E1A. Oncogene 1996, **13**, 1405–12.

238. Ueno NT, Yu D, Hung MC. Chemosensitization of HER-2/neu-overexpressing human breast cancer cells to paclitaxel (Taxol) by adenovirus type 5 E1A. Oncogene 1997, **15**, 953–60.

239. Ring CJ, Harris JD, Hurst HC, *et al*. Suicide gene expression induced in tumour cells transduced with recombinant adenoviral, retroviral and plasmid vectors containing the ERBB2 promoter. Gene Ther 1996, **3**, 1094–103.

240. Ring CJ, Blouin P, Martin LA, *et al*. Use of transcriptional regulatory elements of the MUC1 and ERBB2 genes to drive tumour-selective expression of a prodrug activating enzyme. Gene Ther 1997, **4**, 1045–52.

241. Xing X, Wang SC, Xia W, *et al*. The ets protein PEA3 suppresses HER-2/neu overexpression and inhibits tumorigenesis. Nat Med 2000, **6**, 189–95.

242. Ebbinghaus SW, Gee JE, Rodu B, *et al*. Triplex formation inhibits HER-2/neu transcription *in vitro*. J Clin Invest 1993, **92**, 2433–9.

243. Juhl H, Downing SG, Wellstein A, *et al*. Her-2/neu is rate limiting for ovarian cancer growth. Conditional depletion of HER-2/neu by ribozyme targeting. J Biol Chem 1997, **272**, 29482–6.

244. Colomer R, Lupu R, Bacus SS, *et al*. erbB-2 antisense oligonucleotides inhibit the proliferation of breast carcinoma cells with erbB-2 oncogene amplification. Br J Cancer 1994, **70**, 819–25.

245. Casalini P, Menard S, Malandrin SM, *et al*. Inhibition of tumorigenicity in lung adenocarcinoma cells by c-erbB-2 antisense expression. Int J Cancer 1997, **72**, 631–6.

246. Vaughn JP, Stekler J, Demirdji S, *et al*. Inhibition of the erbB-2 tyrosine kinase receptor in breast cancer cells by phosphoromonothioate and phosphorodithioate antisense oligonucleotides. Nucl Acids Res 1996, **24**, 4558–64.

247. Messerle K, Schlegel J, Hynes NE, *et al*. NIH/3T3 cells transformed with the activated erbB-2 oncogene can be phenotypically reverted by a kinase deficient, dominant negative erbB-2 variant. Mol Cell Endocrinol 1994, **105**, 1–10.

248. Qian X, O'Rourke DM, Zhao H, *et al*. Inhibition of p185neu kinase activity and cellular transformation by co-expression of a truncated neu protein. Oncogene 1996, **13**, 2149–57.

249. Wright M, Grim J, Deshane J, *et al*. An intracellular anti-erbB-2 single-chain antibody is specifically cytotoxic to human breast carcinoma cells overexpressing erbB-2. Gene Ther 1997, **4**, 317–22.

250. Graus Porta D, Beerli RR, Hynes NE. Single-chain antibody-mediated intracellular retention of erbB-2 impairs Neu differentiation factor and epidermal growth factor signaling. Mol Cell Biol 1995, **15**, 1182–91.

251. Alvarez RD, Curiel DT. A phase I study of recombinant adenovirus vector-mediated delivery of an anti-Erbb-2 single chain (sFv) antibody gene for previously treated ovarian and extraovarian cancer patients. Hum Gene Ther 1997, **8**, 229–42.

Targeting the metastatic process

*Lloyd A. Culp, Wen-Chang Lin, Nanette R. Kleinman,
Priit Kogerman, Raymond Judware, Carson J. Miller, and
Julianne L. Holleran*

Recent approaches to dissect tumor progression and metastasis in animal model systems

Metastasis of a tumor to target organ sites is a very complex series of events (1–7). It must involve highly selected primary tumor subpopulations, blood and/or lymphatic vessels, and specific organs amenable to 'receive' the tumor cells. At least six to eight different steps can be envisioned in this migratory sequence, each of which must require specific and specialized gene products to be successful. One of the most impressive aspects of cancer metastasis is the remarkable versatility of tumor cells to generate such sophisticated subpopulations.

Angiogenesis is one critical consideration during metastasis (1, 10, 11). Not only must metastatic tumor subsets intravasate and extravasate currently established blood vessels, they must also secrete the critical factors required at their foreign target sites to induce new blood vessel formation if micrometastases are to grow successfully into overt metastases. Since other chapters in this volume deal with angiogenesis regulation specifically, no further comment will be made on the significance of these specialized gene products and their functions in this chapter.

There are analogies between the evolution of metastatic variants in the primary tumor and some complex events that occur during normal embryonic development (12, 13). For example, development of the neural crest generates multiple cell subsets that migrate to other 'foreign' regions of the embryo where they differentiate into adrenal gland cells, peripheral neurons at many sites, melanocytes throughout the skin, and some facial bones. Developmental biologists have shown that these complex patterns require a shifting in the expression of many genes, not just one or a few genes (13).

Likewise, metastasis to various target organs from the site of the primary tumor must involve a large array of gene activities. This is evident since the primary tumor is embedded in its 'native' cellular environment while all target metastatic sites must be viewed as 'highly foreign' to that particular tumor cell (1–6). This complexity is compounded by intravasation/extravasation of blood vessels and/or lymphatic vessels during these events and by the fact that a particular class of primary tumor does not metastasize to only one target site (although one site might be highly preferred during early events) but to multiple sites.

Targeting multiple tissue sites presumably requires different, but overlapping, gene classes in tumor cell subsets. In support of this hypothesis, evidence is mounting for organ-specific regulation of tumor cell genes (7, 8; see the next two sections on 'Histochemical marker genes' and 'Selection and counterselection for CD44 overexpression'). Furthermore, these new patterns of gene expression in metastatic tumor subsets are a reflection of the genetic instability of cells in the primary tumor, permitting select subsets to be successful and efficient in the multiple steps involved. Therefore, it is highly unlikely that there is a master 'metastasis-control' gene in any tumor type that oversees these complex events (9). Rather, it is genetic instability leading to many subsets of tumor cells that guarantees success in metastasis to lung, liver, bone, bone marrow, brain, and other target organs.

Another consideration in these experimental paradigms of tumor progression and metastasis is the pattern(s) by which genes change their expression. It is highly likely that some genes are turned off to generate metastatic variants, while other gene classes are turned on to execute specialized functions. There is also evidence, reviewed in the section on CD44 overexpression, of reversible expression of at least one gene during progression and metastasis, a concept predicted by Nicolson (4) many years ago.

Our studies, summarized in this review, involve three different tumor systems. The first is the mouse fibrosarcoma system in which Balb/c 3T3 cells are transfected with one of three different oncogenes—the human EJ-H-*ras* oncogene, the mouse Ki-*ras* oncogene, or the human c-*sis* oncogene (14). The second system is human neuroblastoma, with or without N-*myc* oncogene amplification (15). More recently, we have initiated studies of the progression and metastasis of new human prostate carcinoma (PCA) tumor cell systems (16). These PCA studies are particularly significant since so little is known in the human disease and/or model systems regarding its mechanism(s) of metastatic progression. In all cases, *in vivo* studies have been analyzed in athymic nude mice and compared with phenotypes of respective tissue culture cell subpopulations.

These three tumor systems will be reviewed from three different methodological and gene regulatory perspectives that bear directly on metastatic mechanisms. First, the use of histochemical marker genes will be reviewed for genetically tagging tumor cells and following their fate during metastatic spread in virtually any organ of the experimental animal. Single tumor cells can be followed with relative ease by these approaches. We have now used these marker genes in fibrosarcoma, neuroblastoma, and prostate carcinoma experimental models. Second, we will review evidence that modulation of expression of the CD44 gene is a critical factor in metastatic spread of fibrosarcoma, as well as provide some insight into CD44's mechanism of action. Finally, evidence will be summarized for downregulation of specific integrin genes by highly amplified N-*myc* oncogene in the neuroblastoma system. Analyzing these three tumor systems with these and other methodologies will enable us to predict some important advances in metastasis studies during the next decade.

Histochemical marker genes to track micrometastasis formation and subsequent development into overt metastases

Micrometastasis to organs never implicated previously

During early studies of fibrosarcoma and neuroblastoma metastasis in athymic nude mice (14, 15), we had been frustrated by our inability to detect the earliest events in primary tumor formation and, more impor-

tantly, the earliest events during micrometastasis. Following the precedent set by developmental biologists to study single-cell lineages in embryos (12), we transfected the *Escherichia coli lacZ* gene into fibrosarcoma cells to track these tumor cells. Using the X-gal histochemical staining reaction, single tumor cells could be easily detected in virtually any target organ of the animal (17, 18). In later studies (19), we developed the use of Red-gal which stains these cells red, rather than the blue product generated from X-gal. This approach using histochemical marker genes generated the first studies in any tumor system (17, 18). EJ-H-*ras*-transformed Balb/c 3T3 cells were detected undergoing spontaneous metastasis to the lung and liver, as expected from previous low-resolution methods. The sensitivity for detecting tumor cells was so refined that single tumor cells could be detected in sections of lung adherent to the lining of blood vessels, possibly in the act of extravasating; in other cases single tumor cells had already escaped (Fig. 18.1). Moreover, micrometastases were detectable in the brain and kidney, organs never previously implicated in metastasis of fibrosarcoma tumors (6, 17, 18). In the case of the brain, these micrometastases were transient and failed to thrive into overt metastases, possibly indicat-

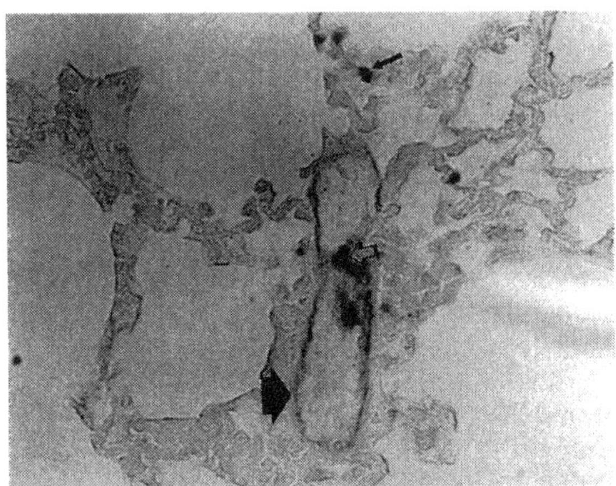

Fig. 18.1 Tumor cell adherence and extravasation in a lung blood vessel. *Ras*-transformed, *lacZ*-tagged 3T3 cells (17, 18) were injected into tail veins of athymic nude mice. Thirty minutes post-injection, an animal was sacrificed and the lung was excised, fixed, and embedded in methyacrylate for cutting into 4 μm thin sections after X-gal staining (6). X-gal-staining tumor cells can be observed after escape from blood vessels in the lung tissue (small arrow). Blood vessels are detectable as red staining (staining red at broad arrow) with alkaline phosphatase reagent while tumor cells are detectable as small clusters of blue staining within the blood vessel (open arrow). Magnification, 400 ×

ing an environment hostile for fibrosarcoma growth promotion (6).

The versatility of this system was enhanced further by genetically tagging a second fibrosarcoma tumor cell class with the histochemical marker gene, placental alkaline phosphatase (PAP) whose enzyme product remains intercalated in intracellular membranes thereby permitting its enzymatic product to remain intracellular (19, 20). The resulting color reflecting PAP enzyme activity could also be manipulated by the chemical nature of the substrate, thereby yielding red, reddish-brown, black, or blue staining cells depending upon which combination of histochemical substrates were used (19). For this system, the PAP gene was transfected into *sis*-transformed 3T3 cells to evaluate their micrometastatic potential from the subcutaneous site (19, 21). In contrast to the excellent metastatic potential of the *ras* transformant, virtually no spontaneous micrometastasis could be detected with the *sis* transformant from the subcutis.

The effectiveness of this approach for evaluating micrometastatic potential in nude mice has been demonstrated for the first time in human prostate carcinoma using PCA cells transfected with *lacZ* (16; C. Miller, J. Holleran, and L. Culp, unpublished data). In the vast majority of animal experimental models of human prostate carcinoma, metastasis can only be observed to the lung and rarely to liver and bone which are high-probability targets of the human disease (22, 23). Using the new human PCA cell line, CWR22R (24), generated from a human xenograft in nude mice and transfected with *lacZ*, we have shown that these cells spontaneously metastasize from the subcutaneous site to lung, liver, and brain (J. Holleran, C. Miller, and L. Culp, unpublished data). In some of these cases, micrometastases gave rise to well-staining overt metastases. This multiplicity of targets for PCA metastasis should markedly improve our ability to quantitatively and qualitatively evaluate the mechanisms by which difficult-to-study PCA tumor cells undergo metastatic processes.

Micrometastases converted into overt metastases

The ease of detecting *lacZ*-tagged fibrosarcoma cells in micrometastases enabled us to monitor the efficiency with which micrometastases became overt metastases. The lung was the ideal site for such a study since an enormous number of micrometastases could be readily detected in this organ, even with spontaneous metasta-

sis from the subcutis as the site of primary tumor development (18,19). Many micrometastases persisted in the lung for days and weeks and failed to expand into overt metastases. Others developed slowly into overt metastases, while a select few grew very rapidly (within 1 week) into metastases. This phenotypic diversity raises question as to the genetic diversity within the *ras*-transformed 3T3 population responsible for these three subsets of tumor cells. Alternatively, there may be special microenvironments within the lung that permit more successful outgrowth of micrometastases or that may be inhibitory for their outgrowth. These issues require much more detailed molecular biological analyses than histochemically tagged tumor cells will now permit.

Using the experimental metastasis model provided by tail-vein injections, the ability to detect single fibrosarcoma tumor cells in the lung permitted us to analyze the time course of events for establishment of micrometastases in this target organ (18, 25). Within 5 minutes after injection, micrometastases were becoming established in the lung, the quantitation of which revealed maximization in number by 1 hour (Table 18.1). Within 24 hours, > 98 per cent of these foci were 'cleared' from the lung while the remaining 1.5 per cent became truly established (18). These results confirm studies from the 1970s of melanoma and other tumor systems for clearance from the lungs of the majority of experimental micrometastases but not all of them (1–4). However, the mechanisms of the selective 'clearance' or 'resistance' of individual micrometastases remain to be determined in terms of molecular and cellular targeting events.

Lin and Culp (25) took a different approach in addressing micrometastatic mechanisms in the lung. They pretreated their *lacZ*/H-*ras*-transformed 3T3 cells with formaldehyde, ^{60}Co irradiation, or mitomycin C to effect any modulation on micrometastasis size, morphology, or stability. Pre-fixation generated micrometastases that were somewhat larger and more rounded in morphology, while the irradiation or mitomycin treatments generated micrometastases that were identical to those of live, untreated cells. However, the irradiated or mitomycin-treated cells were cleared from the lungs completely and more rapidly than live cells, while the fixed cells persisted for much longer periods of time. When untreated cells were mixed with fixed cells and then the mixture injected into the tail vein, all micrometastases were cleared from the lungs, including those containing live cells. These studies indicate the importance of cell surface events (altered by fixation

Table 18.1 Quantitation of pulmonary micrometastases/nodules (taken from reference 21 with permission)*

| Time of sacrifice | APSI injected singly | | | APSI co-injected with LZEJ[†] | | | | |
| | Micrometastases[§] | Nodules[‡] | | Double staining foci[¶] | Nodules[‡] | | | |
		Staining	Non-staining		LZWJ	APSI	Non-staining	Double staining
1 hour	2500–3000 (100)	0	0	500 (100)	0	0	0	0
6 hours	700 (28–23)	0	0	122 (24)	0	0	0	0
24 hours	104 (4.2–3.5)	0	0	24 (5)	0	0	0	0
3 weeks	38 (1.5–1.3)	10	0	3 (0.6)	26	20	7	3
5 weeks	37 (1.5–1.2)	54	17	ND	ND	ND	ND	ND
7 weeks	8 (0.3)	10	5	ND	ND	ND	ND	ND

* Mice (24 for two separate experiments) were given intravenous injection of 1×10^5 APSI cells (*sis*-transformed, placental alkaline phosphatase-tagged 3T3 cells) alone or as a mixture with 1×10^5 LZEF cells (*ras*-transformed, *lacZ*-tagged 3T3 cells) as indicated. At various times post-injection, mice were sacrified. Whole lungs were removed, rinsed with phosphate-buffered saline (PBS), and stained with X-phosphate (or sequentially with X-gal and then with X-phosphate/NBT in the case of co-injections of LZEJ and APSI cells). The values for 1×10^5 LZEJ cells injected alone have been published previously (18).
[†] ND, Not determined.
[‡] Denotes nodules of considerable size (> 100 cells). Nodules that are heterogeneous in their staining of the histochemical marker genes are referred to as non-staining nodules.
[§] Number of micrometastases determined with the use of a dissecting microscope. Values in parentheses represent the number of foci remaining in the lung as a percentage of the 1 hour value.
[¶] These are the number of micrometastases containing both LZEJ and APSI cells in co-localized foci. Values in parentheses represent the number of foci remaining in the lung as a percentage of the 1 hour value. The maximal number of foci of all cell classes (LZEJ-only plus APSI-only plus co-localized foci) observed at any time point was 6000–7000.

but not by the DNA-directed irradiation or mitomycin treatments) for (1) establishing micrometastases long-term in the lung and (2) guaranteeing their survivability in this organ site (25).

Synergy between two genetic classes during metastasis to the lung

We generated two different oncogene derivatives of Balb/c 3T3 cells—one transformed with EJ-H-*ras* and the other with *sis* (the former is spontaneously metastatic and the latter nonmetastatic). Tagging these with two different histochemical marker genes (19, 21)—the former with *lacZ* and the latter with PAP—enabled us to evaluate possible synergistic or interfering mechanisms in mixed populations of the two classes. When equal numbers of the two cell types were mixed and injected into the subcutis (21), primary tumors developed that were regionally concentrated with only one cell type, providing a mosaic of blue-staining or reddish-brown-staining tumor tissue (16). Sectioning revealed that each region was comprised of only one cell type; there was very little intermixing of the two tumor classes except at the margins of two stained regions. This result for all subcutaneous primary tumors indicated that clonal dominance of each tumor class must occur to give rise to this regional pattern (16). These studies also indicate that the two oncogenes change the gene expression pattern differently in the same Balb/c 3T3 parent population such that selective growth patterns can be observed in the earliest primary tumors (16).

When mixtures of these two fibrosarcoma classes were injected into tail veins, synergy between the two classes became evident when quantitating sites and qualitatively analyzing cell distributions in the lung (19, 21) (Table 18.1 and Fig. 18.2). Most micrometastases were comprised of only the *ras* transformant or the *sis* transformant based on homogeneous staining of blue or red sites (both in whole-organ staining as well as in section staining) (Fig. 18.2 (a), (b)). However, a significant fraction (> 7 per cent) of sites that became stably established after 24 hours contained both cell types (Table 18.1; Fig. 18.2 (a), (b)). When *sis*-transformed cells alone were injected into tail veins, all their micrometastases were cleared from the lungs within a few days, demonstrating the absence of a stabilizing set of conditions for these transformants and contrasting with the stability of *ras*-transformed micrometastases (Table 18.1). With mixtures of these two cell classes, the *ras* population provides some unknown stabilizing influence on the *sis* population such that the latter

persist as micrometastases and some develop into overt metastases containing both classes of tumor cells (19, 21) (Fig. 18.2 (c), (d)). There is an enrichment of the two-cell-class of metastases indicating the synergy between the two during their outgrowth (Table 18.1)—the *ras* transformants must be providing environmental cues to neighboring *sis* transformants for stability and subsequent outgrowth. Whether this synergy is mediated by soluble factors secreted selectively by one of these cell types or by extracellular-matrix-mediated events remains to be determined. Having two histochemically tagged cell types permits us to examine gene regulation events in these earliest mixed-cell micrometastases.

Multiple tumor cells in the earliest micrometastases in lung

Injection of *lacZ*-tagged, *ras*-transformed 3T3 cells into tail veins permitted us to evaluate the number of tumor cells in individual micrometastases (18, 25). Sectioning, embedding, and histochemically staining these lungs revealed some surprises (25). Rarely were single cells observed in early micrometastases; the vast majority were comprised of 2–7 cells under conditions where single-cell suspensions were being injected into the tail veins. This indicates that fibrosacroma cells form microaggregates during the first minutes in the animal's circulation or that they aggregate at each site in the smallest blood capillaries of the lung. Cardiac perfusion of fixative during euthanasia also revealed details of the lung's microvessels and demonstrated that micrometastases almost always form in the very smallest capillaries. The same results were observed for *lacZ*-tagged human neuroblastoma cells (26), while our *lacZ*-tagged prostate carcinoma cells remain to be tested in this paradigm. Could multicellularity result from physical entrapment of microaggregates in these sites or are these sites preferentially adhesive for tumor cells? Use of histochemically tagged tumor cells and high-resolution molecular biological approaches (see the section 'Perspectives on "regulating" the metastatic phenotype') should assist better definition of these potential mechanisms.

Angiogenesis during tumor progression

Cardiac perfusion of fixative also permitted us to evaluate the formation of new blood vessels in the vicinity of the developing primary tumor by contrasting red-staining blood vessels with blue-staining tumor cells

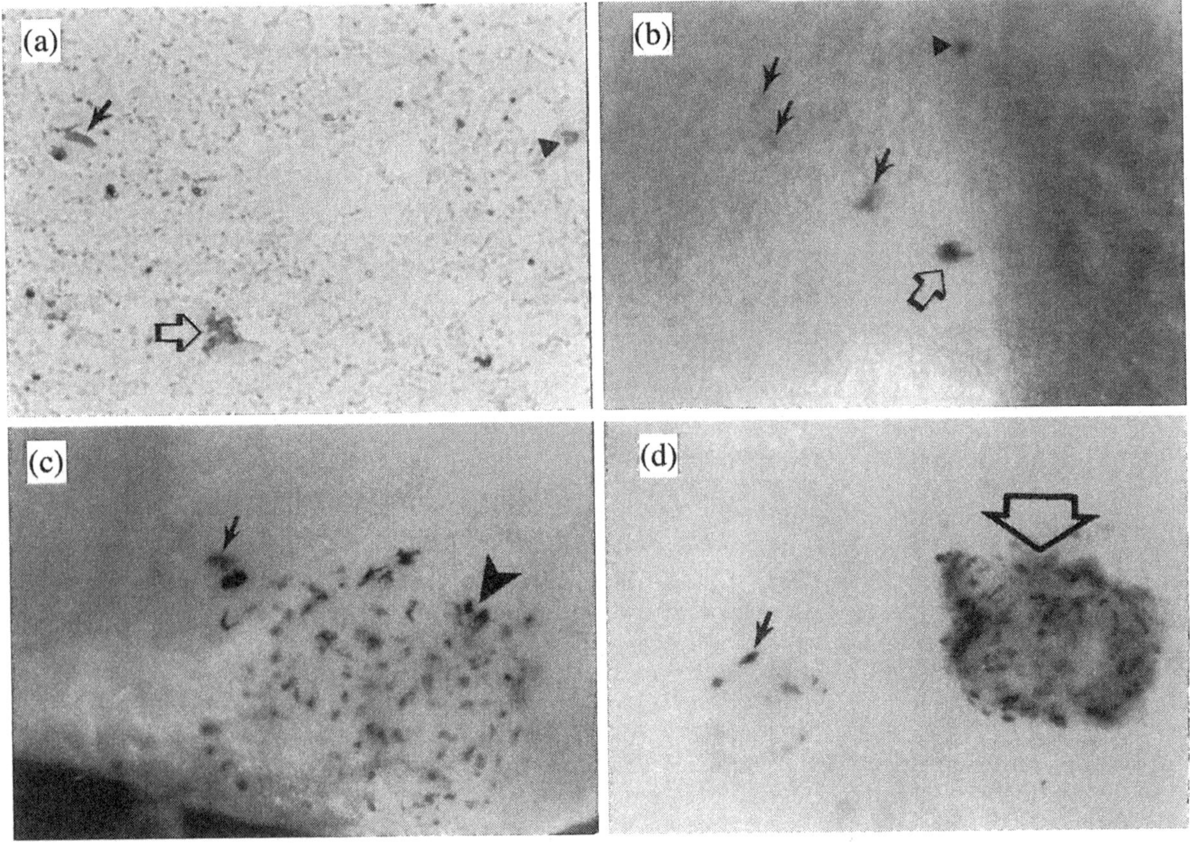

Fig. 18.2 Two genetically different classes of tumor cells establish multiple classes of micrometastases and overt metastases in lung. *Ras*-transformed, *lacZ*-tagged 3T3 cells (LZEJ) were mixed with *sis*-transformed, PAP-tagged 3T3 cells (APSI) after detachment from their respective tissue culture dishes. The equal-number mixture was injected into the tail veins of nude mice and at the specified times animals were sacrificed. Lungs were excised, fixed, and in some cases stained as whole organs or in other cases embedded in methyacrylate and sectioned after dual staining—first for β-galactosidase (red staining using Red-gal) and then for placental alkaline phosphatase activity (blue staining using X-phosphate substrate). Homogeneous micrometastases of LZEJ cells are denoted with small arrows, homogeneous micrometastases of APSI with arrowheads, and micrometastases containing both cell types with broad-open arrow. (a) 1 hour after tail vein co-injection. This is a section of lung in which all three classes of micrometastases could be readily identified, with a sizeable fraction containing both cell types. These are quantitated in Table 18.1. (b) Five hours after co-injection: whole-organ staining. Note that all three classes of micrometastases persist, as detected with whole-organ staining. (c) Three weeks after co-injection: whole-organ staining. Some micrometastases persisted at this late time point (LZEJ cells at small arrow) while others were growing into overt metastases (APSI cells at large arrowhead). (d) Three weeks after co-injection: whole-organ staining. An overt metastasis is shown with both cell types (large open arrow), demonstrating that these two genetically related cell types can contribute to the same overt metastasis. LZEJ micrometastases are also evident (small arrow). All magnifications 220 ×. Also see 'Plates' section.

(26). In the case of *lacZ*-tagged neuroblastoma in the subcutis, staining of the entire subcutaneous site or transverse sections of the primary tumor revealed how quickly angiogenesis is promulgated by tumor cell-secreted factors. New blood vessels were seen developing at the periphery of dense populations of tumor cells within 48–72 hours. Several days postinjection, a few of these microvessels had developed into sizeable blood vessels. By the time the primary tumor had become palpable, one or more of these larger vessels had become a major vessel feeding the central regions of the tumor.

The rapid induction of new blood vessels by tumor cells indicates that a long period of adaptation in the subcutis by tumor cells to secrete angiogenic factors is unlikely. Rather, the tumor cells may be secreting angiogenic factors (10, 11) as cultured populations prior to their injection into the subcutis. Alternatively, induction of angiogenesis genes occurs in tumor cells within the first 24 hours of residence. This system can now be used to assay pro-angiogenic and anti-angiogenic factors in ectopic and orthotopic sites of primary tumor development.

Histochemical markers as indicators of tumor cell genetic instability

Since histochemical marker genes do not provide any selective advantage or disadvantage for tumor cell growth at any site in the experimental animal, their activities can be used quantitatively and qualitatively to monitor the relative genetic instability of tumor cell subsets (6, 16). This instability was noted in our very first fibrosarcoma tumor studies (19, 21). *LacZ*-transfected, *ras*-transformed 3T3 cells retained excellent stainability in culture for > 20 passages and in very large primary tumors grown over a period of weeks in the animal. In contrast, PAP-transfected, *sis*-transformed 3T3 cells began losing stainability within 5–10 passages in culture and virtually all large primary tumors contained regions of nonstaining cells (16, 19, 21).

The same spectrum of stability applied to *lacZ*-transfected human neuroblastoma cells (26). One clone yielded excellent stainability for > 15 passages in culture and throughout large primary tumors in the subcutis. A second clone, by contrast, was losing stainability within 5–10 passages and virtually all primary tumors using this clone contained large regions of non-stainable tumor tissue.

Three different *lacZ* transfectants of the human prostate carcinoma cell line, CWR22R, also demonstrate this gradient of genetic instability in expression (16; C. Miller, J. Holleran, and L. Culp, unpublished data). Clone H cells stain very well for > 25 passages in medium without drug selection and produced excellent staining primary tumors after 6–12 weeks in the subcutis of animals. Clone B steadily lost stainability over 10–20 passages in culture without selective media and invariably gave rise to tumors with large regions of nonstainable tissue. Clone D was so unstable that virtually all stainability was lost after five passages in culture.

The ease of quantitation of histochemical marker gene expression affords us the opportunity to evaluate the molecular mechanisms of this instability and whether it relates to organ-specific metastasis at all. Several mechanisms for loss of reporter gene expression can be envisioned. First, the marker gene may be deleted from the genome or rearranged in such a way

that it has lost integrity. Second, transcriptional downregulation may occur by induction of a new transcriptional-inhibitory factor (*trans*-acting) in tumor subpopulations. Third, the marker gene may be transcriptionally downregulated by a hypermethylation mechanism, which is known to alter regulation of many genes in tumor cells (see the following section on this point). Fourth, transcription of the marker gene may be perfectly normal but there may be induction of a factor(s) that inhibits protein enzymatic activity in the cytoplasm of cells. As discussed more fully in the section 'Perspectives on "regulating" the metastatic phenotype', there are approaches available now that permit resolution of these various possibilities.

Selection and counterselection for CD44 overexpression during progression and metastasis

CD44 is a transmembrane glycoprotein on the surface of many, but not all, cell types in animals (27, 28). It harbors several binding domains—its most external domain binds hyaluronan (HA); a membrane-proximal domain homes lymphocytes; and its cytoplasmic tail binds intracellular cytoskeletal elements. Its pre-mRNA is alternatively spliced into a wide variety of splice products, most of which occur in the membrane-proximal/external portion of the molecule responsible for lymphocyte homing. In contrast to the 'standard' isoform (CD44s), which lacks all spliced sequences and is the only identifiable product in lymphoid cells and fibroblasts, its 'variant' isoforms (CD44v) frequently do not bind HA, have lost lymphocyte-homing ability, and are observed in cell-type-specific distributions among various epithelial cell types (27, 28).

CD44 is a likely gene product with significance for progression and metastasis of some human tumor systems (29). First, many primary tumors of human or experimental animal origin have elevated levels of CD44s or CD44v; in some cases, there are different distributions of CD44v in the tumor population from that of the host tissue (30–33). Second, metastases of tumors express more elevated levels of these CD44 isoforms or a different isoform distribution than that observed in the primary tumor, suggestive of unique functions for the spliced variants (34–37). Third, transfection and overexpression of CD44v (38) induces metastatic potential in normally nonmetastatic carcinoma cells. Transfection/overexpression of CD44s in lymphoma cells (39) also induces metastatic competence. Finally, CD44s on the surface of lymphoid cells with its ability to bind HA is a critical element in the homing of these cells to adhere to blood vessel endothelial cells and their successful extravasation from vessels (40, 41). These processes resemble those undertaken by metastatic tumor cells as they migrate to target organs.

Because of these functional implications for metastasis, we undertook analyses of the significance of CD44s in our fibrosarcoma systems, that is, Balb/c 3T3 cells transformed with either a *ras* oncogene to make them metastatic or with the *sis* oncogene, which does not confer metastatic competence (as described in the previous section). We also analyzed nontumorigenic revertants (IIIA4 cells) of the *ras* transformants that had lost the transforming *ras* oncogene (14). These studies have revealed a remarkable plasticity of expression of CD44s in these cells during progression and metastasis, as delineated below (42–45).

Oncogene-dependent regulation of mouse CD44s gene expression

FACS (fluorescence-activated cell sorting) analysis of Balb/c 33 cells demonstrated that they had modest levels of mouse CD44s (mCD44s) on their surfaces and no detectable CD44v isoforms as expected (42). In contrast, *ras* transformants of these 3T3 cells had very high levels of mCD44s and no CD44v isoforms. *Sis* transformants had levels of mCD44s comparable to those of 3T3 cells while revertant IIIA4 cells had reduced expression levels from the high levels observed in the original *ras*-transformed population. These data indicated correlation of metastatic competence with the elevated levels of mCD44s in the *ras* transformants (42). A second correlation was also made—the high mCD44s-expressing *ras* transformants could bind exogenously added HA very well, while the *sis* transformants and the revertant cells could bind very little HA in a CD44-dependent manner. When a wide variety of nude mouse primary tumors and lung metastases derived from the *ras* transformants were evaluated by FACS and/or Western blotting after transplant back into tissue culture, all demonstrated very high levels of CD44s (42). Therefore, expression of the *ras* oncogene leads to upregulation in mouse CD44s expression, while expression of *sis* is without effect on expression of this gene.

Transfection of human CD44s gene into *sis* transformants—acquisition of metastatic competence and the counterselection model of progression

We then designed a system to artificially elevate levels of CD44s in transformed cells with a molecule that could be differentiated from the endogenous mouse homolog using specific monoclonal antibodies (43). The human CD44s cDNA gene, under regulation of a very active long terminal repeat (LTR) promoter, was transfected into *sis*-transformed 3T3 cells in an effort to test elevation of cell surface CD44s (either hCD44s or mCD44s). Three independent and stable transfectants were isolated. There was no elevation of mCD44s in any transfectants. In contrast, there were very high levels of hCD44s on these cells. Furthermore, exogeneously added HA could bind to the hCD44s on the cell surface but not to the mCD44s, providing further functional discrimination between these two classes of molecules (43).

When the hCD44s-overexpressing transfectants were injected into the subcutis of nude mice (43, very aggressive primary tumors formed within 1–2 weeks. Furthermore, these cells were now highly metastatic to the lung, contrasting with the lack of spontaneous metastasis using the original *sis* transformants. When micrometastatic tumor cells from the lung were isolated back into culture, FACS analyses of their CD44s levels revealed the expected levels of mCD44s and very high levels of hCD44s (Fig. 18.3 (b), (d)), consistent with the hypothesis that overexpressed levels of hCD44s led directly to acquisition of metastatic competence.

Similarly, primary tumors in this series were isolated into culture and evaluated for their CD44s levels. This led to a very surprising finding (43). All large primary tumors from transfectants had lost expression of hCD44s while retaining the modest levels of mCD44s; this loss was observed in > 20 primary tumors examined (Fig. 18.3 (a), (c)). These results indicate that overexpression of the human gene may be counterproductive and/or antagonistic for outgrowth of primary tumor in the subcutis. This counterselection against hCD44s gene expression contrasted with the high expression levels of this gene product in all lung micrometastatic tumor cells.

This led us to examine a third tumor population. Micrometastases of some hCD44s transfectants in the lung invariably grew into large overt metastases (43). When large metastases were transplanted back into

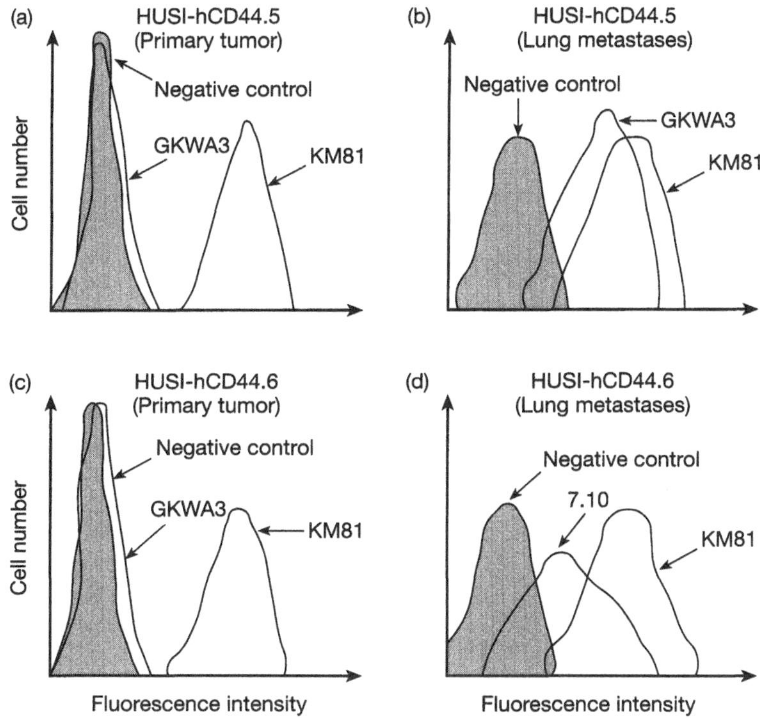

Fig. 18.3   Selection for or against overexpressed hCD44s in tumors from two different transfectants. *Sis*-transformed 3T3 cells were transfected with a cDNA from of hCD44s, regulated by an LTR promoter, on a eukaryotic expression plasmid. Several stable transfectants, expressing high levels of hCD44s, were isolated, two of which are analyzed here. Transfectants HUSI-hCD44.5 or HUSI-hCD44.6 were then injected into the subcutis of nude mice. After 2 weeks, animals were sacrificed and the primary tumor cells grown out in culture, along with lung micrometastatic tumor cells selected in culture based on their drug resistance. These culture populations were then analyzed by FACS for expression of mouse CD44s (using monoclonal antibody KM81) of human CD44s (using monoclonal antibodies GKWA3 or 7.10). (a) Subcutaneous tumor after injection of transfectant 5 cells. There has been loss of expression of hCD44s while mCD44s continues to be expressed at the expected levels. (b) Lung micrometastatic cells from the same animal as in (a). These cells retain high-level expression of hCD44s. (c) Subcutaneous tumor after injection of transfectant 6 cells. Again, hCD44s but not mCD44s has been lost from the surface of these cells. (d) Lung micrometastatic cells from the animal in (c). High levels of hCD44s persist in these cells. (Taken from reference 43 with permission.)

culture and tested by FACS for CD44s levels, they had lost virtually all of their hCD44s while retaining the expected levels of mCD44s. This would indicate that there is not an organ-specific downregulation of this gene in the two tissue sites. Rather, aggressive outgrowth of tumor, whether it be the primary tumor or distant metastases, required downregulation of hCD44s for some inapparent reason, perhaps linked to its HA-binding ability, which is defective in mCD44s.

These important studies led us to hypothesize a selection/counterselection model of tumor progression in this system (43, 46). Elevated levels of hCD44s would be critical to get metastatic spread from the subcutis to the lung. Conversely, outgrowth of the primary tumor and any overt metastases required that the gene be turned off in highly selected subpopulations if aggressive cell division was to be successful.

What is the origin of the lung micrometastatic cells with overexpressed hCD44s (43, 46)? Two alternative models for the origin of lung metastatic cells could be envisioned. Perhaps these cells migrate from the subcutis to the lung soon after injection and prior to downregulation of the hCD44s gene. Alternatively, a small subpopulation of hCD44s-overexpressing cells may exist at all times in the primary tumor; it cannot be readily identified by FACS analyses (or by Western blotting for that matter).

As one approach to address these questions, we undertook a second round of tumor analyses (43). In the first case, primary tumor cells that had lost expression of hCD44s were re-injected subcutaneously into a second group of animals. These cells formed excellent primary tumors, all of which failed to express detectable hCD44s. These primary tumors also gave rise to micrometastatic tumor cells in the lungs of these animals. When these micrometastatic tumor cells were explanted into culture and grown out in drug selection medium to eliminate any mouse lung cells, these micrometastatic tumor populations expressed high levels of hCD44s in all cases. Therefore, metastatic competence correlated again with acquisition of high levels of cell surface hCD44s. In the second case, lung micrometastatic tumor cells from the first round (high hCD44 sexpressers) were injected into a second group of animals—all subcutaneous primary tumors had lost hCD44s expression while lung micrometastatic tumor cells retained high levels of this cell surface protein. These experiments demonstrate the remarkable plasticity of hCD44s expression during progression and metastasis with these *sis* transformants of 3T3 cells.

Possible mechanism of modulation of the hCD44s gene

These studies raised the question of how the elevated levels of hCD44s may facilitate metastatic spread while endogenous mCD44s does not convey this competence (46). It appears likely that the ability of the human protein to bind exogenous HA is the critical characteristic that distinguishes hCD44s from the properties of the mouse protein. To prove this, we must test overexpression of a mutant form of hCD44s that is specifically unable to bind HA but is capable of other binding functions. If such a molecule proves incompetent in conveying metastatic competence, then clearly HA binding is a central issue for metastatic spread of fibrosarcoma tumor cells (also will the mutant gene be downregulated in primary tumor cells if it cannot bind HA?). If HA-nonbinding mutants persist in conveying metastatic competence, then there must be some additional and unknown binding activity in this domain of the molecule that is critical. Further experiments along these lines should prove particularly informative.

Some insight has been provided into the mechanism of modulation of hCD44s expression in these tumor cells (43). Hypermethylation of gene promoter regions has been shown to downregulate a number of genes in tumor cells (47, 48). Testing the hCD44s gene region for sensitivity to digestion with restriction enzymes responding to hypermethylated DA sequences revealed two very different levels of methylation in or proximal to this gene (43). In the original transfectant cells and

lung micrometastatic tumor cells, both of which express considerable hCD44s, there were low levels of methylation in this gene region. In contrast, primary tumor cells and overt metastatic tumor cells that had lost hCD44s protein displayed high levels of DNA methylation in this region. This correlation was further reinforced using aza-deoxycytidine treatment of cells in culture to inhibit DNA methylation (43). This treatment led to high levels of hCD44s in primary tumor cells and only slightly increased the levels in transfectant cells and in lung micrometastatic tumor cells that already had elevated levels. Therefore, it is highly likely that plasticity of expression of this transfected gene in these fibrosarcoma cells is effected by regulation of DNA methylation in this gene's promoter region. To test this hypothesis directly, we can transfect hCD44s gene into these cells under regulation of other active promoters that are much less susceptible to hypermethylation and then test for plasticity of hCD44s expression, aggressiveness of primary tumor development, and acquisition of metastatic competence in this paradigm.

Additional hCD44s expression/plasticity systems

In addition to the *sis* transformants described above, transfection of the hCD44s gene was performed in revertant IIIA4 cells (43). These revertant cells were isolated from a clonal population of K-*ras*-transformed 3T3 cells and were shown to have deleted the *ras* oncogene by some unknown mechanism (14). In doing so, they had lost much of their tumorigenic potential.

Several stable transfectants of IIIA4 cells were isolated after transfecting the hCD44s gene (43). They expressed very high levels of hCD44s protein, which was competent for binding exogenous HA. Upon subcutaneous injection into nude mice, they were much more tumorigenic than parental IIIA4 cells. Of particular interest, they had acquired metastatic competence for the lungs of these animals. Lung micrometastatic tumor cells, explanted into culture, expressed high levels of hCD44s, while the large primary tumors had lost expression.

This led us to test the third biological system (44). The hCD44s gene was transfected into nontumorigenic Balb/c 3T3 cells to determine if their phenotype was altered in any way. Several stable transfectants were isolated with low, intermediate, or high levels of hCD44s on their surface. In all cases, exogenous HA binding was proportional to the amount of cell surface hCD44s and unaffected by mouse CD44s. Of particular note, the highest hCD44s-expressing clone was tumorigenic in the subcutis of nude mice and subpopulations of these cells formed spontaneous micrometastases. In agreement with the other two systems, the primary tumor cells lost expression ofhCD44s while the lung micrometastatic tumor cells retained high levels of hCD44s (44).

This latter 3T3 system was explored further by testing whether these hCD44s levels, observed with tissue cultured populations, could be reflective of tumor populations *in vivo* (44). Using immunohistochemical approaches, we demonstrated that fixed sections of the primary tumor tissue retained immunohistochemical stainability for mouse CD44s but lacked any significant levels of human CD44s. In contrast, small foci of tumor cells in the lung expressed high levels of hCD44s and low levels of mCD44s (44). These experiments confirmed the results of tissue culture analyses of these various tumor populations and discounted an artefact of altered expression upon tissue culturing of these populations.

Experimental metastasis system to evaluate functional significance of overexpressed hCD44s

The results described above suggest that overexpressed hCD44s facilitated metastatic spread of normally nonmetastatic *sis* transformants and other cell types to the lung. One approach for testing this hypothesized mechanism involves injection of tumor cells into tail vein blood vessels to evaluate later steps in metastatic spread but not the initiating events. This approach would not be evaluating the intravasation steps into blood vessels at the site of the primary tumor. Since the plasmid used for transfection of the *sis* oncogene into these transformants also harbored the hygromycin B resistance gene, we could quantitate lung colonization by enumerating drug-resistant colonies grown out in culture after harvesting lungs and dispersing them into single-cell suspensions. This approach yielded some very important mechanistic information for the significance of overexpressed hCD44s in the early events of micrometastatic establishment (45).

Untransfected *sis*-transformed cells generated a low number of micrometastatic foci in lungs at any time point examined after tail vein injection, for example, 1 hour, 24 hours, and 4 weeks (45) (Fig. 18.4). In contrast, hCD44s transfectant cells yielded three times that number of foci at 1 hour, more than tenfold that

number at 24 hours, and tenfold more at 4 weeks (Fig. 18.4). These results indicate that high hCD44s levels: (1) greatly improve initial implantation of micrometastases in the small blood vessels of the lung within the first hour in the circulation; (2) further improve the stabilization of these micrometastases during the clearance mechanisms that operate between 1 and 24 hours. Furthermore, persistence of these micrometastases over the next 4 weeks reveals a lasting effect on their residence in the lungs.

These culture-isolated colonies were also evaluated by FAS for levels of hCD44s and its ability to bind exogenous HA (45). As expected, the lung-colonizing

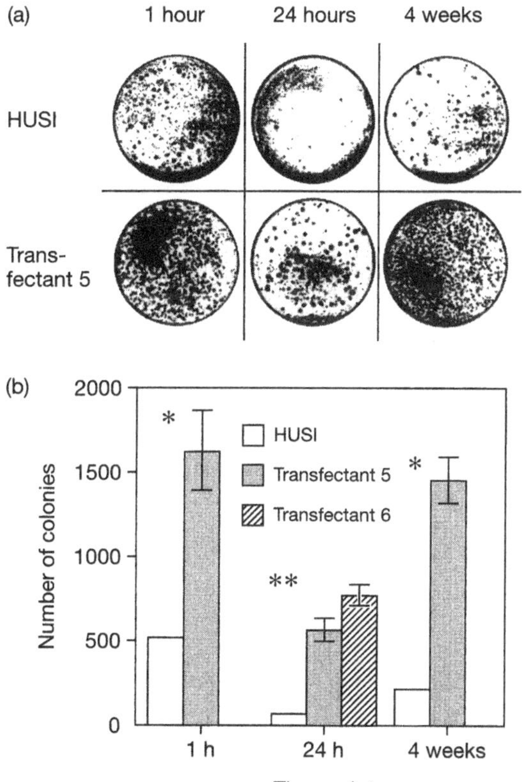

Fig. 18.4 hCD44s promotes the earliest stages of micrometastasis establishment in the lung. Untransfected or hCD44s-transfectant clone 5 or 6 cells were injected into tail vein blood vessels (experimental metastasis assay with three mice per datum point). At the indicated times, mice were sacrificed, their lungs dispersed into culture, and tumor cell colonies were quantitated in a colony growth assay based on their resistance to hygromycin B killing. (a) Colonies were visualized with Coomassie blue staining and (b) enumerated. *, $p < 0.05$; **, $p < 0.005$. (Taken from reference 45 with permission.)

population of transfectant cells had very high levels of hCD44s and excellent ability to bind HA at the 1 and 24 hour time points. In contrast and consistent with plasticity of hCD44s gene expression, the 4 week-harvested cells had lost much of their cell surface hCD44s and their ability to bind HA. These results confirm the importance of cell surface hCD44s in establishing and stabilizing micrometastases but not in promoting their eventual outgrowth in the lung into overt metastases.

The next series of experiments in this paradigm tested the various tumor cell types described in the subsection 'Microstases converted into overt metastases' and harvested after subcutaneous injection of hCD44s-overexpressing transfectants (45). hCD44s-negative primary tumor cells, injected into tail veins, gave colony numbers from the lungs that were not statistically different from those of untransfected *sis*-transformed cells. In contrast, hCD44s-overexpressing lung micrometastatic tumor cells, injected into tail veins, gave colony numbers that were 7–10-fold higher than primary tumor cells and comparable to the numbers observed with the original transfectant cells. FACS analyses revealed very high levels of hCD44s on these cells and excellent binding of exogenous HA as well. These results confirm the correlation of high levels of HA-binding hCD44s on cells with their efficiency at colonizing the lung microvasculature (45, 46).

In the experimental metastasis assays described above using hCD44s-overexpressed cell classes, a large number of overt metastases grew out within 3–5 weeks (45). Re-isolation of these cells into culture, based on their selection using the drug resistance marker on the transfected plasmid, yielded populations that were depleted of cell surface hCD44s and displayed poor HA binding. These results also confirm those of the subsection 'Micrometastases converted into overt metastases' and illustrate the selection against high levels of hCD44s when tumor outgrowth becomes aggressive, whether it is the primary tumor in the subcutis or large metastases in the lung (46).

Two general models for these results can be proposed (45, 46). First, hCD44s and its ability to bind HA could promote formation of small aggregates of tumor cells in the circulation that would subsequently be trapped in the microvessels of the lung, that is promotion of tumor cell: tumor cell adherence. The second model involves more effective adherence of tumor cells to endothelial cells of these blood vessels by overexpressed hCD44s on the tumor cell surface binding to HA on the surface of the endothelium. Such binding may be relatively weak, as suggested by studies of lym-

phoid cell homing to sites of inflammation (40, 41). Because microvessels do not experience the fluid shear stress that occurs in larger vessels, hCD44s: HA interactions in microvessels may be strong enough to hold tumor cell aggregates to the endothelium. This may explain why tumor cell aggregates are only observed in microvessels of the lung.

To test these alternatives, hCD44s transfectant cells were mixed with untransfected cells in varying ratios. Then the mixtures were injected into tail veins to test the 'specific activity' of the overexpressers to colonize lungs in competition with untransfected cells. Hygromycin B was used to select all tumor cell classes in the lung, while puromycin (the drug resistance marker on the hCD44s-bearing plasmid) was used to select transfectant cells specifically. Increasing the proportion of untransfected cells had no adverse effect on the much greater efficiency of colonization by the transfected subset. Consistent with this result, the lung tumor populations re-isolated into culture were tested for levels of cell surface hCD44s and were found to be overwhelmingly high expressers. These results would suggest that tumor cell: tumor cell adhesion is not playing a critical role in this mechanism. They are more consistent with the model of much improved adhesion of transfectant cells to the endothelium, possibly mediated by HA-binding hCD44s (45, 46). This would parallel a similar mechanism of lymphoid cell adhesion to the endothelium at sites of inflammation (40, 41).

To test this model more directly, we can transfect non-HA-binding mutants of the hCD44s gene into these cells and determine if colonization remains low. We can also test whether other cell surface HA-binding receptors (at overexpressed levels) can facilitate the much improved colonization of these cells and whether HA oligosaccharides, co-injected into the circulation at the same time as tumor cells, can hapten-inhibit colonization.

N-myc *amplification in neuroblastoma: its regulation of integrin receptor expression*

Human neuroblastoma is a tumor arising from the malignant conversion of a neural crest cell in the embryo destined to become an adrenal gland, a melanocyte in the skin, a peripheral neuron, or a facial bone (12, 13). It afflicts young children prior to the age of 10 and can arise at many different organ sites

(15, 49, 50). Some neuroblastoma tumor cell lines are neuritogenic in culture and have been studied as models of peripheral neuron differentiation (15).

N-*myc* is a proto-oncogene in the human genome and a member of the *myc* family of proto-oncogenes whose protein products are regulators of transcription of specific genes (51). This proto-oncogene displays a unique correlation with neuroblastoma tumor biology and progression (49–51). It becomes highly amplified in aggressive and metastatic neuroblastomas of stage III or IV, does not display any unique mutations in metastatic tumors, and is not amplified in less-aggressive stage I or II tumors that do not metastasize. In the same tumor populations, the c-*myc* proto-oncogene is unaffected during progression and metastasis, suggesting that N-myc protein is responsible for transcription of genes other than those regulated by c-myc protein and that these N-myc-regulated genes participate in the aggressiveness of this tumor.

Earlier studies had demonstrated that amplification of the N-*myc* oncogene in neuroblastoma cells correlated with downregulation of the major histocompatibility complex (MHC) class 1 gene, protein kinase C signaling, and the neural cell adhesion molecule (NCAM) gene (52–54). Since the class of extracellular matrix receptors, called integrins (55), are critical elements in the altered relationship between tumor cells and their environment (14, 15, 55), we sought to more directly test whether metastatic progression of neuroblastoma, mediated by N-*myc* amplification/overexpression, could be based on altered regulation of integrin genes in these tumor populations. Such evidence was obtained.

Integrin expression in naturally occurring human neuroblastoma cells

Our laboratory undertook analysis of the integrin receptor classes in three human neuroblastoma tumor classes (56, 57). Two of these, IMR-32 and LaN1, display amplified N-*myc* oncogene while the third, SK-N-SH, does not. IMR-32 and LaN1 cells do not display significant amounts of any of the common $\beta1$ integrin family members. When these cells were injected into the subcutis (an ectopic injection site) or the adrenal gland (an orthotopic injection site for neuroblastoma), all primary tumors conserved this pattern of poor integrin expression. The rounded, weakly adherent morphologies of LaN1 and IMR-32 cells in culture were also consistent with poor integrin expression.

In contrast, SK-N-SH cells, harboring a diploid number of N-*myc* genes, expressed significant amounts of $\alpha2\beta1$, $\alpha3\beta1$, and smaller amounts of $\alpha1\beta1$ (56, 57). These levels of integrins were conserved in all subcutaneous and adrenal gland primary tumors derived from this cell line. When these populations were analyzed by FACS, approximately one-half of the parental SK-N-SH cells expressed $\alpha3\beta1$ on their surfaces while the other half did not. Both subcutaneous and adrenal primary tumors conserved this dual-expression pattern, indicating that $\alpha3^+$ or $\alpha3^-$ cells were not clonally dominant during progression of primary tumors. There was also another distinctive pattern change observed in these studies. The parent SK-N-SH cell line did not express $\alpha v\beta1$, nor did the adrenal gland primary tumors; in contrast, all subcutaneous primary tumors expressed $\alpha v\beta1$, suggesting that upregulation of this integrin may be important in the biology of the primary tumor at this site.

These analyses demonstrate several important findings (56, 57). First, integrin expression patterns are generally conserved between the original human tumor population, grown for many passages in culture, and the resultant athymic nude mouse tumors derived from them. Second, this conservation of expression is maintained at both ectopic and orthotopic injection sites. Third, induction of $\alpha v\beta1$ in the subcutaneous primary tumors may indicate an important function that is specific to this site, possibly for angiogenesis as suggested from other αv-expressing tumor populations (26, 58). Finally, clonal heterogeneity for $\alpha3\beta1$ expression is conserved in all primary subcutaneous or adrenal gland tumors, indicating that expression of this integrin is not essential for primary tumor expansion. These studies raise question as to how N-*myc*-amplified tumor cells interact with extracellular matrices, since they lack common fibronectin- and collagen-binding integrins and since these are the more aggressive and metastatic classes of this tumor. The weak adherence of these cells in culture is certainly consistent with this poor integrin expression pattern.

Transfection/overexpression of N-*myc* oncogene in SK-N-SH cells

To test more directly hypotheses relating N-*myc* oncogene overexpression with altered regulation of integrin subunit expression, we transfected an episomal plasmid, pREP4, harboring the human N-*myc* oncogene under regulation of a very active LTR promoter, into SK-N-SH cells which have a diploid number of N-*myc* genes and express a basal level of N-myc protein (59). Using the episomal plasmid for transfection permitted us to raise the concentration of N-*myc* onco-gene in these cells by selection with increasing concentrations of hygromycin, the drug-resistance marker on this plasmid (59).

Several notable changes were identified in N-*myc* transfectant cells (59). They displayed an altered morphology in culture from that of well-spread SK-N-SH—they were rounded and easily detachable from the substratum, resembling IMR-32 or LaN1 cells in this regard. Selection with higher concentrations of hygromycin generated a higher percentage of rounded cells and much higher levels of N-myc protein. The level of N-myc protein in these transfectants was directly related to the dosage of the N-*myc* oncogene in these cells. Conversely, higher concentrations of hygromycin led to cell populations with greatly decreased amounts of β1 integrin subunit. Plotting the levels of N-myc protein against the levels of β1 integrin subunit in many different transfectants and at many hygromycin selection concentrations demonstrated the inverse relationship between the levels of these two gene products (Fig. 18.5) (59). Transfection of

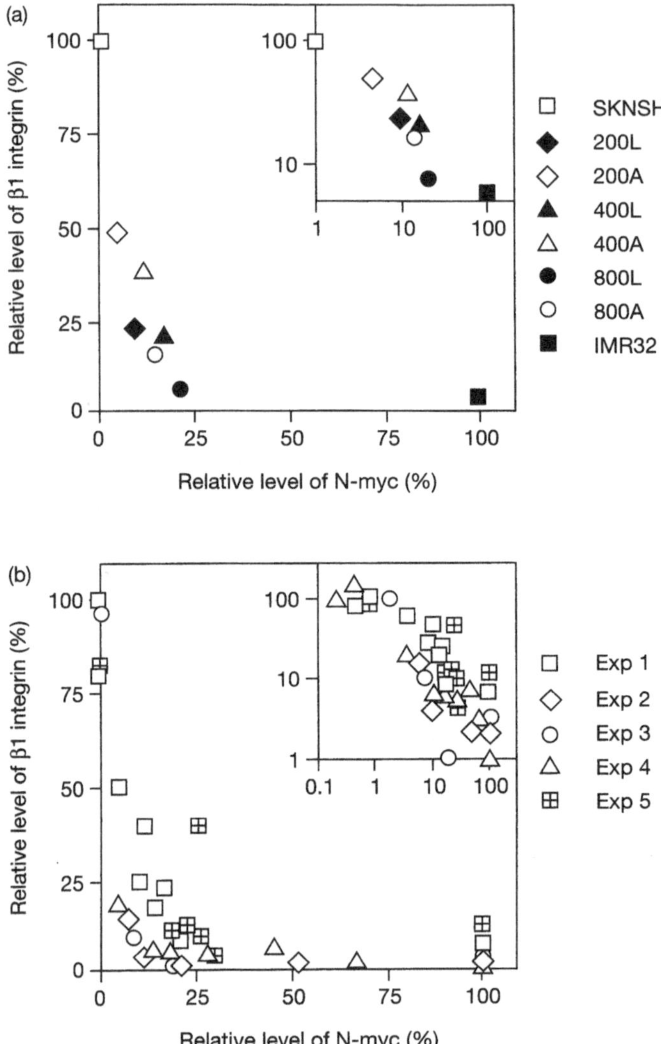

Fig. 18.5   Quantitation of relationships between increased hygromycin B selection with N-myc and β1 integrin subunit levels. (a) SKMYC2 transfectant cells (59) were grown in the indicated concentrations of hygromycin B and the resultant attached (A) or loosely adherent (L) populations isolated. N-myc and β1 integrin proteins were quantitated by fluorography and scanning densitometry. The inset is a log:log plot of the same data showing inverse relationship between the levels of the two proteins. (b) Five independent experiments were quantitated as described in (a). (Taken from reference 59 with permission.)

SK-N-SH cells with an antisense construct of N-*myc* failed to generate these changes. Therefore, these experiments directly relate higher dosages of N-myc protein in neuroblastoma cells to decreasing levels of $\beta1$ integrin subunit and are consistent with either direct or indirect regulation of the $\beta1$ integrin gene by the N-myc protein.

Two different mechanisms for down-regulating integrin expression by N-*myc*

The studies described above left open the issue whether integrin subunits $\alpha2$ or $\alpha3$ were also altered in N-*myc* transfectants. This was shown to be the case with the discovery that two different molecular mechanisms are operating (60).

Increasing concentrations of hygromycin, to select for increased levels of N-myc protein, led to cells with decreased levels of both $\alpha2$ and $\alpha3$ integrin subunits (60). In contrast, the modest levels of $\alpha1$ subunit observed in these cells were unaffected by higher N-myc levels, dissociating regulation of this subunit from those of the other two (61). Very little $\alpha2\beta1$ or $\alpha3\beta1$ were observed at the cell surface in N-*myc* over-expressers (60) while the levels of cell surface $\alpha1\beta1$ was unaffected (61). Evaluation of the levels of mRNAs for these subunits by RNAase protection assay showed that levels of $\alpha2$ and $\alpha3$ mRNAs were greatly reduced (> 85 per cent) in N-*myc* overexpressers while the level of $\beta1$ mRNA was reduced only 40–50 per cent (Fig. 18.6) (60). Of significance as well, the levels of *max* mRNA were unaltered in these cells (Fig. 18.6), demonstrating that this co-effector of N-myc transcriptional regulation was not being co-regulated by the much higher levels of N-myc protein (Fig. 18.6). Metabolic radiolabeling of proteins in these cells, in concert with pulse-chase analyses, revealed that the half-life of $\beta1$ was greatly reduced in transfectants while those of the α subunits were unaffected. Therefore, it is likely that the greatly reduced amounts of $\alpha2$ and $\alpha3$ subunits in these cells lead to uncomplexed $\beta1$ which then undergoes degradation (60). The exception to this fate is the modest amount of $\alpha1$ subunit that does complex with small amounts of $\beta1$ and successfully gets to the cell surface (61).

Overall, these studies indicate three different regulatory patterns of integrin genes in neuroblastoma tumor cells with highly overexpressed N-*myc* oncogene. First, there appears to be transcriptional downregulation of the integrin $\alpha2$ and $\alpha3$ genes by an N-myc protein-dependent pathway; the *max* co-regulator is unaffected in these cells. Second, downregulation of $\beta1$ levels are

effected at the posttranscriptional level, probably by protein instability caused by insufficient amounts of α subunit for complexing. Finally, the expression of the $\alpha1$ integrin gene is unaffected by N-*myc*, consistent with levels of $\alpha1\beta1$ that persist in high-metastatic, N-*myc*-amplified tumor populations. It remains to be seen how tumorigenic and how metastatic the N-*myc* transfectants are in nude mice. Do they display the same progression and metastasis patterns as the naturally-occurring N-*myc*-amplified IMR-32 and LaN-1 tumor cells? Both ectopic and the orthotopic (adrenal gland) injection sites must be tested in these regards (56, 57).

Is N-*myc* downregulation of integrins tumor-specific?

These analyses questioned whether N-myc protein regulation of integrins was specific to neuroblastoma tumors because one or more unknown factors in these tumor cells conveyed tumor specificity. To address this question, we transfected the same overexpressing episomal plasmid of N-*myc* into human Saos-2 osteosarcoma cells, a tumor cell line whose biology and lineage are very different from that of neuroblastoma having been derived from a connective tissue cell type (62).

Several transfectants of Saos-2 were isolated that had greatly elevated levels of N-myc protein (62). While parental Saos-2 cells were well-spread on the substratum and expressed considerable $\alpha2\beta1$ and $\alpha3\beta1$ integrins, the transfectant cells displayed very little of these integrins on their surfaces and displayed very rounded, easily detachable morphologies. When mRNA levels and protein turnover patterns were analyzed, the same changes were found to occur in these cells (62) as shown above for N-*myc*-overexpressing neuroblastomas (59, 60). There was transcriptional downregulation of $\alpha2$ and $\alpha3$ genes while $\beta1$ transcription was minimally altered. In contrast, $\beta1$ protein turned over much more rapidly, probably because of lack of a partners and resulting in much lower basal levels of this subunit (62). *Max* mRNA levels were unaltered in transfectant cells, again casting the regulatory role on excess amounts of the N-myc protein. These results indicate that N-*myc* regulatory mechanisms can apply to a different cell and tumor types and are not neural lineage-specific. However, the osteosarcoma system is artificial in that there is no evidence for N-*myc*-dependent regulation or N-*myc* amplification in this tumor under naturally occurring conditions.

These analyses of N-*myc*-overexpressing neuroblastoma and osteosarcoma cells prompt more extensive study of the interactions (or lack thereof) of N-myc

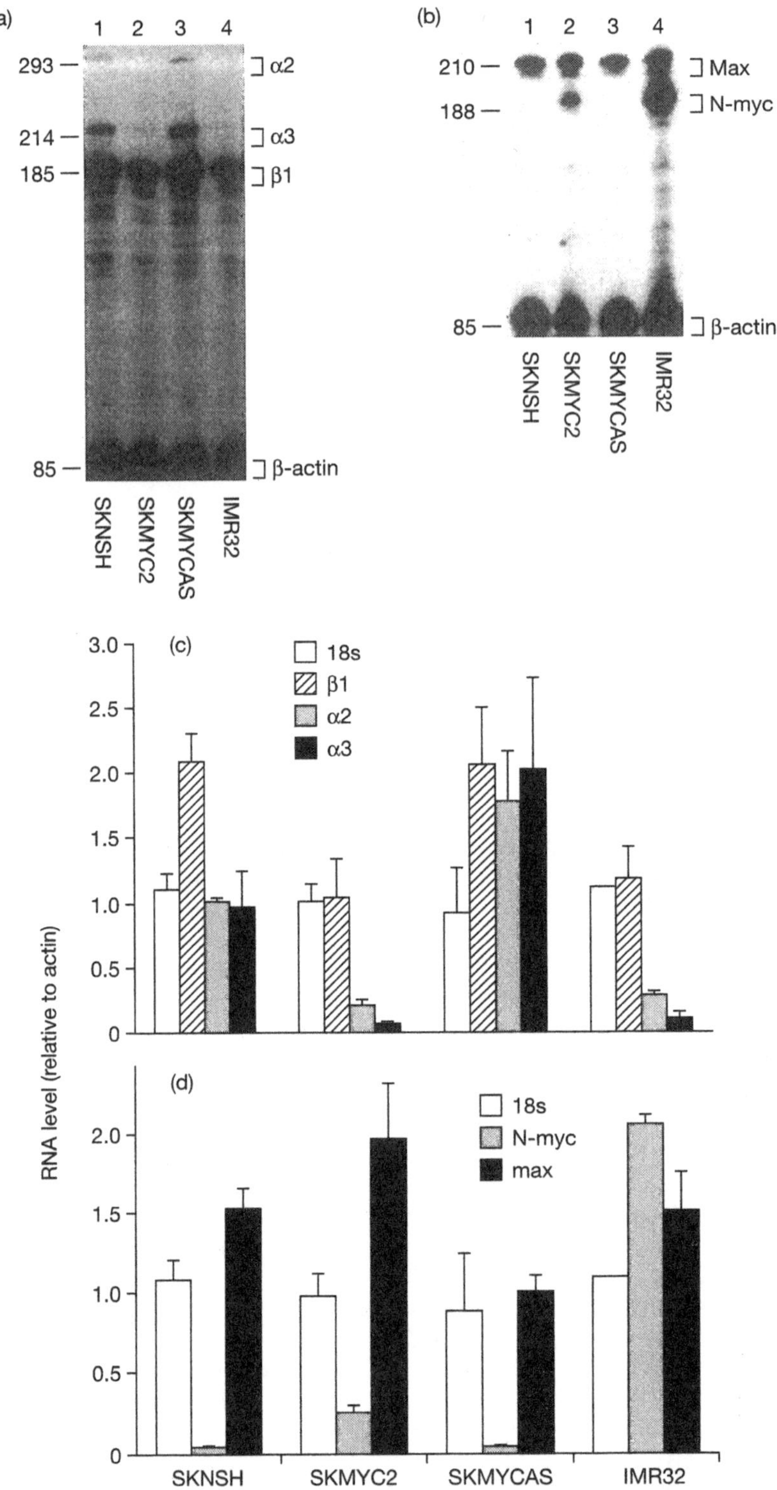

Fig. 18.6 RNAase protection assay for levels of various mRNAs in several neuroblastoma cell lines. SK-N-SH, IMR-32, transfectant SKMYC2, and antisense transfectant SKMYCAS (60) cells were grown in culture and total cellular RNAs prepared. Five micrograms of RNA from each sample were analyzed by RNase protection. In (a), probe sequences analyzed levels of α2, α3, and β1 integrins, as well as β-actin as a control. In (b), probes included those for max, N-*myc*, and β-actin genes. Migration positions of protected fragments are shown on the right of the panels and their sizes (nucleotides) are shown on the left of these autoradiograms. (c), (d) Quantitation of these autoradiograms from several experiments by scanning densitometry. 18s rRNA is included as an internal control for RNA levels. (Taken from reference 60 with permission.)

protein, complexed with max protein, with the promoter regions of these three integrin genes. Unfortunately, these promoters have not been well-studied or their *cis-* or *trans*-acting sequences deciphered completely (63). If N-myc protein regulates transcription of specific genes, including α2 and α3 integrin genes, in ways that are independent of c-myc protein, then these N-myc mechanisms may be targetable for interfering with metastatic competence of these tumor cells.

Perspectives on 'regulating' the metastatic phenotype

The findings described in the preceding sections, when combined with new high-resolution methodologies, enable us to speculate on future directions in deciphering and possibly interfering with metastasis. First, we will be able to more precisely define the small cell subpopulations in which metastatic competence is being acquired as a consequence of altered regulation of genes such as CD44 and integrin receptors. Second, by defining which genes are critical for metastatic competence, clinicians will be afforded much more powerful molecular tools for predicting when and where metastasis occurs. A corollary of this is that we should be able to generate reagents that specifically disrupt the functions of these metastasis-conveying gene products while minimally interfering with their 'normal' functions in well-behaved cell populations. Finally, if we are able to define organ-specific regulation of some genes in tumor subpopulations, interference with the functions of these genes may permit us to inhibit metastasis specifically to that organ. Some examples of these approaches are offered below. Angiogenesis may be a particularly important target for antagonizing the metastatic process, and other chapters in this volume deal with this issue specifically.

Histochemical marker gene-tagged cells for drug screening studies

As shown in the second section of this chapter, 'Histochemical marker genes to track micrometastasis formation and subsequent development into overt metastases', tumor cells tagged with histochemical marker genes can be easily visualized and quantitated in lung and other organs during experimental metastasis. Co-injection of marker gene-tagged tumor cells and candidate metastasis-inhibiting drugs will facilitate identification of useful drugs in several ways. Many drugs can be screened for metastasis-interfering properties using fewer animals and much shorter assay times. In addition, different routes for introducing these drugs into animals can be monitored for the potential to interfere with spontaneous metastasis after either ectopic or orthotopic injections of tumor cells.

Laser-capture microdissection—a high-resolution tool to analyze gene expression patterns in single tumor cells

The recent development of laser-capture microdissection (LCM) of tissue sections (64–66) permits investigators to select one or a few tumor cells in a tissue environment to analyze. Gene products may be detected in these select cells by immunohistochemistry or by their specific functions (65, 66). Expression of any gene may also be analyzed at the transcriptional level by reverse transcriptase polymerase chain reaction (RT-PCR) or *in situ* hybridization (64, 66). Furthermore, use of histochemical marker genes will greatly facilitate the identification of tumor cells, to be selected by LCM, in experimental animal models as discussed in the second section of this chapter. These markers discriminate the tagged tumor cells from untagged neighboring host-organ cells, whose gene expression pattern must also be considered. Therefore, LCM in combination with histochemical tags should be effective at determining whether 'normal' host-organ cells, adjacent to the primary tumor or metastatic cells, have altered gene regulation programs from their distant counterparts. Conversely, the possible altered regulation of tumor cell genes by neighboring host cells can be addressed.

LacZ- or PAP-tagged tumor cells can be detected in fixed sections by first performing histochemical staining and then identifying the appropriate small subset of cells for subsequent laser capture. When two genetically different tumor classes are tagged with different marker genes as shown in the second section of this chapter, this approach becomes particularly beneficial in addressing clonal dominance of one cell type over another in specific regions of the primary tumor and in potential metastatic target sites. These dual approaches should prove particularly effective in deciphering the gene expression patterns in micrometastases as they form.

LCM, in combination with histochemical markers, can be used to determine when and where the CD44 gene is being upregulated (or different isoforms expressed) with RT-PCR and primers recognizing specific CD44 splice products. Does this regulation occur early in primary tumor formation or is it occurring in small subpopulations at later stages of the primary tumor? These approaches will permit us to determine whether selected tumor subpopulations, with altered expression of CD44, occur randomly throughout the primary tumor or only in regions adjacent to larger blood vessels, the latter possibly predicting more effective intravasation into blood vessels for eventual metastatic spread.

As reviewed in the previous section on N-*myc* amplification in neuroblastoma, neuroblastoma metastasis correlates with N-*myc* amplification and subsequent downregulation of $\alpha2\beta1$ and $\alpha3\beta1$ integrin receptors, but not the $\alpha1\beta1$ receptor. Using LCM in combination with marker-tagged neuroblastoma cells, we can test a variety of hypotheses relating the absence of the two integrins to acquisition of metastatic competence. As an example, *lacZ*-tagged/N-*myc*-amplified neuroblastoma cells can be mixed with PAP-tagged/N-*myc*-amplified neuroblastoma in which $\alpha2$ integrin subunit expression is upregulated by transfection with an $\alpha2$ gene under control of a very active promoter. Do both cell types contribute to formation of the primary tumor or does one cell type clonally dominate? By LCM and by following the two histochemical tags, we can determine the relative distributions of the two cell types near major blood vessels in the primary tumor and near other host tissue sites that may be synergistic. Do both cell types metastasize to the same or differing organs? These experiments may reveal some level of synergy between two classes of tumor cells. LCM could be used to examine the gene expression patterns in the earliest micrometastases of these different organs.

Interfering with the functions of genes critical for metastasis

The studies of the two previous sections on CD44 overexpression and N-*myc* amplification, respectively, indicate the relative importance of two different gene classes in the progression of two different tumors in apposing regulation schemes—CD44s in the case of fibrosarcoma metastasis and integrin receptors for neuroblastoma metastasis. In the former, overexpression of the CD44s appears important for conveying metastatic competence while for neuroblastoma downregulation of integrin expression appears important. The identification of such genes raises the issue as to whether antagonists can be identified that inhibit metastasis effectively, based on the structure and function of the metastasis-targeting molecule(s). Hopefully, such an antagonist would not inhibit the normal functions of this molecular class in host organ cells.

An early indication of the possible success in this approach was the demonstration of small synthetic peptides, containing the Arg—Gly—Asp—Ser (RGDS) sequence, to effectively inhibit colonization of the lung when they were co-injected with melanoma and other tumor cells injected into the tail veins of experimental animals (67, 68). This approach proved successful because some integrins on tumor cells recognize an RGDS sequence in target extracellular matrix ligands, such as fibronectin, laminin, and certain collagens. These target ligands in the lungs of the animal would be the 'natural' adherence site for tumor cells and provide the stabilization mechanism for eventual extravasation into lung tissue to establish micrometastases. Remarkably, there was very little toxicity to other tissues of the animal when high dosages of these synthetic peptides were injected.

Histochemical marker gene-tagged cells will provide much more facile and quantitative approaches for testing inhibition of metastasis by other haptens or antagonists of specific molecular domains. As examples, specific spliced sequences of CD44v on the surfaces of some carcinoma cells may provide binding sites for as-yet unidentified receptors on the surfaces of endothelial cells, thereby facilitating development of micrometastases (27–30). Synthetic peptides may be identified that inhibit this specific binding function while leaving the other generic binding functions of CD44v unaffected. These peptides would be ideal candidates for specific inhibition of metastatic spread of some carcinoma tumor types while being minimally toxic to other cell and tissue types.

CD44s is the simplest member of the CD44 family and has been shown important in metastasis of fibrosarcoma, as reviewed in the section on overexpression of CD44, via improved colonization of the lung once tumor cells entered the circulation. Some monoclonal antibodies to specific epitopes of CD44s may be identified that interfere with metastatic spread while having limited inhibition of normal lymphocyte or connective cell functions. Alternatively, the HA-binding function of CD44s appears very important in the lung colonization function of this molecule. Therefore, small oligosaccharides of HA may hapten-inhibit this colonization process and afford a complementary therapeutic approach with other drug modalities. As much more molecular information becomes available on the multiple binding functions of this complex class of cell surface receptors, we may be able to design dominant-negative inhibitors of one or more of these specific functions and greatly improve the tumor-targeting potential of such antagonists.

Molecular biological approaches may also prove useful for interfering with metastatic processes. An antisense gene for CD44s may inhibit metastatic spread of lymphoma (39) or fibrosarcoma (46) if it could be expressed in a retroviral construct that infects tumor cells more effectively than any neighboring host tissue cells. A similar and more specific approach might be considered for CD44v isoforms—use of antisense constructs with sequences targeting specifically the alternatively spliced domains to inhibit carcinoma metastasis (46). In the case of integrin receptors where downregulation occurs commensurate with metastatic spread of neuroblastoma, retroviral infection with an $\alpha2$ or $\alpha3$ integrin subunit gene, regulated by a high-activity promoter, may improve extracellular matrix adhesion of the primary tumor population and subsequently inhibit any spreading potential of these cells by other adhesion mechanisms. This is comparable to the overexpression of transfected E-cadherin gene in some carcinoma cells, thereby inhibiting their invasion and metastatic behavior (69, 70).

Will genetic instability in tumor populations help or hinder in targeting the metastatic phenotype?

It is fair to say that one characteristic of malignant cells is their ability to generate many genetically different subpopulations as the primary tumor expands, thereby providing the versatility that permits metastatic spread for highly selected subpopulations (1–5). The small number of these subpopulations may provide greater efficiency at inhibiting their functions but may require weeks or months of patient treatment to do so because metastatic-competent subpopulations may be generated in the primary tumor on a regular basis. If there were some way to specifically kill such subpopulations by inhibiting their metastatic-competence functions, chances for success in treating the patient may be greatly improved. Greater knowledge of apoptotic and other cell death mechanisms in tumor cells, some of which may be tumor- or cell-type-specific, may afford the complementary treatment approach that will ultimately prove successful. In response, however, the versatility in generating many different subpopulations

may also lead to antagonist-resistant variants within the primary tumor that can overcome the treatment modality and still metastasize to various target organs. In any case, greater knowledge of the various mechanisms for generating genetic instability in tumor populations will be a prerequisite for more effective targeting of the metastatic phenotype.

Acknowledgements

The authors acknowledge partial support for some of these studies from NIH grants to LAC (CA27755 and NS17139), from the Comprehensive Cancer Center of the Ireland Cancer Center at Case Western Reserve University (NCI-supported via P30-CA43703) for pilot studies on prostate carcinoma metastasis, and research grant DAMD 17-98-1-8587 from the US Army on prostate carcinoma metastasis (LAC). Athymic nude mouse experiments were conducted in the Athymic

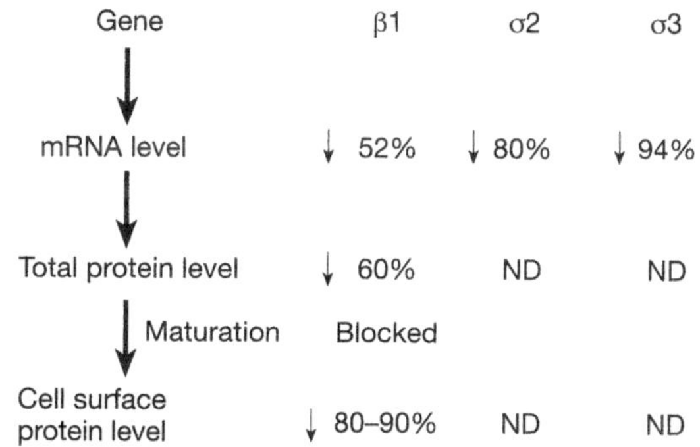

Fig. 18.7 Model for regulation of integrin expression by N-*myc* amplification in neuroblastoma tumors. The various levels of regulation of three different integrin subunit genes—α2, α3, and β1—are shown, as well as their decreased amounts when high levels of N-myc protein are observed both in naturally occurring tumors with N-*myc* amplification, as well as transfectant populations where N-myc protein is elevated artificially (59, 60). Transcription of integrin subunit genes produces mRNA, which is translated into immature proteins. Immature αs and β1 then associate, mature, and translocate to the cell surface. While β1 mRNA levels are reduced approximately twofold in high-N-myc cells, α2 is reduced to less than 20 per cent and α3 to less than 6 per cent of levels observed in the absence of N-myc protein. While very little (ND) α2 or α3 protein are detectable in these cells, the reduced amount of β1 protein produced is incapable of maturation and appearance at the cell surface, undoubtedly because of its inability to partner with an α subunit. Therefore, only approximately 10 per cent of β1 produced actually shows up at the cell surface, partnered with small amounts of α1 subunit produced in these cells, and whose production is unaffected by N-myc protein (61).

Animal Facility (AAALAC-I-approved) of the Case Western Reserve University/Ireland Cancer Center and approved by the Animal Care and Use Committee of this University. One of the authors (NK) was supported by the Animal Resource Center of Case Western Reserve University. The authors thank Drs Thomas and Theresa Pretlow of the Department of Pathology for assistance with tumor and organ tissue sectioning and immunohistochemistry protocols, as well as pathology consultation. Special gratitude is extended to Dr James Jacobberger of the Ireland Cancer Center for the donation of tissue culture-adapted CWR22R prostate carcinoma cells.

References

1. Fidler IJ, Ellis LM. The implications of angiogenesis for the biology and therapy of cancer metastasis. Cell 1994, **79**, 185–8.
2. Fidler IJ, Gersten DM, Hart IR. The biology of cancer invasion and metastasis. Adv Cancer Res 1978, **28**, 149–250.
3. Heppner GH, Miller BE. Tumor heterogeneity: biological implications and therapeutic consequences. Cancer Metastasis Rev 1983, **2**, 5–23.
4. Nicolson GL. Cancer progression and growth: relationship of paracrine and autocrine growth mechanisms to organ preference of metastasis. Exp Cell Res 1993, **204**, 171–80.
5. Nowell PC. Mechanisms of tumor progression. Cancer Res 1986, **46**, 2203–7.
6. Lin W-C, Culp LA. New insight into micrometastasis development using ultrasensitive marker genes. In: Current perspectives on molecular and cellular oncology, Vol. 1, Part B (ed. DA Spandidos). JAI Press, London, 1992, 261–309.
7. Radinsky R. Modulation of tumor cell gene expression and phenotype by the organ-specific metastatic environment. Cancer Metastasis Rev 1995, **14**, 323–38.
8. Singh RK, Tsan R, Radinsky R. Influence of the host microenvironment on the clonal selection of human colon carcinoma cells during primary tumor growth and metastasis. Clin Exp Metastasis 1997, **15**, 140–50.
9. Fidler IJ, Radinsky R. Search for genes that suppress cancer metastasis. J Natl Cancer Inst 1996, **88**, 1700–3.
10. Blood CH, Zetter B. Tumor interactions with the vasculature: angiogenesis and tumor metastasis. Biochim Biophys Acta 1990, **1032**, 89–118.
11. Folkman J. Angiogenesis in cancer, vascular, rheumatoid and other disease. Nat Med 1995, **1**, 27–31.
12. Sanes JR, Rubenstein JLR, Nicolas J-F. Use of a recombinant retrovirus to study post-implantation cell lineages in mouse embryos. EMBO J 1986, **5**, 3133–42.
13. LeDouarin NM, Teillet MA, Catala M. Neurulation in amniote vertebrates: a novel view deduced from the use of quail-chick chimeras. Int J Dev Biol 1998, **42**, 909–16.
14. Culp LA, Radinsky R, Lin W-C. Extracellular matrix interactions with neoplastic cells: tumor- vs. cell type-specific mechanisms. In: Aspects of the biochemistry and molecular biology of tumors (ed. TG Pretlow II and TP Pretlow). Academic Press, Orlando, 1991, 99–149.
15. Culp LA, Barletta E. Matrix adhesion of neuroblastoma and related neuronal derivative cells: cell type versus tumor-specific mechanisms. Sem Dev Biol 1990, **1**, 437–52.
16. Culp LA, Lin W-C, Kleinman NR, Campero NM, Miller CJ, Holleran JL. Tumor progression, micrometastasis, and genetic instability tracked with histochemical marker genes. Prog Histochem Cytochem 1998, **33**, 329–50.
17. Lin W-C, Pretlow TP, Pretlow TG, Culp LA. Bacterial *lacZ* gene as a highly sensitive marker to detect micrometastasis formation during tumor progression. Cancer Res 1990, **50**, 2808–17.
18. Lin W-C, Pretlow TP, Pretlow TG, Culp LA. Development of micrometastases: earliest events detected with bacterial *lacZ* gene-tagged tumor cells. J Natl Cancer Inst 1990, **82**, 1497–503.
19. Lin W-C, Pretlow TP, Pretlow TG, Culp LA. High resolution analyses of two different classes of tumor cells *in situ* tagged with alternative histochemical marker genes. Am J Pathol 1992, **141**, 1331–42.
20. Lin W-C, Culp LA. Selectable plasmid vectors with alternative and ultrasensitive histochemical marker genes. BioTechniques 1991, **11**, 344–51.
21. Lin W-C, O'Connor KL, Culp LA. Complementation of two related tumour cell classes during experimental metastasis tagged with different histochemical marker genes. Br J Cancer 1993, **67**, 910–21.
22. Pretlow TG, Pelley RJ, Pretlow TP. Biochemistry of prostatic carcinoma. In: Biochemical and molecular aspects of selected cancers, Vol. 2 (ed. TG Pretlow, II and TP Pretlow). Academic Press, San Diego, 1994, 169–237.
23. Lalani E-N, Lanaido ME, Abel PD. Molecular and cellular biology of prostate cancer. Cancer Met Rev 1997, **16**, 29–66.
24. Sramkoski RM, Pretlow TG, Giaconia JM, Pretlow TP, Schwartz S, Sy M-S, Marengo SR, Zhang D, Jacobberger J. A new human prostate carcinoma cell line, 22Rv1. In Vitro Cell Dev Biol Anim 1999, **35**, 403–09.
25. Lin W-C, Culp LA. Altered establishment/clearance mechanisms during experimental micrometastasis with live and/or disabled bacterial *lacZ*-tagged tumor cells. Invasion Metastasis 1992, **12**, 197–209.
26. Kleinman NR, Lewandowska K, Culp LA. Tumour progression of human neuroblastoma cells tagged with a *lacZ* marker gene: earliest events at ectopic injection sites. Br J Cancer 1994, **69**, 670–9.
27. Lesley J, Hyman R, Kincade PW. CD44 and its interaction with extracellular matrix. Adv Immunol 1993, **54**, 271–335.
28. Knudson CB, Knudson W. Hyaluronan-binding proteins in development, tissue homeostasis, and disease. FASEB J 1993, **7**, 1233–41.
29. Tarin D, Matsumura Y. Deranged activity of the CD44 gene and other loci as biomarkers for progression to metastatic malignancy. J Cell Biochem 1993, **17G**, 173–85.

30. Matsumura Y, Tarin D. Significance of CD44 gene products for cancer diagnosis and disease evaluation. Lancet 1992, **340**, 1053–8.

31. Heider K-H, Hofmann M, Hors E, van den Berg F, Ponta H, Herrlich P, Pals S. A human homologue of the rat metastasis-associated variant of CD44 is expressed in colorectal carcinomas and adenomatous polyps. J Cell Biol 1993, **120**, 227–33.

32. Iida N, Bourguignon LYW. New CD44 splice variants associated with human breast cancers. J Cell Physiol 1995, **162**, 127–33.

33. Heider K-H, Dammrich J, Skroch-Angel P, Muller-Hermelink H-K, Vollmers HP, Herrlich P, Ponta H. Differential expression of CD44 splice variants in intestinal- and diffuse-type human gastric carcinomas and normal gastric mucosa. Cancer Res 1993, **53**, 4197–203.

34. Hofmann M, Rudy W, Gunthert U, Zimmer SG, Zawadzki V, Zoller M, Lichtner RB, Herrlich P, Ponta H. A link between *ras* and metastatic behavior of tumor cells: *ras* induces CD44 promoter activity and leads to low-level expression of metastasis-specific variants of CD44 in CREF cells. Cancer Res 1993, **53**, 1516–21.

35. Jamal HH, Cano-Gauci DF, Buick RN, Filmus J. Activated *ras* and *src* induce CD44 overexpression in rat intestinal epithelial cells. Oncogene 1994, **9**, 417–23.

36. Wielenga VJM, Heider K-H, Offerhaus GJA, Adoft GR, van den Berg FM, Ponta H, Herrlich P, Pals ST. Expression of CD44 variant proteins in human colorectal cancer is related to tumor progression. Cancer Res 1993, **53**, 4754–6.

37. Li H, Hamou M-F, de Tribolet N, Jaufeerally R, Hofmann M, Diserens AC, van Meir EG. Variant CD44 adhesion molecules are expressed in human brain metastases but not in glioblastomas. Cancer Res 1993, **53**, 5345–9.

38. Gunthert U, Hofmann M, Rudy W, Reber S, Zoller M, Haussmann I, Matzku S, Wenzel A, Ponta H, Herrlich P. A new variant glycoprotein CD44 confers metastatic potential to rat carcinoma cells. Cell 1991, **65**, 13–24.

39. Sy M-S, Guo YJ, Stamenkovic I. Distinct effects of two CD44 isoforms on tumor growth *in vivo*. J Exp Med 1991, **174**, 859–66.

40. DeGrendele HC, Estess P, Picker LJ, Siegelman MH. CD44 and its ligand hyaluronate mediate rolling under physiologic flow: a novel lymphocyte—endothelial cell primary adhesion pathway. J Exp Med 1996, **183**, 1119–30.

41. DeGrendele HC, Estess P, Siegelman MH. Requirement for CD44 in activated T cell extravasation into an inflammatory site. Science 1997, **278**, 672–5.

42. Kogerman P, Sy M-S, Culp LA. Oncogene-dependent expression of CD44 in Balb/c 3T3 derivatives: correlation with metastatic competence. Clin Exp Metastasis 1996, **14**, 73–82.

43. Kogerman P, Sy M-S, Culp LA. Counter-selection for over-expressed human CD44s in primary tumors versus lung metastases in a mouse fibrosarcoma model. Oncogene 1997, **15**, 1407–16.

44. Kogerman P, Sy M-S, Culp LA. Over-expression of human CD44s in murine 3T3 cells: selection against during primary tumorigenesis and selection for during micrometastasis. Clin Exp Metastasis 1998, **16**, 83–93.

45. Kogerman P, Sy M-S, Culp LA. Overexpressed human CD44s promotes lung colonization during micrometastasis of murine fibrosarcoma cells: facilitated retention in the lung vasculature. Proc Natl Acad Sci, USA 1997, **94**, 13233–8.

46. Culp LA, Kogerman P. Plasticity of CD44s expression during progression and metastasis of fibrosarcoma in an animal model system. Frontiers Bioscience 1998, **3**, d672–83.

47. Lengauer C, Kinzler KW, Vogelstein B. DNA methylation and genetic instability in colorectal cancer cells. Proc Natl Acad Sci, USA 1997, **94**, 2545–50.

48. Smith SS. Stalling of DNA methyltransferase in chromosome stability and chromosome remodelling. Int J Mol Med 1998, **1**, 147–56.

49. Brodeur GM, Seeger RC, Barrett A, *et al.* International criteria for diagnosis, staging, and response to treatment in patients with neuroblastoma. J Clin Oncol 1988, **6**, 1874–81.

50. Thiele CJ. Biology of pediatric peripheral neuroectodermal tumors. Cancer Met Rev 1991, **10**, 311–19.

51. Marcu KB, Bossone SA, Patel AJ. *myc* function and regulation. Annu Rev Biochem 1992, **61**, 809–60.

52. van't Veer LJ, Beijersbergen RL, Bernards R. N-*myc* suppresses major histocompatibility complex class I gene expression through down-regulation of the p50 subunit of NF-kB. EMBO J 1993, **12**, 195–200.

53. Bernards R. N-*myc* disrupts protein kinase C-mediated signal transduction in neuroblastoma. EMBO J 1991, **10**, 1119–25.

54. Akeson R, Bernards R. N-*myc* downregulates neural cell adhesion molecule expression in rat neuroblastoma. Mol Cell Biol 1990, **10**, 2012–16.

55. Albelda SM. Role of integrins and other cell adhesion molecules in tumor progression and metastasis. Lab Invest 1993, **68**, 4–17.

56. Flickinger KS, Judware R, Lechner R, Carter WG, Culp LA. Integrin expression in human neuroblastoma cells with or without N-*myc* amplification and in ectopic/orthotopic nude mouse tumors. Exp Cell Res 1994, **213**, 156–63.

57. Judware R, Lechner R, Culp LA. Inverse expressions of the N-*myc* oncogene and β1 integrin in human neuroblastoma: relationships to disease progression in a nude mouse model system. Clin Exp Metastasis 1995, **13**, 123–33.

58. Brooks PC, Clark RAF, Cheresh DA. Requirement of vascular integrin αvβ3 for angiogenesis. Science 1994, **264**, 569–71.

59. Judware R, Culp LA. Over-expression of transfected N-*myc* oncogene in human SKNSH neuroblastoma cells down-regulates expression of ß1 integrin subunit. Oncogene 1995, **11**, 2599–607.

60. Judware R, Culp LA. Concomitant down-regulation of expression of integrin subunits by N-*myc* in human neuroblastoma cells: differential regulation of α2, α3, and ß1. Oncogene 1997, **14**, 1341–50.

61. Judware, R, Culp LA. Persistent α1 integrin subunit expression in human neuroblastoma cell lines which

overexpress N-*myc* and downregulate other integrin subunits. Oncology Rep 1997, **4**, 433–7.

62. Judware R, Culp LA. N-*myc* over-expression downregulates α3ß1 integrin expression in human Saos-2 osteosarcoma cells. Clin Exp Metastasis 1997, **15**, 228–38.

63. Boudreau N, Bissell MJ. Extracellular matrix signaling: integration of form and function in normal and malignant cells. Curr Opin Cell Biol 1998, **10**, 640–6.

64. Emmert-Buck MR, Bonner RF, Smith PD, Chuaqui RF, Zhuang Z, Goldstein SR, Weiss RA, Liotta LA. Laser capture microdissection. Science 1996, **274**, 998–1001.

65. Schutze K, Lahr G. Identification of expressed genes by laser-mediated manipulation of single cells. Nat Biotechnol 1998, **16**, 737–42.

66. Simone NL, Bonner RF, Gillespie JW, Emmert-Buck MR, Liotta LA. Laser-capture microdissection: opening the microscopic frontier to molecular analysis. Trends Gene 1998, **14**, 272–6.

67. Humphries MJ, Yamada KM, Olden K. Investigation of the biological effects of anti-cell adhesive synthetic peptides that inhibit experimental metastasis of B16-F10 murine melanoma cells. J Clin Invest 1988, **81**, 782–90.

68. Saiki I, Iida J, Murata J, Ogawa R, Nishi N, Sugimura K, Tokura S, Azuma I. Inhibition of the metastasis of murine malignant melanoma by synthetic polymeric peptides containing core sequences of cell-adhesive molecules. Cancer Res 1989, **49**, 3815–22.

69. Frixen UH, Behrens J, Sachs M, Eberle G, Voss B, Warda A, Lochner D, Birchmeier W. E-cadherin-mediated cell-cell adhesion prevents invasiveness of human carcinoma cells. J Cell Biol 1991, **113**, 173–85.

70. Vleminckx K, Vakaet J, Mareel M, Fiers W, van Roy F. Genetic manipulation of e-cadherin expression by epithelial tumor cells reveals an invasion suppressor role. Cell 1991, **66**, 107–19.

Index

Note: 'f' after a page number indicates a reference to a figure and 't' indicates a reference to a table.

The manufacturer's authorised representative in the EU for product safety is Oxford
University Press España S.A. of El Parque Empresarial San Fernando de Henares,
Avenida de Castilla, 2 – 28830 Madrid (www.oup.es/en or product.safety@oup.com).
OUP España S.A. also acts as importer into Spain of products made by the manufacturer.

Printed in the USA/Agawam, MA
May 28, 2025

888208.012